WITHDRAWN

DIAGNOSTIC AUDIOLOGY

DIAGNOSTIC AUDIOLOGY

Edited by

JOHN T. JACOBSON, Ph.D.

Director of Audiology,
University of Texas Health Science Center, Houston

JERRY L. NORTHERN, Ph.D.

Head, Audiology Division, University Hospital,
University of Colorado Health Science Center, Denver

pro·ed

8700 Shoal Creek Boulevard
Austin, Texas 78758

© 1991 by John T. Jacobson and Jerry L. Northern

Library of Congress Cataloging in Publication Data
Main entry under title:

Diagnostic audiology / [edited by] John T. Jacobson, Jerry L.
    Northern.
        p.   cm.
    Includes bibliographical references.

    ISBN 0-89079-297-6

    1. Hearing disorders — Diagnosis. 2. Audiometry.   I. Jacobson,
John T., 1943–   .   II. Northern, Jerry L.
    [DNLM: 1. Hearing Disorders — diagnosis. 2. Hearing Tests.   WV
270 D5365]
RF294.D49   1989
617.8'075 — dc20
DNLM/DLC   89-12799
for Library of Congress   CIP

Printed in the United States of America

pro·ed

8700 Shoal Creek Boulevard
Austin, Texas 78758

1 2 3 4 5 6   95 94 93 92 91

Contents

Contributing Authors

Peter W. Alberti, M.B., Ph.D., F.R.C.S.(C)

Professor and Chairman, Faculty of Medicine, Department of Otolaryngology, University of Toronto; Otolaryngologist-in-Chief, Mount Sinai Hospital, Toronto

M. Jean Davidson, M.D.

Faculty of Medicine, Department of Otolaryngology, University of Toronto, Toronto

J. Michael Dennis, Ph.D.

Professor and Vice Head, Department of Otorhinolaryngology, University of Oklahoma Health Sciences Center; Director and Section Head, Audiology and Speech-Language Pathology, Oklahoma Memorial Hospital, Oklahoma City

John D. Durrant, Ph.D.

Professor of Otolaryngology and Communication, University of Pittsburgh School of Medicine; Director, Center for Audiology, Eye and Ear Hospital of Pittsburgh, Pittsburgh

Gerald M. English, M.D., F.A.C.S.

Clinical Professor of Otolaryngology, University of Colorado Health Sciences Center, Denver

Bechara Y. Ghorayeb, M.D.

Assistant Professor, Department of Otolaryngology, University of Texas Medical School, Houston

James W. Hall III, Ph.D.

Associate Professor, Division of Hearing and Speech Sciences, Department of Otolaryngology, Vanderbilt University School of Medicine; Director of Audiology, Vanderbilt Hospital, Nashville

Martyn L. Hyde, Ph.D.

Associate Professor of Otolaryngology, University of Toronto Faculty of Medicine; Director, Silverman Audiology Research Laboratory, Mount Sinai Hospital, Toronto

Deborah Hayes, Ph.D.

Director, Audiology, Speech Pathology, and Learning Services, The Children's Hospital, Denver

John T. Jacobson, Ph.D.

Director of Audiology, Division of Audiology, Department of Otolaryngology, University of Texas Health Science Center, Houston

James F. Jerger, Ph.D.

Professor, Department of Otorhinolaryngology and Communicative Sciences, Baylor College of Medicine; Head, Department of Audiology and Speech Pathology, The Methodist Hospital, Houston

Susan Jerger, Ph.D.

Associate Professor, Department of Otorhinolaryngology and Communicative Sciences and Director, Children's Hearing Center, Baylor College of Medicine, Houston

Robert W. Keith, Ph.D.

Professor and Director, Division of Audiology and Speech Pathology, University of Cincinnati College of Medicine, Cincinnati

John L. Kemink, M.D.

Associate Professor, Department of Otolaryngology-Head and Neck Surgery, University of Michigan Medical School, Ann Arbor

Paul R. Kileny, Ph.D.

Associate Professor, Department of Otolaryngology-Head and Neck Surgery, University of Michigan Medical School, Ann Arbor

Paul R. Lambert, M.D.

Associate Professor, Department of Otolaryngology-Head and Neck Surgery, University of Virginia School of Medicine; Director of Otology-Neurotology, University of Virginia Medical Center, Charlottesville

Jean M. Lovrinic, Ph.D.

Professor of Speech-Language-Hearing, Temple University School of Communication and Theater, Philadelphia

Michele D. Morris, M.S.

Electrophysiologist, Division of BioelectroDiagnosis and Neural Monitoring, University of Pennsylvania Medical Center, Philadelphia

J. Gail Neely, M.D.

Professor and Head, Department of Otorhinolaryngology, University of Oklahoma School of Medicine, Oklahoma City

Jerry L. Northern, Ph.D.

Head, Audiology Division, University Hospital, University of Colorado Health Science Center, Denver

Wayne O. Olsen, Ph.D.

Consultant in Audiology and Professor, Department of Otorhinolaryngology, Mayo Clinic, Rochester

Nigel R. T. Pashley, M.B., B.S.,
F.R.C.S.(C), F.A.A.P.

Chairman, Department of Pediatric Otolaryngology-Head and Neck Surgery, The Children's Hospital, Denver

Roger A. Ruth, Ph.D.

Associate Professor of Otolaryngology, University of Virginia School of Medicine; Director, Division of Communicative Disorders, University of Virginia Medical Center, Charlottesville

Daniel M. Schwartz, Ph.D.

Director, Division of BioelectroDiagnosis and Neural Monitoring, University of Pennsylvania Medical Center, Philadelphia

Neil T. Shepard, Ph.D.

Assistant Professor and Director, Vestibular Testing Center, Department of Otolaryngology, University of Michigan Medical School, Ann Arbor

Brad A. Stach, Ph.D.

Director of Audiology and Speech Pathology Service, The Methodist Hospital; Baylor College of Medicine, Houston

Steven A. Telian, M.D.

Assistant Professor, Department of Otolaryngology-Head and Neck Surgery, University of Michigan Medical School, Ann Arbor

Preface

The profession of audiology continues in a state of emerging metamorphosis. As this evolutionary process enters its fifth decade, recent developments in computer technology and clinical medicine present tangible opportunities to the audiologist that were never before realized. How aggressively our profession accepts these new challenges will undoubtedly shape our future into the twenty-first century.

To date, one of the more rewarding professional developments has been the role audiology has established in the overall diagnosis and management of patients with auditory pathology. This acceptance has been brought about by our ability to provide improved audiologic test protocol and increased diagnostic accuracy with regard to hearing impairment, vestibular abnormality, and neurologic deficits.

In today's rapidly changing health care delivery systems, practitioners are expected to maintain certain levels of professional standards, stay abreast of current clinical methodology, and continually update new improved techniques into daily practice. Unfortunately, our collective experience has shown that, all too often, audiologists are resistant to change. For whatever reasons, clinicians seem reluctant to incorporate new procedures, approaches, and diagnostic schemes into their daily operational routines. In an attempt to allay previous bias, *Diagnostic Audiology* offers an alternative perspective to the current clinical literature.

Contributors have been selected because of their established expertise in specific clinical areas, and individual chapters are designed to reflect new and progressive attitudes in patient diagnosis, management, and professional cooperation. In 1977, Alford and Jerger editorialized the importance of a "partnership" between otolaryngology and audiology. In an attempt to further establish this relationship, whenever feasible, chapters have been coauthored by an audiologist and an otolaryngologist. We strongly feel that input from both disciplines has enhanced this text by providing a diverse perspective to common medical and (re)habilitative problems. Our clinical experience suggests that the diagnosis and management of a patient population are not the sole domain of any single discipline, and the highest level of patient care results from a team approach.

The intended readership includes any hearing health professional who may benefit from a practical and logical approach to auditory assessment, but specifically graduate students in audiology, residents in otolaryngology, and other practicing professionals working in the area of audition. This book is not designed for the introductory audiology student. The material presented is based on the assumption that the reader has acquired a basic knowledge of the anatomy and physiology of the auditory system, hearing sciences, and a general orientation to various disorders of the hearing and vestibular mechanism. In addition, the reader is expected to have an understanding and experience with the basic hearing tests including air and bone conduction, masking, and speech audiometry. A review of immittance audiometry and other various physiologic tests will be helpful in the integration of advanced clinical techniques and decision analysis.

Prior to committing to the development of a new textbook, we surveyed a substantial number of our colleagues who were associated with university programs and had taught various aspects of clinical audiology. In general, their responses indicated that a textbook that focused on clinical assessment, diagnosis, prognosis, and ultimate outcome for hearing-impaired patients would be a welcome addition to the current literature. That is, a need existed for a textbook that concentrated on methods of evaluating hearing impairment from a diagnostic strategy rather than a series of isolated test procedures. It became obvious from their feedback that a "gestalt" approach to clinical audiology was required. The design and development of *Diagnostic Audiology* reflect those aspirations.

The structure of this textbook is intended to accommodate typical university course offerings in clinical audiology. In Part I, Fundamentals, our intent was to provide a series of chapters that offers a basic clinical foundation laying the groundwork for the remainder of the text. Chapter 1, Overview of Auditory Diagnosis, offers the clinical and philosophic direction of this textbook. Chapter 2, Special Auditory Tests, A Historical Perspective, is a review of the classic historical development reflecting growth and change in clinical audiology with a description of conventional tests. Many changes in clinical activity have been established from advances in instrumentation and technology. These developments are described in Chapter 3, Audiologic Instrumentation. Chapter 4, Otologic Evaluation, and Chapter 5, Otoneurologic Diseases and Associated Audiologic Profiles, discuss direct medical relationships of audiology and neurotology that are germane to the following sections.

The essence of *Diagnostic Audiology* lies in the specific methodologies of test protocol and decision analysis found in Part II, Auditory Assessment. Chapter 6, Immittance Measures in Auditory Disorders, and Chapter 7, Strategies for Optimizing the Detection of Neuropathology from the Auditory Brainstem Response, provide the basic principles and clinical applications of these special electrophysiologic test entities as they apply to normal, hearing-impaired, and retrocochlear patients. The remaining four chapters, Diagnosis of Middle Ear Pathology and Evaluation of Conductive Hearing Loss (Chapter 8), Evaluation and Diagnosis of Cochlear Disorders (Chapter 9), Acoustic Neuroma: Diagnosis and Management (Chapter 10), and Central Auditory Disorders (Chapter 11), deal with assessment procedures and strategies de-

signed to evaluate disorders of the auditory system as they relate to site of lesion pathology.

Part III, Special Considerations, provides information dealing with unique populations such as evaluating hearing in infants, young children, and pediatric multi-handicapped groups (Chapter 12, Assessment of Infants for Hearing Impairment), and vestibular abnormalities (Chapter 13, Balance Disorders: The Dizzy Patient). The final chapter (Chapter 14, Auditory Test Strategy) introduces the concepts of operating characteristics and their overall application in the diagnostic decision analysis model. This chapter is pivotal to the understanding of clinical diagnostic assessment and attempts to coalesce auditory test strategies into practical clinical application.

Acknowledging that this organizational approach to diagnostic audiology represents a unique view to auditory assessment, it is our wish that the culmination of this textbook will provide students and practicing clinicians with a new perspective on auditory assessment. Hopefully, the hearing evaluation of each patient will be viewed with renewed enthusiasm and a feeling of challenge supported by a strong basic understanding of the strengths and limitations of audiologic test protocol. The final diagnostic outcome is not simply a recount of scores from individual tests, but the integration of results from a well-conceived cross-check principle that takes into account all aspects of each auditory impaired patient.

J.T.J.
J.L.N.

PART I

Fundamentals

CHAPTER 1

Overview of Auditory Diagnosis

John T. Jacobson • *Jerry L. Northern*

DIAGNOSTIC AUDIOLOGY

As our knowledge and understanding of the complexities of the auditory system have increased during the past 30 years, technologic and medical advances have kept pace to provide the means by which we accurately identify etiology and locus of hearing disorders. The successful application of various auditory testing strategies has confirmed the important contribution of audiology in the diagnostic process. By definition, *diagnostic audiology* is the advanced psychoacoustic and electrophysiologic study of the auditory response (Sanders, 1988). Audiologic results based on highly developed test strategies, when properly interpreted, often provide the key to successful management of hearing-impaired children and adults.

According to Sanders (1988) the audiologist's role is to seek understanding of aberrant auditory behavior through specialized test procedures and then interpret these findings to provide specific diagnostic information. Obviously, results from *all* hearing tests contribute to the ultimate diagnosis of the hearing disorder; however, the term *diagnostic audiology* is usually reserved for those advanced tests, techniques, and procedures applied beyond the traditional pure tone screening or threshold test that are used in their entirety to assess the auditory system from "pinna to cortex."

The term *diagnosis* is historically linked to the domain of the medical profession. Contemporary usage of the term, however, has been broadened considerably over the years to include a wide variety of applications wherein one seeks the underlying basis of any problem. Thus we have *diagnostic* automobile repair, *diagnostic* reading and learning centers, *diagnostic* marketing strategies, *diagnostic* financial assessment, and even *diagnostic* astrologic interpretation! Webster's (1981) defines the noun *diagnosis* quite liberally to mean (1) the art or act of identifying a disease from its signs and symptoms; (2) the investigation or analysis of the cause or nature of a condition, situation, or problem; and (3) a statement or conclusion concerning the cause of some phenomenon. Clearly, this term is no longer within the single purview of medicine.

Considerable concern, debate, and careful maneuvering has centered around the use of the term *diagnosis* as it relates to the practice of audiology. Many discussions and debates have been held about this issue for as long as the profession of audiology has been in existence. Are these concerns factual or has the audiology profession developed an unnecessary paranoia? What is this much maligned term *diagnosis* and how has it influenced our development? Finally, what are the implications for the future and what role will the audiology community serve in the diagnosis and management of the hearing-impaired population?

Let us consider the following hypothetical illustration: Will the application of auditory cross-check principles contribute to the pathognomonic nature of a disease process? Take, for example, a patient with middle ear effusion who is examined by an otolaryngologist. The use of tuning forks and visual inspection of the external auditory canal and tympanic membrane are equally important to the basic hearing test battery in reaching a diagnostic conclusion. Although subjective, those otologic components add significant weight to the eventual interpretation and medical management of the patient. The use of these techniques in the hands of an experienced physician is invaluable. Yet, can they be described as more *diagnostic* than a basic hearing evaluation? Or simply, do they add to the overall impression of pathology that presents with specific signs and symptoms? Is the hearing evaluation any less important to the eventual confirmation?

As early as 1948, Dix, Hallpike, and Hood published a paper dealing with the differential diagnosis of inner ear and eighth nerve hearing disorders. In the early 1960s, the audiologic research group from Northwestern University led by Carhart and Jerger were developing a number of diagnostic audiologic tests to be used in differentiating site of lesion in hearing disorders. In a chapter entitled, "Diagnostic Audiometry," Jerger (1973) wrote that "all audiometry is diagnostic since it contributes, in some sense, to the ultimate localization of the auditory disorder" (p. 75).

Sanders (1988) stated that "special auditory tests" are qualitative in that they seek the pathogenesis and not necessarily just the degree of hearing impairment. Although minor differences of interpretation may exist concerning the contribution of various audiologic tests, it is clear that the term *diagnostic* is well embedded in our approach to the complete evaluation of hearing.

This tenet, however, is not shared by all. In fairness, it must be mentioned that some authors prefer to avoid this term. Konkle and Rintelmann (1979) wrote that *diagnostic audiology* is not an appropriate descriptor to apply to the test battery concept. Their rationale was that "audiologic tests do not identify the disease process responsible for a lesion, but simply provide information that may be compatible with a particular type of disorder" (p. 532). Instead, Konkle and Rintelmann argued for the use of *differential audiologic assessment*, coined earlier by Olsen and Matkin (1978).

Suffice it to say that the ultimate medical diagnosis of any disease is the responsibility of the physician. However, physicians use all available information to determine this final diagnosis, and in the specialty of otolaryngology, the audiologic evaluation is an important part of this fact-collecting analysis. To continue the debate serves no good purpose; the controversy has been reduced to a matter of simple semantics. As a point in fact, *diagnostic audiology* describes the culmination of a professional collaboration, including test result analysis, leading to the accurate identification and confirmation of an individual's hearing impairment.

SCOPE OF PRACTICE: DEFINED

Recently, a number of organizations have established a "scope of practice" statement for the audiology profession. These statements usually include a definition of an audiologist and the roles and responsibilities of the profession. For example, the U.S. Department of Labor (1977) defines an audiologist as one who "specializes in *diagnos-* tic evaluation of hearing, prevention, habilitative and rehabilitative services for auditory problems, and research related to hearing and attendant disorders; determines range, nature, and degree of hearing function related to patient's auditory efficiency [and] differentiates between organic and nonorganic hearing disabilities through evaluation of total response pattern and use of acoustic tests." According to the American Speech-Language-Hearing Association (ASHA) (1984), "audiologists are specialists in prevention, identification, and assessment of hearing impairment, and in the habilitation and rehabilitation of persons with hearing impairments, including the fitting and dispensing of hearing aids." The scope of practice encompasses "a continuum of services including prevention, identification, *diagnosis*, consultation, and treatment of patients regarding ... hearing and balance. Services include, but are not limited to, ... evaluating and *diagnosing* auditory and vestibular competencies" (ASHA, 1985). The Joint Commission for Accreditation of Health Care Organizations' description of audiology services has adopted into their scope of practice the ASHA (1985) statement "evaluating and *diagnosing* auditory and vestibular competencies."

More recently, a new professional organization, the American Academy of Audiology (AAA), has been established to represent all segments of the audiology community. In recognition of the importance of instituting a broad statement of professional practice, the Academy created an ad hoc committee on the scope of practice. As of this publication, the committee has submitted a draft proposal on the scope of practice to the advisory board of the Academy. As stated, the purpose of the document is to serve as a reference for issues of service delivery, third-party reimbursement, legislation, consumer education, regulatory action, state and professional licensure, and interprofessional relations. Further, the AAA ad hoc committee has defined an audiologist as expert in the *diagnosis* of normal and disordered auditory and vestibular function. Consistent with previously cited definitions, it is clear that this new organization also identified and acknowledges the importance of *diagnosis* as an intricate part of current philosophy.

Even the discussion of audiology scope of practice brings out dissenting points of view while emphasizing the diversity of audiologists' roles. Jerger (Mahon, 1988) has expressed reservations over the role of the audiologists' involvement in two areas he believes are "peripheral" to our field: electronystagmography and intraoperative monitoring. Although Jerger admits that audiologists are most familiar with the equipment and the tasks involved, and that both peripheral areas measure attributes of the eighth cranial nerve, he asks, "At what point do we define the boundaries of our field?"

Clearly the evolution and development of the scope of the audiology profession have not yet been set in concrete, and we can expect further refinement, expansion, and reorganization to occur in future years.

PROFESSIONAL RELATIONSHIPS

In 1977, Alford and Jerger editorialized the importance of a "continuing partnership" between the professions of otolaryngology and audiology. Because of the clinical and research expertise that the audiologist brought to this partnership, the end result was mutually beneficial to both parties as well as the hearing-impaired community. The authors point out, however, that this partnership had yet to reach a satisfactory level of acceptance from all practitioners. The instability of the working relationship was due, in part, to undefined roles and responsibilities. The concern from both groups of specialists has resulted in a "keep your distance" attitude, as well as a lack of understanding about the goals of each group in relation to care and management of the hearing-impaired patient population. In describing their role as intermediaries, Alford and Jerger suggested a number of recommendations to increase the mutual working relationship, including that (1) hearing problems are potential health problems, and as such, the otolaryngologist is the responsible party for primary care of the hearing disorder; (2) medical and surgical treatment take precedence whenever possible in the care of a hearing-impaired patient; (3) the otolaryngologist must recognize that the audiologist is professionally trained and should not be considered to be working in a subservient role; (4) the audiologist is best suited to perform audiologic evaluations, and the otolaryngologist should discourage the use of audiometric testing by technicians; and (5) once medical or surgical treatment, or both, is completed, otolaryngologists must accept the principle that the audiologist should coordinate rehabilitative management of the hearing-impaired patient. It should be noted that more than a decade has passed since this editorial was published, and although the personal relationships between individuals of both professions have improved significantly, on a national scope ample room still exists for mutual cooperation and progress.

PROFESSIONAL ORGANIZATIONS

Several professional organizations lend themselves to the interests of audiology. Most are eclectic and self-motivated. Regardless of personal concern, active participation by members is a necessary prerequisite for the successful perpetuation and evolution of any profession. Organizations such as the Academy of Dispensing Audiologists, the Academy of Rehabilitation Audiology, the American Academy of Audiology, the American Auditory Society, and the American Speech-Language-Hearing Association are well known to the audiology community. Audiologists must appreciate the need for diversity and not limit themselves to any single professional entity or philosophy lest they lose the importance of multidisciplinary collaboration. The contribution of other professional affiliations takes on new importance in light of this embracing *diagnostic* revolution. For instance, organizations such as the American Academy of Pediatrics, the American Academy of Otolaryngology, Head and Neck Surgery, the Acoustical Society of America, and the Association for Research in Otolaryngology offer unique opportunities for audiologists to become involved with other disciplines that contribute both directly and indirectly to the audiology profession and the hearing impaired. In one facet or another, all of these groups influence the role and responsibility of audiology as a clinical diagnostic component.

HISTORICAL PERSPECTIVE

Lineage

As a neophyte in the area of biologic science, audiology was once referred to as "a young but lusty infant" (Jerger, 1963, p. xv). Whereas Jerger's portrayal of a lusty infant provided an accurate account of the profession during its second decade, the metamorphosis of audiology has changed considerably over the past 25 years. Audiology has grown rapidly from its early rehabilitative role to one of great diversity. This expansion has paralleled, or surpassed, other emerging allied health professions over the past few years. The advent of computer-based technology and improved recording and testing techniques have given audiology a viable and meaningful role in auditory diagnosis. Audiology is no longer developing in a period of prepubescence, but rather has reached the stage of adolescence wherein substantial contributions are continuing to emerge. Nevertheless, a number of the controversial characteristics associated with this developmental period remain.

Audiology, as a specialty field of study, evolved from a number of established physical and social sciences. Davis (1970) pointed out that the word *audiology* is a strange configuration of Latin root and Greek suffix, although its meaning is explicitly clear — "the study of hearing." Hearing is a biologic phenomenon, which for humans is the cornerstone of communication. The study of hearing and the understanding of hearing dysfunction require a strong underpinning in the basic physical and life sciences as well as a comprehension of human psychology and human development. Each of these pieces of elemental knowledge contributes substantially to the complex relationship of hearing, speech, and language in the important role of social communication.

It is difficult to identify a single locus of time or place as the exact origin of the science of audiology. In general, audiology developed as a rehabilitative service following World War II, when thousands of military personnel returned home with significant acquired hearing impairments. Raymond Carhart, a speech pathologist, and Norton Canfield, an otolaryngologist, were designated by the military to develop a program in aural rehabilitation so that the armed forces medical service could provide appropriate clinical treatment to return the hearing-impaired veteran to useful civilian life. The efforts of Carhart and Canfield resulted in the establishment of several aural rehabilitation centers associated with large military hospitals located around the United States. These programs provided tests of hearing function, selection and distribution of hearing aids, as well as rehabilitative therapy in the form of auditory training, speech reading, and counseling. The goal of the programs was to provide veterans with the means to perform normally in their daily life in spite of their hearing deficits. These military aural rehabilitation centers were to be the focus of development of audiologic testing and clinical management of hearing disorders, which would pervade our growing profession for the years ahead. These military clinics became the training and testing ground for many of our leading clinicians and scientists in the understanding and treatment of hearing dysfunction.

The genealogy of audiology is complex and includes influences from many other specialty fields. Audiology continues to have a close relationship to many medical, surgical, and nonmedical disciplines. From specialties in medicine the audiologist must be prepared to work with pediatrics, family practice, neurology, infectious disease, genetics, neonatology, anesthesiology, internal medicine, gerontology, rehabilitative medicine, radiology, and psychiatry. Several surgical specialties may require audiologic testing or electrophysiologic evaluation of their patients prior to, during, or following surgery. These surgical specialties include otolaryngology, neurosurgery, trauma surgery, orthopedics, nephrology, general surgery, ophthalmology, and plastic surgery as well as oral surgery and even dentistry.

Influence on the development and conduct of audiology also comes from nonmedical disciplines. Certainly a number of areas within psychology such as sensory, clinical, experimental, and developmental psychology all contribute to our daily activities. Other social sciences such as sociology, family relations, social work, and group dynamics have impact on the way we interact with hearing-impaired patients and their families. Finally, there must be recognition for the basic science areas that gave audiology its beginning — physics, acoustics, and electronics. Certainly, one of the most appealing aspects of working in the area of audiology is the constant involvement with the wide fields of knowledge that contribute to our particular area of expertise.

Technological Development

The most complete history of the development of the audiometer was prepared by Glorig and Downs (1965), and much of the following material is based on their report. Glorig and Downs pointed out that the audiometer could not have been possible until "all the pieces of an acoustic and electronic jigsaw puzzle fell together at a point of time when medical needs demanded such an instrument." The point of time was 1875 when Alexander Graham Bell invented the electric telephone as an aid for his wife's hearing impairment. The basic components of the early telephone, including the microphone and the earphone, were essential precursors to the audiometer. By 1878, Arthur Hartmann, an otolaryngologist in a Berlin hospital, reported that he had devised an "acoumeter" that used a telephone receiver for the purpose of testing hearing. In the early attempts to build electronic devices for testing hearing, the basic system was to place a tuning fork in the primary circuit of an induction coil, and to use an "interrupter switch" to induce an alternating current to produce a tone corresponding to the frequency of the vibrating tuning fork.

However, these early instruments were of little use because they were too limited, bulky, and difficult to use. Of special interest is the work of Seashore (1899, 1920) at the University of Iowa, who coined the term *audiometer* and built a special circuit in which the secondary windings were arranged as a series of coils in which the loudness of the stimulus corresponded to the Weber–Fechner law, which was the rage of the field of experimental psychology at the turn of the century.

In 1914, Stefanini of Italy constructed an audiometer with an electric generator and an alternating current that could produce a complete range of test frequencies for hearing measurement. In 1919, Lee Dean, the head of the Department of Otolaryngology at the University of Iowa, and Corida C. Bunch, his research assistant, applied this electric generator to the first clinically useful audiometer. The audiometer built by Dean and Bunch was never actually commercially available, but these researchers published a collection of studies describing the clinical application of their audiometric tests to the practice of otology. They published graphs of the test results, which they called "hearing fields." Bunch (1943) produced a seminal textbook, *Clinical Audiometry*, which described a series of fundamental techniques for assessing auditory function, and set the stage for the expansion of this fledgling field following World War II.

Glorig and Downs' (1965) historical accounting of audiometer development identifies a second important period as 1921 to 1940, when the vacuum tube was developed and used in audiometers to produce oscillating electric currents of almost any frequency. In 1922 (a, b), an otologist and physicist, Fowler and Wegel, respectively, reported on the clinical use of the Western Electric 1A audiometer developed by Fletcher and Wegel (1922) for the Bell Telephone Laboratories. Glorig and Downs credit Fowler and Wegel for applying the name *audiogram* to the chart of auditory thresholds. The Western Electric 1A audiometer was not widely used because it was very expensive, giving way to the Western Electric 2A model, which was eventually adopted by otolaryngologists for office use.

The limitations of the pure tone hearing test were obvious early in the era of audiometer development. The earliest speech audiometers were not available until 1904 and then used Edison's phonograph with speech stimuli presented through stethoscope tubes (Bryant, 1904). In 1920, Seashore published his classic studies on testing music abilities using phonograph records as discrimination tests for pitch and intensity. The technique of phonograph recording speech audiometric testing was used in the Western Electric 4A audiometer with 20 to 40 sets of earphones for group hearing testing in school children (McFarlan, 1927).

In 1947, George von Bekesy invented an automatic, self-recording audiometer in which the patient tracked his own auditory threshold. The Bekesy audiometer had a tremendous influence on more than a decade of research and clinical applications in diagnostic audiology. Jerger (1960) described Bekesy "patterns," which were highly related to specific site of lesions in the auditory pathway, thereby opening the door for research activity in developing tests for advanced audiologic evaluation. For an in-depth description of the historical development of clinical audiology, refer to Chapter 2.

Each subsequent decade has seen the rapid development of additional procedures related to diagnostic audiology. The 1960s were the years of speech audiometry growth with tests to identify central auditory lesions, speech tests with competing messages, dichotic procedures, and forced-choice speech tests, to name a few. During the 1970s, the audiologic community quickly embraced the application of clinical immittance audiometry. This technique, developed in Scandinavia, brought a new level of accuracy in audiometric diagnosis previously deemed impossible. A treatise on acoustic immittance measures may be found in Chapter 6.

During the late 1970s and early 1980s, the electrophysiologic evaluation of the auditory system became a reality as the use of computerized signal averagers became commonplace in nearly every clinical setting. Short-latency, middle, and cortical auditory evoked potentials (AEPs) have been the focus of audiologic diagnosis. They shed light on more rostral levels of auditory function and integrity, as well as providing an objective means to evaluate hearing, in all age groups of patients — from infants to geriatrics. A detailed account of clinical AEP application may be found in Chapter 7.

The advent of new technology in audiology seems to have no end. The use of personal computer technology in audiology has been incorporated into clinical practice, hearing aid evaluation and dispensing, office management, data storage, microprocessor-based controlled auditory tests, and refinement of measurement analysis (Stach and Jerger, 1986).

Audiologic diagnosis represents a professional level of expertise not easily attained without substantial academic preparation and extensive clinical experience. Proper use of the high-tech instrumentation currently available requires professionally trained individuals dedicated to the challenge of searching out and decoding the complexities of the impaired auditory system. Numerous subtle, but nonetheless significant, auditory dysfunctions may now be identified with a high rate of accuracy not realized in earlier years.

AUDIOLOGIC ASSESSMENT

A significant role of the clinician in the assessment of hearing impairment is to quantify and qualify auditory pathology based on perceptual and physiologic response to acoustic stimuli. The psychophysical principles of audition and the development of the "transistor age" supported through various commercial enterprises have helped the basic audiologic evaluation diversify to its current state of behavioral and electrophysiologic indices. In this section, we develop clinical ground rules that set the theme for the remainder of the text.

TERMINOLOGY

For editorial consistency throughout the text, we have attempted to establish an acceptable terminology that reflects today's educational and clinical environment. After an extensive review of the literature including established standards (ANSI, 1970; 1973; 1978; 1986), proposed ASHA guidelines (1974; 1978; 1979; 1988a and b), and a general consensus of contributing authors, the following terms have been adopted in this text. Only those terms that are frequently (mis)used in clinical practice or a matter of controversy will be cited here.

It should be noted that three regulatory agencies currently write standards for audiometric calibration. They include the American National Standards Institute (ANSI), the International Electro-technical Commission, and the International Standards Association. Although not legally bound, manufacturers usually adhere to ANSI standards, and organizations such as ASHA and the American Academy of Otolaryngology, Head and Neck Surgery endorse their application.

Acoustic immittance Although the terms *impedance* and *immittance* have been used interchangeably, in recent years, the term *immittance* has gained clinical popularity and is now found ubiquitously throughout the current literature. *Immittance* has gained international acceptance denoting either acoustic impedence or acoustic admittance and is consistent with terminology recommendations of the proposed Standard for Aural, Acoustic Immittance Instruments under development by ANSI (1986). The term *immittance* will be used hereafter.

Sensory hearing loss The term *sensorineural* has been used similarly to describe hearing loss from which the cochlea, acoustic nerve, or more rostral regions of the auditory pathway or any combination thereof contributed. Despite evidence to suggest that auditory pathology may be isolated to either the receptor end organ or the neural pathway, these combined anatomic loci (sensory and neural) remain an acceptable term in clinical practice. As Katz (1985) correctly points out, the use of *sensorineural* is a serious overgeneralization. We encourage and have adopted the following throughout the remainder of the text. Hearing impairment of a congenital or acquired nature that can be attributed exclusively to cochlear damage resulting in either partial or total destruction of the sensory receptor site is best described as a *sensory hearing loss (SHL)*. Any decrease in hearing sensitivity that represents neurogenic damage, that is, limited to the acoustic nerve and more rostral brainstem regions, should be described as *retrocochlear* or *neural*. When undisputed evidence exists that both cochlea and neural mechanisms contribute to a reduction in hearing sensitivity, the term *sensorineural* is acceptable.

Speech audiometry Recently, the ASHA Committee on Audiologic Evaluation (1988a) developed a new set of *Guidelines for Determining the Threshold Level for Speech*. The intent of the new *Guidelines* is to provide a standard procedure allowing interclinician and interclinic data comparisons. In their document, ASHA recommends the use of the term *speech recognition threshold (SRT)* (rather than *speech reception threshold*) as the preferred term because it more accurately describes the listener's task. The term *speech threshold* should not be used because it does not adequately describe recognition or reception of the material. The term *speech detection threshold (SDT)*, defined as the minimum hearing level for speech at which an individual can just discern the presence of speech material 50 percent of the time, is suggested in place of the term *speech awareness threshold,* which is also recognized as a synonymous expression but similarly does not accurately describe the listener's task. The terms *speech recognition threshold* and *speech detection threshold* will be used when appropriate in this text.

In speech audiometry, a number of terms have been used to describe an individual's ability to perceive and correctly identify words in isolation or in context. They include *articulation, discrimination, intelligibility, identification, recognition, PB "max,"* and *performance intensity* to name just a few. Clinically, open-ended monosyllabic word lists and to a lesser degree, nonsense syllables, closed set words, and sentences have been employed to measure speech perception. Unlike the term *speech recognition threshold,* ASHA has not recommended a term to describe this function, and as a consequence, *speech discrimination* has gained favor throughout historical use; however, *speech discrimination* implies an ability to differentiate among stimuli as "same or different" (Olsen and Matkin, 1979). Given that routine speech tasks do not require the listener to make decisions between two speech stimuli, the term *discrimination* used in conventional speech audiometry is inaccurate. The expression *speech recognition (SR)* is a more correct description and is used throughout the text to express an individual's ability to identify speech material at a suprathreshold level.

Auditory evoked potentials *Auditory evoked potentials (AEPs)* is a generic term that implies a series of objective, electrophysiologic procedures that attempt to assess auditory function and neurologic integrity. Currently, no standard classification system has been accepted, but generally AEPs can be considered either receptor (originating in the cochlea) or neurogenic (generated for the acoustic nerve or neuronal populations within the auditory central nervous system) potentials. AEPs have also been described by their response latency, anatomic origin, stimulus-response relationship, or electrode placement (Jacobson, 1985). An example of the response-time domain or "epoch" is the short-latency AEPs, which consist of the electrocochleograph (ECochG; ≤ 2 msec), the auditory brainstem response (ABR; ≤ 10 msec),

and perhaps the middle latency response (MLR; ≤ 60 msec).

Within the framework of auditory assessment, AEPs offer an objective method of audiogram approximation. In doing so, several AEPs and numerous techniques may be used to complete an audiometric evaluation. Unfortunately to date, no independent response or series of procedures has accomplished this goal with the same accuracy as behavioral pure tone measures. Nevertheless, for populations that are difficult to test with behavioral protocol, AEPs have proved to be the most reliable of objective techniques for estimating threshold sensitivity.

Short-latency AEPs, particularly the ECochG and the ABR, present a major application in the detection and localization of disorders affecting the cochlear nerve and higher elements in the auditory pathway. AEPs provide a diagnostic measure that reveals normal or abnormal neural function in certain types of central disorders such as acoustic tumors and other space-occupying lesions of the posterior cranial fossa, detection of more rostral lesions in the brainstem, differentiating structural from metabolic causes of coma secondary to closed head injury, and monitoring neural function during surgery. AEPs are a complementary investigative mode; with their noninvasive character, high-level operating characteristics, and relative low cost, their role is established in otoneurologic investigation.

THE AUDIOGRAM

The audiogram provides a means of recording audiometric data for permanent display and minimally includes pure tone threshold sensitivity as a function of frequency and speech test results. The basic specifications of an audiogram have been recommended by ASHA (1974; 1988b) and adopted by ANSI (S3.21–1978, R–1986). ASHA recommends that frequency (in Hertz [Hz]) plotted on the abscissa is graphed on a logarithmic scale whereas hearing level (HL) (in decibels [dB]) on the ordinate is expressed linearly. Further, they recommend that a division of one octave on the frequency scale is equivalent to 20 dB on the ordinate or HL scale.

Typically, audiometric data can be recorded in two ways. They are graphic, that is, the symbol plotting of audiometric thresholds by frequency, and tabular, the numeric representation of threshold sensitivity. The graphic illustration is found most typically although some clinic facilities including the Veterans Administration use the tabular form almost exclusively.

Both forms have advantages. The graphic form offers a visual comparison between ears and is perhaps the easiest method of describing hearing status to a patient. The tabular form has been used successfully when a series of audiometric records are to be performed on the same patient. Industrial and school screening programs tend to favor this latter approach.

Audiometric symbols adopted by ASHA (1988b) appear in Figure 1-1A (Response) and Figure 1-1B (No Response); however, as indicated by Jerger (1976), when plotted on one audiogram, the number of ASHA-recommended symbols for the right and left ears under various conditions presents a confusing dilemma at best. This is particularly true in bilateral symmetric conductive or mixed hearing loss. As an alternative, Jerger (1976) proposed a simplification to the ASHA guidelines (Figure 1-1C). The primary advantages are the use of two graphs, one for each ear, and the use of only two audiometric symbols. Masking is indicated by shading in the existing air and bone conduction (open) symbols. The result is a less cluttered visual representation of audiometric data. This is clearly demonstrated in Figure 1-2 by a hypothetical example of an asymmetric bilateral hearing loss typically found in patients presenting with sensory pathology. The advantages of the Jerger method are vividly evident from the obtained audiometric results. Based on our support of this audiometric symbol concept, we recommend the adoption and use of the Jerger symbols and have incorporated them throughout the remainder of *Diagnostic Audiology*.

An example of an audiometric record that incorporates both graphic and tabular format is illustrated in Figure 1-3. Audiometric symbols may be used to graphically display the first audiometric test; thereafter, tabular data are compiled for each test session. This allows a serial comparison of each patient visit collected on a single audiometric sheet. The format has been found to save space in the patient's chart, reduce the time and confusion searching for any one particular test result, and is considerably less expensive than generating a single audiogram per visit.

With the advent of more complex diagnostic tests that are used routinely in the audiologic evaluation, the audiogram offers a convenient form to record various test results. Figure 1-4 presents an audiogram that uses the Jerger graphic symbol system, allows for conventional and nonconventional speech testing, and provides an area for illustrative acoustic immittance audiometry.

Regardless of the audiogram adopted, an audiometric record should best suit the primary audiologic activities and the department needs as an integrated part of the diagnostic process. Elaborate audiograms as illustrated have little application in a school screening environment where the audiologist or speech pathologist may be limited to a portable audiometer. On the other hand, in teaching institutions, the opportunity of visual supplementation for students learning how to *read* audiometric configurations and interpret the audiogram (e.g., acoustic immittance and nonstandard speech results) may provide the necessary transition from theory to practical application.

Figure 1-1. Audiometric symbols adopted by ASHA (A and B) and those recommended by Jerger (C).

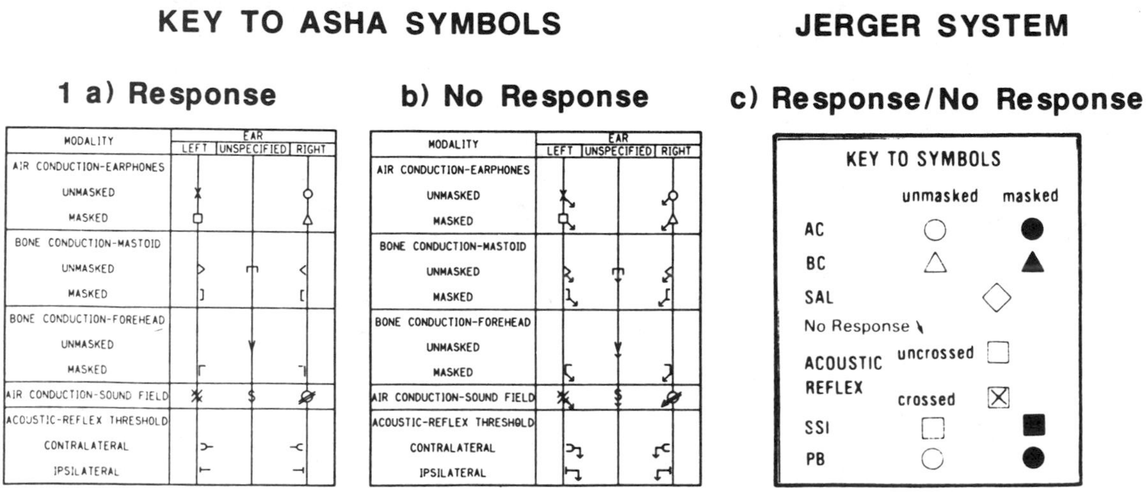

KEY TO ASHA SYMBOLS

JERGER SYSTEM

1 a) Response

b) No Response

c) Response/No Response

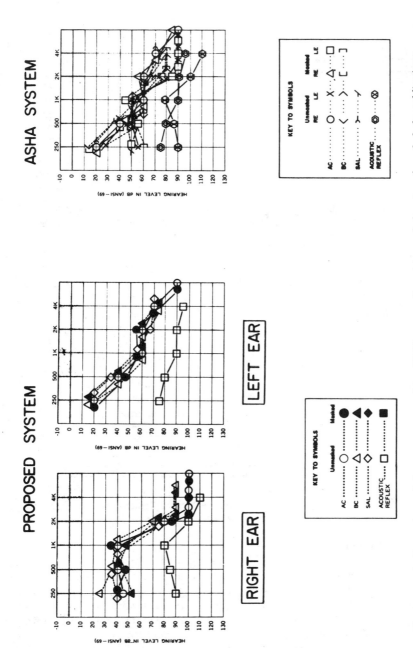

Figure 1-2. Audiometric symbol system proposed by ASHA and Jerger (1976) for a hypothetical case of bilateral sensory hearing loss. (From Jerger, J. [1976]. A proposed audiometric symbol system for scholarly publications. *Archives of Otolaryngology, 102,* 33–36. Copyright 1976, American Medical Association. With permission.)

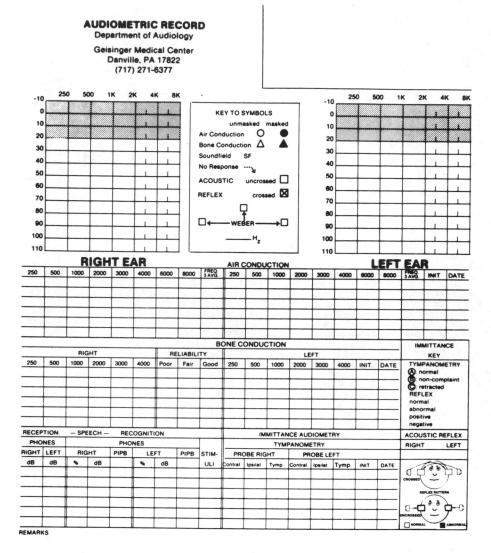

Figure 1-3. Audiometric record using both pictorial and numeric data entry.

Clinical Application

A hearing evaluation should include in its armamentarium a series of tests that leads to an accurate assessment of the degree of hearing loss and site of lesion in the most efficient and economic means possible. In recent years, the basic auditory test battery has consisted of pure tone threshold measures, conventional speech (SRT and SR), and immittance audiometry.* Based on initial test result outcome, a test strategy, conducted in either serial or parallel, could be generated to demonstrate threshold sensitivity and existing pathophysiology. The introduction of sensitized speech material and objective electrophysiologic measures, which bring improved operating characteristics, particularly as they relate to retrocochlear and central processing disorders, has done much to change the attitudes toward and the rationale for current test strategy.

In a profession that is ever increasing its dependence on objective measures, it is important to remember that the pure tone audiogram remains

---

* Because basic principles and clinical application of acoustic immittance are detailed in Chapter 6 and examples are delineated in various case studies throughout the text, a discussion of acoustic immittance will be omitted in this section. Suffice it to say that since the seminal report by Jerger (1970), the impact of acoustic immittance on the auditory evaluation of normal and pathologic patients has been unprecedented in the field of audiology.

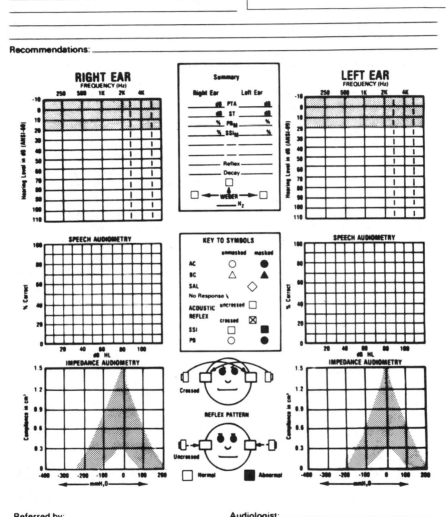

Figure 1-4. Audiology report providing a recording of pure tone, speech, and immittance audiometry for each ear.

the cornerstone of the audiologic evaluation. Whereas the primary goal of pure tone audiometry is to define auditory threshold sensitivity as a function of frequency, the employment of air and bone conduction testing provides additional information concerning a patient's hearing status. Pure tone measures offer insight into (1) the type of hearing impairment (e.g., conductive, sensory);

(2) the degree of severity; (3) the possible site of lesion, which may include the external, middle, and inner ear, or acoustic nerve and caudal regions of the auditory mechanism; and (4) rehabilitative needs of the patient including hearing aid benefit and aural (re)habilitative measures.

Interpretation

Superficially, the interpretation of pure tone audiometry appears to be a simple and straightforward exercise. If auditory instrumentation is routinely calibrated and standardized testing protocol is followed, the assumption is made that the interpretation of an audiometric configuration should provide sufficient information to make a reasonably accurate estimate of the peripheral hearing status in most patients. It is important to recognize that several sources of variability exist in basic audiometry that may confuse and even mislead the examiner from the true measure of auditory status. This is most evident in the medical environment. Here, pathologic patients with subclinical findings are frequently misidentified because clinical evaluation may be limited to only basic pure tone and conventional speech audiometry.

0 Take for example a patient who presents with normal pure tone sensitivity (less than or equal to 20-dB HL from 250–8000 Hz) and a speech recognition score of about 86 percent or better to a phonetically balanced word list. Is this sufficient information to confirm normal auditory function? The findings of several publications (Antonelli, 1970; Bocca and Calearo, 1963; Jerger, 1964, 1973; Keith, 1977) have pointed out that significant central auditory dysfunction may exist in the presence of normal audiometric findings. Jerger and Jordan (1980) and more recently Hedley, Jerger, and Stach (1987) have described a series of 40 patients who met "normal" conventional criteria, yet presented with auditory disorders of the acoustic

nerve and brainstem pathway. Through the use of improved sensitive speech measures (phonetically balanced words and synthetic sentence index rollover functions), they were able to accurately demonstrate abnormal test findings that led to the identification and eventual confirmation of retrocochlear pathology in all 40 patients.

Because much of test protocol is based on empiric evidence, patient history, physical examination, and audiologic environment, a diagnostic evaluation should be a synthesis of sound clinical judgment. Most often, the results of a basic auditory test battery (i.e., pure tones, speech, and immittance audiometry) will predicate further diagnostic strategy. Given the complexity of auditory pathology, this basic test battery should be conceived of as a first-level auditory evaluation. A suggested flow chart for this initial auditory assessment is displayed in Figure 1-5. Ideally, immittance measures are the first component of any auditory evaluation since they provide key insight into auditory integrity and function. A comprehensive diagnostic flow chart for middle ear and sensory pathology is illustrated in Chapter 8 and Chapter 9, respectively.

If components within the initial screen suggest abnormal findings, a second-level evaluation of more specific site of lesion tests is in order. What

Figure 1-5. Flow chart for an ideal basic hearing evaluation.

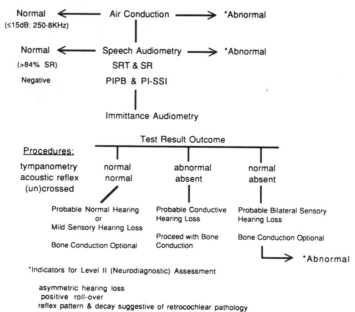

BASIC HEARING EVALUATION: LEVEL I

*Indicators for Level II (Neurodiagnostic) Assessment

  asymmetric hearing loss
  positive roll-over
  reflex pattern & decay suggestive of retrocochlear pathology

tests are most appropriate is dictated by initial test results, suspected pathology, environment, and patient status. Although specific tests for second-level evaluation remain undefined, the use of decision matrix analysis is beginning to provide a reasonable justification for specific test battery protocol (Turner, 1988).

Common sense argues that a test battery is only as efficient as the individual components that compose it. Test procedures must undergo constant scrutiny to ensure that their ability to correctly identify auditory pathology and, for that matter, normal hearing, remains uncompromised. This becomes clear with the recent proliferation of articles emphasizing the importance of operating characteristics (sensitivity, specificity, and predictive values) in the diagnostic evaluation (Jacobson and Jacobson, 1987; J. Jerger, 1983; S. Jerger, 1983; Murray, Javel, and Watson, 1985; Schwartz, 1987; Turner, Frazer, and Shepard, 1984; Turner and Nielsen, 1984; Turner, Shepard, and Frazer, 1984). A comprehensive description of the basic principles of clinical decision analysis may be found in Chapter 14.

WORK ENVIRONMENT

In the early stages of the communicative disorders profession, the type of work environment in which to pursue a career was limited; however, as the profession of audiology began to expand in both clinical and research settings, a wide variety of opportunities became available (Northern, 1986). As surveyed from recent audiology graduates, the largest increase in occupational activity has been found in clinical services, which have tripled over the past 4 decades (Shewan, 1987). It has been estimated that approximately 85 percent

of the ASHA profession is currently involved in some aspect of clinical service (Shewan, 1988a). Table 1-1 lists the primary employment settings of audiologists and the activities of all ASHA members currently in the profession. As expected, the precise activities of individual ASHA members are most often dictated by the primary site of employment. Interestingly, almost one-fourth of the profession holds a second position in addition to their current site of primary employment (Shewan, 1988a). Although most audiologists maintain some direct contact with hearing-impaired clients, a very small percentage of professionals are engaged in full-time research activities (about 1%; see Table 1-1) to develop a better understanding of normal and abnormal auditory function and the mechanisms that cause hearing impairment.

MEDICAL CENTERS AND HOSPITALS

Most medical centers, hospitals, and rehabilitative agencies employ audiologists to perform hearing testing services, including the pre- and postoperative evaluation of otologic surgical patients. The audiologist receives referrals from a variety of medical specialists and surgeons including otolaryngologists, neurologists, neurosurgeons, pediatricians, family practitioners, and internists. In hospitals with active neonatal and pediatric intensive care nurseries, the audiologist may be administratively responsible for directing and supervising a hearing screening program for at-risk infants who may be suspect for hearing loss. Recently, audiologists have begun to provide electrophysiologic monitoring in pediatric and adult intensive care units as well as other sensory evoked potential monitoring in the operating room. An increasing number of audiology-based hospital clinics dispense hearing aids as part of

TABLE 1-1. PRIMARY EMPLOYMENT SETTINGS (AUDIOLOGISTS) AND ACTIVITIES (AUDIOLOGISTS AND SPEECH PATHOLOGISTS) OF ASHA MEMBERS

Primary employment setting (%)[a]		Primary employment activity (%)[b]	
College/university	12.1	Administration	7.4
School	9.7	College/university teaching	4.4
Hospital/clinic and rehabilitation facility	25.8	Consultation	2.5
Government health service	4.6	Clinical service	70.1
Private practice	8.8	Research	1.3
Other setting	11.1	Special education teaching	4.6
Unknown	27.9	Supervisor of clinical activity	3.1
		Other activity	6.5

[a] Adapted from Punch, J. (1983). Characteristics of ASHA members. *ASHA, 25*(10), 31.
[b] From Demographic profile of the ASHA membership. (1988). ASHA Research Division.

their routine services. The Veterans Administration Hospital and Medical Centers employ audiologists to work with the large number of military service veterans who have hearing loss. Caseloads are diverse and commonly include, but are not limited to, diagnostic assessment, compensation examinations, hearing aid dispensing, and adult rehabilitation.

MEDICAL OFFICES

Many audiologists are employed in private practice medical offices or group medical clinics. The audiologists in these work environments spend most of their time in direct patient contact conducting a full battery of diagnostic audiologic hearing tests, vestibular evaluations, and hearing aid dispensing. Usually the audiologist in a medical practice works in cooperation with a physician who specializes in disease of the ears, nose, and throat.

PRIVATE PRACTICE

A growing trend continues with more and more audiologists establishing themselves in private practice offices. The number of full-time employees has risen to 11 percent with an additional 19 percent who work part-time in private practice (Shewan, 1988b). Audiologists venturing into this marketplace usually have previous work experience (median, 5 years) before embarking into this challenging area (Shewan, 1988a). This increase has, for the most part, been attributed to the changing attitude toward dispensing hearing aids and personal gains found in private practice. Thus, these audiologists are primarily involved with the retail dispensing of hearing aids directly to hearing-impaired consumers. In this employment setting, the audiologist, in addition to drawing on special knowledge of hearing, auditory pathology, and hearing aids, must possess additional skills in business-related activities such as financial planning, marketing, and public relations.

UNIVERSITIES

According to the 1985 *Guide to Graduate Education,* the number of accredited (110) and nonaccredited (37) programs has grown substantially over the past 4 decades; however, the number of professionals working in this environment has decreased to about 5 percent of the recently graduated ASHA membership (Shewan, 1987). Audiologists who work in college and university set-

tings are primarily involved in teaching and preparing students to become professional audiologists or speech-language pathologists. In conjunction with the educational aspects, most training programs incorporate some type of clinical service as a practicum site for graduate clinicians. The practicum experiences vary greatly and depend on the expertise of the staff (Jacobson, Kileny, and Ruth, 1988). University personnel are usually expected to supervise student practicum and direct research projects that culminate in advanced degrees for their students.

COMMUNITY HEARING AND SPEECH CENTERS

Each community hearing and speech center employs audiologists to work with adults and children with hearing impairments. In this employment setting, the audiologist is primarily a rehabilitation specialist rather than a medical-oriented diagnostician. The audiologist performs hearing tests, selects and fits hearing aids, and guides the rehabilitation of hearing-impaired individuals fitted with personal amplification. Many such facilities include special education programs for hearing-impaired children who benefit from the audiologist's special training and understanding of pediatric problems. The audiologist's duties may include helping individuals use their hearing aids better, working to improve speechreading skills, or assisting in community public service health education programs.

HEARING CONSERVATION

Excessive environmental noise and acoustic abuse in the work place contribute substantially to employee hearing loss. The audiologist plays a major role in dealing with hearing problems related to overexposure to such noises. Governmental influences through the Occupational Safety and Health Act and the Workman's Compensation Program require that employers with noisy work environments provide for employee hearing protection. Many industries conduct periodic employee hearing tests, develop noise reduction plans, and issue and maintain effective personal hearing protection for employees.

SCHOOLS

With the enactment of Public Law 94-142, the number of school audiologists has increased substantially. Today, most states mandate some sort of hearing screening program in public and private schools. These school hearing programs are usually directed and supervised by audiologists. Children receive hearing tests at various times during their primary and secondary school years to identify educationally handicapping hearing loss. The children with hearing loss are referred for medical attention to improve their hearing problem or are fitted with hearing aids if their hearing loss is not amenable to medical treatment.

FUTURE DIRECTIONS

The transformation of a profession is usually impacted by those most closely associated with its internal organizational structure. In retrospect, however, a review of the historical developments of audiology reflects influence over the decades by several medical and nonmedical disciplines. Given the influx of diverse backgrounds and views, it is not surprising that audiology is often accused of suffering from an "identity crisis." Heterogeneous input, on the other hand, offers a number of compelling advantages. For example, the explosion of hearing aid technology has been greatly influenced by the engineering community, computer experts have written programs to support virtually every aspect of diagnostic and rehabilitative audiology, and biomedical manufacturers have provided new methods of recording electrophysiologic responses now commonplace in the clinic setting. These innovations, which have modified our behavior, have occurred through the efforts of individuals not necessarily directly associated with audiology or the hearing-impaired community.

Audiology is rapidly expanding its clinical service component and, in many instances, necessitating professional subspecialization. Examples are prolific: The private practitioner, (re)habilitation with cochlear implant patients, hearing aid dispensing, intensive care and operative monitoring, and industrial litigation are a few of the new challenges that face our profession. Keeping abreast of change is not only essential but required. Nonetheless, with such rapidly developing technology, can audiologists maintain expertise in every aspect of the field? Review the number of articles published on a monthly basis in audiology and other medical journals that are specifically related to audition and the answer becomes self-evident. The 1990s will develop as an era of expansion that will dictate specialization for most clinicians in order to maintain improved services to the hearing-impaired community.

Where does the profession go from here? If the past 2 decades have taught us anything, future change must be expected and anticipated. Meeting this continued developmental evolution may be our biggest challenge of the future.

REFERENCES

Alford, B. R., & Jerger, J. (1977). Audiology and otolaryngology: A continuing partnership. *Archives of Otolaryngology, 103,* 249–250.

Antonelli, A. R. (1970). Sensitized speech tests in aged people. In C. Rojskjar (Ed.), *Speech audiometry.* Second Danavox Symposium, Odense, Denmark.

American Academy of Audiology. (1989). *Scope of practice.* Houston.

American National Standards Institute. (1970). *Specifications for audiometers* (ANSI S3.6–1969 [R–1973]). New York.

American National Standards Institute. (1973). *American National Standards psychoacoustical terminology* (ANSI S3.20). New York.

American National Standards Institute. (1978). *Methods for manual pure-tone threshold audiometry* (ANSI S3.21 [R–1986]). New York.

American National Standards Institute. (1986). *Proposed American National Standards specifications for instruments to measure aural acoustic impedance and admittance (aural acoustic immittance)* (ANSI S3.39–1986). New York.

American Speech and Hearing Association. Committee on Audiometric Evaluation. (1974). Guidelines for audiometric symbols. *ASHA, 17*(5), 260–264.

American Speech and Hearing Association. Committees on Audiometric Evaluation. (1978). Guidelines for manual pure-tone threshold audiometry. *ASHA, 20*(4), 297–301.

American Speech-Language-Hearing Association. Committees on Audiometric Evaluation. (1979). Guidelines for determining the threshold levels for speech. *ASHA, 21*(5), 353–355.

American Speech-Language-Hearing Association. (1984). ASHA National Office letter from Steven C. While, Ph.D., Director, Reimbursement Policy Division, to the Health Insurance Assocation of America.

American Speech-Language-Hearing Association. (1985). ASHA National Office staff for Rehabilitation Standards Division, Department of Standards, Joint Commission on Accreditation of Hospitals.

American Speech-Language-Hearing Association. (1988a). Guidelines for determining threshold level for speech. *ASHA, 30*(3), 85–88.

American Speech-Language-Hearing Association. Committee on Audiometric Evaluation. (1988b). Guidelines for audiometric symbols. *ASHA, 30*(12), 39–42.

Bocca, E., & Calearo, C. (1963). Central hearing processes. In J. Jerger (Ed.), *Modern developments in audiology.* New York: Academic Press.

Bryant, W. S. (1904). A phonographic acoumeter. *Archives of Otolaryngology, 33,* 438.

Bunch, C. C. (1943). *Clinical audiometry.* St. Louis: C.V. Mosby.

Davis, H. (1970). Audiology. In H. Davis & S. R. Silverman (Eds.), *Hearing and deafness* (3rd ed.). New York: Holt, Rinehart & Winston.

Dean, L., & Bunch, C. C. (1919). The use of the pitch range audiometer in otology. *Laryngoscope, 29,* 453.

Dix, M. R., Hallpike, C. S., & Hood, J. D. (1948). Observations upon the loudness recruitment phenomenon, with special reference to the differential diagnosis of disorders of the internal ear and VIIIth nerve. *Journal of Laryngology and Otology, 62,* 671–686.

Fletcher, H., & Wegel, R. L. (1922). The frequency sensitivity of normal ears. *Physiology Review, 19,* 553.

Fowler, E. P., & Wegel, R. L. (1922a). Presentation of a new instrument for determining the amount and character of auditory sensation. *Transactions of the American Otology Society, 16,* 105–123.

Fowler, E. P., & Wegel, R. L. (1922b). Audiometric methods and their applications. *Transactions of the American Laryngology, Rhinology, and Otolaryngology Society, 28,* 96.

Glorig, A., & Downs, M. (1965). Introduction to audiometry. In A. Glorig (Ed.), *Audiometry: Principles and practices* (pp. 1–14). Baltimore: Williams & Wilkins.

Hartmann, A. (1878). Eine Nene Methode der Horprufung mit Hulfe Elektrischer Strone. *Archives of Physiology, 155.*

Hedley, A. J., Jerger, J. F., & Stach, B. A. (1987). Normal audiometric findings revisited. (Abstract). *ASHA, 29,* 125.

Jacobson, J. T. (1985). An overview of the auditory brainstem response. In J. T. Jacobson (Ed.), *The auditory brainstem response* (pp. 3–12). Boston: College-Hill Press.

Jacobson, J. T., & Jacobson C. A. (1987). Principles of decision analysis in high risk infants. *Seminars in Hearing, 8,* 133–141.

Jacobson, J. T., Kileny, P. R., & Ruth, R. A. (1988). Auditory evoked potentials: A survey of educational and practice patterns. *ASHA, 30,* 49–52.

Jerger, J. (1960). Bekesy audiometry in analysis of auditory disorders. *Journal of Speech and Hearing Research, 3,* 275.

Jerger, J. (Ed.). (1963). *Modern developments in audiology.* New York: Academic Press.

Jerger, J. (1964). Auditory tests for disorders of the central auditory mechanism. In B. R. Alford & W. S. Fields (Eds.), *Neurological aspects of auditory and vestibular disorders* (pp. 77–86). Springfield, IL: Charles C Thomas.

Jerger, J. (1970). Clinical experiences with impedance audiometry. *Archives of Otolaryngology, 92,* 311–324.

Jerger, J. (1973). Diagnostic audiometry. In J. Jerger (Ed.), *Modern developments in audiology* (pp. 75–115). New York: Academic Press.

Jerger, J. (1976). A proposed audiometric symbol system for scholarly publications. *Archives of Otolaryngology, 102,* 33–36.

Jerger, J. (1983). Strategies for neuroaudiological evaluation. *Seminars in Hearing, 4,* 109–120.

Jerger, J., & Jordan, C. (1980). Normal audiometric findings. *American Journal of Otology, 1,* 157–159.

Jerger, S. (1983). Decision matrix and information theory analyses in the evaluation of neuroaudiological tests. *Seminars in Hearing, 4,* 121–132.

Katz, J. (1985). Clinical audiology. In J. Katz (Ed.), *Handbook of clinical audiology.* Baltimore: Williams & Wilkins.

Keith, R. (1977). Synthetic sentence identification. In R. W. Keith (Ed.), *Central auditory dysfunction.* New York: Grune & Stratton.

Konkle, D. F. & Rintelmann, W. F. (1979). Peripheral and central auditory systems: Test battery interpretation. In W. F. Rintelmann (Ed.), *Hearing assessment.* Baltimore: University Park Press.

Mahon, W. J. (1988). ADA focuses on the future. *The Hearing Journal, 41,* 22–25.

McFarland, D. (1927). The voice test of hearing. *Archives of Otolaryngology, 5,* 1.

Murray, A., Javel, E., & Watson, C. (1985). Prognostic validity of auditory brainstem evoked response screening in newborn infants. *American Journal of Otolaryngology, 6,* 120–131.

Northern, J. L. (1986). Auditory overview. In J. Van Cleve (Ed.), *Encyclopedia of deaf people and deafness.* New York: McGraw-Hill.

Olsen, W., & Matkin, N. (1978). Differential audiology. In D. Rose (Ed.), *Audiology assessment.* Englewood Cliffs, NJ: Prentice-Hall.

Olsen, W., & Matkin, N. (1979). Speech audiometry. In W. F. Rintelmann (Ed.), *Hearing assessment.* Baltimore: University Park Press.

Sanders, J. (1988). Diagnostic audiology. In N. J. Lass, L. V. McReynolds, J. L. Northern, & D. E. Yoder (Eds.), *Handbook of speech-language pathology and audiology* (p. 1123). Toronto: B.C. Decker.

Schwartz, D. M. (1987). Neurodiagnostic audiology: Contemporary perspectives. *Ear & Hearing, 8,* (Suppl. 4), 43S–48S.

Seashore, C. E. (1899). An audiometer. *University of Iowa Studies in Psychology* (No. 2). Iowa City: University of Iowa Press.

Seashore, C. E. (1920). *University of Iowa Studies in Psychology* (No. 36, Vols. 1 and 2). Iowa City: University of Iowa Press.

Shewan, C. M. (1987). ASHA Members: You are a changin! Part II. *ASHA, 29,* 41.

Shewan, C. M. (1988a). 1988 Omnibus survey. *ASHA, 30*(8), 27–30.

Shewan, C. M. (1988b). ASHA members at work. *ASHA, 30*(1), 49.

Stach, B., & Jerger, J. (1986). Microcomputer applications in audiology. In J. Northern (Ed.), *The personal computer for speech, language and hearing professionals* (pp. 113–134). Boston: Little, Brown.

Stefanini, A. (1914). Alternatore pendolare electromagnetico. *Il Nuovo cimento, Series VI, 7,* 261.

Turner, R. G. (1988). Techniques to determine test protocol performance. *Ear & Hearing, 9,* 177–189.

Turner, R. G., & Nielsen, D. W. (1984). Application of clinical decision analysis to audiological tests. *Ear & Hearing, 5,* 123–133.

Turner, R. G., Frazer, G. J., & Shepard, N. T. (1984). Formulating and evaluating audiological test protocols. *Ear & Hearing, 5,* 321–330.

Turner, R. G., Shepard, N. T., & Frazer, G. J. (1984). Clinical performance of audiological and related diagnostic tests. *Ear & Hearing, 5,* 187–194.

U.S. Department of Labor. (1977). *Dictionary of occupational titles* (4th ed.). Washington, DC.

von Bekesy, G. (1947). A new audiometer. *Acta Oto-laryngologica* (Stockholm), *35,* 441–422.

Webster's new collegiate dictionary. (1981). Springfield, MA: G.C. Merriam.

CHAPTER 2

Special Auditory Tests: A Historical Perspective

Wayne O. Olsen

This chapter will review various audiologic tests from a historical perspective. Other chapters review these tests in terms of their clinical integration, interpretation of results, and operating characteristics.

To facilitate this discussion, the material is organized according to sites of involvement within the auditory system. Hence, one section is directed at tests for conductive hearing losses, another section is concerned with audiologic procedures to help differentiate retrocochlear from cochlear pathology, a third section deals with audiologic assessment of central auditory dysfunction, and the final section considers tests for pseudohypacusis. Obviously not all references or tests can be cited, but, insofar as possible, some historical background, representative studies for common or more popular test procedures, and some recent developments are reviewed.

CONDUCTIVE HEARING LOSSES

Cardano's description in 1550 of sound transmission to the ear by means of a rod held between one's teeth is the first description of sound reception via bone conduction. A few years later Capivocci employed like means of stimulation to differentiate disorders of the tympanic membrane and nerve (Feldmann, 1960/1970). "Historically speaking, bone conduction is of such importance ... that one may consider this to be the time of birth of the functional diagnosis of hearing disorders" (Feldmann, 1960/1970, p. 14). Observations of lateralization of responses by hearing-impaired subjects to tuning forks applied to the skull by Weber in 1834 suggested the diagnostic potential of such tests. Rinne's comparison of responses to tuning forks applied to the skull and then held near the ear for normal and hearing-impaired

individuals was described by him in 1855. Thirty years later, Schwabach summarized comparisons of responses to tuning forks by hearing-impaired persons relative to those with normal hearing. Thus in the latter part of the 1800s, the origins of the standard audiologic test battery, comparing responses to air-conducted and to bone-conducted stimuli for a given individual (Rinne), and against a "normal standard" (Schwabach), were described.

PURE TONE AUDIOMETRY

Fowler and Wegel (1922a, b) described the first electronic audiometer produced commercially. The Western Electric 1A generated 20 octave and semioctave frequencies from 32 through 16,384 Hz and had a logarithmic attenuator. They also described charts called *audiograms* for plotting hearing sensitivity relative to a straight line for "normal hearing." "Hearing loss" was plotted on the ordinate and frequency, in octave intervals, on the abscissa. A less expensive Western Electric 2A, covering the frequency range of 64 through 8192 Hz, followed and gained considerable attention and acceptance by the otologists at that time (Bunch, 1941).

In 1943, Bunch published a book entitled *Clinical Audiometry*. Many of the 74 figures in his publication show air conduction audiograms for patients with various pathologies including congenital atresia, otitis media, "traumatic deafness" from intense noise, syphilis, diphtheria, and "hearing loss accompanying advanced age."

As of 1928, Western Electric audiometers routinely were equipped with bone vibrators calibrated empirically from 64 through 8192 Hz. This calibration proved to be quite accurate according to Greenbaum, Kerridge, and Ross (1939). They tested bone conduction thresholds for 100 sub-

19

jects aged 18 to 25 years with two Western Electric audiometers and compared their normal bone conduction curves to the curve suggested by the manufacturer.

Despite pioneering work by, among others, Fowler (1925) and Dean (1930) on "audition by bone conduction," and Guild's (1936) anatomic study of sound transmission by bone conduction, audiometric bone conduction testing did not gain wide acceptance until the early 1950s. In 1946 Lierle and Reger reported air and bone conduction audiograms for patients with otosclerosis, active otitis media, and after recovering from otitis media, as well as for patients with "inner ear lesions." They defined the air-bone threshold relationships associated with middle ear lesions, inner ear lesions, and "mixed lesions," that is, "simultaneous middle and inner ear involvement" (pp. 221–222).

General acceptance of bone conduction audiometry came about with Carhart's article entitled "Clinical Applications of Bone Conduction Audiometry" in 1950. Among other topics addressed in that publication, Carhart described the mechanical shift (decrease) in bone conduction sensitivity observed for patients with stapes fixation. His observation of 5, 10, 15, and 5 dB depression in bone conduction thresholds at 500, 1000, 2000, and 4000 Hz, respectively ("Carhart notch"), was observed for patients found to have stapes fixation due to otosclerosis. This decrease in bone conduction sensitivity disappeared following successful middle ear surgery (fenestration surgery at that time, stapes surgery a few years later). This information allowed surgeons to predict cochlear sensitivity and therefore hearing sensitivity following successful middle ear surgery. These observations, along with the findings of enhanced bone conduction sensitivity for 250 and 500 Hz and slightly elevated bone conduction thresholds at 2000 and 4000 Hz for patients with otitis media (also observed by Lierle and Reger in 1946), as well as interweaving air and bone conduction thresholds for patients with sensory hearing losses demonstrated the diagnostic significance of air and bone conduction threshold tests. Henceforth, audiograms indicating responses to air and bone conduction stimuli became routine evaluations for patients with suspected hearing losses.

SPEECH AUDIOMETRY

Just as pure tone air and bone conduction audiometry have become routine audiologic procedures for patients with hearing impairments, speech audiometry is almost equally routine. The time span over which systematic use of speech stimuli for assessment of auditory deficits developed is also relatively brief.

In 1804 Pfingsten categorized hearing disorders relative to which of three categories of speech sounds a given patient heard: vowels, voiced consonants, and voiceless consonants. Schmalz, in 1846, classified hearing impairments on the basis of the distance that speech was understood when spoken at "normal" and "moderate" levels. Wolf reported further refinements of these methods in 1871. He classified speech sounds according to their frequency content and determined the distances at which different speech sounds could be heard. He also noted that large differences in the audibility of various speech sounds disappeared when speech was whispered (Feldmann, 1960/1970).

Edison's invention of the phonograph in 1877 led to the development of the first recorded test materials by Lichtwitz in 1889. Intensity of the materials was adjusted by speaking at a constant level but at different distances from the sound pickup. Based on Wolfe's work, Lichtwitz devised an acumetric scale and suggested that equivalent lists in all languages would be developed and recorded, allowing "uniform" tests in all countries (Feldmann, 1960/1970).

Tests for recognition or identification of single phonemes in German were developed by Barany in 1910. In his "phoneme substitution words," one phoneme at a time was changed while the others remained constant. Lempert carried Barany's work further in 1923 when he reported tests with sets of words in which, again, only one phoneme changed, but the difference could be the vowel or the initial or final consonants (Feldmann, 1960/1970). Obviously Barany's and Lempert's tests were early forerunners of subsequently developed closed response sets.

During the same time, Campbell and Crandall, in 1910, developed "articulation lists" of 50 nonsense syllables, 5 consonant-vowel, 5 vowel-consonant, and 40 consonant-vowel-consonant items per list to test telephone circuits (O'Neill and Oyer, 1966). In 1924 Jones and Knudsen incorporated circuitry for speech tests into their pure tone audiometer.

Egan's development of 20 lists of monosyllables, each with 50 words per list, phonetically balanced and representative of English speech (Egan, 1948) led to recordings of some of these lists and their early application in clinical settings by Carhart (1946b) and by Thurlow, Davis, Silverman, and Walsh (1949). The latter investigators administered these Harvard Psychoacoustic Laboratory Phonetically Balanced Word Lists (PAL PB 50) as recorded by Rush-Hughes to patients considered to be candidates for middle ear surgery. They stated that "the maximum PB score varies with clinical diagnosis. It is higher in conductive deafness, slightly lower in conductive deafness with some nerve involvement causing high tone hearing loss, and still lower if the nerve involvement predominates" (Thurlow et al., 1949, p. 127). Thus, scores for the Rush-Hughes recording of monosyllabic word lists were viewed as providing diagnostic information in a clinical setting; however, recordings of other test materials such as CID W-22 lists (Hirsh et al., 1952) were less difficult; that is, yielded higher scores than did the materials recorded by Rush-Hughes. This delineation in the continuum of scores noted by Thurlow et al. is not seen with other less difficult test materials (Carhart, 1965). Therefore, differential results obtained from most currently used word recognition test materials presented at sufficiently high suprathreshold levels with good quality reproduction are, at best, only generally suggestive of the nature of the hearing involvement. Individuals with hearing losses due to middle ear pathologies generally yield word recognition scores of 90 percent or better when undistorted test materials are presented at sensation levels of 25 dB or greater. Scores of 80 percent or poorer for like sensation levels usually indicate some sensory or neural involvement, but scores better than 80 percent should not be considered to preclude sensory or neural hearing loss.

IMMITTANCE TESTS

In his classic publication, "The Acoustic Impedance Measured on Normal and Pathological Ears," Metz (1946) credits West in 1928, Troger in 1930, Shuster in 1934, Robinson in 1937, and Waetzmann in 1938 for making early measurements of the acoustic impedance of human ears. But it was Metz' work with normal and pathologic ears that served as the impetus for further development of measurements of middle ear impedance, now more popularly labeled as *immittance*.

According to the comprehensive review of immittance tests prepared by Shallop (1976), the first commercially available immittance unit was introduced in Denmark in 1957. Terkildsen and Thomsen published the first tympanograms for normal and pathologic ears using an electroacoustic immittance unit in 1959. The following year Terkildsen and Nielsen (1960) described an "electroacoustic impedance bridge for clinical use." Zwislocki described his mechanical bridge for measuring middle ear impedance in 1960 followed 2 years later by further description (Zwislocki, 1963), and its application to pathologic ears (Feldman, 1963). The more easily used electroacoustic immittance units and tympanometry became the popular choice clinically. Classification of tympanograms by Liden (1969), Jerger (1970), Liden, Peterson, and Björkman (1970), and Liden, Harford, and Hallen (1974) further demonstrated the clinical utility of immittance measurements.

Liden (1969), Jerger (1970), and Liden and associates (1970, 1974) classified tympanograms indicating normal tympanic membrane and ossicular mobility in conjunction with normal middle ear air pressure as *type A*. Tympanograms showing virtually no movement of the tympanic membrane were associated with otitis media with effusion, that is, fluid-filled middle ears, and were labeled *type B*. A *type C* designation was given to tympanograms revealing mobility of the eardrum and middle ear chain, but with maximum mobility at considerably less than atmospheric pressure. Usually the inferred middle ear pressure had to be more negative than -100 daPa to be called type C associated with abnormal eustachian tube function.

Modifying terms have been added to the type A and type C labels to describe the tympanograms further. Type A_s (shallow) describes tympanograms showing normal middle ear pressure but less mobility than normal as often observed for unusually stiff or thick tympanic membranes, or decreased mobility of the ossicular chain. The letter *d* is appended to type A designation for unusually deep tympanograms seen for flaccid eardrums or interrupted ossicular systems. Type C tympanograms may show a sharp peak (type C_p) when only less than normal middle ear pressure is altering eardrum mobility, or be rounded (type C_r) if the middle ear cavity is partially filled with fluid.

Appropriate diagnostic interpretation of tympanometric results necessitates consideration of air and bone conduction audiometric data also. For example a type A_d tympanogram in conjunction with little or no difference in thresholds for air and bone conduction stimuli suggests a flaccid eardrum, whereas in association with a large air-bone gap, ossicular interruption should be considered. It must be remembered, however, that whatever pathology affects the tympanic membrane mobility most directly will be reflected in the tympanogram. Several problems may coexist in a given ear, but the tympanometric results will suggest the most peripheral involvement. Therefore, the most meaningful interpretations of tympanograms are based on information gleaned from medical history and air and bone conduction audiograms.

Currently immittance units are available in almost all clinical settings. Tympanometry is considered almost routine for patients having conductive hearing losses, or for patients reporting ear complaints of "blocked," "plugged," or "fullness" sensations. Tympanometry is precluded, of course, if medical history contraindicates this test procedure due to previous middle ear surgery, or if it is clear that tympanometry is not necessary for appropriate diagnosis and management of the ear problem.

In his 1946 publication, Metz observed that although contractions of the stapedius muscle could be detected for patients with normal middle ears, conductive hearing losses obliterated such observations on the affected side. Using an electroacoustic immittance unit, Klockhoff (1961) confirmed Metz' observations, noting that even a slight middle ear involvement abolished measurement of the acoustic reflex response in the involved ear. Basing their observations on a large sample of patients, Jerger, Anthony, Jerger, and Mauldin (1974) reported that no reflex response was found in the affected ear 75 percent of the time even when the air-bone gap was only 10 dB.

Slight changes in middle ear impedance just at the onset and offset of an intense acoustic stimulus presented contralaterally were reported by Flottorp and Djupesland (1970) for ears with otosclerosis. They labeled these momentary negative-going deflections at stimulus onset and offset as "diphasic" reflex responses. Terkildsen, Osterhammel, and Bretlau (1973) noted that in their experience, diphasic reflex responses were observed for 16 of 17 patients with symptoms of clinical otosclerosis for less than 5 years, but for none of the 13 patients with clinical otosclerosis for a duration of 10 years or more.

These reports demonstrate that absence of acoustic reflex responses can help confirm even a mild conductive hearing loss in some instances, and diphasic reflex responses can assist in establishing a diagnosis in other cases.

In summary, combinations of air and bone conduction thresholds, word recognition scores, tympanograms, and acoustic reflex results yield considerable diagnostic information for patients having conductive hearing losses. In some clinical settings word recognition tests are bypassed when conductive hearing losses are found because a high score is anticipated and almost always observed. Tympanometry and acoustic reflex testing for such cases, unless medically contraindicated, or deemed unnecessary by a clear medical history, can yield relatively definitive diagnostic information.

COCHLEAR VERSUS EIGHTH NERVE HEARING LOSS

Over the years since Fowler's (1937a, b) description of the recruitment phenomenon, a variety of test procedures have been devised to assess abnormal sensory and neural function, particularly to differentiate neural from sensory involvement. This section reviews early descriptions of those test procedures that came to be incorporated into "audiologic test batteries." Word recognition tests are reviewed first in order to present various tests designed to assess recruitment in sequence.

WORD RECOGNITION

Following Fowler's description of recruitment in 1937, investigators became interested in relating word recognition scores to recruitment. In 1948 Huizing stated that recruitment limited the dynamic range for speech intelligibility and that hearing aids should be fitted on the basis of the patient's "loudness curve." Dix, Hallpike, and Hood (1949) noted that word recognition improved as a function of intensity to a point but then declined at higher intensities for two patients with Ménière's disease and recruitment but continued to improve at higher intensities for two patients with eighth nerve lesions and no recruitment. Eby and Williams (1951) made similar observations for larger samples of Ménière's disease and eighth nerve tumor patients.

Liden (1954) was the first to note unusually poor word recognition scores for patients with eighth nerve tumors. Based on observations for seven patients with eighth nerve tumors, he wrote, "All of the tumor cases showed conspicuously poor discrimination, the ... score usually being worse than might be supposed from the pure tone audiogram" (p. 110). Schuknecht and Woellner (1955) supported Liden's observations in their report of two patients with eighth nerve tumors. They concluded that "a small number of cochlear nerve fibres are adequate to conduct an impulse of threshold magnitude, but that greater numbers of nerve fibres are needed to conduct the complex neural patterns of speech" (p. 97). Similarly, Walsh and Goodman (1955) found very poor word recognition scores for three patients having cerebellopontine angle lesions, but they concluded that "discrimination for speech does not differentiate between auditory lesions in the cochlea and those central to the cochlea" (p. 8).

The latter comments have been substantiated many times, for example, by Johnson (1979) and Bess (1983), so that it is now widely recognized that word recognition scores do not differentiate sensory (cochlear) from neural (eighth nerve) involvements. Although some eighth nerve lesion patients attain very poor word recognition scores, many do not. Similarly, some patients with cochlear hearing losses yield very low word recognition scores whereas others, revealing like audiometric configurations and etiologies, achieve considerably higher scores. Bess (1983) clearly shows that word recognition scores vary widely across various sizes of eighth nerve tumors and degrees of hearing loss; only when the hearing loss reaches 80 dB hearing level (HL) are word recognition scores consistently very low (0%) in his sample (Figure 2-1).

Figure 2-1. Word recognition scores in percentage correct for eighth nerve tumor patients as a function of tumor size and hearing loss. Heavy bar, one standard deviation; light bar, two standard deviations. (Adapted from F. H. Bess [1983]. From Olsen, W. O. [1984]. Audiologic test battery results for cochlear and for VIIIth nerve lesions. *Audiology Journal for Continuing Education, 9,* 147–163. With permission.)

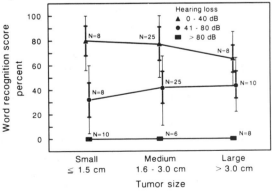

In contrast to the continued improvement in word recognition scores at higher presentation levels for patients with eighth nerve tumors noted above, Jerger and Jerger (1971) observed a marked decrease in performance at high-intensity levels for patients with eighth nerve lesions. The reduction in scores at the same intensity levels was less for patients with cochlear pathologies. Their procedure was to present lists of monosyllabic words (half lists of Harvard PB 50 words) at successively higher intensity levels until a maximum score (PBmax) was reached, then determine the "roll over" as additional lists were presented at still higher levels up to a maximum of 110 dB sound pressure level. A "rollover ratio" was calculated by subtracting the poorest score (PBmin) obtained above the rollover point from the best score (PBmax) and dividing the result by the PBmax score.

$$\text{Rollover ratio} = (\text{PBmax} - \text{PBmin})/\text{PBmax}$$

The highest rollover ratio found by Jerger and Jerger for cochlear hearing loss patients was 0.40; the lowest rollover ratio they obtained for eighth nerve lesion patients was 0.45. On this basis, Jerger and Jerger defined rollover ratios of 0.45 or greater as being suggestive of retrocochlear involvement. Dirks, Kamm, Bower, and Bettsworth (1977) also used Harvard PB 50 word lists and confirmed the findings of Jerger and Jerger, but cautioned that the accuracy of the PBmax score is critical; near PBmax intensity increments of 4 or 6 dB rather than 10 dB should be used to establish the PBmax score as accurately as possible. Further, Dirks et al. strongly recommended that each facility establish its own differential rollover rates for the specific test materials being used. Bess, Josey, and Humes (1979) and Meyer and Mishler (1985) confirmed the latter recommendations of Dirks et al. Bess et al. reported that a rollover ratio of 0.25 for their Northwestern University Auditory Test No. 6 materials separated most of the cochlear and eighth nerve tumor patients in their sample. Meyer and Mishler found that a rollover ratio of 0.35 for their Auditec version of Northwestern University Auditory Test No. 6 best separated the eighth nerve tumor patients from the cochlear hearing loss patients in their sample.

These early reports indicated excellent sensitivity and specificity for this test procedure; however, a recent report by Turner, Shepard, and Frazer (1984) indicated poorer overall sensitivity than observed in the studies cited here. (Sensiti-

vity and specificity for this and other test procedures are reviewed in Chapter 14).

LOUDNESS BALANCE TESTS

As early as 1924 Pohlman and Kranz noted that
despite loss of threshold sensitivity in some frequency regions, their listener reported normal
loudness sensation when the tone was raised to
suprathreshold levels. Fowler (1928) noted the
necessity for higher sensation levels in the normal
ear to equal the loudness of a lower sensation
level tone in the impaired ear of some patients
with unilateral hearing losses. Eight years later he
described the alternate binaural loudness balance
(ABLB) test, hoping at that time to identify early
otosclerosis (Fowler, 1936). Fowler's procedure
compared the loudness of a tone in the impaired
ear to the same tone, or possibly a different tone,
in the other ear. The stimuli were presented alternately to the two ears. In the same year, Reger
(1936) described a procedure in which the loudness of a signal at one frequency where there is
some hearing loss is compared to the loudness of
a tone at a different frequency for which hearing
sensitivity is normal in a single ear — the monaural bifrequency loudness balance test.

The term *recruitment* was used by Fowler
(1937a) to describe the loudness phenomenon
noted earlier by Pohlman and Kranz (1924) and
Fowler (1928). In another publication Fowler
(1937b) reported ABLB test results for a number
of patients showing recruitment, including one
patient with an eighth nerve tumor.

Interest in recruitment, and the ABLB test procedure in particular, was heightened following the
1948 publication of Dix, Hallpike, and Hood. They
reported ABLB results for 30 Ménière's disease
patients and for 20 eighth nerve tumor patients.
All of the Ménière's disease patients demonstrated recruitment. Fourteen of the eighth nerve tumor patients revealed absence of recruitment, and
six showed "incomplete" recruitment. Specific criteria for the stimuli, administration of the loudness
balance procedure, and interpretation of the test
results were not published until 1962 by Jerger.
Hood (1969) took exception to Jerger's recommendations as being quite different from Fowler's
procedure and that used by Hood and coworkers.
Just as Fowler observed recruitment for an eighth
nerve patient in his early publication, and Dix et al.
noted partial recruitment for 6 of 20 eighth nerve
patients in their samples, other investigators have
found that ABLB test results suggesting recruit-

ment do not rule out eighth nerve lesions. Tillman
(1969) reported that all 22 of the labyrinthine hydrops subjects in his sample demonstrated recruitment, but 10 of 21 eighth nerve tumor patients did
too. Similarly, Johnson (1979) found that 75 of 148
eighth nerve tumor patients showed recruitment.
Sanders, Josey, and Glasscock (1974) observed recruitment for 61 of 72 cochlear hearing loss patients and for 5 of 15 eighth nerve tumor patients.
Thus, from the outset, it has been demonstrated
that the vast majority of patients with cochlear
pathologies reveal recruitment, but about one-half
of the patients in the above samples with eighth
nerve lesions did too. Such findings limit the utility of loudness balance tests as a single procedure
for raising suspicion of eighth nerve involvement
on the basis of absence of recruitment.

METZ TEST — ACOUSTIC REFLEX

In 1952 Metz reported that ears that revealed
recruitment as measured by the ABLB test could
also be shown to elicit acoustic reflex responses
when stimulated at hearing levels similar to the
levels that elicited reflexes in normal ears. These
observations were made for patients with hearing
losses attributed to the organ of Corti. This relationship between results for loudness balance
tests and acoustic reflex testing was strengthened
by Metz' findings for two eighth nerve tumor patients who demonstrated absence of recruitment
according to the ABLB test and absence of acoustic reflexes in response to intense acoustic stimulation. Metz pointed out that, unlike the loudness
balance procedures, it was not necessary for the
patient to have normal hearing in one ear or at
one or more test frequencies to administer and
interpret acoustic reflex test results; it was merely
necessary to determine whether or not acoustic
reflexes could be elicited (for ears with no conductive involvement) at levels similar to those
yielding reflex responses in normal ears. Acoustic
reflexes usually are obtained at 70 to 100 db HL,
or 75 to 85 dB sensation levels across the 500 to
4000 Hz frequency range. Elicitation of acoustic
reflexes at lower sensation levels was interpreted
as indicative of recruitment.

Recently, Silman and Gelfand (1981) reported
a further evaluation of the levels at which acoustic
reflexes are elicited for patients with sensory
hearing losses. They reviewed audiograms and
acoustic reflex thresholds at 500, 1000, and 2000
Hz for a large sample of patients with hearing
losses attributed to cochlear pathologies. From

TABLE 2-1. NINETIETH PERCENTILE
LEVELS FOR ACOUSTIC REFLEX
THRESHOLDS AS A FUNCTION
OF HEARING LOSS

Hearing level	500	1000	2000
0–5	95	100	95
10–15	95	100	100
20–25	95	100	100
30–35	100	100	105
40–45	100	105	105
50–55	105	105	110
60–65	105	110	115
70–75	115	115	125
80–85		125	125
>85		125	125

Data from Silman, S., & Gelfand, S. A. (1981). The relationship between magnitude of hearing loss and acoustic reflex threshold levels. *Journal of Speech and Hearing
Disorders, 46,* 312–316.

their analysis of these data, they derived ninetieth
percentile levels for acoustic reflexes as a function
of hearing loss (Table 2-1). They suggested that
these levels be considered as the upper limits of
acoustic reflex thresholds for patients with sensory
hearing losses, and that acoustic reflex thresholds
at higher levels might suggest neural pathology.

In a follow-up to the work of Silman and Gelfand (1981), Olsen, Bauch, and Harner (1983)
compared acoustic reflex results for 30 patients
with cochlear hearing losses and for 30 patients
with cerebellopontine angle tumors (subsequently confirmed surgically). The degree and configuration of the hearing loss for each patient in the
eighth nerve lesion group were matched in degree and configuration by a patient in the cochlear
hearing loss group. Only one patient with a sensory hearing loss of 85 dB HL or less yielded an
acoustic reflex threshold above the ninetieth per-
centiles of Silman and Gelfand; 25 of the neural
lesion patients yielded no reflex response or reflexes only at levels above the ninetieth percentile
levels at one or more frequencies. Thus application of the ninetieth percentile criteria of Silman
and Gelfand to the acoustic reflex results for these
two groups of patients matched for hearing loss
correctly identified 97 percent of the sensory
hearing loss patients and 83 percent of the eighth
nerve lesion patients. Recall that ABLB test results
reviewed earlier were less successful in raising
suspicion of neural involvement for patients subsequently found to have cerebellopontine angle tumors.

SHORT INCREMENT
SENSITIVITY INDEX

Interest in the difference limens for intensity
(DLI) for hearing-impaired persons developed
following Bekesy's (1947) observation of very
narrow tracings when patients with sensory hearing losses traced their threshold for continuous
tones. Very narrow excursions in threshold tracings were not obtained for persons with conductive hearing losses (Figure 2-2). Bekesy concluded that the reduced excursions in threshold
tracings observed for persons with sensory hearing impairments reflected recruitment and a concomitant enhancement in DLI.

In 1949 Luscher and Zwislocki described their
DLI test based on abrupt changes in the intensity of continuous pure tones. These abrupt
changes occurred at a rate of about two per
second on signals presented at 40 dB sensation
level. The subjects simply indicated when they
heard a change in the intensity of the stimulus.
Subjects with normal hearing detected changes
on the order of 10 to 16 percent (0.9–1.6 dB).
Patients with sensory hearing losses of 30 dB HL
or greater, and recruitment, detected intensity
changes of 8 percent (0.7 dB) or smaller. In a
follow-up article, Luscher (1951) stated that "a
normal difference limen is met with in retrolabyrinthine deafness. . . . Consequently the decrease
in the difference limen . . . characterizes peripheral damage to the sound receptor, i.e., the organ
of Corti, and appears to be in evidence when the
sensory cells are damaged" (p. 507). He noted
normal DLI for two patients with cerebellopontine angle tumors.

At about the same time Denes and Naunton
(1950) described a different clinical procedure
measuring DLI. Two stimuli, each 1.7 seconds in
length, were presented in succession separated
by 0.33 seconds. The task of the listener was to
judge whether the second signal was louder or
softer than the first stimulus. Just noticeable differences in intensity were determined at 4, 24,
and 44 dB sensation levels; however, they recommended 4 and 44 dB sensation levels as being sufficient. Their rationale for DLI measurements at
two levels was that the difference limen is relatively large at low sensation levels and much
smaller at higher levels for normal hearing persons. Thus, if the DLI becomes smaller at the higher sensation levels, recruitment was assumed to
be absent; if, on the other hand, the DLI was small
at the low sensation level and remained unchanged

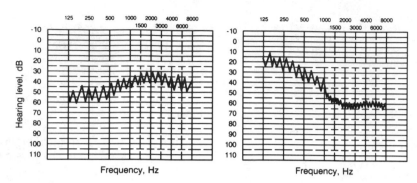

Figure 2-2. Threshold tracings (Bekesy method) for continuous tone for a patient with a conductive hearing loss (left) and for a patient with a cochlear hearing loss (right). Note narrowing of excursions above 1000 Hz in right tracing.

or only slightly larger at the higher sensation level, recruitment was judged to be present.

Publications by Lund-Iverson (1952) and Hirsh, Palva, and Goodman (1954) cast doubt on the relationship between recruitment and DLI as measured by the Luscher and Zwislocki method and Denes and Naughton procedure, respectively. Lund-Iverson (1952) was unable to demonstrate a clear relationship between recruitment as measured by ABLB tests and the DLI test of Luscher and Zwislocki. He noted considerable variability in DLIs across subjects with various etiologies. With or without recruitment, the mean DLIs were about the same for both groups. He stated that "the [DLI] values in those cases in which recruitment has been demonstrated by the [alternate binaural loudness] balance test do not differ appreciably neither from normal cases nor from those in which recruitment has not been demonstrable" (p. 233). In support of their argument that loudness and DLIs are not related, Hirsh et al. (1954) pointed out inconsistencies in loudness and DLI behavior. For example, for normal-hearing subjects, loudness growth is more rapid for low-frequency tones than for mid-frequency tones, but DLIs are larger for low-frequency signals than for mid-frequency stimuli. Further, when results of loudness balance tests and Denes and Naunton's DLI tests from 44 patients and 18 normal-hearing subjects were analyzed, they concluded, "The difference limen can not distinguish recruiting and nonrecruiting cases, nor can the difference limen distinguish hard of hearing listeners from normal listeners" (p. 538).

Work by Jerger (1952, 1953) with a modification of the Luscher and Zwislocki DLI procedure at 15 dB sensation level (1952) and at 10 and 40 dB sensation levels (1953) led to the development of the Short Increment Sensitivity Index (SISI) by Jerger, Shedd, and Harford (1959). Rather than

measure DLI size, their procedure assessed the percentage of 1 dB intensity increments heard when superimposed on a continuous tone. Twenty such increments were presented with the continuous tone remaining constant at 20 dB sensation level. Given the publications of Lund-Iverson (1952) and Hirsh et al. (1954), the interest was not in DLI as an indirect test of recruitment, but whether sensitivity to small changes in stimulus intensity was related to site of lesion within the auditory system. Early experience reported by Jerger (1961) showed that 20 Ménière's disease patients detected a majority of 1 dB increments, but 11 patients with eighth nerve tumors heard few, if any, of the small-intensity changes. Scores for the SISI of 70 to 100 percent were considered high, suggestive of cochlear involvement, scores of 0 to 30 percent low, indicative of eighth nerve pathology, and scores of 35 to 65 percent were in a nondescript questionable category. Others considered scores of 0 to 55 percent low and 60 to 100 percent high. Sanders et al. (1974) used the former categories whereas Tillman (1969) and Owens (1971) used the latter classification scheme when finding that the majority of their sensory hearing loss patients attained high scores; however, they found that many of the eighth nerve lesion patients attained high scores too, as did Johnson (1979) (Table 2-2). Approximately one-half of the patients with eighth nerve tumors in the studies of Tillman (1969), Sanders et al. (1974), and Johnson (1979) yielded high scores on the SISI test. These findings indicated that an ability to detect 1 dB increments superimposed on a continuous tone is not lost by many patients with eighth nerve lesions; therefore, results from the SISI test do not

TABLE 2-2. SHORT-INCREMENT SENSITIVITY INDEX SCORES FOR
PATIENTS WITH SENSORY AND NEURAL LESIONS FROM FOUR STUDIES

	N	0–30	0–55	35–65	60–100	70–100
Tillman (1969)						
Labyrinthine hydrops	22		2 (9)		20 (91)	
Eighth nerve tumor	22		11 (50)		11 (50)	
Owens (1971)						
Cochlear	101		2 (2)		99 (98)	
Retrocochlear	78		62 (79)		16 (21)	
Sanders et al. (1974)						
Cochlear	92	22 (24)		0 (0)		70 (76)
Eighth nerve tumor	25	12 (48)		2 (8)		11 (44)
Johnson (1979)						
Eighth nerve tumor	340	190 (56)		29 (8)		121 (36)

Percentage of sample is in parentheses.

effectively differentiate patients with eighth nerve tumors from those with cochlear lesions.

It should be noted that Thompson (1963) advocated administration of the SISI test at 75 dB HL (approximately 85 dB HL for current HL reference levels) rather than at 20 dB sensation level. Review of the literature by Turner et al. (1984) indicates similar results for the SISI test in differentiating cochlear versus eighth nerve lesions whether administered at 20 dB sensation level or at 75 to 85 dB HL.

TONE DECAY

As early as 1893 Gradenigo explored the "exhaustibility" of the auditory nerve. He studied exhaustibility of the ear in two ways. In one approach he determined threshold with his "telephone audiometer," then stimulated that ear at the maximum output of the device for 1 minute, followed by a sharp decrease in stimulus level to the previously established threshold. He noted that the normal ear continued to perceive the tone, but "in cases of great exhaustibility this perception either ceases for several seconds or is lost entirely" (p. 215). His other method of examination was to find threshold and then continue to present the tone at that level for some time. He found that some patients failed to perceive the tone after a few seconds, and that it was necessary to increase the intensity of the stimulus from time to time "in order to renew the perception." Gradenigo "found this symptom of exhaustibility in cases of neuritis" and suggested that "in cases of beginning neuritis of intracranial origin . . . the . . . test can be of great value" (p. 215).

An early report of excess adaptation for a patient with a subsequently confirmed eighth nerve tumor was provided by Reger and Kos (1952). Using a Bekesy audiometer (von Bekesy, 1947) Reger and Kos observed 25 to 30 dB threshold shifts over periods of 3 minutes or less when the patient traced his threshold for a continuous tone. In 1955 Lierle and Reger reported even more dramatic threshold shifts for an eighth nerve tumor patient. Jerger, Carhart, and Lassman (1958) compared threshold tracings with a Bekesy-type audiometer for interrupted and continuous tones. They confirmed the observations of Reger and coworkers in noting marked threshold shifts for the continuous tone but not for the interrupted tone for a patient with an eighth nerve tumor. Such marked threshold shifts were not observed for patients with cochlear lesions by Reger and Kos (1952), Lierle and Reger (1955), or Jerger et al. (1958).

Jerger's (1960a) classification of Bekesy audiograms followed his earlier observations (Jerger et al., 1958). Tracings in which the thresholds for the interrupted and continuous tones overlapped one another throughout the frequency range of 100 to 10,000 Hz were observed for normal-hearing persons, and those with conductive hearing losses were labeled *type I*. A *type II* designation was assigned to the threshold tracings in which the thresholds for the continuous tones were slightly poorer than thresholds for the interrupted tone; such patterns were obtained for patients with cochlear hearing losses. Tracings in which thresholds for the continuous tone continued to shift to levels beyond the output limits of the audiometer noted for patients with eighth nerve tumors were called *type III*. Other patients with eighth nerve tumors yielded threshold tracings for interrupted and continuous tones with considerable separation across the whole frequency range, but the continuous tone was heard at levels within the limits of the audiometer; these tracings were assigned a *type IV* label. Hughes, Winegar, and Crabtree (1967) clarified the criteria for type II and type IV tracings in their recommendations that tracings that reveal 20 dB or less separation between thresholds for interrupted and continuous tones be labeled *type II*, and those that show more than 20 dB difference between the two tracings, *type IV*.

A method for measurement of adaptation with a conventional pure tone audiometer was described by Carhart in 1957. In Carhart's procedure continuous tone presentation begins 10 to 15 dB below threshold and increases the intensity in 5 dB steps until the patient responds; at this point timing of the duration of the response is initiated. If the listener maintains perception of the tone at that level for 1 minute, the test is complete and 0 dB of threshold tone decay is noted. When the tone is not heard for 60 seconds, the stimulus is increased 5 dB without interrupting the tone, and a new minute of timing is begun each time the patient indicates loss of perception of the tone. This procedure continues until the signal is heard at one level for a full minute or equipment limits are reached. The difference between the hearing level of the initial response and the level at which the tone was heard for 1 minute is reported as the amount of threshold tone decay.

Yantis (1959) observed tone decay as great as 40 dB for a patient with a noise-induced hearing loss, and as great as 50 dB for a Ménière's disease patient, but three patients with eighth nerve tumors demonstrated excess adaptation beyond the limits of the audiometer. Yantis concluded that "abnormal auditory adaptation . . . seems indicative of poor functional integrity of retrocochlear aspects" (p. 786). Since Carhart's original description of the threshold tone decay test, various modifications have been suggested (Green, 1963; Jerger and Jerger, 1975a; Olsen and Noffsinger,1974; Owens, 1964; Rosenberg, 1958; Sorenson, 1960), but generally it has been accepted that 30 dB or less tone decay re threshold is associated with sensory involvement; 35 dB or greater adaptation suggests retrocochlear pathology (Olsen and Noffsinger, 1974; Sanders et al., 1974; Tillman, 1969).

Over the years results for tone decay tests and Bekesy audiometry have been compared (Olsen and Noffsinger, 1974; Parker and Decker, 1971; Sanders et al., 1974; Tillman, 1969). There is general agreement that the threshold tone decay test of Carhart, or those very similar to it, are more sensitive in revealing excess adaptation and thereby raising suspicion of retrocochlear involvement than is Bekesy audiometry. Correct identification of retrocochlear involvement was usually on the order of 70 percent or better for tone decay tests whereas Bekesy tracings were classified as type III or type IV for about one-half of the eighth nerve tumor patients.

During the 1960s and early 1970s, the pure tone auditory test battery commonly used to help differentiate sensory from neural involvements consisted of two suprathreshold tests, loudness balance and SISI, and two tests at threshold levels, threshold tone decay and Bekesy audiometry. Interpretation of findings relative to cochlear versus neural indications was based on a composite of test results because it was well accepted that none of the tests was sufficiently sensitive or specific to the site of lesion to be considered singly.

ACOUSTIC REFLEX DECAY

A new test was added to the audiologic armamentarium in 1969 with the report of Anderson, Barr, and Wedenberg. They noted that when stimulating ears with eighth nerve lesions for 10 seconds at 10 dB above the acoustic reflex threshold, the amplitude of the reflex response in the contralateral ear decreased to one-half or less amplitude within 5 seconds. Of 17 such cases, Anderson et al. noted that acoustic reflexes were "pathologically elevated" (criteria for elevated were not given) for all, and no reflexes could be elicited for 7. Reflex decay as described above was observed for the other 10 patients. Such decay was observed for only about 1 percent of a larger sample of patients not having eighth nerve tumors. Support for the observations of Anderson et al. was provided by Jerger, Harford, Clemis, and Alford (1974); Olsen, Noffsinger, and Kurdziel (1975a); Sheehy and Inzer (1976); Hall (1977); Sanders, Josey, Glasscock and Jackson (1981); Olsen, Stach, and Kurdziel (1981); and Olsen et al. (1983). In all of these investigations, the occurrence of absent or elevated acoustic reflexes was more common than reflex decay, but for some patients reflex decay served as a second

TABLE 2-3. ACOUSTIC REFLEX TEST RESULTS FOR PATIENTS
WITH SENSORY AND NEURAL LESIONS FROM FIVE STUDIES

	Cochlear			Retrocochlear		
	N	Normal	Abnormal	N	Normal	Abnormal
Olsen et al. (1975a)	100	79 (79)	21 (21)	28	4 (14)	24 (86)
Hall (1977)	464	390 (84)	74 (16)	63	12 (19)	51 (81)
Olsen et al. (1981)	58	42 (72)	16 (27)	58	3 (5)	55 (95)
Sanders et al. (1981*)	74	62 (84)	12 (16)	162	13 (8)	149 (92)
Olsen et al. (1983)	30	27 (90)	3 (10)	30	5 (17)	25 (83)

*Taken from Table III of Sanders et al. Absent or elevated acoustic reflex thresholds or reflex decay, or combination of these, considered abnormal for patients with threshold sensitivity less than 80 dB HL.

indication of retrocochlear involvement in conjunction with elevated reflex thresholds. For a few, reflex decay alone raised suspicion of eighth nerve pathology. The combination of acoustic reflex and reflex decay results correctly raised suspicion of retrocochlear involvement for 80 percent or more of the eighth nerve tumor patients evaluated in these studies.

As mentioned, the report of Anderson et al. indicated that very few patients with cochlear hearing losses yielded acoustic reflex results suggestive of retrocochlear involvement; however, follow-up studies have shown about a 10 to 20 percent incidence of abnormal acoustic reflex results for such patients (Hall, 1977; Olsen et al., 1975; Olsen et al., 1981; Olsen et al., 1983; Sanders et al., 1981) (Table 2-3).

Given that the acoustic reflex and reflex decay tests are more sensitive to retrocochlear lesions than other tests heretofore reviewed and are more economical in terms of time and expense to the patient, ABLB or monaural bifrequency loudness balance, SISI, Bekesy audiometry, and threshold tone decay have fallen into relative disuse. In fact acoustic reflex and reflex decay tests have taken on sufficient importance to devote a book solely to these topics (Silman, 1984).

AUDITORY BRAINSTEM RESPONSE

Measurements of neural activity in response to sound stimuli have been of interest since the work of Davis (1939). In that investigation electrical activity from awake humans in response to tonal stimuli was recorded from electrodes attached to the scalp. "On effects" in the form of diphasic or triphasic waves of about 300-msec duration were observed 30 to 40 msec after the onset of the stimulus. Measurement of electrical activity from the eighth nerve and brainstem is more recent.

Sohmer and Feinmesser (1967) offered the first reports of auditory evoked responses from the eighth nerve and brainstem with electrodes not penetrating the eardrum. With an active electrode attached to the earlobe, an indifferent electrode on the nose, and a ground electrode on the wrist, they recorded four waves they attributed to the cochlear action potentials and possible brainstem auditory nuclei. The publication of Jewett and Williston (1971) conclusively demonstrated the feasibility of measurement of auditory evoked potentials from the eighth nerve and brainstem. They assigned Roman numerals to the seven waves elicited within the first 10 msec following stimulus presentation. Jewett and Williston also suggested that waves I through VI were observed with sufficient reliability that clinical and experimental norms could be established. Further, they stated that "wave V will probably be the best basis of comparison across individuals and between different laboratories because its amplitude makes it the easiest to record and it can be recorded in only 100 seconds at repetition rates of 20 stimuli/sec" (p. 694). These comments set the stage for excitement and enthusiasm directed at the study of auditory brainstem response (ABR) and its application in clinical settings. This interest and enthusiasm is reflected in the fact that at least five books on this topic have been published since 1981 (Glasscock, Jackson, and Josey, 1981; Glattke, 1983; Hood and Berlin, 1986; Jacobson, 1985; Moore, 1983).

Selters and Brackmann (1977) presented the first analysis of ABR results for a relatively large sample of patients with eighth nerve tumors. They found that wave V could not be observed for 21 of 46 patients with cerebellopontine angle tumors. For the other patients with eighth nerve lesions, abnormalities in the latencies were found for all but three patients. Other ABR findings considered abnormal were wave V latency greater than 6.0 msec, differences in the latencies of wave V at the two ears of a given patient greater than 0.2 msec for normal hearing ears or for hearing losses at 4000 Hz up to 50 dB HL, greater than 0.3 msec when hearing losses at 4000 Hz were 55 to 65 dB HL, and 0.4 msec for hearing losses at 4000 Hz greater than 65 dB HL. These criteria identified 94 percent of the retrocochlear patients in this sample. Applying these guidelines to the interpretation of ABR results for 54 other patients not having cerebellopontine angle tumors led to a judgment of abnormal ABR waveforms for 12 percent of them. A later publication by Selters and Brackmann (1979) for 266 nontumor patients and 142 eighth nerve tumor patients was even more impressive; abnormal ABR findings for 96 percent of the eighth nerve tumor patients, and for 8 percent of the nontumor patients. Other investigators also have found ABR testing to be very sensitive to eighth nerve lesions, but some have obtained abnormal waveforms more frequently from patients with cochlear hearing losses (Bauch, Olsen, and Harner, 1983; Bauch, Rose, and Harner, 1982) (Table 2-4). Some of these differences in observation of abnormal ABR waveforms for patients with sensory hearing losses may be due to the severity of the hearing losses of the patients tested.

To investigate this factor, Bauch et al. (1983) compared ABR results for 30 patients having cerebellopontine angle tumors and 30 patients with cochlear hearing losses. The patients in the two groups were matched for degree and configuration of hearing losses. For the eighth nerve tumor group, reproducible waveforms could not be elicited from 15, wave V latencies were ex-

cessively different between ears (Selters and Brackmann criteria) for 13, and wave V latency was delayed (>6.2 msec) for one. In other words, ABR results were abnormal for 29, or 97 percent, of the eighth nerve lesion patients in this sample. For the cochlear hearing loss group, no repeatable responses were found for three, wave V latencies between ears were abnormally different for three, and wave V latency was delayed for one. Thus, 7 or 23 percent, of this sample of cochlear hearing losses yielded ABR results judged to be abnormal. The absence of ABR response for two of these patients could be explained by the severity of their hearing losses, 50 dB HL or greater at 1000 Hz, 90 dB HL or greater at 2000 and 4000 Hz; however, severity and configuration of hearing loss could not explain the ABR abnormalities for the other five cochlear hearing loss patients because other patients in this group with similar or greater hearing losses demonstrated normal ABR waveforms. Therefore, other factors such as specific etiologies or pathologies responsible for some cochlear hearing losses, stability or progression of hearing loss, duration of hearing loss, and so forth probably influence ABR waveforms. More clinical data from relatively large samples of patients are necessary in order to sort out one or more of these and other possible factors as being associated with abnormal ABR results when eighth nerve lesions have been ruled out by other examinations. Such information will lead to better understanding and interpretation of ABR results.

It is clear, however, that ABR testing is a very powerful tool for differentiating between sensory and neural lesions. Surgical intervention is not undertaken on the basis of ABR findings alone, but ABR test results certainly can provide useful information in raising suspicion of eighth nerve lesions for many patients and in helping to rule out retrocochlear involvement for others. Never-

TABLE 2-4. AUDITORY BRAINSTEM RESPONSE DATA FOR PATIENTS WITH SENSORY AND WITH NEURAL LESIONS FROM FIVE STUDIES

	Cochlear			Retrocochlear		
	N	Normal	Abnormal	N	Normal	Abnormal
Selters and Brackman (1979)	266	245 (92)	21 (8)	142	6 (4)	136 (96)
Glasscock et al. (1981)	409	382 (93)	27 (7)	55	1 (2)	54 (98)
Terkildsen et al. (1981)	71	66 (93)	5 (7)	56	2 (4)	54 (96)
Bauch et al. (1982)	229	172 (75)	57 (25)	26	1 (4)	25 (96)
Bauch et al. (1983)	30	23 (77)	7 (23)	30	1 (3)	29 (97)

Percentage of sample is in parentheses.

theless, definitive diagnosis of mass lesions in the internal auditory meatus or cerebellopontine angle rests on sophisticated radiographic techniques, such as computed axial tomography or magnetic resonance imaging, and ultimately on surgical excision of the lesion.

SUMMARY

Over the years a number of auditory test procedures have been developed for the purpose of differentiating between hearing deficits due to cochlear pathologies and those attributable to eighth nerve involvement. During that same time, radiographic techniques for detecting mass lesions have improved considerably. Consequently, smaller and less symptomatic tumors of or near the eighth nerve have been found and removed surgically. The auditory manifestations of these smaller lesions are often very subtle. For this reason auditory tests that seemed relatively successful in raising suspicion of eighth nerve involvement a few years ago no longer seem sufficiently sensitive to eighth nerve pathology. It is encouraging to note that developments in audiology have tended to keep pace with the times. Acoustic reflex tests that can be completed relatively quickly and with relatively inexpensive apparatus currently raise suspicion of retrocochlear involvement for about 85 percent of patients having eighth nerve tumors or mass lesions in the cerebellopontine angle. Similarly, acoustic reflex and reflex decay test results correctly suggest cochlear involvement for 85 percent of the patients for whom other medical and radiographic examinations rule out mass lesions affecting the eighth nerve. ABR testing, which is more expensive in terms of time and equipment, correctly identifies 95 percent of patients with space-occupying lesions affecting the eighth nerve and yields responses judged to be normal for 90 percent of patients for whom medical and radiographic evaluations indicate absence of mass lesions of the internal auditory meatus or cerebellopontine angle (Turner et al., 1984). It should be kept in mind that not only space-occupying lesions can influence eighth nerve function. Obviously some cochlear hearing losses and vascular and other insults to the eighth nerve can disrupt neural function too; however, definitive substantiation of such other insults is more tenuous and usually inferential at best.

Appropriately, acoustic reflex and reflex decay tests and ABR tests have been and are being used more frequently than other tests for differentiating between sensory and neural involvements. The literature review of Turner et al. (1984) revealed published research reports of acoustic reflex results for more than 4000 patients and ABR results for more than 2000 patients with sensory or neural involvements. Data for tone decay tests, the third most popular test in their review, were available for less than 2000 patients. Further investigation, modification, and refinement of test procedures and interpretation of results, along with development of other methods, will continue to provide a role for audiology in heightening suspicion of retrocochlear involvement for patients in whom the possibility of retrocochlear pathology should be considered.

CENTRAL AUDITORY NERVOUS SYSTEM DISORDERS

Given the multiplication in the number of neurons throughout the afferent portions of the auditory nervous system beginning with multiple synapses within the cochlear nuclei, ipsilateral and contralateral tracts, innervation between tracts and between cortical hemispheres, detecting lesions within this system requires tasks more difficult than those discussed above (Lundborg, Rosenhamer, Murray, and Zwetnow, 1975). As early as 1928, Bunch demonstrated that removal of one cortical hemisphere did not result in any marked changes in hearing sensitivity in either ear. Further, patients having had one cortical hemisphere removed have not shown any significant decrement in word recognition scores for undistorted monosyllables presented to either ear (Goldstein, Goodman, and King, 1956; Goldstein, 1961; Hodgson, 1967). Only for unusual cases with bilateral damage to the temporal lobes have losses in hearing sensitivity for conventional pure tone stimuli been demonstrated (Graham, Greenwood, and Lecky, 1980; Jerger, Lovering, and Wertz, 1972; Jerger, Weikers, Sharbrough, and Jerger 1969). More difficult tasks are necessary to evaluate unilateral temporal lobe lesions.

BRIEF TONES

It should be noted that Gersuni, Baru, Karaseva, and Tonkonghii (1971) have observed marked abnormalities in thresholds for very brief tonal

stimuli presented to patients having temporal
lobe lesions. That is, compared to threshold patterns as a function of stimulus duration observed
for normal-hearing persons, such patients required inordinate increases in stimulus intensity
to detect stimuli shorter than 7 msec delivered to
the ear contralateral to the temporal lobe lesion.
Stephens (1976) obtained similar results for 2 of
12 patients with temporal lobe lesions. Similarly,
Cranford, Stream, Rye, and Slade (1982) observed
sharp increases in intensity for threshold response to stimuli shorter than 20 msec for two of
seven patients with temporal lobe lesions in their
study; however, the difference limen for frequency for 1000 Hz signals of equally brief durations
was abnormally large for all seven of these patients.

TEMPORAL ORDERING

Just as threshold sensitivity or frequency discrimination may be abnormal for some patients
with temporal lobe lesions, temporal ordering of
tonal or click stimuli may be impaired for such patients. Efforts along this line follow the early work
of Hirsh (1959) and Swisher and Hirsh (1972).
Hirsh found that trained subjects require only 2
msec time differences to detect separate sounds
but 15 to 20 msec to determine which of two
overlapping sounds occurred first in time, that is,
low tone or high tone, tone or noise, tone or click,
and so forth. Untrained subjects needed 60 msec
of asynchrony in stimulus onset of overlapping
signals in order to judge temporal order but could
be trained to achieve better performance (Efron,
1963). Swisher and Hirsh (1972) found that brain-
injured patients required greater onset asynchrony of two tonal stimuli to report temporal order.
Patients with left hemisphere brain damage had
most difficulty when the stimuli were presented to
the same ear, whereas patients with right hemisphere lesions had greater difficulty when the
stimuli were presented independently to the two
ears. Similarly, Efron (1963) noted that patients
who experienced some difficulty on a temporal
ordering task also had some degree of aphasia.
Lackner and Teuber (1973) observed that patients
with left hemisphere damage and some dysphasia
required a longer gap between dichotic clicks in
order to sequence them than did patients with
damage to the right cortical hemisphere.

Efron, Yund, and Crandall (1985) noted poorer
gap detection for 4 msec gaps in noise presented
to the ear contralateral to a temporal lobectomy.
Such patients also demonstrated poorer localiza-

tion of tape-recorded environmental stimuli for
the side contralateral to the partial temporal lobectomy according to Efron, Crandall, Koss, Divenyi, and Yund (1983). Both of these observations held regardless of whether the right or left
temporal lobe had undergone excision of its anterior portion.

Pinheiro (1977) described a pitch pattern test
consisting of three tone presentations of 200 msec
each with 150 msec separating each of the stimuli,
delivered monaurally. Two of the signals are of
one frequency, and the other tone is at a slightly
different frequency. The two frequencies used are
880 Hz and 1122 Hz. The task of the listener is to
indicate the pitch pattern of the three stimuli; for
example, 880, 1122, and 880 Hz stimuli would be
reported as low, high, low; 1122, 880, 1122 Hz as
high, low, high. Some patients with lesions of
either hemisphere and patients with lesions of the
corpus callosum reveal difficulty with this task
when asked to indicate the pattern with verbal
labels of high, low, high, and so on. Interestingly,
some of these same patients can hum the se-
quences correctly; their difficulty is not associated
with identifying the pitch pattern but in accurately attaching labels to them (Musiek, Kibby, and
Baran, 1984; Musiek, Pinheiro, and Wilson, 1980).
(For a thorough review of temporal ordering by
the central nervous system [CANS], see Pinheiro
and Musiek, 1985.)

Obviously, in order to assess dysfunction within the CANS, it has been necessary to devise tasks
that pose some difficulty even for those with
wholly normal auditory function. Speech stimuli
readily lend themselves to such tasks because
speech is a complex acoustic stimulus that can be
distorted, masked, or delivered in various listening paradigms to render accurate comprehension
or identification of a specific stimulus quite difficult. The intent is to reduce the redundancy of
the cues available to the listener, or to ask the listener to attend to only one or to both ears when
stimuli are presented bilaterally. The recency in
virtually all of these developments is reflected in
the dates of the references cited above and those
that follow. Bocca, Calearo, Cassinari, and Bocca,
Calearo, Cassinari, and Magliavacca first reported
their work in 1954 and 1955, respectively. The
first chapter on this topic to appear in an audiology text was in 1963 by Bocca and Calearo. Since
then, however, books have been devoted to these
tests, including Sullivan (1975), Keith (1977,
1981), Lasky and Katz (1983), and Pinheiro and
Musiek (1985).

DISTORTED SPEECH

Bocca et al. (1954, 1955) were the first to demonstrate that temporal lobe disorders could be detected by speech stimuli that had been low-pass filtered to reduce the inherent redundancy in speech. In 1955 they reported that of 18 patients with temporal lobe lesions, 13 demonstrated sharply decreased performance for the ear contralateral to the temporal lobe lesion. The following year, Goldstein et al. (1956) reported pre- and postsurgical test results for four patients with right infantile hemiplegia who underwent left hemispherectomies. Despite normal hearing sensitivity and word recognition scores for CID W-22 word lists judged to be essentially normal, their word recognition scores for Rush-Hughes recordings of Harvard PB-50 word lists were considerably poorer than observed for other normal-hearing subjects. Scores for the right ear, contralateral to the left hemispherectomy, were substantially reduced. Goetzinger and Angell (1965) and Goetzinger (1972) have made similar observations for patients with temporal lobe lesions.

Speech that had been low-pass filtered below 1000 Hz, usually 500 Hz, was used most commonly in the 1960s and 1970s to assess temporal lobe function (Jerger, 1960b, 1964; Korsan-Bengsten, 1973; Lynn and Gilroy, 1977). The most common finding was decreased performance via the ear contralateral to the temporal lobe lesion. Lynn and Gilroy (1977) showed that 25 patients (74%) in their sample of 34 patients with temporal lobe lesions yielded abnormal scores via the ear contralateral to the pathology for their low-pass filtered speech materials; 8 obtained normal scores, and 1 revealed decreased performance for the ear ipsilateral to the lesion. Twenty (74%) of 27 patients with parietal lobe tumors achieved normal scores on this task; one revealed abnormal scores for the ipsilateral ear, and six did so for the ear contralateral to the parietal lobe tumor. They observed abnormal scores via contralateral, ipsilateral, or both ears for patients with brainstem lesions.

Korsan-Bengsten (1973) noted deficits in performance on filtered speech tests only for those patients with temporal lobe lesions in the area she called the "auditory cortex," Wernicke's area. Patients with temporal lobe lesions located in the temporal pole, that is, the anterior portion of the temporal lobe distant from the auditory cortex, did not demonstrate excess difficulty with the filtered speech test materials. The four brainstem lesion patients in her sample showed decreased scores for these materials when delivered to the ear ipsilateral to the lesion.

Another means of degrading speech intelligibility is a procedure in which time segments of the speech signal are periodically eliminated, so-called interrupted speech (Miller and Licklider, 1950). Bocca (1958) suggested use of such test materials as a challenge for patients with temporal lobe lesions. Korsan-Bengsten (1973) found that speech (Swedish sentences) chopped at rates of 4, 7, and 10 interruptions per second, 50 percent on-time, seemed quite sensitive to lesions affecting the auditory cortex. The differences between scores for the ears ipsilateral and contralateral to the involved side exceeded 50 percent.

Accelerating the rate of speech is another test procedure that decreases speech intelligibility (Calearo and Lazzaroni, 1957). Accelerated speech may be accomplished simply by having a talker speak at rates greater than the normal rate of about 140 words per minute; a more popular procedure, however, is to use tape recorders that eliminate small time segments of speech, without silent intervals as in interrupted speech, via electromechanical or electronic means, without changing the pitch characteristics of the speech. Speech processed by one of these methods is usually called *time-compressed speech.* Calearo and Lazzaroni (1957), deQuiros (1961/1964), and Korsan-Bengsten (1973) have reported that performance via the ear contralateral to the temporal lobe lesion is reduced considerably for time-compressed sentence materials. Korsan-Bengsten found that scores were decreased about 50 percent via the contralateral ear relative to the ear ipsilateral to the temporal lobe lesion when sentence test materials were delivered at a rate of 290 words per minute. In addition, she noted that the brainstem patients in her sample attained poorer scores for both the interrupted and time-compressed sentences for the ear ipsilateral to the lesion.

Time-compressed speech materials in the United States generally have consisted of lists of monosyllables rather than sentences and have been described in terms of percentage time compression rather than words per minute (Beasley, Schwimmer, and Rintelmann, 1972). Using such materials with 40 percent and 60 percent time compression, Kurdziel, Noffsinger, and Olsen (1976) found that patients with diffuse temporal lobe lesions due to cerebrovascular accidents experienced considerable difficulty, particularly with the 60 percent time-compressed version of the test. Average performance via the ear contralateral to the diffuse temporal lobe lesion was 28 percent poorer than the average score for the ipsilateral ear. Patients with discrete lesions, that is, they had undergone surgery to remove the anterior portion of the temporal lobe (up to 52 mm of the left, or up to 70 mm of the right temporal lobe) to control seizures, or to remove a tumor, yielded similar scores for both ears; differences between ears did not exceed 10 percent for the 60 percent time-compressed materials. These findings are in accord with those of Korsan-Bengsten (1973).

MASKED SPEECH

Sinha (1959) noted abnormal breakdown in word recognition scores for monosyllables mixed with white noise presented monaurally to the contralateral ears of patients who underwent partial temporal lobectomies to remove tumors or other abnormal brain tissue. These results were obtained for pre- and postsurgical tests and were noted regardless of whether or not the lesion involved Heschl's gyrus. Olsen, Noffsinger, and Kurdziel (1975b) found that 9 of 10 patients with cerebrovascular accidents experienced excess breakdown (>40%) in word recognition scores for speech in white noise (0 dB signal-to-noise ratio) compared to their scores in quiet. None of the 11 patients who had undergone unilateral partial temporal lobectomies encountered such difficulties. Further, 2 of 3 patients with hemispherectomies revealed excess difficulty with the speech in white noise task. The other hemispherectomy patient attained normal word recognition scores in quiet and in white noise bilaterally.

Jerger and Jerger (1975b) presented third-order synthetic sentences developed by Speaks and Jerger (1965) mixed with competing speech at message-to-competition ratios of +10 to −20 dB to patients with temporal lobe lesions. They found decreased performance via the contralateral ear or both ears.

Just as Lynn and Gilroy (1977) and Korsan-Bengsten (1973) observed that patients with brainstem lesions revealed decreased performance for low-pass filtered speech, interrupted speech, and time-compressed speech, Noffsinger, Olsen, Carhart, Hart, and Sahgal (1972) and Jerger and Jerger (1974) observed poor word recognition scores in white noise and poor synthetic sentence identification in competing speech for

one or both ears of patients with brainstem involvement. Given the close proximity of the auditory nuclei and auditory tracts for the two ears within the brainstem and thalamus, this variety of results for patients with brainstem lesions is not surprising.

It must be kept in mind that hearing losses associated with peripheral sensory or neural pathologies can disrupt performance on these tests (Speaks, 1980). The statement of Olsen et al. (1975b) regarding their results for the speech in white noise test — "It is apparent that lesions at any point in the auditory system from the cochlea through the temporal lobe can result in marked reduction in speech discrimination in white noise . . . results from speech in . . . white noise . . . may have some usefulness in revealing abnormalities in auditory function but not in suggesting a particular site of involvement as being responsible for the dysfunction" (pp. 381–382) — applies to filtered speech, interrupted speech, and time-compressed speech tests too.

DICHOTIC STIMULI

"Dichotic refers to the condition in which the sound stimulus presented at one ear differs from the sound stimulus presented to the other ear. . . . The stimuli may differ in sound pressure, frequency, phase, time, duration, bandwidth, etc. Diotic refers to the condition in which the sound stimulus presented to each ear is identical" (Sonn, 1969, p. 12).

A number of investigators have employed various dichotic and sometimes diotic stimuli to assess function or dysfunction within the CANS. One approach presents two similar speech stimuli to the two ears simultaneously and requires a response to both. This procedure follows the early work of Broadbent (1954). He found that when normal-hearing individuals heard six digits, three sets of pairs presented simultaneously to the two ears, subjects generally reported all digits heard in one ear before reporting digits heard in the other ear.

Kimura (1961) presented like stimuli to patients with seizures whose focus was in one of the temporal lobes and who subsequently underwent partial temporal lobectomies. As might be expected, decreased performance was observed for the ear contralateral to the damaged temporal lobe. Oxbury and Oxbury (1969) observed poorer scores on dichotic digit tasks following temporal lobe surgery when Heschl's gyrus was removed; error rates were essentially unchanged postsurgically when Heschl's gyrus was spared.

Based on their experience with patients having cortical lesions, Sparks, Goodglass, and Nickel (1970) developed a model of the central auditory pathways to explain most of their findings (Figure 2-3). This model suggests that the final processing of speech stimuli occurs in the posterior portion of the left temporal lobe, but that some preliminary processing occurs anteriorly also, in the right temporal lobe for speech stimuli heard via the left ear, and in the left temporal lobe for speech stimuli delivered to the right ear. They observed both contralateral and ipsilateral ear deficits in processing dichotic digits or words. Abnormal scores for the contralateral ear could be explained by lesions in the anterior portions of either temporal lobe; abnormal scores bilaterally might suggest posterior temporal lobe involvement on the left side. Ipsilateral ear deficits alone were noted more frequently for patients with left temporal lobe lesions than for patients with right temporal lobe involvement. Sparks et al. (1970) and Speaks (1975) suggested that damage in the left temporal lobe at the point where crossing cortical tracts from the right temporal lobe enter the left temporal lobe could explain decreased performance in the ipsilateral ear (left) in some cases. It should be noted, however, that Sparks et al. (1970) also observed decreased performance for the ipsilateral (right) ear for 2 of 20 patients with right hemisphere lesions.

Support for final processing of speech in the left temporal lobe for speech messages delivered to the left ear is obtained from patients who have

undergone section of the corpus callosum. In such cases performance is markedly decreased for the left ear (Musiek and Wilson, 1979; Musiek, Wilson, and Pinheiro, 1979; Sparks and Geschwind, 1968). Interestingly, pre- and postsurgical scores for patients who have had only the anterior portion of the corpus callosum sectioned do not reveal greater left ear deficits following surgery (Baran, Musiek, and Reeves, 1986).

The development of the Staggered Spondaic Word (SSW) test also using a dichotic mode of presentation was reported by Katz (1962, 1968). Spondaic words with onsets such that the last half of a spondee in one ear occurs at the same time as the first word of a spondee in the other ear are the test items. Extensive scoring systems for SSW test results have been described, most recently by Lukas and Genchur-Lukas (1985). Keith (1983) and Mueller (1987) have questioned the validity and reliability of interpretation of SSW test results scored on the basis of corrected scores, ear effects, order effects, and reversals. The competing portion of the stimulus paradigm is most difficult for patients and most meaningfully scored simply as percentage correct or incorrect responses.

A more difficult test using six nonsense syllables (voiceless and voiced plosives /p, t, k, b, d, g/ followed by the vowel /a/) was described by Lowe, Cullin, Berlin, Thompson, and Willett in 1970. The stimuli on each channel of the two-channel tape recording were controlled precisely for the stimulus onsets to be simultaneous or separated by specified durations. A report by Berlin, Lowe-Bell, Jannetta, and Kline (1972) demonstrated marked contralateral ear deficits in performance for four patients who had undergone anterior temporal lobectomies on either the right or left side. Since these reports, dichotic nonsense syllables have served as stimuli to investigate "cerebral dominance" (Berlin et al., 1973; Speaks, Niccum, and Carney, 1982), "stimulus dominance" (Speaks et al., 1981), "the effect of age on performance" (Gelfand et al., 1980; Mirabile et al. 1978), "the effects of amplification on the auditory system" (Jacobson, McCandless, and Mahoney, 1979), as well as patients with disorders of the CANS. Note should be taken of the data of Speaks and Niccum (1977) and Bingea and Raffin (1986), which demonstrated that inference of hemispheric dominance on the basis of right ear and left ear scores for dichotic nonsense syllables is very tenuous. Also recent reports (Collard et al., 1986; Olsen, 1983) indicate that not all patients with

Figure 2-3. Block diagram of the auditory pathways suggested by Sparks et al. (1970). Heavy lines indicate contralateral tracts, light lines ipsilateral paths from brainstem.

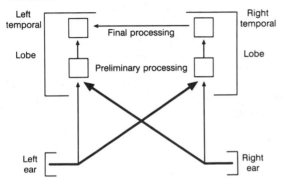

TABLE 2-5. PATTERNS OF DICHOTIC NONSENSE SYLLABLE TEST
RESULTS BEFORE AND AFTER TEMPORAL LOBE SURGERY FOR 33 RIGHT
TEMPORAL LOBE SEIZURE AND 34 LEFT TEMPORAL LOBE SEIZURE PATIENTS

	Right temporal lobe		Left temporal lobe	
	Presurgery	Postsurgery	Presurgery	Postsurgery
C Normal I Normal	14 (43)	18 (55)	14 (42)	10 (29)
C Abnormal I Normal	9 (27)	11 (33)	7 (20)	10 (29)
I Abnormal C Normal	5 (15)	1 (3)	7 (20)	8 (24)
C Abnormal I Abnormal	5 (15)	3 (9)	6 (18)	6 (18)

Note: C, contralateral ear; I, ipsilateral ear. Percentage of sample is in parentheses.
Source: Data from Olsen, W. O. (1983). Dichotic test results for normal subjects and temporal lobectomy patients. *Ear & Hearing, 4,* 324–330.

temporal lobe seizures and subsequent temporal lobectomies reveal abnormal performance. Table 2-5 summarizes Olsen's (1983) test results for dichotic nonsense syllables administered to 67 patients prior to and following temporal lobectomies. Some yielded normal scores, some revealed decreased performance for both ears, some demonstrated contralateral ear deficits, and others showed abnormally low scores for the ear ipsilateral to the involved temporal lobe. In agreement with the observations of Sparks et al. (1970), Table 2-5 shows that ipsilateral ear deficits were more common for left temporal lobe lesions than for right temporal lobe disorders. Nevertheless, as stated by Speaks (1980), "The existence of the ipsilateral ear effect dictates that results of dichotic tests, by themselves, should not be used to determine the side of neurologic lesions that affect central auditory processing" (p. 1850).

Given the minimal redundancy in the nonsense syllable, these test materials are considerably more difficult than tests using longer, more redundant stimuli such as the SSW test. Of 14 patients in Olsen's 1983 sample who yielded abnormally low scores for dichotic nonsense syllables, only 3 obtained scores below 90 percent on the SSW test before surgery and 5 after surgery. Because the latter test is not as difficult as the dichotic nonsense syllable test, it is not as sensitive to cortical lesions. Lynn and Gilroy (1977) have reported similar findings.

Niccum, Rubens, and Speaks (1981) have presented a logical developmental hierarchy of dichotic tests in terms of difficulty. Nonsense syllables are the most difficult, followed by words in which only the initial consonant differs for two sets of three words each in a group of six words, vowel words in which six words use two of the consonants but different vowels, high-contrast words with different consonants and vowels, and single digits, in that order.

Tests using competing sentences of six to seven words in length have been described by Willeford (1985a, b). Repetition of sentences heard at both ears proves to be a difficult task. Scoring is not straightforward in that it "is based on the degree to which the language in, and meaning of, each test item is preserved without being adversely influenced by the competing sentences" (Willeford, 1985b, pp. 249–250). Two errors per sentence such as borrowing from a competing sentence, omitting or adding a word, substituting a word not found in either sentence, or altering a word that changes the meaning of the sentence constitutes an incorrect response.

Identifying 2 synthetic sentences from a list of 10 presents a less difficult task (Fifer et al., 1983). Developed to overcome problems associated with administration and interpretation of dichotic tests for patients with peripheral hearing losses, this test seems to be influenced very little by hearing losses up to 39 dB HL. Interestingly, Mueller, Beck, and Sedge (1987) found that results from this test compared favorably to the other dichotic tests they used in their study of Viet Nam veterans who had sustained head injuries during combat (Mueller and Sedge, 1987).

Rather than requiring responses to dichotic stimuli at both ears, test procedures directing attention to one ear while ignoring the signal at the other ear have been used in a variety of forms. Competing sentences (Lynn and Gilroy, 1977), synthetic sentences at one ear with continuous discourse at the other ear (Jerger and Jerger, 1975b), and monosyllabic test items at one ear with meaningful sentences at the opposite ear (Jerger, 1964; Korsan-Bengsten, 1973) have been used. Such tasks are less difficult than dichotic tests requiring responses to stimuli delivered to both ears.

A different dichotic paradigm was suggested by the early work of Bocca et al. (1955) and followed by Jerger (1960b). Undistorted speech at a very low sensation level was presented to one ear while simultaneously the same words but low-pass filtered were delivered to the other ear at a considerably higher sensation level. Scores from dichotic presentation were compared to scores for monaural presentation of the faint and the filtered stimuli. Persons with normal auditory function combined the two signals for an improved score whereas patients with temporal lobe pathology attained scores similar to the higher monaural score (Jerger, 1960b).

Speech filtered in such a way that a relatively narrow band of low-frequency speech energy is delivered to one ear while the same test items but filtered so that a relatively narrow band of high-frequency speech spectra is presented to the other ear has been used (Matzker, 1959; Smith and Resnick, 1972). Diotic and dichotic modes of stimulation were used by these investigators. In the diotic mode, both the low- and high-pass bands of speech were delivered simultaneously to both ears; one band was presented to each ear for the dichotic condition. Matzker (1959) tested a large sample of patients, but interpretation of his results is difficult. Interpretation of the findings of Smith and Resnick (1972) for filtered monosyllabic word lists is straightforward. Dichotic scores equalled diotic scores for normal-hearing subjects and patients with sensory hearing losses. Similarly, three patients with temporal lobe lesions achieved equivalent scores (within 8%) for the diotic and dichotic conditions, but four patients with brainstem lesions attained scores 18 to 34 percent lower for the dichotic than for the diotic presentation of these test materials. These results suggest that resynthesis of the test items as required in this task is altered by brainstem abnormality rather than temporal lobe dysfunction.

Another test that compares diotic to dichotic stimuli assesses the *masking level difference* (MDL) phenomenon. First observed by Licklider (1948) and by Hirsh (1948), this procedure most commonly alters the phase of either the stimulus or the masking noise by 180 degrees at the two ears for the dichotic conditions (Figure 2-4). Compared to the diotic condition, masked thresholds for low-frequency signals and for speech improve considerably when the phase of the signal or

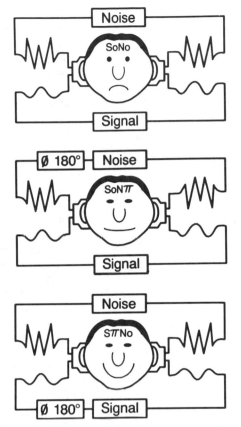

Figure 2-4. Three conditions for masking level difference tests. Signal in phase, noise in phase at two ears (SoNo) homophasic (diotic) condition; signal in phase, noise 180° out of phase (SoNπ) at two ears, antiphasic (dichotic) condition; signal 180° out of phase, noise in phase at two ears, (SπNo) antiphasic (dichotic) condition. (Adapted from Olsen, W. O., & Noffsinger, D. [1976]. Masking level differences for cochlear and brainstem lesions. *Annals of Otology, Rhinology & Laryngology, 86,* 820–825.)

noise is reversed at the two ears. These improvements in masked threshold are the MLD. Schoeny and Carhart (1971); Quaranta and Cervellera (1974); Olsen, Noffsinger, and Carhart (1976); and Jerger, Brown, and Smith (1984) established that MLDs are reduced for patients having peripheral hearing losses. Noffsinger et al. (1972) observed smaller than normal MLDs to be relatively common for a sample of patients with multiple sclerosis, despite normal hearing sensitivity. Cullen and Thompson (1974) reported normal MLDs for four patients who had undergone temporal lobectomies. In agreement with Cullen and Thompson, Olsen et al. (1976) found normal MLDs for all but 1 of 20 patients with temporal lobe lesions. All of these findings indicate the need for bilateral integrity of the peripheral auditory system, but not necessarily for the temporal lobes for normal MLDs to be observed. However, brainstem lesions such as associated with multiple sclerosis often disrupt the processing within the CANS necessary for attaining normal MLDs. Additional evidence from the work of Noffsinger, Kurdziel, and Applebaum (1975); Lynn, Gilroy, Taylor, and Leiser (1981); Noffsinger, Martinez, and Schaefer (1982); and Hannley, Jerger, and Rivera (1983) indicate that lesions at the lower levels of the brainstem are more likely to affect MLDs than are lesions in the upper pontine, midbrain, or thalamic levels of the CANS.

A procedure presenting different time segments of speech alternately to the two ears was described by Cherry and Taylor in 1954. They found a slight dip in the performance of normal hearing subjects when the speech alternated between ears at a rate of four times per second. Calearo and Antonelli (1968) observed a decrease in performance for 9 of 22 patients with brainstem lesions when the speech materials switched from ear to ear 3 to 8 times per second. Only 6 of 48 patients with brainstem lesions demonstrated difficulty with this task in the study of Lynn and Gilroy (1977) when they presented 300 msec time segments of speech alternating between ears to their subjects. Bocca and Calearo (1963) observed no breakdown on this task for patients with temporal lobe lesions. Thus this task too seems to be one that, for some patients, taxes the integrity of the CANS at the level of the brainstem.

PHYSIOLOGIC TESTS

Two other procedures that can assess the integrity of the CANS at the level of the brainstem are the acoustic reflex test and ABR test discussed earlier. In the absence of peripheral pathology, comparisons of acoustic reflex responses for contralateral and ipsilateral stimulation can be used to evaluate the acoustic reflex arc within the brainstem. Griesen and Rasmussen (1970) first reported observations of acoustic reflexes for ipsilateral stimulation but not for contralateral stimulation of each ear for two patients with brainstem lesions. Observations of ipsilaterally elicited reflexes demonstrated normal middle ear, eighth nerve, and seventh nerve function on each side, but the brainstem lesion interrupted the crossing neural paths necessary for elicitation of the contralateral reflex response. Jerger, Neely, and Jerger (1975) and Jerger and Jerger (1977) have presented additional documentation of such findings and a detailed account of recent acoustic reflex applications can be found in Chapter 6.

Given inferred sites for the generation of waves in the ABR to acoustic stimuli (Figure 2-5), relatively specific sites of involvement within the brainstem have been suspected on the basis of waveform abnormalities. Early reports of ABR abnormalities associated with brainstem disorders were provided by Starr and Achor (1975) and Stockard, Stockard, and Sharbrough (1977). Increased latencies of later waves, absence of

Figure 2-5. (A) ABR waveform and (B) probable generator sites. (Adapted from Moeller, A. R., & Jannetta, P. J. [1985]. Neural generators of the auditory brainstem reponse. In J. T. Jacobson [Ed.], *The auditory brainstem response* [pp. 13–31]. Boston: College-Hill Press.)

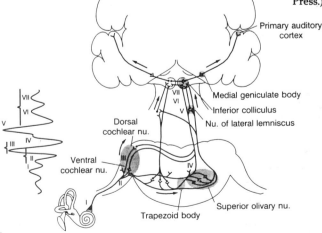

A

SIMPLIFIED SUMMARY OF PROBABLE GENERATOR SITES (ABR)

Wave I	Distal auditory nerve (N_1)
Wave II	Proximal auditory nerve
Wave III	Cochlear nucleus
Wave IV	Superior olivary complex
Wave V	Lateral lemniscus
Wave VI	Inferior colliculus
Wave VII	Inferior colliculus

B

some waves or all waveforms after wave I, and unusual changes in conjunction with increased repetition rates of click stimuli are among the observed ABR abnormalities. Chiappa, Harrison, Brooks, and Young (1980) observed abnormal ABR tracings for 57 percent of the multiple sclerosis patients in their sample who had other symptoms indicating brainstem involvement. These findings were confirmed, particularly at high repetition rates, by Jacobson, Murray, and Duppe (1987).

Patterns of results from ABR and acoustic reflex tests can be used very nicely to suggest specific sites of involvement within the brainstem. Hayes and Jerger (1981) reported six case studies in which acoustic reflex and ABR testing suggested side and possible site of involvement at low levels within the brainstem. Similarly, Noff-singer et al. (1982), Hannley et al. (1983), and Jerger, Oliver, Chmiel, and Rivera (1986) have demonstrated relationships between MLDs, acoustic reflexes, and waveforms obtained from ABR tests. In particular, it appears that when abnormalities in ABR waveforms beginning at wave III are observed, MLDs are smaller than normal and acoustic reflex results may be abnormal too.

Patients having multiple sclerosis have been included in many of the studies cited above designed to assess auditory abnormalities arising from lesions in the brainstem. Because plaques of multiple sclerosis demyelination can occur at isolated or multiple sites in the myelinated portions of the central nervous system, and remiss or exacerbate from time to time, findings for groups of such patients are variable across and within studies (Jacobson, Duppe, and Murray, 1983). For these reasons a variety of patterns of test results are obtained from them. Nevertheless much has been learned about auditory function and dysfunction in the lower levels of the CANS through administration of MLD, acoustic reflex, and ABR tests to such patients.

Recent technological advances have allowed "mapping" of activity within the human brain of awake subjects responding to various stimuli, or when they are performing various mental tasks. For example, metabolic activity in circumscribed regions of an intact human brain is measured in terms of increased blood flow in a given region. Movement of radioisotopes injected into the bloodstream (Lassen, Ingvar, and Skinhoj, 1978) or inhaled from gases (Stump and Williams, 1980) is traced with sensors placed near the head, processed by a computer, and displayed on a television monitor. This technique assesses increased blood flow in a given region associated with a specific mental task. With such methods, Knopman, Rubens, Klassen, Meyer, and Niccum (1980) reported increased blood flow in the vicinity of Wernicke's area in the left temporal lobe when subjects were instructed to discriminate between loud and soft noise bursts, or to recognize a noun in a list of monosyllables. Maximilian (1982) also observed increased blood flow in the temporo-parietal region in the right hemisphere in response to speech stimuli to either ear.

Three-dimensional mapping of brain activity with positron emission tomography (Alavi et al., 1981) also has been used to search for the loci of brain activity in response to auditory stimuli. A radioactive tracer is injected via the radial artery in awake subjects. The tracer is taken up in the brain at a rate proportional to that of glucose, and the radioactive metabolic products remain trapped in the brain tissue long enough to be detected by positron emission tomography. Three-dimensional images are reconstructed by computer to display areas of brain activated by specific stimuli presented to awake humans. Using this technique Greenberg et al. (1981) observed increased metabolic rate in the temporal lobe contralateral to the ear in which a factual story was presented.

Brain electrical activity mapping electroencephalogram (EEG) electrodes is another recent development for mapping cortical activity (Finitzo and Pool, 1987). For example, 2 seconds of EEG tracings can be analyzed in 4 msec segments, allowing sharper analyses of ongoing EEG activity. Fast Fourier transforms can be applied to the electrical waveforms to determine the frequency content of the electrical activity at the different electrodes. Topographic mapping of evoked potentials in response to stimuli can be accomplished with this technique also. The electrical activity analyzed by these means is projected in different colors on a monitor to display ongoing events at various electrodes attached to the scalp.

No doubt further investigations in cerebral blood flow, positron emission tomography, and brain electrical activity mapping will lead to further refinements in the techniques and analyses of normal and abnormal patterns of activity. Such information will lead to a better understanding of cortical function, including the auditory cortex, and, in time, should allow assessment of specific cortical sites of involvement in cases of auditory dysfunction.

SUMMARY

Over the years, a variety of behavioral and physiologic tests have been devised to assess the function of the CANS. Tasks that prove to be 4somewhat difficult even for normal hearing persons must be used if subtle breakdowns in a highly redundant CANS are to be detected. To this end, behavioral tests for thresholds, frequency discrimination, and temporal ordering of brief tonal or click stimuli, recall and labeling of pitch patterns, understanding or identification of distorted speech, masked speech, and dichotic speech stimuli have been used. The complexity and redundancy of the central nervous system is such that even though these procedures may detect abnormal auditory function, they generally cannot specify site or side of involvement. Patterns of results from physiologic measures such as contralateral and ipsilateral acoustic reflexes and ABR may be more site specific for brainstem regions given the anatomy of the reflex arc and inferred generator sites for waves I through V of the ABR. Recent developments in noninvasive techniques for mapping metabolic and electrical activity at the level of the cortex may provide more definitive localization of disorders at the cortical level in the future.

PSEUDOHYPACUSIS

That some patients respond to stimuli only at levels well above their true thresholds during tests for hearing sensitivity has long been recognized. Only recently, however, has the term *pseudohypacusis* for such "hearing losses" been used. *Pseudo neural hypacusis* was coined by Brockman and Hoversten (1960) in the title of their publication reporting observations for a small sample of children who were less than accurate in their responses to threshold stimuli. Carhart (1961) modified their term to *pseudohypoacusis*, and Goldstein (1966) advocated the term *pseudohypacusis* for "false hearing loss." Prior to the 1960s a variety of terms such as *nonorganic hearing loss, functional hearing impairment, hysterical deafness, psychogenic hearing disorder, simulated hearing problems,* and *malingering* were among the descriptive terms found in the literature. These terms are found in more recent publications also, but *pseudohypacusis* is used here because it does not imply an underlying causal factor as do some of the other labels. Although a variety of tests have been devised to detect pseudohypacusis, the purpose of these tests

is to demonstrate the inaccuracy of the obtained threshold data, not to identify causal factors.

Pseudohypacusis may take virtually any form: unilateral, bilateral, mild to profound in degree. The audiometric configuration also may vary widely depending on the "true" hearing sensitivity of the patient; individuals having a bona fide hearing impairment may superimpose some degree of pseudohypacusis on their actual hearing loss. The astute clinician must be alert to the possibility of pseudohypacusis, be sensitive to clues raising suspicion of such problems, use tests to support or deny such suspicions, ascertain as accurately as possible actual hearing status, and assist in the management of the patient.

Early clues to the possbility of pseudohypacusis are very subjective; for example, seemingly exaggerated efforts to hear or lip-read, hearing complaints inconsistent with ease of communication during the initial interview. Similarly, during initial testing the patient may exhibit excess strain to hear and respond; responses may be absent or inconsistent and may not be in accord with impressions of hearing for communication gained during the interview and instructions for the test procedures. At this point, clinical observations and tests developed over the years to demonstrate the presence of pseudohypacusis and to assess as accurately as possible the actual hearing status are initiated.

PURE TONE AVERAGES AND SPEECH RECEPTION THRESHOLDS

As early as 1940, Steinberg and Gardner reported good agreement between the average of pure tone thresholds for 512, 1024, 2048, and 4096 Hz and the level at which hearing-impaired subjects attained 40 percent correct for lists of monosyllables. Hughson and Thompson (1942) demonstrated a direct correlation between hearing loss for pure tones and thresholds for Bell Telephone intelligibility sentences (Fletcher and Steinberg, 1929) using a descending and bracketing approach to establish threshold. They found this procedure to be accurate within 1 to 2 dB and coined the term *speech reception threshold* (SRT). Carhart (1946a), having access to materials described by Hudgins, Hawkins, Karlin, and Stevens (1947), found threshold relationships between pure tones and Bell Telephone intelligibility sentences, and between pure tones and spondaic words to be essentially equivalent. Since that time spondees generally have been used to establish SRTs, and agreement between pure tone averages and SRTs has been considered a vital indicator of the accuracy of initial pure tone thresholds. Various pure tone averages have been proposed, for example, for 500, 1000, and 2000 Hz (Fletcher, 1929; Carhart, 1946a), two best thresholds for the octave frequencies of 500 through 2000 Hz (Fletcher, 1950), or thresholds for 500 and 1000 Hz minus 2 dB (Carhart, 1971) are among pure tone averages suggested for comparison to SRTs.

Carhart (1952) first reported marked discrepancies between the pure tone averages and SRTs with the thresholds for speech indicating considerably better hearing sensitivity for cases of pseudohypacusis. Since then his observations have been confirmed (Brockman and Hoversten, 1960; Menzel, 1960; Ventry and Chaiklin, 1965). Menzel (1960) found pure tone average and SRT discrepancies of 6 dB or greater for 91 percent of a large sample of patients demonstrating pseudohypacusis; Ventry and Chaiklin (1965) reported that speech thresholds were at least 12 dB better than the pure tone averages for 70 percent of their patients revealing pseudohypacusis. Menzel noted that completion of SRT tests before beginning pure tone testing significantly reduced the observation of differences between thresholds for pure tones and for speech. The basis for the discrepancies in thresholds for the two types of stimuli seems to be the greater loudness experience for speech than for pure tones at the same hearing levels (Ventry, 1976). The important point is that unexplained differences greater than 6 dB between one of the above mentioned pure tone averages and SRT warrant further investigation, reinstruction, and further testing to resolve the discrepancy. Because of the expected close relationship between SRTs and pure tone thresholds, it is vital that both sets of thresholds be established in a systematic manner using predetermined criteria to specify threshold levels. (Caution should be noted in that even though some patients deliberately may exaggerate their hearing losses, others simply may fail to understand the instructions to respond to even the softest tones they hear but do make efforts to guess at the soft speech stimuli they hear. For the latter, reinstruction and retesting usually resolve the discrepancy.)

DOERFLER-STEWART TEST

One of the earliest tests developed specifically for detection of bilateral pseudohypacusis using speech stimuli was described by Doerfler and Stewart (1946). The test procedure consists of comparing two SRTs (SRT_1 and SRT_2), noise interference level (NIL) (the level at which noise interferes with perception of spondees presented at 5 dB sensation level), and noise detection threshold (NDT) (the acknowledged presence of the masking noise). Comparisons are made between SRT_1 and SRT_2, NDT and SRT_1 and SRT_2, NIL and SRT_1 + 5 dB, and NDT and NIL. Although comparisons between SRT_1 and SRT_2 are straightforward, criteria for other comparisons depend on the type of noise used. Because the effectiveness of this test procedure seems limited (Hattler and Schuchman, 1971; Menzel, 1960; Ventry and Chaiklin, 1965), it has fallen into disuse.

ASCENDING AND DESCENDING THRESHOLDS

Given suspicion of pseudohypacusis, or inconsistencies in threshold responses, Harris (1958) suggested comparisons of thresholds for stimuli presented at successively higher levels (ascending) and thresholds obtained when stimulus presentations are begun at high levels and then presented at successively lower levels (descending). Based on his evaluation, Harris stated that "results showing the descending threshold to be higher than the ascending threshold should be considered suspicious if the difference exceeds 5 d.b. [sic] ... a difference of 10 d.b. [sic] or greater between the two thresholds is highly indicative of inorganic involvement" (p. 769).

BEKESY AUDIOMETRY

In 1961, Jerger and Herer added a type V classification to the original four classifications of Bekesy audiograms described by Jerger (1960a). In contrast to types I through IV Bekesy tracings in which the threshold tracings overlap one another, or the threshold for the continuous tone is traced at higher intensity levels than for the pulsed tone, the threshold tracings for the continuous tone were at levels lower than for the pulsed tone for three patients demonstrating pseudohypacusis. Jerger and Herer designated this pattern as a type V Bekesy audiogram. Support for their observations has been provided by Resnick and Burke (1962) and Stein (1963) for adults and by Peterson (1963) and Rintelmann and Harford (1963) for children. Based on investigations in which normal-hearing subjects were instructed to trace comfortable loudness levels, or levels akin to a reference tone using pulsed and continuous tones, Rintelmann and Carhart (1964) concluded that listeners judged the pulsed tone to be less loud than a continuous tone at the same sensation levels. Melnick (1967) attributed the difference to ambiguity in the listener's loudness standard. In any event, tracings at lower levels for continuous tones than for pulsed tones were found in both investigations.

Hattler (1970) sought to enhance the difference between tracings for pulsed and continuous tones with his development of the lengthened off-time (LOT) test. Rather than the conventional 50 percent duty cycle for the pulsed signal (200 msec on, 200 msec off), the LOT procedure uses the 200 msec on-time but an 800 msec off-time for the signals. Threshold tracings for the conventional pulsed signals, LOT stimuli, and continuous tones are compared. The LOT stimulus increased the separation between the pulsed and continuous tones to at least 5.5 dB for patients demonstrating pseudohypacusis, but not for normal-hearing subjects or patients with bona fide hearing losses. Hattler (1970) reported excellent success in identifying pseudohypacusis with the LOT test (95% or higher); however, Citron and Reddell (1976) reported less success for a smaller sample of patients.

A procedure similar to the Harris test described earlier but using a Bekesy audiometer was described by Hood, Campbell, and Hutton in 1964. Thresholds for fixed-frequency Bekesy tracings are compared for a continous tone begun at levels well below threshold, for a pulsed tone begun at subthreshold levels, and for a pulsed tone begun at levels well above the previously obtained threshold tracing for the pulsed tone in that sequence. This procedure was labeled *BADGE* for "Bekesy ascending descending gap evaluation." Hood et al. found this procedure "to be about 70% efficient in differentiating between organic and nonorganic hearing loss" (p. 131).

DELAYED AUDITORY FEEDBACK

Observations by Lee (1950) and Black (1951) that hearing one's own speech via air conduction when delayed by about 200 msec at the two ears disrupted a talker's ability to self-monitor the fluency and intensity of one's speech production led Tiffany and Hanley (1952) to propose this technique for detection of pseudohypacusis. The patient's task is to read aloud a selected passage several times while the length of time taken to read the passage as well as the reader's rate, fluency, and intensity of speech are determined by the examiner. The patient continues to read the same material when the examiner activates the delayed auditory feedback system at output levels below the obtained speech thresholds. (Delays of about 200 msec are available on commercial tape recorders with independent record and playback heads that can be activated simultaneously. The microphone input to the record head stores the speech on magnetic tape, which then passes across the playback head a short time later. The output from the playback head is delivered to the reader via earphones about 200 msec after the utterance.) If the speech is not heard at sufficiently intense levels via the earphones, the reader continues without disruption; when the reader increases vocal intensity, exhibits dysfluencies, or decreases reading rate, then the delayed speech is sufficiently loud to disrupt the patient's normal speech pattern. For various reasons, including hearing one's own speech simultaneously via bone conduction, delayed feedback speech tests cannot estimate actual hearing sensitivity for speech (Hanley and Tiffany, 1956a, b; Harford and Jerger, 1959).

Rather than using one's speech under delayed feedback conditions, Chase, Harvey, Standfast, Rapin, and Sutton (1959) and Chase, Sutton, Fowler, Fay, and Ruhm (1961) used simultaneous or delayed click stimuli associated with a key-tapping paradigm to assess disruption in performance due to delayed auditory feedback. Short tone pulses were substituted for clicks by Ruhm and Cooper (1962, 1963, 1964a, b); Billings and Stokinger (1975); Cooper and Stokinger (1976); and Cooper, Stokinger, and Billings (1976, 1977). The patient taps out simple patterns (for example, four taps, pause, two taps) with an electromechanical key that triggers a short tone burst delivered to the patient's ear with each tap. It is important that the movement of the hand tapping the pattern be very minimal to limit kinesthetic feedback, that the patient not be able to see the hand and key to eliminate visual feedback, and that the key does not produce any mechanical noise in order to limit the feedback to only the desired tonal signal. The tone duration is 50 msec and is first delivered simultaneously with each key tap while the patient establishes a rhythm and pattern for the key tapping recorded by strip chart recorder. Switching to a 200 msec delay between the key tap and tone presentation disrupts the rhythm and pattern of the key tapping. Thus a change noted in the pattern of key tapping when the feedback stimuli are switched from simultaneous to delayed indicates that the tones were heard; when the tones are inaudible, the key-tapping pattern is unchanged in the simultaneous and delayed conditions. Delayed signals at levels as low as 5 to 10 dB sensation level have been shown to disrupt the key-tapping pattern. Furthermore, the effects of delayed feedback on key tapping persist despite practice and sophistication (Martin and Shipp, 1982; Monro and Martin, 1977). Therefore, although the delayed auditory feedback test using the patient's own speech as the stimulus cannot estimate hearing sensitivity, key tapping and delayed auditory feedback with pure tone stimuli can provide an estimate of hearing sensitivity for pure tones within about 10 dB.

STENGER TEST

As early as 1900 Stenger demonstrated that detection of pseudohypacusis could be accomplished with two tuning forks of the same frequency presented to each ear. This procedure takes advantage of the fact that with very similar signals at each ear, the listener perceives only the louder stimulus. Hinsberg performed the Stenger test with pure tones and speech using electroacoustic instrumentation in 1928, and Frenzel was the first to use an audiometer for this test in 1932 (Feldmann, 1960/1970). The usual procedure is to present a tone at a sensation level of about 10 dB to the better ear and simultaneously to the "poorer" ear at a level below its previously attained threshold. Pseudohypacusis is demonstrated if the patient fails to respond because the stimulus is heard at the poorer ear and she or he is unaware that the same signal is being delivered to the other ear at suprathreshold levels also; if the signal is at subthreshold levels in the poorer ear, the patient immediately responds to the suprathreshold signal in the better ear. Through manipulation of the stimulus intensities for pure tones or speech in the poorer ear, estimates of its hearing sensitivity are gained from observations of the levels at which responses cease. The Stenger test can be used very successfully to detect pseudohypacusis and to gain some information on hearing sensitivity for unsophisticated listeners (Kinstler, Phelan, and Lavender, 1970; Kinstler, Phelan, and Lavender, 1972; Peck and Ross, 1970); however, substantial errors in estimation of hearing sensitivity can occur with

sophisticated listeners (Martin and Shipp, 1982; Robinette and Gaeth, 1972).

ELECTROPHYSIOLOGIC TESTS

In the late 1940s, Michels and Randt (1947) and Doerfler (1948) demonstrated that presentation of auditory stimuli resulted in measurable psychogalvanic skin responses in the form of slight changes in skin resistance to current flow. These changes were sensed with electrodes attached to the hand and arm and were recorded on a strip chart recorder. Such responses, however, often extinguished quickly after a few presentations of the same signal. Bordley and Hardy (1949) overcame the problem of extinction by pairing an electric shock with the auditory stimulus. In their approach, which ultimately came to be called *electrodermal audiometry*, a conditioning paradigm is used in which a conditioned pure tone stimulus (or speech [Ruhm and Carhart, 1958; Ruhm and Menzel, 1959]) is paired with an unconditioned stimulus, a mild electric shock delivered via electrodes. A set of measurement electrodes is attached to an area rich in sweat glands, usually the tips or pads of fingers on one hand, to record the reaction of autonomic nervous system in the form of a reduction in skin resistance. Initial conditioning to the combination of auditory signals and electric shock, and occasional reinforcement with electric shock following an observed psychogalvanic skin response to the auditory stimulus alone maintain the desired response while threshold is sought. For patients who do respond to such conditioning, thresholds established with electrodermal audiometry are remarkably close, within 5 dB, to actual thresholds (Burk, 1958; Doerfler and McClure, 1954), but not all patients can be conditioned (Citron and Reddell, 1976; Goldstein, 1956). Because this procedure is unpleasant, it was used sparingly except in Veterans Administration clinics where it was part of the routine in cases with claims for compensation due to hearing losses associated with military duty. Fortunately other less noxious electrophysiologic measures for assessment of hearing sensitivity have been developed.

As mentioned earlier, electrical activity of the auditory nervous system at the level of the cortex in response to acoustic stimuli was described as early as 1939 by Davis. Measurement of these responses to repeated stimuli with the aid of a special purpose summing and averaging computer was reported by Lowell, Troffer, Warburton, and

Rushford (1960) and Lowell, Williams, Ballinger, and Alvig (1961). Subsequent reports by McCandless and Best (1964) and Davis, Hirsch, Shelnutt, and Bowers (1967) demonstrated that such averaged responses to acoustic stimuli, including short tone bursts, could be observed within 5 dB of voluntary threshold. McCandless and Lentz (1968) reported application of this technique for assessment of hearing sensitivity for patients yielding inconsistent responses or indications of pseudohypacusis on other tests. Rose, Keating, Hedgecock, Miller, and Schreurs (1972) have cautioned that close agreement between thresholds for evoked response audiometry and voluntary thresholds is not always observed, even for cooperative patients.

Obviously measurement of ABR to brief acoustic stimuli as mentioned earlier also lends itself to estimation of hearing sensitivity. Although hearing sensitivity for click stimuli generally can be observed to within 10 to 20 dB of behavioral thresholds for such stimuli, inferences relative to audiometric configuration cannot be made on the basis of such measurements (Jerger and Mauldin, 1978; Moeller and Blegvad, 1976). ABR to brief tone bursts has been used, but data for hearing impaired subjects are sparse (Davis and Hirsch, 1976; Mitchell and Clemis, 1977). Similarly reports of middle latency responses to tonal stimuli when averaging electrical activity of the auditory nervous system within the first 50 to 100 msec after each stimulus (rather than just within the first 10 msec as for ABR) for hearing-impaired patients are limited (Dauman, Szyfter, deSauvage, and Cazals, 1984; McFarland, Vivion, and Goldstein, 1977). Although estimates of hearing sensitivity can be obtained from measurements of electrical activity in the auditory nervous system, such observations should not be viewed as precise indicators of hearing status.

OTHER TESTS

A number of other tests developed over the years can demonstrate pseudohypacusis but do not estimate hearing sensitivity. For example, observation of acoustic reflexes when stimulating at levels below thresholds obtained during conventional audiometry has been cited in a number of reports as an obvious indication of pseudohypacusis (Feldman, 1963; Jepsen, 1953; Lamb and Peterson, 1967; Thomsen, 1955). Absence of acoustic reflexes does not rule out pseudohypacusis, however; as discussed earlier, absence of reflex responses can be due to many middle ear, sensory, or neural abnormalities and could be concomitant with pseudohypacusis.

The Lombard test takes advantage of the Lombard effect in which the talker increases the intensity level of speech in response to strong background noise. Although there is some dispute as to whether the observation was first described by Barany or by Lombard, Lombard's name has been attached to it (Feldmann, 1960/1970; Lane and Tranel, 1971). For the Lombard test, masking is introduced to the ears while the patient is reading aloud. When the reader increases vocal intensity in response to gradual introduction of masking noise, it demonstrates that the noise is at suprathreshold levels, but the sensation level of the masking noise cannot be estimated (Heller and Lindenberg, 1953; Taylor, 1949).

Application of the alternating speech test (described earlier) as a test for unilateral pseudohypacusis is based on the inability of the listener to maintain separate recall of the words or parts of words heard in each ear, thus better hearing in the "impaired" ear can be revealed with this procedure. This concept is expanded in the swinging story tests in which the meaning of the sentences or questions changes depending on the segments heard (Davis and Goldstein, 1960; Martin, 1985; Newby, 1958).

A speech-reading test in which the patient is encouraged to watch and listen to homophonous monosyllabic word lists has been described by Falconer (1966). Consistently correct responses indicate hearing the stimuli because many words have the same articulatory gestures in their production, for example, "plaid, plant, plan, bland." Correct responses to presentation of such homophonous words while gradually decreasing the intensity level can support a suspicion of pseudohypacusis when a number of correct responses are obtained for levels at or below previously established SRTs.

SUMMARY

A number of tests for detection of pseudohypacusis have been developed, but initial suspicion of the possibility of pseudohypacusis often is based on patient behavior or history, and SRTs at levels considerably better than pure tone thresholds. In order to observe such discrepancies, it is vital that systematic approaches and specific criteria be used for establishing thresholds for pure tones and speech. Haphazard methodology or failure to apply predetermined criteria for threshold determination, or simply failure to compare pure tone and speech thresholds routinely can lead to perfunctory misses of pseudohypacusis. Although simply reinstructing the patient and retesting sometimes resolve discrepancies between test results, retesting by a second examiner often is the preferred option; psychologically the patient does not "lose face" when responding consistently and accurately for the second examiner. Most tests for pseudohypacusis merely demonstrate such behavior. Delayed auditory feedback with pure tone stimuli and Stenger tests (pure tones or speech) can estimate thresholds, but it must be remembered that since almost all of the tests reviewed require some form of voluntary response, they can be defeated by total refusal to cooperate. Only acoustic reflex and evoked response tests do not require voluntary response, and of these, only evoked response testing can estimate thresholds.

FINAL COMMENT

From the preceding review it is obvious that through cognizance of activities in other disciplines, audiology, during its few short years of existence, has applied, adapted, expanded, and developed a variety of methods for the assessment and study of hearing and hearing disorders. Given its brief history and notable accomplishments to date, it is critical that audiologists keep pace with developments within their own and other disciplines in order to continue to increase the knowledge and skills that are required with the expanding technology and demand for understanding of hearing and hearing problems.

REFERENCES

Alavi, A., Reivich, M., Greenberg, J., Hand, P., Rosenquist, A., Rintelmann, W., Christman, D., Fowler, J., Goldman, A., MacGregor, R., & Wolf, A. (1981). Mapping of functional activity in the brain with ^{18}F-fluoro-deoxyglucose. *Seminars in Nuclear Medicine, 11,* 24–31.

Anderson, H., Barr, B., & Wedenberg, E. (1969). Intra-aural reflexes in retrocochlear lesions. In C. A. Hamberger & J. Wersall (Eds.), *Nobel symposium 10, Disorders of the skull base region* (pp. 48–54). Stockholm: Almqvist & Wikell.

Baran, J. A., Musiek, F. E., & Reeves, A. G. (1986). Central auditory function following anterior sectioning of the corpus callosum. *Ear & Hearing, 6,* 359–362.

Bauch, C. D., Olsen, W. O., & Harner, S. G. (1983). Auditory brain stem response and acoustic reflex test results for patients with and without tumor matched for hearing loss. *Archives of Otolaryngology, 109,* 522–525.

Bauch, C. D., Rose, D. E., & Harner, S. G. (1982). Auditory brain stem response results from 255 patients with suspected retrocochlear involvement. *Ear & Hearing, 3,* 83–86.

Beasley, D. S., Schwimmer, S., & Rintelmann, W. F. (1972). Intelligibility of time-compressed CNC monosyllables. *Journal of Speech and Hearing Research, 15,* 340–350.

Bekesy, G. V. (1947). A new audiometer. *Acta Oto-laryngologica* (Stockholm), *45,* 411–422.

Berlin, C. I., Lowe-Bell, S. S., Cullen, J. K., Jr., Thompson, C. L., & Loovis, C. F. (1973). Dichotic speech perception: On interpretation of right ear advantage and temporal offset effects. *Journal of the Acoustical Society of America, 53,* 699–709.

Berlin, C. I., Lowe-Bell, S. S., Jannetta, P. J., & Kline, D. G. (1972). Central auditory deficits after temporal lobectomy. *Archives of Otolaryngology, 96,* 4–10.

Bess, F. H. (1983). Clinical assessment of speech recognition. In D. F. Konkle & W. F. Rintelmann (Eds.), *Principles of speech audiometry* (pp. 127–201). Baltimore: University Park Press.

Bess, F. H., Josey, A. F., & Humes, L. E. (1979). Performance intensity functions in cochlear and eighth nerve disorders. *American Journal of Otolaryngology, 1,* 27–31.

Billings, B. L., & Stokinger, T. E. (1975). A comparison of pure-tone thresholds as measured by delayed feedback audiometry, electrodermal response audiometry and voluntary response audiometry. *Journal of Speech and Hearing Research, 18,* 754–764.

Bingea, R. L., & Raffin, M. J. M. (1986). Normal performance on a dichotic CV test across nine onset-time-asynchrony conditions: Application of a binomial distribution model. *Ear & Hearing, 7,* 246–254.

Black, J. W. (1951). The effect of delayed side-tone upon vocal rate and intensity. *Journal of Speech and Hearing Disorders, 16,* 56–60.

Bocca, E. (1958). Clinical aspects of cortical deafness. *Laryngoscope, 68,* 301–309.

Bocca, E., & Calearo, C. (1963). Central hearing processes. In J. Jerger (Ed.), *Modern developments in audiology* (pp. 337–370). New York: Academic Press.

Bocca, E., Calearo, C., & Cassinari, V. (1954). A new method for testing hearing in temporal lobe tumors. *Acta Oto-laryngologica* (Stockholm), *44,* 219–221.

Bocca, E., Calearo, C., Cassinari, V., & Migliavacca, F. (1955). Testing "cortical" hearing in temporal lobe tumors. *Acta Oto-laryngologica* (Stockholm), *45,* 289–304.

Bordley, J., & Hardy, W. (1949). A study in objective audiometry with the use of psychogalvanometric response. *Annals of Otology, Rhinology, and Laryngology, 58,* 751–760.

Broadbent, D. E. (1954). The role of auditory localization in attention and memory span. *Journal of Experimental Psychology, 47,* 191–196.

Brockman, S. J., & Hoversten, G. H. (1960). Pseudo neural hypacusis in children. *Laryngoscope, 70,* 825–839.

Bunch, C. C. (1928). Auditory acuity after removal of the entire right cerebral hemisphere. *Journal of the American Medical Association, 90,* 2102.

Bunch, C. C. (1941). The development of the audiometer. *Laryngoscope, 51,* 1100–1118.

Bunch, C. C. (1943). *Clinical audiometry.* St. Louis: C.V. Mosby.

Burk, K. (1958). Traditional and psychogalvanic skin response audiometry. *Journal of Speech and Hearing Research, 1,* 175–278.

Calearo, C., & Antonelli, A. R. (1968). Audiometric findings in brain stem lesions. *Acta Oto-laryngologica* (Stockholm), *66*, 305–319.

Calearo, C., & Lazzaroni, A. (1957). Speech intelligibility in relation to the speed of the message. *Laryngoscope, 67*, 410–419.

Carhart, R. (1946a). Monitored live voice as a test of auditory acuity. *Journal of the Acoustical Society of America, 17*, 339–349.

Carhart, R. (1946b). Tests for selection of hearing aids. *Laryngoscope, 56*, 780–794.

Carhart, R. (1950). Clinical application of bone conduction audiometry. *Archives of Otolaryngology, 51*, 798–808.

Carhart, R. (1952). Speech audiometry in clinical evaluation. *Acta Oto-laryngologica* (Stockholm), *41*, 18–42.

Carhart, R. (1957). Clinical determination of abnormal auditory adaptation. *Archives of Otolaryngology, 65*, 32–40.

Carhart, R. (1961). Tests for malingering. *Transactions of the American Academy of Ophthalmology and Otolaryngology, 65*, 437.

Carhart, R. (1965). Problems in the measurement of speech discrimination. *Archives of Otolaryngology, 82*, 253–260.

Carhart, R. (1971). Observations on relations between thresholds for pure tones and for speech. *Journal of Speech and Hearing Disorders, 36*, 476–483.

Chase, R. A., Harvey, S., Standfast, S., Rapin, I., & Sutton, S. (1959). Comparison of the effects of delayed auditory feedback on speech and keytapping. *Science, 29*, 903–904.

Chase, R. A., Sutton, S., Fowler, E. P., Jr., Fay, T. H., & Ruhm, H. B. (1961). Low sensation level delayed clicks and keytapping. *Journal of Speech and Hearing Research, 4*, 73–78.

Cherry, E. C., & Taylor, W. K. (1954). Some further experiments upon the recognition of speech with one and with two ears. *Journal of the Acoustical Society of America, 26*, 554–559.

Chiappa, K. H., Harrison, J. L., Brooks, E. B., & Young, R. R. (1980). Brainstem auditory evoked responses in 200 patients with multiple sclerosis. *Annals of Neurology, 7*, 135–143.

Citron, D., III, & Reddell, R. C. (1976). A comparison of EDR, LOT, pure-tone DAF, and conventional pure-tone threshold audiometry for medical-legal audiological assessment. *Archives of Otolaryngology, 102*, 204–206.

Collard, M. E., Lesser, R. P., Luders, H., Dinner, D. S., Morris, H. H., Hahn, J. F., & Rothner, A. D. (1986). Four dichotic speech tests before and after temporal lobectomy. *Ear & Hearing, 7*, 363–369.

Cooper, W. A., Jr., & Stokinger, T. E. (1976). Pure tone delayed auditory feedback: Effect of prior experience. *Journal of the American Audiology Society, 1*, 164–168.

Cooper, W. A., Jr., Stokinger, T. E., & Billings, B. L. (1976). Pure tone delayed auditory feedback: Development of criteria of performance deterioration. *Journal of the American Audiology Society, 1*, 192–196.

Cooper, W. A., Jr., Stokinger, T. E., & Billings, B. L. (1977). Pure tone delayed auditory feedback: Effect of hearing loss on disruption of tapping performance. *Journal of the American Audiology Society, 3*, 102–107.

Cranford, J. L., Stream, R. W., Rye, C. V., & Slade, T. L. (1982). Detection v discrimination of brief-duration tones. *Archives of Otolaryngology, 108*, 350–356.

Cullen, J. K., Jr., & Thompson, C. L. (1974). Masking release for speech in subjects with temporal lobe resection. *Archives of Otolaryngology, 100*, 113–116.

Dauman, R., Szyfter, W., deSauvage, R., & Cazals, Y. (1984). Low frequency thresholds assessed with 40 Hz MLR in adults with impaired hearing. *Archives of Otorhinolaryngology, 240*, 85–89.

Davis, H., & Goldstein, R. (1960). Special auditory tests. In H. Davis & S. R. Silverman (Eds.), *Hearing and deafness* (pp. 218–241). New York: Holt, Rinehart & Winston.

Davis, H., & Hirsh, S. K. (1976). The audiometric utility of brainstem response to low frequency sounds. *Audiology, 15*, 181–195.

Davis, H., Hirsh, S. K., Shelnutt, J., & Bowers, C. (1967). Further validation of evoked response audiometry (ERA). *Journal of Speech and Hearing Research, 10*, 717–732.

Davis, P. A. (1939). Effects of acoustic stimuli on the waking human brain. *Journal of Neurophysiology, 2*, 494–499.

Dean, C. E. (1930). Audition by bone conduction. *Journal of the Acoustical Society of America, 2*, 281–296.

Denes, P., & Naunton, R. F. (1950). The clinical detection of auditory recruitment. *Journal of Laryngology and Otology, 64*, 375–398.

deQuiros, J. B. (1964). *Accelerated speech audiometry, an examination of test results.* (J. Tonndorf, Trans., for Beltone Institute for Hearing Research, No. 17.) (Reprinted from Interpretacion de los resultados obtenidos con logoaudiometria acelerada. *Revista Fonoaudiologica*, 1961, Tomo VII, 128–164.)

Dirks, D. D., Kamm, C., Bower, D., & Bettsworth, A. (1977). Use of performance intensity functions for diagnosis. *Journal of Speech and Hearing Disorders, 42*, 408–415.

Dix, M. R., Hallpike, C. S., & Hood, J. D. (1948). Observations upon the loudness recruitment phenomenon with especial reference to the differential diagnosis of disorders of the internal ear and VIIIth nerve. *Journal of Laryngology and Otology, 62*, 671–686.

Dix, M. R., Hallpike, C. S., & Hood, J. D. (1949). Nerve deafness: Its clinical criteria, old and new. *Proceedings of the Royal Society of Medicine, 42*, 527–536.

Doerfler, L. G. (1948). Neurophysiological clues to auditory acuity. *Journal of Speech and Hearing Disorders, 13*, 227–232.

Doerfler, L. G., & McClure, C. (1954). A study in objective audiometry with the use of psychogalvanometric response. *Journal of Speech and Hearing Disorders, 19*, 184–189.

Doerfler, L. G., & Stewart, K. (1946). Malingering and psychogenic deafness. *Journal of Speech Disorders, 11*, 181–186.

Eby, L. G., & Williams, H. L. (1951). Recruitment of loudness in differential diagnosis of end organ and nerve fibre deafness. *Laryngoscope, 61*, 400–414.

Efron, R. (1963). Temporal perception, aphasia and deja vu. *Brain, 86*, 405–424.

Efron, R., Crandall, P. H., Koss, D., Divenyi, P. L., & Yund, E. W. (1983). Central auditory processing III. The "cocktail party" effect and anterior temporal lobectomy. *Brain & Language, 19*, 254–263.

Efron, R., Yund, E. W., & Crandall, P. H. (1985). An ear asymmetry for gap detection following anterior temporal lobectomy. *Neuropsychologica, 23*, 43–50.

Egan, J. (1948). Articulation testing methods. *Laryngoscope, 58*, 955–991.

Falconer, G. (1966). A "lipreading test" for nonorganic deafness. *Journal of Speech and Hearing Disorders, 31*, 241–247.

Feldman, A. S. (1963). Impedance measurements at the eardrum as an aid to diagnosis. *Journal of Speech and Hearing Research, 6*, 315–327.

Feldmann, H. (1960). A history of audiology, a comprehensive report and bibliography from the earliest beginnings to the present [Die geschichliche Entwicklung der Horprufungmethoden, kurze Darstellung und Bibliographie von der Anfangen biz zur Gegenwart]. (J. Tonndorf, Trans., for Beltone Institute for Hearing Research, No. 22, 1970.) In H. Leicher, R. Mittmaier, & G. Theissing (Eds.), *Zwanglose Abhandlugen aus dem Gebiet der Hals-Nasen-Ohren-Heilkunde.* Stuttgart: Georg Thieme Verlag.

Fifer, R. C., Jerger, J. F., Berlin, C. I., Tobey, E. A., & Campbell, J. C. (1983). Development of a dichotic sentence identification test for hearing impaired adults. *Ear & Hearing, 4,* 300–305.

Finitzo, T., & Pool, K. D. (1987). Brain electrical activity mapping. *ASHA, 29,* 21–25.

Fletcher, H. (1929). *Speech and hearing.* Princeton: Van Nostrand Reinhold.

Fletcher, H. (1950). A method for calculating hearing loss for speech from an audiogram. *Acta Oto-laryngologica. Supplement* (Stockholm), *90,* 26–37.

Fletcher, H., & Steinberg, J. C. (1929). Articulation testing methods. *Bell Systems Technical Journal, 7,* 806–854.

Flottorp, G., & Djupesland, G. (1970). Diphasic impedance change and its applicability in clinical work. *Acta Oto-laryngologica. Supplement* (Stockholm), *263,* 200–204.

Fowler, E. P. (1925). Fundamentals of bone conduction. *Archives of Otolaryngology, 2,* 529–542.

Fowler, E. P. (1928). Marked deafened areas in normal ears. *Archives of Otolaryngology, 8,* 151–156.

Fowler, E. P. (1936). A method for the early detection of otosclerosis. *Archives of Otolaryngology, 24,* 731–741.

Fowler, E. P. (1937a). The diagnosis of diseases of the neural mechanism of hearing by aid of sounds well above threshold. *Transactions of the American Otological Society, 27,* 207–219.

Fowler, E. P. (1937b). Measuring the sensation of loudness. *Archives of Otolaryngology, 26,* 514–521.

Fowler, E. P., & Wegel, R. L. (1922a). Audiometric methods and the applications. *Transactions of the 28th Annual Meeting of the American Laryngological, Rhinological and Otological Society,* 98–132.

Fowler, E. P., & Wegel, R. L. (1922b). Presentation of a new instrument for determining the amount and character of auditory sensation. *Transactions of the American Otology Society, 16,* 105–123.

Gelfand, S. A., Hoffman, S., Watzman, S. B., & Piper, N. (1980). Dichotic C.V. recognition at various interaural temporal onset asynchronies: Effect of age. *Journal of the Acoustical Society of America, 68,* 1258–1261.

Gersuni, G. V., Baru, A. V., Karaseva, T. A., & Tonkongii, I. M. (1971). Effects of temporal lobe lesions on perception of sounds of short duration. In G. V. Gersuni (Ed.) (J. Rose, Trans.), *Sensory processes at the neuronal and behavioral levels* (pp. 287–300). New York: Academic Press.

Glasscock, M. E., Jackson, C. G., & Josey, A. F. (1981). *Brain stem electric response audiometry.* New York: Grune & Stratton.

Glattke, T. J. (1983). *Short latency auditory evoked potentials.* Baltimore: University Park Press.

Goetzinger, C. P. (1972). Word discrimination testing. In J. Katz (Ed.), *Handbook of clinical audiology* (pp. 157–179). Baltimore: Williams & Wilkins.

Goetzinger, C. P., & Angell, S. N. (1965). Audiological assessment in acoustic tumors and cortical lesions. *Eye, Ear, Nose, and Throat Monthly, 44,* 39–49.

Goldstein, R. (1956). Effectiveness of conditioned electrodermal response (EDR) in measuring pure tone thresholds in cases of nonorganic hearing loss. *Laryngoscope, 66,* 119–130.

Goldstein, R. (1961). Hearing and speech follow-up of left hemispherectomy. *Journal of Speech and Hearing Disorders, 26,* 126–129

Goldstein, R. (1966). Pseudohypacusis. *Journal of Speech and Hearing Disorders, 31,* 341–352.

Goldstein, R., Goodman, A. G., & King, R. B. (1956). Hearing and speech in infantile hemiplegia before and after left hemispherectomy. *Neurology, 6,* 869–875.

Gradenigo, G. (1893). On the clinical signs of the affections of the auditory nerve. *Archives of Otology, 22,* 213–215.

Graham, J., Greenwood, R., & Lecky, B. (1980). Cortical deafness: A case report and review of the literature. *Journal of Neurological Sciences, 48,* 35–49.

Green, D. S. (1963). The modified tone decay test (MTDT) as a screening procedure for eighth nerve lesions. *Journal of Speech and Hearing Disorders, 28,* 31–36.

Greenbaum, A., Kerridge, P., & Ross, E. (1939). Normal hearing by bone conduction. *Journal of Laryngology and Otology, 59,* 88–92.

Greenberg, J. H., Reivich, M., Alavi, A., Hand, P., Rosenquist, A., Rintelmann, W., Stein, A., Tusa, R., Dann, R., Christman, D., Fowler, J., MacGregor, R., & Wolf, A. (1981). Metabolic mapping of functional activity in human subjects with the [18F] fluorodeoxyglucose technique. *Science, 212,* 678–680.

Griesen, O., & Rasmussen, P. E. (1970). Stapedius muscle reflexes and otoneurological examination in brainstem tumors. *Acta Oto-laryngologica* (Stockholm), *70,* 366–370.

Guild, S. R. (1936). Hearing by bone conduction: The pathways of transmission of sound. *Annals of Otology, Rhinology, and Laryngology, 45,* 736–754.

Hall, C. M. (1977). Stapedial reflex decay in retrocochlear and cochlear lesions. *Annals of Otology, Rhinology, and Laryngology, 86,* 219–222.

Hanley, C. N., & Tiffany, W. R. (1954a). An investigation into the use of electro-mechanically delayed side-tone in auditory testing. *Journal of Speech and Hearing Disorders, 19,* 367–374.

Hanley, C. N., & Tiffany, W. R. (1954b). Auditory malingering and psychogenic deafness. *Archives of Otolaryngology, 60,* 197–201.

Hannley, M., Jerger, J., & Rivera, V. M. (1983). Relationships among auditory brainstem responses, masking level differences and acoustic reflexes in multiple sclerosis. *Audiology, 22,* 20–33.

Harford, E. R., & Jerger, J. F. (1959). Effect of loudness recruitment on delayed speech feedback. *Journal of Speech and Hearing Research, 2,* 361–368.

Harris, D. A. (1958). A rapid and simple technique for the detection of non-organic hearing loss. *Archives of Otolaryngology, 68,* 758–760.

Hattler, K. W. (1970). Lengthened off-time: A self-recording screening device of nonorganicity. *Journal of Speech and Hearing Disorders, 35,* 113–122.

Hattler, K. W., & Schuchman, G. (1971). Efficiency of Stenger, Doerfler-Stewart and lengthened off-time Bekesy tests. *Acta Oto-laryngologica* (Stockholm), *72,* 252–267.

Hayes, D., & Jerger, J. (1981). Patterns of acoustic reflex and auditory brainstem response abnormality. *Acta Oto-laryngologica* (Stockholm), *92,* 199–209.

Heller, M. R., & Lindenberg, P. (1953). Evaluation of deafness of nonorganic origin. *Archives of Otolaryngology, 58,* 575–581.

Hirsh, I. J. (1948). The influence of interaural phase on interaural summation and inhibition. *Journal of the Acoustical Society of America, 20,* 536–544.

Hirsh, I. J. (1959). Auditory perception of temporal order.

Journal of the Acoustical Society of America, 31, 759–767.

Hirsh, I. J., Davis, H., Silverman, S. R., Reynolds, E. G., Eldert, E., & Benson, R. W. (1952). Development of materials for speech audiometry. *Journal of Speech and Hearing Disorders, 17,* 321–337.

Hirsh, I. J., Palva, T., & Goodman, A. (1954). Difference limen and recruitment. *Archives of Otolaryngology, 60,* 525–540.

Hodgson, W. R. (1967). Audiologic report of a patient with left hemispherectomy. *Journal of Speech and Hearing Disorders, 32,* 39–45.

Hood, J. D. (1969). Basic audiologic requirements in neurootology. *Journal of Laryngology and Otology, 83,* 695–711.

Hood, L. J., & Berlin, C. I. (1986). *Auditory evoked potentials.* Austin, TX: Pro-Ed.

Hood, W. H., Campbell, R. A., & Hutton, C. L. (1964). An evaluation of the Bekesy ascending descending gap. *Journal of Speech and Hearing Research, 7,* 123–132.

Hudgins, C. V., Hawkins, J. E., Jr., Karlin, J. E., & Stevens, S. S. (1947). The development of recorded auditory tests for measuring hearing loss for speech. *Laryngoscope, 57,* 57–89.

Hughes, R. L., Winegar, W. J., & Crabtree, J. A. (1967). Bekesy audiometry: Type 2 versus type 4 patterns. *Archives of Otolaryngology, 86,* 424–430.

Hughson, W., & Thompson, E. A. (1942). Correlation of hearing acuity for speech with discrete frequency audiograms. *Archives of Otolaryngology, 36,* 526–540.

Huizing, H. C. (1948). The symptom of recruitment and speech intelligibility. *Acta Oto-laryngologica* (Stockholm), *36,* 346–355.

Jacobson, J. T. (Ed.). (1985). *The auditory brainstem response.* Boston: College-Hill Press.

Jacobson, J. T., Duppe, U., & Murrey, J. (1983). Dichotic test paradigms in multiple sclerosis. *Ear & Hearing, 4,* 311–317.

Jacobson, J. T., McCandless, G., & Mahoney T. (1979). Influence of amplification on the discrimination of dichotic consonant-vowel syllables in a population with sensorineural hearing loss. *Audiology, 18,* 1–15.

Jacobson, J. T., Murrey, J., & Duppe, U. (1987). The effects of ABR rate presentation in multiple sclerosis. *Ear & Hearing, 8,* 115–120.

Jepson, O. (1953). Intratympanic muscle reflexes in psychogenic deafness (impedance measurement). *Acta Oto-laryngologica. Supplement* (Stockholm), *109,* 61–69.

Jerger, J. (1952). A difference limen recruitment test and its diagnostic significance. *Laryngoscope, 62,* 1316–1332.

Jerger, J. (1953). DL difference test: An improved method for the clinical measurement of recruitment. *Archives of Otolaryngology, 57,* 490–500.

Jerger, J. (1960a). Bekesy audiometry in analysis of auditory disorders. *Journal of Speech and Hearing Research, 3,* 275–287.

Jerger, J. (1960b). Observations on auditory behavior in lesions of the central auditory pathways. *Archives of Otolaryngology, 71,* 797–806.

Jerger, J. (1961). Recruitment and allied phenomena in differential diagnosis. *Journal of Auditory Research, 1,* 145–151.

Jerger, J. (1962). Hearing tests in otologic diagnosis, *ASHA, 4,* 139–145.

Jerger, J. (1964). Auditory tests for disorders of the central auditory mechanism. In B. R. Alford & W. S. Fields (Eds.), *Neurological aspects of auditory and vestibular disorders* (pp. 77–86). Springfield, IL: Charles C. Thomas.

Jerger, J. (1970). Clinical experience with impedance audi-ometry. *Archives of Otolaryngology, 92,* 311–324.

Jerger, J., & Herer, G. (1961). Unexpected dividend in Bekesy audiometry. *Journal of Speech and Hearing Disorders, 26,* 390–391.

Jerger, J., & Jerger, S. (1971). Diagnostic significance of PB word functions. *Archives of Otolaryngology, 93,* 573–580.

Jerger, J., & Jerger, S. (1974). Auditory findings in brainstem disorders. *Archives of Otolaryngology, 99,* 342–350.

Jerger, J., & Jerger, S. (1975a). A simplified tone decay test. *Archives of Otolaryngology, 101,* 403–407.

Jerger, J., & Jerger, S. (1975b). Clinical validity of central auditory tests. *Scandinavian Audiology, 4,* 147–163.

Jerger, J., & Jerger, S. (1977). Diagnostic value of crossed versus uncrossed acoustic reflexes. Eighth nerve tumor and brainstem disorders. *Archives of Otolaryngology, 103,* 445–453.

Jerger, J., & Mauldin, L. (1978). Prediction of sensorineural hearing level from brainstem evoked response. *Archives of Otolaryngology, 104,* 456–461.

Jerger, J., Anthony, L., Jerger, S., & Mauldin, L. (1974). Studies in impedance audiometry III. Middle ear disorders. *Archives of Otolaryngology, 99,* 165–171.

Jerger, J., Brown, D., & Smith, S. (1984). Effect of peripheral hearing loss on masking level difference. *Archives of Otolaryngology, 110,* 290–296.

Jerger, J., Carhart, R., & Lassman, J. (1958). Clinical observations on excessive threshold adaptation. *Archives of Otolaryngology, 68,* 617–623.

Jerger, J., Harford, E., Clemis, J., & Alford, B. (1974). The acoustic reflex in eighth nerve disorders. *Archives of Otolaryngology, 99,* 409–413.

Jerger, J., Lovering, J., & Wertz, M. (1972). Auditory disorder following bilateral temporal lobe insult — report of a case. *Journal of Speech and Hearing Disorders, 37,* 523–535.

Jerger, J. F., Oliver, T. A., Chmiel, R. A., & Rivera, V. M. (1986). Patterns of auditory abnormalities in multiple sclerosis. *Audiology, 25,* 193–209.

Jerger, J., Shedd, J. L., & Harford, E. (1959). On the detection of extremely small changes in sound intensity. *Archives of Otolaryngology, 69,* 200–211.

Jerger, J., Weikers, N. J., Sharbrough, F. W., III, & Jerger, S. (1969). Bilateral lesions of the temporal lobe. *Acta Oto-laryngologica. Supplement* (Stockholm), *258.*

Jerger, S., Neely, G., & Jerger, J. (1975). Recovery of crossed reflexes in brainstem auditory disorders. *Archives of Otolaryngology, 101,* 329–332.

Jewett, D. L., & Williston, J. S. (1971). Auditory evoked far fields averaged from the scalp of humans. *Brain, 94,* 681–696.

Johnson, E. W. (1979). Results of auditory tests in acoustic tumor patients. In W. F. House & C. M. Luetje (Eds.), *Acoustic tumors: Vol. 1. Diagnosis* (pp. 209–224). Baltimore: University Park Press.

Jones, I. H., & Knudsen, V. O. (1924). Functional tests of hearing. *Transactions of the 30th Annual Meeting of the American Laryngological, Rhinological, and Otological Society,* 121–136.

Katz, J. (1962). The use of staggered spondaic words for assessing the integrity of the central auditory nervous system. *Journal of Auditory Research, 2,* 327–337.

Katz, J. (1968). The SSW test: An interim report. *Journal of Speech and Hearing Disorders, 33,* 132–146.

Keith, R. W. (Ed.). (1977). *Central auditory dysfunction.* New York: Grune & Stratton.

Keith, R. W. (Ed.). (1981). *Central auditory dysfunction and language disorders in children.* Boston: College-Hill Press.

Keith, R. W. (1983). Interpretation of the staggered spondaic word test. *Ear & Hearing, 4*, 287–292.

Kimura, D. (1961). Some effects of temporal-lobe damage on auditory perception. *Canadian Journal of Psychology, 15*, 156–165.

Kinstler, D. B., Phelan, J. G., & Lavender R. W. (1970). Efficiency of the Stenger tests in identification of functional hearing loss. *Journal of Auditory Research, 10*, 118–123.

Kinstler, D. B., Phelan, J. G., & Lavender, R. W. (1972). The Stenger and speech Stenger tests in functional hearing loss. *Audiology, 11*, 187–193.

Klockhoff, I. (1961). Middle ear muscle reflexes in man. *Acta Oto-laryngologica. Supplement* (Stockholm), *164*.

Knopman, D. S., Rubens, A. B., Klassen, A. C., Meyer, M. W., & Niccum, N. (1980). Regional cerebral blood flow patterns during verbal and nonverbal activation. *Brain & Language, 9*, 93–122.

Korsan-Bengsten, M. (1973). Distorted speech audiometry: A methodological and clinical study. *Acta Oto-laryngologica. Supplement* (Stockholm), *310*.

Kurdziel, S., Noffsinger, D., & Olsen, W. O. (1976). Performance by cortical lesion patients on 40 and 60% time-compressed materials. *Journal of the American Audiology Society, 2*, 3–7.

Lackner, J., & Teuber, H.-L. (1973). Alterations in auditory fusion thresholds after cerebral injury in man. *Neuropsychologica, 11*, 409–415.

Lamb, L. E., & Peterson, J. L. (1967). Middle ear reflex measurements in pseudohypacusis. *Journal of Speech and Hearing Disorders, 32*, 46–51.

Lane, H., & Tranel, B. (1971). The Lombard sign and the role of hearing in speech. *Journal of Speech and Hearing Research, 14*, 677–709.

Lasky, E. Z., & Katz, J. (Eds.). (1983). *Central auditory processing disorders*. Baltimore: University Park Press.

Lassen, M. A., Ingvar, D. H., & Skinhoj, E. (1978). Brain function and blood flow. *Scientific American, 239*, 62–71.

Lee, B. (1950). Some effects of side-tone delay. *Journal of the Acoustical Society of America, 22*, 639–640.

Licklider, J. C. R. (1948). The influence of interaural phase relations upon the masking of speech by white noise. *Journal of the Acoustical Society of America, 20*, 150–159.

Liden, G. (1954). Speech audiometry. *Acta Oto-laryngologica. Supplement* (Stockholm), *114*.

Liden, G. (1969). The scope and application of current audiometric tests. *Journal of Laryngology and Otology, 83*, 507–520.

Liden, G., Harford, E., & Hallen, O. (1974). Automatic tympanometry in clinical practice. *Audiology*, 126–139.

Liden, G., Peterson, J., & Björkman, G. (1970). Tympanometry. *Archives of Otolaryngology, 92*, 248–257.

Lierle, D. M., & Reger, S. (1946). Correlations between air and bone conduction measurements with wide frequency ranges in different types of hearing impairments. *Laryngoscope, 56*, 187–224.

Lierle, D. M., & Reger, S. N. (1955). Experimentally induced temporary threshold shifts in ears with impaired hearing. *Annals of Otology, Rhinology, and Laryngology, 64*, 263–277.

Lowe, S. S., Cullen, J. K., Berlin, C. I., Thompson, C. L., & Willett, M. (1970). Perception of simultaneous dichotic and monotic monosyllables. *Journal of Speech and Hearing Research, 13*, 812–822.

Lowell, E. L., Troffer, C. I., Warburton, E. A., & Rushford, G. M. (1960). Temporal examination: A new approach in diagnostic audiology. *Journal of Speech and Hearing Disorders, 25*, 340–345.

Lowell, E. L., Williams, C. T., Ballinger, R. M., & Alvig, D. P. (1961). Measurement of auditory threshold with a special purpose analog computer. *Journal of Speech and Hearing Research, 4*, 105–112.

Lukas, R. A., & Genchur-Lukas, J. (1985). Spondaic word tests. In J. Katz (Ed.), *Handbook of clinical audiology* (pp. 383–403). Baltimore: Williams & Wilkins.

Lundborg, T., Rosenhamer, H., Murray, T., & Zwetnow, N. (1975). Information abundance of speech and distorted speech testing in topical diagnosis within the C.N.S. *Scandinavian Audiology, 4*, 9–16.

Lund-Iverson, L. (1952). An investigation on the difference limen determined by the method of Luscher and Zwislocki in normal hearing and in various forms of deafness. *Acta Oto-laryngologica* (Stockholm), *42*, 219–224.

Luscher, E. (1951). The difference limen of intensity variations of pure tones and its diagnostic significance. *Journal of Laryngology and Otology, 65*, 486–510.

Luscher, E., & Zwislocki, J. (1949). A simple method for indirect monaural determination of the recruitment phenomenon (difference limen in intensity in different types of deafness). *Acta Oto-laryngologica. Supplement* (Stockholm), *78*, 156–168.

Lynn, G. E., & Gilroy, J. (1977). Evaluation of central auditory dysfunction in patients with neurological disorders. In R. W. Keith (Ed.), *Central auditory dysfunction* (pp. 177–221). New York: Grune & Stratton.

Lynn, G. E., Gilroy, J., Taylor, P. C., & Leiser, R. P. (1981). Binaural masking-level differences in neurological disorders. *Archives of Otolaryngology, 107*, 357–362.

Martin, F. N. (1985). The pseudohypacusic. In J. Katz (Ed.), *Handbook of clinical audiology* (pp. 742–765). Baltimore: Williams & Wilkins.

Martin, F. N., & Shipp, D. B. (1982). The effects of sophistication and three threshold tests for patients with simulated hearing loss. *Ear & Hearing, 3*, 34–36.

Matzker, J. (1959). Two new methods for the assessment of central auditory function in cases of brain disease. *Annals of Otology, Rhinology, and Laryngology, 68*, 1185–1196.

Maximilian, V. A. (1982). Cortical blood flow asymmetries during monaural verbal stimulation. *Brain & Language, 15*, 1–11.

McCandless, G. A., & Best, L. (1964). Evoked responses to auditory stimuli in man using a summing computer. *Journal of Speech and Hearing Research, 7*, 193–202.

McCandless, G. A., & Lentz, W. E. (1968). Evoked response audiometry in nonorganic hearing loss. *Archives of Otolaryngology, 87*, 123–128.

McFarland, W. H., Vivion, M. C., & Goldstein, R. (1977). Middle components of AER to tone pips in normal-hearing and hearing-impaired subjects. *Journal of Speech and Hearing Research, 20*, 781–798.

Melnick, W. (1967). Comfort level and loudness matching for continuous and interrupted signals. *Journal of Speech and Hearing Research, 10*, 99–109.

Menzel, O. J. (1960). Clinical efficiency in compensation audiometry. *Journal of Speech and Hearing Disorders, 25*, 49–54.

Metz, O. (1946). The acoustic impedance measured on normal and pathological ears. *Acta Oto-laryngologica. Supplement* (Stockholm), *63*.

Metz, O. (1952). Threshold of reflex contractions of muscles of middle ear and recruitment of loudness. *Archives of Otolaryngology, 55*, 536–543.

Meyer, D., & Mishler, E. T. (1985). Rollover measurements with Auditec NU-6 word lists. *Journal of Speech and Hearing Disorders, 50,* 356–360.

Michels, M. W., & Randt, C. T. (1947). Galvanic skin response in differential diagnosis of deafness. *Archives of Otolaryngology, 45,* 302–311.

Miller, G. A., & Licklider, J. C. R. (1950). The intelligibility of interrupted speech. *Journal of the Acoustical Society of America, 22,* 167–173.

Mirabile, P. J., Porter, R. J., Hughes, L. F., & Berlin, C. L. (1978). Dichotic lag effect in children. *Developmental Psychology, 14,* 277–285.

Mitchell, C., & Clemis, J. D. (1977). Audiograms derived from the brainstem response. *Laryngoscope, 87,* 2016–2022.

Moeller, A. R., & Janetta, P. J. (1985). Neural generators of the auditory brainstem response. In J. T. Jacobson (Ed.), *The auditory brainstem response* (pp. 13–31). Boston: College-Hill Press.

Moeller, K., & Blegvad, B. (1976). Brainstem potentials in subjects with sensorineural hearing loss. *Scandinavian Audiology, 5,* 115–127.

Monro, D. A., & Martin, F. N. (1977). Effects of sophistication on four tests for nonorganic hearing loss. *Journal of Speech and Hearing Disorders, 42,* 528–534.

Moore, E. (Ed.). (1983). *Bases of auditory brain-stem evoked responses.* New York: Grune & Stratton.

Mueller, H. G. (1987). The staggered spondaic word test: Practical use. *Seminars in Hearing, 8,* 267–277.

Mueller, H. G., & Sedge, R. K. (Eds.). (1987). Audiological aspects of head trauma. *Seminars in Hearing, 8*(3).

Mueller, H. G., Beck, W. G., & Sedge, R. K. (1987). Comparison of the efficiency of cortical level speech tests. *Seminars in Hearing, 8,* 279–298.

Musiek, F. E., & Wilson, D. H. (1979). SSW and dichotic digit results pre- and post-commissurotomy: A case report. *Journal of Speech and Hearing Disorders, 44,* 528–533.

Musiek, F. E., Kibby, K., & Baran, J. A. (1984). Neuroaudiological results from split brain patients. *Seminars in Hearing, 5,* 219–229.

Musiek, F. E., Pinheiro, M. L., & Wilson, D. H. (1980). Auditory pattern perception in "split brain" patients. *Archives of Otolaryngology, 106,* 610–612.

Musiek, F. E., Wilson, D. H., & Pinheiro, M. L. (1979). Audiological manifestations in split-brain patients. *Journal of the American Audiology Society, 5,* 25–29.

Newby, H. A. (1958). *Audiology: Principles and practices.* New York: Appleton-Century-Crofts.

Niccum, N., Rubens, A. B., & Speaks, C. (1981). Effects of stimulus material on the dichotic listening performance of aphasia patients. *Journal of Speech and Hearing Research, 24,* 526–534.

Noffsinger, D., Kurdziel, S., & Applebaum, E. L. (1975). Value of special auditory tests in the latero-medial inferior pontine syndrome. *Annals of Otology, Rhinology, and Laryngology, 84,* 384–390.

Noffsinger, D., Martinez, C. D., & Schaefer, A. B. (1982). Auditory brainstem responses and masking level differences from persons with brainstem lesions. *Scandinavian Audiology. Supplementum, 15,* 81–93.

Noffsinger, D., Olsen, W. O., Carhart, R., Hart, C. W., & Sahgal, V. (1972). Auditory and vestibular aberrations in multiple sclerosis. *Acta Oto-laryngologica. Supplement* (Stockholm), *303.*

Olsen, W. O. (1983). Dichotic test results for normal subjects and temporal lobectomy patients. *Ear & Hearing, 4,* 324–330.

Olsen, W. O. (1984). Audiologic test battery results for cochlear and for VIIIth nerve lesions. *Audiology Journal for Continuing Education, 9,* 147–163.

Olsen, W. O., & Noffsinger, D. (1974). Comparison of one new and three old tests of auditory adaptation. *Archives of Otolaryngology, 99,* 94–99.

Olsen, W. O., & Noffsinger, D. (1976). Masking level differences for cochlear and brain stem lesions. *Annals of Otology, Rhinology, and Laryngology, 86,* 820–825.

Olsen, W. O., Bauch, C. D., & Harner, S. G. (1983). Application of Silman and Gelfand 90th percentile levels for acoustic reflex thresholds. *Journal of Speech and Hearing Disorders, 48,* 330–332.

Olsen, W. O., Noffsinger, D., & Carhart, R. (1976). Masking level differences encountered in clinical populations. *Audiology, 15,* 287–301.

Olsen, W. O., Noffsinger, D., & Kurdziel, S. (1975a). Acoustic reflex and reflex decay occurrence in patients with cochlear and eighth nerve lesions. *Archives of Otolaryngology, 101,* 622–625.

Olsen, W. O., Noffsinger, D., & Kurdziel, S. (1975b). Speech discrimination in quiet and in white noise by patients with peripheral and central lesions. *Acta Otolaryngologica* (Stockholm), *80,* 375–382.

Olsen, W. O., Stach, B., & Kurdziel, S. (1981). Acoustic reflex decay in 10 seconds and in 5 seconds for Ménière's disease patients and for VIIIth nerve tumor patients. *Ear & Hearing, 2,* 180–181.

O'Neill, J. J., & Oyer, H. J. (1966). *Applied audiometry.* New York: Dodd, Mead.

Owens, E. (1964). Tone decay in eighth nerve and cochlear lesions. *Journal of Speech and Hearing Disorders, 29,* 14–22.

Owens, E. (1971). Audiologic evaluation in cochlear versus retrocochlear lesions. *Acta Oto-laryngologica. Supplement* (Stockholm), *283,* 1–45.

Oxbury, J. M., & Oxbury, S. M. (1969). Effect of temporal lobectomy on the report of dichotically presented digits. *Cortex, 5,* 3–14.

Parker, W., & Decker, R. L. (1971). Detection of abnormal auditory adaptation. *Archives of Otolaryngology, 94,* 1–7.

Peck, J. E., & Ross, M. (1970). A comparison of ascending and descending modes for administration of the puretone Stenger test. *Journal of Auditory Research, 10,* 218–220.

Peterson, J. L. (1963). Nonorganic hearing loss in children and Bekesy audiometry. *Journal of Speech and Hearing Disorders, 28,* 153–158.

Pinheiro, M. L. (1977). Tests of central auditory function in children with learning disabilities. In R. W. Keith (Ed.), *Central auditory dysfunction* (pp. 223–254). Baltimore: Grune & Stratton.

Pinheiro, M. L., & Musiek, F. E. (1985). Sequencing and temporal ordering in the auditory system. In M. L. Pinheiro & F. E. Musiek (Eds.), *Assessment of central auditory dysfunction foundations and clinical correlates* (pp. 219–238). Baltimore: Williams & Wilkins.

Pinheiro, M. L., & Musiek, F. E. (Eds.). (1985). *Assessment of central auditory dysfunction foundations and clinical correlates.* Baltimore: Williams & Wilkins.

Pohlman, A. G., & Kranz, F. W. (1924). Binaural minimum audition in a subject with ranges of deficient acuity. *Proceedings of the Society of Experimental Biology and Medicine, 21,* 335–337.

Quaranta, A., & Cervellera, G. (1974). Masking level difference in normal and pathological ears. *Audiology, 13,* 428–431.

Reger, S. N. (1936). Differences in loudness response of the normal and hard of hearing ears at intensity levels slightly above threshold. *Annals of Otology, Rhinology, and Laryngology, 45,* 1024–1039.

Reger, S. N., & Kos, C. M. (1952). Clinical measurements and implications of recruitment. *Annals of Otology, Rhinology, and Laryngology, 61,* 810–820.

Resnick, D. M., & Burke, K. S. (1962). Bekesy audiometry in non-organic auditory problems. *Archives of Otolaryngology, 76,* 38–41.

Rintelmann, W. F., & Carhart, R. (1964). Loudness tracking by normal hearers via Bekesy audiometer. *Journal of Speech and Hearing Research, 7,* 93–109.

Rintelmann, W. F., & Harford, E. R. (1963). The detection and assessment of pseudohypoacusis among school-age children. *Journal of Speech and Hearing Disorders, 28,* 141–152.

Robinette, M. S., & Gaeth, J. H. (1972). Diplacusis and the Stenger test. *Journal of Auditory Research, 12,* 91–100.

Rose, D. E., Keating, L. W., Hedgecock, L. D., Miller, K. E., & Schreurs, K. K. (1972). A comparison of evoked response audiometry and routine clinical audiometry. *Audiology, 11,* 238–243.

Rosenberg, P. E. (1958). *Rapid clinical measurement of tone decay.* Paper presented at the annual convention of the American Speech and Hearing Association, New York, NY.

Ruhm, H. B., & Carhart, R. (1958). Objective speech audiometry: A new method based on electrodermal response. *Journal of Speech and Hearing Research, 1,* 169–178.

Ruhm, H. B., & Cooper, W. A., Jr. (1962). Low sensation level effects of pure-tone delayed auditory feedback. *Journal of Speech and Hearing Research, 5,* 185–193.

Ruhm, H. B., & Cooper, W. A., Jr. (1963). Some factors that influence pure-tone delayed auditory feedback. *Journal of Speech and Hearing Research, 6,* 225–237.

Ruhm, H. B., & Cooper, W. A., Jr. (1964a). Delayed feedback audiometry. *Journal of Speech and Hearing Disorders, 29,* 448–455.

Ruhm, H. B., & Cooper, W. A., Jr. (1964b). Influence on motor performance of simultaneous delayed and synchronous pure-tone auditory feedback. *Journal of Speech and Hearing Research, 7,* 175–182.

Ruhm, H. B., & Menzel, O. (1959). Objective speech audiometry in cases of nonorganic hearing loss. *Archives of Otolaryngology, 69,* 212–219.

Sanders, J. W., Josey, A. F., & Glasscock, M. E. (1974). Audiologic evaluation in cochlear and eighth nerve disorders. *Archives of Otolaryngology, 100,* 283–293.

Sanders, J. W., Josey, A. F., Glasscock, M. E., & Jackson, C. G. (1981). The acoustic reflex in cochlear and eighth nerve pathology ears. *Laryngoscope, 91,* 787–793.

Schoeny, Z. G., & Carhart, R. (1971). Effects of unilateral Ménière's disease on masking level differences. *Journal of the Acoustical Society of America, 50,* 1143–1150.

Schuknecht, H. F., & Woellner, R. C. (1955). An experimental and clinical study of deafness from lesions of the cochlear nerve. *Journal of Laryngology and Otology, 69,* 75–97.

Selters, W. A., & Brackmann, D. E. (1977). Acoustic tumor detection with brainstem electric response audiometry. *Archives of Otolaryngology, 103,* 15–34.

Selters, W. A., & Brackmann, D. E. (1979). Brainstem electric response audiometry in acoustic tumor detection. In W. F. House & C. M. Leutje (Eds.), *Acoustic tumors: Vol. 1. Diagnosis* (pp. 225–235). Baltimore: University Park Press.

Shallop, J. K. (1976). The historical development of the study of middle ear function. In A. S. Feldman & L. A. Wilber (Eds.), *Acoustic impedance and admittance* (pp. 8–48). Baltimore: Williams & Wilkins.

Sheehy, J., & Inzer, B. (1976). Acoustic reflex in neuro-otologic diagnosis. *Archives of Otolaryngology, 102,* 647–653.

Silman, S. (1984). *The acoustic reflex basic principles and clinical applications.* New York: Academic Press.

Silman, S., & Gelfand, S. A. (1981). The relationship beween magnitude of hearing loss and acoustic reflex threshold levels. *Journal of Speech and Hearing Disorders, 46,* 312–316.

Sinha, S. P. (1959). *The role of the temporal lobe in hearing.* Unpublished master's thesis, McGill University, Montreal.

Smith, B., & Resnick, D. M. (1972). An auditory test for assessing brain stem integrity: Preliminary report. *Laryngoscope, 82,* 414–424.

Sohmer, H., & Feinmesser, M. (1967). Cochlear action potentials recorded from the external ear in man. *Annals of Otology, Rhinology, and Laryngology, 76,* 427–438.

Sonn, M. (1969). *Psychoacoustical terminology.* Portsmouth, RI: Raytheon.

Sorenson, H. (1962). A threshold tone decay test. *Acta Otolaryngologica. Supplement* (Stockholm), *158,* 356–360.

Sparks, R., & Geschwind, N. (1968). Dichotic listening in man after section of neocortical commissures. *Cortex, 4,* 3–16.

Sparks, R. H., Goodglass, H., & Nickel, B. (1970). Ipsilateral versus contralateral extinction in dichotic listening resulting from hemispheric lesions. *Cortex, 6,* 248–260.

Speaks, C. (1975). Dichotic listening: A clinical or research tool. In M. D. Sullivan (Ed.), *Central auditory processing disorders* (pp. 10–25). Omaha: University of Nebraska Press.

Speaks, C. (1980). Evaluation of disorders of the central auditory system. In M. M. Paperella & D. A. Shumrick (Eds.), *Otolaryngology: Vol. 2. The ear* (pp. 1846–1860). Philadelphia: W. B. Saunders.

Speaks, C., & Jerger, J. (1965). Method for measurement of speech identification. *Journal of Speech and Hearing Research, 8,* 185–194.

Speaks, C., & Niccum, N. (1977). Variability of the ear advantage in dichotic listening. *Journal of the American Audiology Society, 3,* 52–57.

Speaks, C., Carney, C., Niccum, N., & Johnson, C. (1981). Stimulus dominance in dichotic listening. *Journal of Speech and Hearing Research, 24,* 430–437.

Speaks, C., Niccum, N., & Carney, E. (1982). Statistical properties of responses to dichotic listening with CV nonsense syllables. *Journal of the Acoustical Society of America, 72,* 1185–1194.

Starr, A., & Achor, J. L. (1975). Auditory brain stem response in neurological diseases. *Archives of Neurology, 32,* 761–768.

Stein, L. (1963). Some observations on type V Bekesy tracings. *Journal of Speech and Hearing Research, 6,* 339–348.

Steinberg, J. C., & Gardner, M. B. (1940). On the auditory significance of the term hearing loss. *Journal of the Acoustical Society of America, 11,* 270–277.

Stephens, S. D. G. (1976). Auditory temporal summation in patients with central nervous system lesions. In S. D. G. Stephens (Ed.), *Disorders of auditory function II* (pp. 231–242). New York: Academic Press.

Stockard, J. J., Stockard, J. E., & Sharbrough, F. W. (1977). Detection and localization of occult lesions with brain stem auditory responses. *Mayo Clinic Proceedings,* *52,* 761–769.

Stump, D. A., & Williams, R. (1980). The noninvasive measurement of regional cerebral circulation. *Brain & Language, 9,* 35–45.

Sullivan, M. D. (Ed.). (1975). *Proceedings of a Symposium on Central Auditory Processing Disorders.* Omaha: University of Nebraska Medical Center.

Swisher, L., & Hirsh, I. J. (1972). Brain damage and the ordering of two temporally successive stimuli. *Neuropsychologica, 10,* 137–152.

Taylor, G. J. (1949). An experimental study of tests for the detection of auditory malingering. *Journal of Speech and Hearing Disorders, 14,* 119–130.

Terkildsen, K., & Nielsen, S. (1960). An electroacoustic impedance measuring bridge for clinical use. *Archives of Otolaryngology, 72,* 339–346.

Terkildsen, K., & Thomsen, K. A. (1959). The influence of pressure variations on the impedance of the human eardrum. *Journal of Laryngology, 73,* 409–418.

Terkildsen, K., Osterhammel, P., & Bretlau, B. (1973). Acoustic middle ear reflexes in patients with otosclerosis. *Archives of Otolaryngology, 98,* 152–155.

Terkildsen, K., Osterhammel, P., & Thomsen, J. (1981). The ABR and MLR in patients with acoustic neuromas. *Scandinavian Audiology. Supplementum, 13,* 103–107.

Thompson, G. A. (1963). A modified SISI technique for selected cases with suspected acoustic neurinoma. *Journal of Speech and Hearing Disorders, 28,* 299–302.

Thomsen, K. A. (1955). Case of psychogenic deafness demonstrated by measuring impedance. *Acta Oto-laryngologica* (Stockholm), *45,* 82–85.

Thurlow, W. R., Davis, H., Silverman, S. R., & Walsh, T. E. (1949). Further statistical study of auditory tests in relation to the fenestration operation. *Laryngoscope, 59,* 113–129.

Tiffany, W. R., & Hanley, C. N. (1952). Delayed speech feedback as a test for auditory malingering. *Science, 115,* 59–60.

Tillman, T. W. (1969). Special hearing tests in otoneurologic diagnosis. *Archives of Otolaryngology, 89,* 51–56.

Turner, R. G., Shepard, N. T., & Frazer, G. J. (1984). Clinical performance of audiological and related tests. *Ear & Hearing, 5,* 187–194.

Ventry, I. M. (1976). Pure tone-spondee threshold relationships in functional hearing loss. *Journal of Speech and Hearing Disorders, 41,* 16–22.

Ventry, I. M., & Chaiklin, J. B. (1965). The efficiency of audiometric measures used to identify functional hearing loss. *Journal of Auditory Research, 5,* 196–211.

Walsh, T. E., & Goodman, A. (1955). Speech discrimination in central auditory lesions. *Laryngoscope, 65,* 1–8.

Willeford, J. A. (1985a). Sentence tests of central auditory dysfunction. In J. Katz (Ed.), *Handbook of clinical audiology* (pp. 404–420). Baltimore: Williams & Wilkins.

Willeford, J. A. (1985b). Assessment of central auditory disorders in children. In M. L. Pinheiro & F. E. Musiek (Eds.), *Assessment of central auditory dysfunction foundations and clinical correlates* (pp. 239–255). Baltimore: Williams & Wilkins.

Yantis, P. A. (1959). Clinical applications of the temporary threshold shift. *Archives of Otolaryngology, 70,* 779–787.

Zwislocki, J. (1961). Acoustic measurement of middle ear function. *Annals of Otology, Rhinology, and Laryngology, 70,* 599–606.

Zwislocki, J. (1963). An acoustic method for clinical examination of the ear. *Journal of Speech and Hearing Research, 6,* 303–314.

CHAPTER 3

Audiologic Instrumentation

Jean M. Lovrinic • John D. Durrant

The measurement of a given individual's hearing is the product of inferences based on his or her responses to auditory stimuli presented in a prescribed manner by an examiner. Furthermore, hearing often is described in terms of the magnitude, frequency content, and other physical characteristics of the stimulus that evoke the response. Thus, it is imperative that the audiologist use quantifiable and reproducible auditory stimuli. Only well-designed instrumentation that is frequently and completely calibrated can provide the generation, shaping, and control of signals that can be repeated from test to retest, from one listener to another, from one clinic to the next, as required for the clinical assessment of auditory function and hearing.

Audiometry involves the application of psychoacoustic methods and instrumentation in the assessment of hearing, but the measurement of auditory function via electroacoustic immittance or evoked electrical response measurement places equally stringent demands on stimulus generation and control. Additionally, there may be requirements for additional equipment for data analysis, data reduction, and storage, as well as printout devices to provide hard copy. All must function properly in order for the examiner to obtain reliable results.

In short, clinical audiology is an equipment-intensive endeavor. Thus, the practicing audiologist must have a working knowledge of instrumentation, requirements for calibration, and an awareness of possible malfunctioning of the devices involved. These matters are the subject of this chapter.

BASIC CONCEPTS

SIGNALS — THEIR ANALYSIS AND CHARACTERIZATION

Before diving directly into instrumentation, a few basics concerning the signals used to create sound stimuli are in order. In the most general terms, signals are time-varying voltages (*voltage* being a forcelike electrical quantity). The most familiar of such signals is the sinusoid (Figure 3-1A), which, when amplified and transduced, becomes a pure tone. Any such signal can be analyzed to determine its spectral content; that is, the magnitude of the component frequencies composing the signal or sound created. The spectrum of the familiar pure tone is discrete, appearing as a single line at $f = 1/T$ (where T is the period of the tone; that is, the duration of one cycle), of root = mean = square amplitude A_{RMS}. Complex tones also have line spectra, as does any periodic signal (for example, the square wave in Figure 3-1B). Random noise (Figure 3-1C) and transients (Figure 3-1D), on the other hand, have continuous spectra; however, their spectra may reflect concentrations of signal power into more or less narrow regions or bands. Additionally, a broad-band signal may be shaped via filtering (Figure 3-1E). Filters reject or reduce the amplitude of signals above (low pass) or below (high pass) the cutoff frequency. Low- and high-pass filters can be cascaded (that is, connected in tandem) to create a passband (Figure 3-1E) or stopband/band-reject filter (not illustrated). Filters of the same low-, high-, or band-pass characteristics also may be cascaded to increase the rolloff or rate of attenuation.

The shaping of signals in the frequency domain always has consequences in the time domain (compare Figure 3-1C and Figure 3-1E) and vice versa (compare Figure 3-1A and Figure 3-1D). Shaping in the time domain illustrated by Figure 3-1D is accomplished via electronic switching. Relevant parameters include rise/fall time and plateau duration and the shape of the amplitude envelope. Other temporal manipulations include amplitude (Figure 3-1F) and frequency modulation (Figure 3-1G). Both lead to the creation of

54

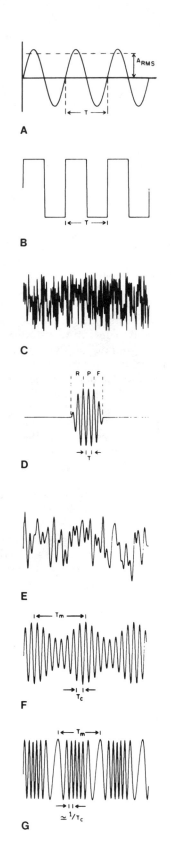

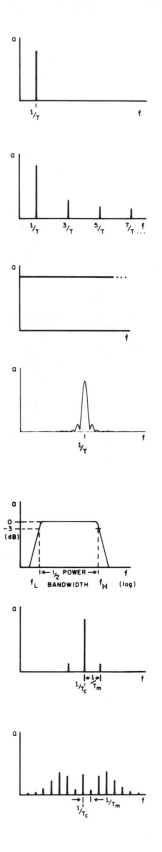

sidebands of energy above and below the carrier frequency (the frequency component that is being modulated). The details of the resulting spectra depend on the modulation frequency and depth of modulation. For a more in-depth discussion of many of these concepts, the reader is referred to Durrant and Lovrinic (1984).

SIGNAL ROUTING

Much of what is involved in audiometric instrumentation is the routing of signals destined to be the test stimuli. Figure 3-2 illustrates the most basic audiometer, typical of portables used for screening purposes. Some details have been omitted for simplicity. Two signal sources (sinusoids and random noise) are routed through attenuators and then to earphones through a mechanical, manually operated switch. Other switches activate one or both signal sources. The signal paths and modes of operation are conveniently represented by a block diagram, as shown in Figure 3-2. Even the most complex electronic instrument can be broken down into basic functional components. In this chapter, whether by diagram or words, we will delve into the components of audiometric and related instruments and consider the nature of signals used in audiometry, their routing, and control.

AUDIOMETERS

Audiometer is the name given to the equipment used to present auditory signals to listeners to elicit behavioral responses. Although some audiometers have quite limited function (e.g., an instrument that presents one or two types of sounds for purposes of screening infants), most equipment appropriate for clinical evaluation can be used to present a variety of signals to the listener with the capability of conveniently switching between various transducers. Audiometers used in clinics frequently contain two independent and al-

most totally redundant systems referred to as *channels*. Regardless of how simple or complex a given audiometer is, all equipment of this type can be described in terms of the electronic components that compose it or the functions involved.

INPUT SIGNALS AND DEVICES

The signals commonly employed in audiometry are pure tones, speech, and various types of noises. Pure tone generators usually are referred to as *oscillators*. In audiometry, these devices are used to generate either a finite number of fixed (discrete) frequencies or continuously variable frequencies spanning a given range. Most audiometer oscillators are of the fixed type yielding pure tones at octave intervals of 125 through 8000 Hz and interoctave frequencies of 750, 1500, 3000, and 6000 Hz. These are close to, but not equal to, the half-octave frequencies, namely 707, 1414, 2828, and 5656 Hz, respectively. The practice of using 125 Hz and the six-octave frequencies has a long history in audiometry, dating back to tuning fork testing before electronic audiometers. Although these limited sampling points seem well accepted by the audiologic and otologic communities, only two factors actually bespeak their virtue: Using these frequencies, a great deal of information has been obtained over the past 5 decades of clinical work, and fairly copious and carefully garnered data allowed normative values to be established by the American National Standards Institute (ANSI) and the International Standards Organization; however, some rather obvious problems exist. For example, the clinical adherence to the octave concept has led to the common misconception that 4000 Hz invariably shows the maximum sensitivity change in noise-induced hearing loss, but this is subject to individual variability. Variable frequency audiometers allow clinicians to probe hearing sensitivity in more detail. Such audiometers also permit the examiner to detect narrow regions of hearing loss, so-called tonal islands. The conventional frequency range has also been established rather arbitrarily. A given etiology may have more profound effects at frequencies below 125 Hz (e.g., perhaps in the case of endolymphatic hydrops) or above 8000 Hz (e.g., drug ototoxicity), yet no ANSI or International Standards Organization standard now exists for audiometers for frequencies below 125 Hz and above 8000 Hz. Admittedly, there are compelling technical problems with stimulus generation and control for very low or

Figure 3-1. Sample time histories or waveforms (amplitude, a, versus time, t; shown in left-hand panels) and corresponding amplitude spectra (amplitude, a, versus frequency, f; shown in right-hand panels). A_{RMS}, root-mean-square amplitude; T, period; R, P, F, rise, plateau, and fall durations, respectively; f_L, f_H, low- and high-frequency cutoffs of filtering; T_c, T_m, periods of carrier and modulating frequencies. (Note: Spectra of noise samples are actually idealized long-time average spectra.)

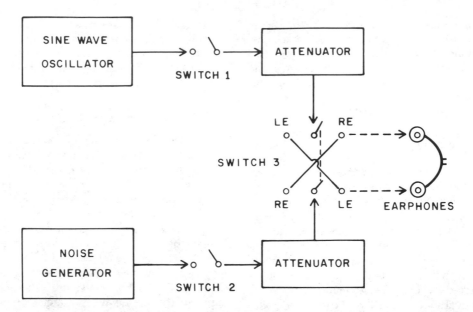

Figure 3-2. Rudimentary pure tone audiometer with broad-band noise-masking capability. Switches 1 and 2 control presentation of the tone and noise; switch 3 controls the routing of these signals to the right versus left earphones.

high frequencies. Nevertheless, high-frequency audiometry is finally beginning to gain attention and respect, and more audiometers now are including some limited high-frequency capability.

In equipment being manufactured today, all pure tone signals are actually generated via integrated circuit devices, yet audiometers with only discretely, rather than continuously, variable frequencies remain the more economical to build and calibrate. Modern "oscillators," on the other hand, are exceedingly reliable and usually vary from their stated values by no more than 1 percent even though the applicable ANSI standard (1969) allows deviations of ±3 percent for discrete frequency oscillators. Thus, for a stimulus of 4000 Hz, outputs of from 3880 to 4120 Hz would be within tolerance. All instruments available today appear to use the single oscillator design even in two-channel audiometers; that is, audiometers that permit two outputs to one or both ears with totally independent control of each channel. Since human listeners are inherently sensitive to small differences in frequency between two signals, this design is preferable over the use of separate oscillators for each channel.

A second major signal used in audiometry is speech. This signal may be generated by at least two sources: live voice via a microphone, or tape recorded via cassette or reel-to-reel transport. Frequently, two channels of taped signals are used simultaneously, for example, the target message on one channel with a competing message on the other channel.

Noises are the third signal type used in hearing evaluation. Most frequently, at least three types of noises are available: narrow-band white noise, broad-band white noise, and speech spectrum noise. Broad-band white noise contains all frequencies at equal spectrum level for a passband of at least 10,000 to 12,000 Hz in width. Half-power points of as low as 60 Hz and as high as 15,000 Hz are available in some units. Audiometric narrow bands have various widths that depend on the test frequency. Conceptually, these noises may be envisioned as white noise bandpass filtered to produce bandwidths typically one-third octave wide or less. In practice, there are various methods of producing such noises; the details will not be presented here. One-third octave approximates the critical bandwidth and has a number of virtues as a masking signal. The most important is that it is not unnecessarily loud for the listener but wide enough to mask a pure tone without listener confusion. Speech spectrum noise is another shaped white noise designed for speech masking. This noise usually contains equal spectrum level up to 1000 Hz with a 12 dB/octave rolloff above this point, mimicking the average spectrum of speech.

It is customary for clinical audiometers to allow additional inputs to be connected to its circuitry, and phonograph inputs may be found, particularly on older instruments. These auxillary inputs are useful for allowing the examiner to use nonstandard or additional stimuli such as that for an external function generator or an additional tape recorder.

COMPENSATION NETWORKS

Minimum audibility for various input signals differs, so it is necessary for the stimulus or input section of the audiometer to be followed by a compensation or "calibration" network. Recall that the flat 0 dB HL line on the audiogram is the product of using the normative threshold values in dB sound pressure level (SPL) as the reference for each frequency. Therefore, this portion of the equipment automatically adjusts the signal selected to conform to the minimum audibility curve for the desired standard. Current ANSI standard values for the TDH-39 earphone (1969) are given for pure tones from 125 to 8000 Hz in Table 3-1 along with accepted values for two other earphones commonly encountered clinically. The compensation network thus adds these values to the attenuator settings to produce the desired hearing levels. Yet another value is required for speech because it is a complex signal whose spectrum covers numerous critical bands. The calibration value used for speech is 12.5 dB greater than the specific earphone calibration value for a 1000 Hz pure tone (7.5 dB SPL), or 20 dB SPL for the TDH-49 earphone.

There is no recommended calibration value for noises. Manufacturers usually calibrate their equipment to yield effective masking level at the dial reading. For passbands in the vicinity of one-third octave wide, this can be approximated fairly readily by adjusting the overall SPL of the noise to yield 3 dB more than the spectrum level of the frequency at the center of the band, that is to say, the frequency to be masked. Thus, to mask a 1000 Hz tone at 50 dB HL through a TDH-49 earphone when calibrated to the 1969 ANSI values, the one-third octave noise would be adjusted to 60.5 dB

SPL (50 + 7.5 + 3). Speech spectrum noise is adjusted by the network for effective masking for speech whereas wide-band white noise may be adjusted for effective masking for either pure tone or speech signals. In several audiometers, however, programming does not allow pure tone masking with wide-band white noise. Others, especially modern microprocessor-based audiometers, do permit flexible stimulus routing allowing any signal on one channel to be paired with any appropriate signal on the other channel.

In older equipment, variable resistor screw adjustments (trimpots) were available for each stimulus and each transducer allowing changes in the compensation network to bring outputs into calibration. Especially with age, internal adjustments were often too limited, requiring the examiner to add correction factors to obtain correct threshold values. The next generation of equipment allowed a single trimpot adjustment that changed the level for all stimuli by the same amount and in the same direction. Presumably the underlying assumption was that all changes would occur simultaneously for all frequencies and in the same direction. Today, only portable audiometers use trimpots whereas larger clinical units are microprocessor based with the calibration data stored in memory. Until approximately 1985 in some of these units, the memory backup was battery powered (random access memory). Thus the calibration data were lost in the event of battery failure. More recent designs have overcome this problem by memory established in firmware (electrically erasable programmable read only memory). Although these stored data are user accessible, changing the audiometer's calibration data is recommended only for knowledgeable individuals.

STIMULUS PRESENTATION AND CONTROL

Various timing and gating functions can be obtained for pure tones in most audiometers. For ex-

TABLE 3-1. REFERENCE EQUIVALENT THRESHOLD SOUND PRESSURE LEVELS AND TOLERANCES FOR THREE EARPHONES USED CLINICALLY

Transducer	125	250	500	1000	1500	2000	3000	4000	6000	8000 Hz	Speech
TDH-39[a]	45	25.5	11.5	7	6.5	9	10	9.5	15.5	13	19.5
TDH-49 and 50[b]	47.5	26.5	13.5	7.5	7.5	11	9.5	10.5	13.5	13	20
Tolerances	±5	±3						±4	±5	±5	±3

[a] ANSI S3.6–1969 (R 1973). Phone contained in MX41/AR cushion.
[b] Source: From Wilber, L. A. (1985). Calibration: Puretone, speech and noise signals. In J. Katz (Ed.), *Handbook of clinical audiology*. Baltimore: Williams & Wilkins. With permission.

ample, the operator may select among steady tones, frequency-modulated (warble) tones, tones that pulse alternately between channels, and automatically pulsed tones of various durations. Durations of 200 to 500 msec are ideal for audiometry since threshold power integration is complete for most conventionally used frequencies by approximately 200 msec. The duty cycle or percentage on-time usually is 50 percent. In some cases, durations of 20 msec are offered for brief tone evaluation, and in at least two of the more elaborate clinical instruments on the market, this can alternate with a 980-msec off-time for lengthened off-time evaluation. In the case of frequency-modulated stimuli, the depth of modulation may be adjustable by as much as 5 percent, and the frequency of modulation is usually 5 Hz.

The short-increment sensitivity index adaptor network also falls under the category of stimulus presentation and control. A steady tone is incremented in intensity for 200 msec by an amount adjustable between less than or equal to 1 dB and 5 dB. The intensity pedestal occurs every 2 seconds.

In some of the more comprehensive clinical audiometers, phase-shifting capabilities for signals in one channel relative to the other channel are provided for the measurement of the binaural masking level difference. This protocol is a bit more complex than required by most binaural tests in that one signal is presented in phase at the two ears (e.g., noise) while the test signal (e.g., tone or speech) is presented out of phase. Thus, not only is it necessary to have two independent channels, but it must be possible to mix the signals within channels while separately controlling the level of each. Automatic (Bekesy) threshold tracking is also desirable for tests such as the masking level difference.

The interruptor switch is used to manually control the presentation of a signal. This switch must operate silently, meaning that it must not generate noise that can be carried through the electronic circuitry or radiated acoustically. In addition, it must function so that in the off position, the output is attenuated by a prescribed amount. Current ANSI requirements (ANSI, 1969) mandate this level to be 50 dB below the dial setting or −10 dB HL, whichever is greater. The rise/fall durations of the output signal are also determined by the characteristics of the interruptor switch and are also subject to calibration standards. The object is to minimize spectral splattering that might cause clicks or other spurious sounds. Currently ANSI standards differ for rise and decay times, but it is

anticipated that the next standard will recommend 20 to 50 msec for both. In most equipment, this portion of the circuit is designed so that closing the switch either turns on the test stimulus or interrupts otherwise continuous presentation. This interruptor control on the audiometer receives more use than any other single component. For this reason, most interruptor switches are designed to function with minimum pressure and to have contact areas that are quite large and that can survive extensive use.

SIGNAL AMPLIFICATION

The minute electrical voltages provided by the signal generators — oscillator, noise generator, tape deck, and microphone — must be amplified by a power amplifier in order to drive the transducers at suitable levels. This component is rated for its signal-to-noise ratio, which must be high enough to prevent any significant masking of the test signals by background noise (hum and thermal noise). In addition, the amplifier can be a source of distortion. The 1969 ANSI requirements mandate that all overtones of the discrete frequencies used for pure tone tests be at least 30 dB below the level of the fundamental frequency or less than 3.2 percent harmonic distortion. For testing listeners in a sound field, that is, via loudspeakers, additional power amplification is typically required; however, due to limits imposed by additional noise and distortion from this stage of amplification, this power amplifier may not be switched into the circuitry until levels of 50 dB HL or higher are needed. For such purposes, an external stereo hi-fidelity audio power amplifier typically is used.

COMMUNICATION AND SIGNAL MONITORING

Auditory monitoring of signals emanating from the audiometer is provided using either a small internal or external loudspeaker or by earphone. A volume control can be used to adjust the signal amplitude at the operator's ear. The earphone must be used whenever a feedback loop can be established with an open microphone. In addition, most audiometers allow visual monitoring of tones via the volume unit meter. The volume unit meter is always used for microphone-introduced signals, such as speech, and for taped stimuli. This monitoring device is a type of volt meter calibrated in dB of power, often relative to 1 mW, and responds to the RMS amplitude of the driving electrical signal. It indicates gains and losses from the attenuator setting used, which must be added to the presentation level of the stimulus; however, a control generally is provided whereby the level of the input signal can be adjusted. Such adjustments have to be made with the ballistics of the needle movement in mind, that is, the meter can only follow the more slowly fluctuating epochs of speech. Visual monitoring of signal on/off and duration is given usually with small lights or light-emitting diodes mounted on the audiometer faceplate or display panel. This same display often gives the oscillator and attenuator levels as well as indicating the transducer and stimulus selected.

Intercommunication between listener and operator is facilitated by a special system called the *talkover-talkback circuit.* The talkover circuit allows the examiner to talk to the listener at several calibrated or continuously adjustable levels. Ordinarily, the talkover will occur via whichever transducer is being used at the output section of the audiometer. The input to this circuit is provided by the same microphone used for testing. The talkback circuit allows the examiner to hear the listener and any other sounds occurring in the listener test area. The input source for this circuit is a microphone placed in the examination room. The gain of the talkback usually is continuously adjustable. Sound quality must be good if listeners use oral responses in speech recognition tasks.

In more elaborate systems, a special auxiliary communication network is included, enabling the operator to talk with an assistant seated with the listener. Such systems can be fabricated from inexpensive intercom devices adapted for earphone use.

ATTENUATORS

The voltage range of the electrical signal used to drive the output transducer encompasses a range over a millionfold. Control of this voltage, and therefore the SPL produced, is accomplished with attenuators that can be of either the step or continuously variable type. The steps commonly used are 2.5 and 5 dB, and in some equipment, the operator may select from between these two options. Other audiometers may provide 2 or 1 dB options directly or via an auxiliary control. Step attenuators generally provide proprioceptive feedback to the operator, making the process of setting the hearing level dial less demanding in terms of precision of hand motion and visual vigilance.

Continuously variable attenuators require careful visual monitoring and precise hand coordination at all times. Because hearing sensitivity is usually given in signal magnitude, precision in attenuation setting is necessary. The current ANSI standard (1969) allows deviations of three-tenths of the step size used or 1 dB, whichever is larger, but it is anticipated that subsequent standards will tighten this tolerance to the smaller of the two options.

As shown in Table 3-1, minimum audibility changes with frequency; however, the threshold of feeling is fairly constant across frequency at approximately 120 dB SPL. These two facts taken together indicate the maximum output in dB HL should vary with frequency being less for frequencies where minimum audibility is poorer (below 500 Hz and above 4000 Hz) and greater where sensitivity is best. Such output limitations exist for all audiometers although there does appear to be a trend toward providing outputs in the vicinity of 120 dB HL in the 500 to 4000 Hz passband. Such a move seems unwise for several reasons. Levels of 130 dB SPL cause extreme discomfort for many individuals, and naive use of such high levels seems to be a prime target for future personal liability claims. No output limit standards exist for audiometers at present. Nevertheless, users of instruments with such high outputs should exercise caution.

It is usual for audiometers to provide a visual indication, usually by light-emitting diode display, when maximum output for any stimulus has been exceeded. Some instruments also require activation of another switch to allow testing over the upper 10 to 20 dB range of output. Customarily, signal strength decreases at attenuator settings beyond this point, if the dial permits further adjustment at all.

Because attenuators receive a great deal of use in routine testing, they tend to be designed for ease of manipulation and situated near the signal interruptor switch. In some cases, it is possible to move both of these controls with one hand, which certainly is highly desirable for the most efficient examiner.

OUTPUT ROUTING AND TRANSDUCERS

Sounds are presented to listeners via earphones, bone vibrators, and loudspeakers, devices that are known as *transducers.* These transducers serve to change the electrical signals generated by the audiometer into an energy form to which the listener can respond. In the case of earphones and loud-speakers, this is acoustic energy; in the case of bone vibrators, the energy is mechanical in nature. Each of these transducers has its own frequency response characteristics, power-handling capabilities, transient response, and impedance. Even within transducer type (e.g., different makes or models), considerable differences exist. A quick perusal of Table 3-1 reveals the differences in frequency responses between the TDH-39 and TDH-49 earphones, which result in minimum audibility for otologically normal, young adult listeners. The frequency responses of the TDH-49 and TDH-50 earphones are the same, but these two phones differ in load impedance with the TDH-49 being a 10 ohm phone and the TDH-50 having an impedance of 50 ohms.

Calibration of an audiometer is done for the complete audiometer-transducer system, implying that transducers cannot be changed without altering the calibration. All earphones are mounted in cushions that either fit on the auricle (supra-aural) or around the auricle (circumaural). Critical differences exist between these cushion-earphone combinations. The circumaural ensemble provides less occlusion of the canal and better attenuation of ambient sounds, but it weighs more and cannot be calibrated to the ANSI standards at this time because no standard coupler (i.e., a reasonable model of the ear) has been developed to accommodate it. The supra-aural ensemble is lighter, provides some attenuation of ambient sounds, but has several shortcomings. These include the creation of a sizable occlusion effect, which is most troublesome when doing masked bone conduction testing, and the potential for causing ear canal collapse. There also may be a fair amount of variability in air volume under the earphone as a function of the subject's age or size. Still, the supra-aural earphone mounting will continue in clinical use for the foreseeable future because well-established standards exist for it (Zwislocki et al., 1988).

Regardless of the earphone-cushion configuration used, the phones are mounted on a spring headband and held in place on the auricles by metal yokes. This headband is designed to hold the phones in place with adequate pressure and should not be stretched unnecessarily. In addition, it seems advisable to have available a variety of headbands if one evaluates listeners who differ markedly in head circumference since the pressure exerted by the phones will vary with head size.

Although earphones are quite hardy, they can be damaged by dropping, being poked with sharp instruments, extreme levels of moisture (such as cleaning with liquids), and the like. On the whole, occasional swabbing of the cushion carefully with a gauze sponge sparingly moistened in a mild antiseptic is all that is needed, and this should be done regularly, both for aesthetic and health reasons.

There is also growing interest in the use of insert earphones, particularly since the development of the tubal insert by Killion (1984). The transducer, per se, is contained in a small case normally clipped to the listener's shirt collar or held by a Velcro headband. Sound is delivered to the external auditory meatus by a plastic tube, usually fitted at the end to a compressible and disposable foam earplug, sealing the assembly in the ear canal. Alternatively, plastic plugs of the type used for immittance testing may be used.

Insert earphones increase interaural attenuation, reducing the need for masking, have good ambient sound reduction, circumvent the problem of collapsing external meati, and are quite comfortable. One of these insert transducers, the Etymotic ER-3A, has a frequency response quite similar to that of the TDH-39 earphone; two others, the ER-1 and ER-2, have extended high-frequency responses but much lower power-handling capabilities. Although use of these transducers necessitates some threshold corrections due to the differences between the inserts, the TDH-39, and the now more frequently used TDH-40 earphones, the many testing dilemmas resolved via the use of the tubal insert earphones merit their more frequent usage. To date, these transducers have received widespread use in auditory evoked potential testing, not only for the reasons previously cited but also because the probe tube creates a time delay that places the stimulus artifact well ahead of the recorded response. Nevertheless, no standard for calibration has been established.

Earphones can change their response over time, thus periodic calibration checks are essential. A regimen of checking reference equivalent threshold SPLs, attenuator linearity, frequency accuracy, and harmonic distortion every 3 months is considered desirable with a more thorough calibration yearly. Tolerances (ANSI, S3.6–1969 [R 1973]) for earphone SPLs are given in Table 3-1.

If earphones are driven beyond their power-handling capabilities, they become nonlinear in their responses. This means that the function of SPL output versus input voltage saturates, and peak clipping of the output waveform occurs, resulting, for example, in the production of complex rather than sinusoidal signals in pure tone testing. This can be quantified as harmonic distortion. In general, the greatest harmonic distortion is observed at maximum output levels, and accordingly, the ANSI standard (1969) recommends measurement of distortion at these attenuator settings.

A third transducer is the *bone vibrator*, sometimes erroneously called a *bone oscillator*. Present-day audiometers are supplied with either Radioear B-71 or B-72 vibrators, which have a 1.75 cm^2 circular contact area. It is applied to the mastoid and held in place by a specially designed steel headband (the P-3333), or to the forehead using an appropriately designed band. Because the pressure at the skull bone–vibrator interface is crucial and must be relatively high, a well-fitting headband is necessary. Hopefully at some time in the future, headbands for both mastoid and forehead placement for various skull circumferences will be available. For now, a common spring-type band is all that one can purchase, the aforementioned P-3333, meaning there is likely to be considerable pressure variability among listeners according to head size. The use of a bone vibrator applied to the skull to stimulate hearing represents a much less efficient system than that involved in earphone testing. Thus, more power is needed to achieve minimum audibility for bone conduction than for air conduction. Practically speaking, this further limits the maximum output achievable with the audiometer, namely by approximately 40 dB as compared to the earphone; however, as with the earphone, the output limits are frequency dependent and are shown for both of these transducers in Table 3-2.

The frequency response of bone vibrators is also poorer than that of the earphone. Because of this, bone conduction stimuli usually are available only for frequencies in the 250 to 4000 Hz range. Even then, harmonic distortion is quite high, especially at 250 and 500 Hz. Although a comprehensive ANSI standard for bone conduction has yet to be adopted, it is likely that higher harmonic distortion than with earphones — possibly as much as 12 percent — will be allowable at these frequencies.

Calibration of the bone vibrator presents some formidable problems. First, no commercially available artificial mastoid conforms to the current ANSI (1972) guidelines for mastoids. This standard is currently in the revision process however, and some inconsistences in one mastoid model have been eliminated with modifications (Dirks et al., 1979). ANSI S3.26–1981 does provide reference equivalent threshold force levels for the B-71 vibrator used with a P-3333 headband on a Bruel and Kjaer 4930 artificial mastoid conforming to this new design and corrections for forehead placement.

Loudspeakers are the fourth transducer used in clinical hearing assessment. It is interesting that no standard loudspeaker exists analogous to the standard TDH-39 earphone or the B-71 bone vibrator. The primary requirement for good loudspeakers for audiometric purposes in the authors' opinions is a flat frequency response ($\pm$ 5 dB from 200–8000 Hz). Speakers also should have sufficient power-handling capabilities to provide outputs up to 110 dB SPL and good response characteristics for brief, transient signals. Quality loudspeakers or speaker systems (since often more than one transducer and an enclosure are involved) intended for hi-fidelity listening generally meet these requirements.

In the usual clinical situation, loudspeakers are situated at 45-degrees azimuth relative to the listener's head with a distance of approximately 1 m separating the listener from the speakers. The exact distance required depends on the speaker diameter (i.e., larger distances for larger diameters) and limits imposed by the dimensions of the sound room. Because of the acoustics of a sound field, maintaining a calibrated signal at the listener's ear is immensely difficult. Although suggested reference levels for frequency-modulated tones in the sound field are available (Morgan, Dirks, and Bower, 1979; Tillman, Johnson, and Olsen, 1966) and are shown in Table 3-3, no ANSI standard is yet available. Considering the multiple variables that must be specified and controlled, it is unlikely that such a standard will be forthcoming.

Steady pure tones cannot be used with confidence in the sound field due to the possible for-

TABLE 3-2. TYPICAL MAXIMUM OUTPUTS FOR EARPHONES AND BONE VIBRATORS

Transducer	125	250	500	1000	2000	3000	4000	6000	8000 Hz	Speech
Earphone	80	100	120	120	120	120	120	100	100	100 dB HL
Bone vibrator (mastoid)	NR	50	60	70	70	70	70	50	NR	50 dB HL

TABLE 3-3. LOUDSPEAKER REFERENCE SOUND PRESSURE LEVELS FOR FREQUENCY-MODULATED TONES

Azimuth	250[a]	500[a]	1000[a]	2000[a]	3000[a]	4000[a]	6000[a]	Speech[b]
45 degrees	20	8	4	4	−3	−4.5	3.5	12.5
0 degrees	15	11.5	8	2.5	NA	2.5	NA	NA

NA, not available.
[a] Source: From Morgan, D. E., Dirks, D. D., & Bower, D. R. (1979). Suggested threshold sound pressure levels for frequency-modulated (warble) tones in the sound field. *Journal of Speech and Hearing Disorders, 44,* 37–54. With permission.
[b] Source: From Tillman, T., Johnson, R., & Olsen, W. O. (1966). Earphone versus sound-field threshold sound-pressure levels for spondee words. *Journal of the Acoustical Society of America, 39,* 125–133. With permission.

mation of interference patterns, which can cause wide sound level variability at various locations and frequencies making precise calibration difficult and the SPL at the ear excessively sensitive to head movement. Therefore, frequency-modulated tones, narrow bands of noise, and speech are the stimuli of choice for sound-field testing.

AUDIOMETRY BEYOND THE CONVENTIONAL FREQUENCY RANGE

Although human hearing abilities span a frequency range of more than 10 octaves (from 20–20,000 Hz), as pointed out earlier, the conventional audiometer provides stimuli covering only six octaves in the center of this range. The restricted frequencies available reflect the assumption that hearing for sound outside this range contributes negligibly to communication, coupled with the belief that only minimal diagnostic information can be obtained from an examination of hearing at these extremes.

Valid and reliable high-frequency audiometry presents problems both in the production of adequate SPLs at frequencies above 8000 Hz and accurate calibration of these sounds. The wavelengths of these sounds are very short (ranging from 4.3–1.7 cm), thereby contributing to the formation of standing waves in both ear canals and in calibration devices such as 6 cc couplers. Thus, the SPL may be highly variable for these sounds whether presented via standard or insert earphones. If the true minimum audible pressure is deemed to be of secondary importance for clinical purposes, calibration methods are available that provide acceptable tolerances (Fausti et al., 1979; Stelmachowicz, Gorga, and Cullen, 1982).

Two recent developments facilitating high-frequency audiometry deserve mention. The first is a commercially available instrument that relies on bone vibration via the electrophonic effect (electrical driving signals applied to the electrodes on the scalp result in a force developed through capacitive coupling). This device, based on work by Tonndorf and Kurman (1984), eliminates the problems of acoustic stimulation but has limited application. More recently a device has been developed under contract for the National Institute of Neurological and Communicative Disorders and Stroke, which uses a probe sound delivery system with a miniature microphone. This device, which is undergoing clinical trials now, is calibrated on a subject-by-subject basis (Stelmachowicz et al., 1988).

Low-frequency audiometry has received less attention, and its major technical difficulty involves achieving substantial SPLs with very low harmonic distortion. The low distortion is mandated lest the harmonics of the test stimuli reach threshold levels before threshold can be reached at the intended frequency. This is due to the sharply rising low-frequency slope of the minimum audibility curve. Durrant, Fung, and Ronis (1983) have suggested that low-frequency hearing screening can be accomplished for frequencies as low as 45 Hz using conventional earphones and an audiometer connected to a low-distortion audio oscillator; however, the maximum undistorted output is quite limited.

ACOUSTIC IMMITTANCE INSTRUMENTS

Immittance test instruments provide valuable information about some functions of the auditory periphery and brainstem pathways (see Chapter 6). These instruments are sometimes referred to as *impedance/admittance audiometers*, but the authors feel that this is an inappropriate term because they do not actually provide a measure of hearing.

Immittance instruments can be divided into two major categories: diagnostic units and screening units. Diagnostic units use a headband or shoulder-held probe arrangement, often provide a choice of probe frequencies, always allow a choice of reflex activators, and offer a selection of functions to be performed. Screening units, on the other hand, most frequently use a hand-held probe, use only one probe frequency, provide only one or very limited reflex activator frequencies, and invariably perform only preprogrammed functions. In spite of their limitations, this type of instrument is very efficient at what it does because most, if not all, operations beyond inserting the probe are automatic. Either type of unit provides numeric readouts via meters or digital display or graphic displays of the results, including hard copies via a printer/plotter.

The input section of immittance instruments consists of separate air pressure and probe tone systems. The air pressure system is composed of a pump, which in diagnostic test units can be manually or automatically manipulated at various speeds and in either direction to regulate air pressure in the closed external meatus above and below atmospheric pressure. These induced pressures, in decaPascals (daPa) are monitored via a visual analog meter or digital display and may extend from $+600$ to -800 daPa. For most clinical purposes, the range of $+200$ to -400 daPa is commonly used. Units of air pressure form the x axis on the tympanogram plot, that is, the graph of admittance versus air pressure (Chapter 6). Various pressure release and checking mechanisms are available. The probe tone system invariably supplies a low-frequency tone, in the vicinity of 226 Hz at 85 to 95 dB SPL, although the new ANSI standard (1987) mandates the probe shall not exceed 90 dB SPL as measured in a 2 cc coupler. Obviously the probe must be at a level that does not cause a stapedial reflex or other significant changes in the tonus of the middle ear muscles, but it must be at a level that facilitates noise-free measurement. Some machines also provide probes in the 600 to 1000 Hz range. Because the ambient noise involved in the measurement is more substantial in the low frequencies and the reflex-eliciting level is lower in the mid frequencies, appropriate levels for higher-frequency probes are lower in SPL than that for the 226 Hz probe.

Measurement via immittance test instruments consists of monitoring sound by a pickup microphone located in the probe assembly. Because this microphone "sees" both incident and reflected sound pressures, amplitude and phase differences will occur between the output voltage signal of the microphone and a reference signal associated with the driving voltage applied to the probe-earphone transducer. By means of mathe-matical relationships, the probe-driving voltage and measured voltage are translated into admittance units specified either in cubic centimeters (cc) or milliliters (ml) of equivalent volumes of air (a measure specifically of compliance), or milli-mho (mmho) of admittance or its components, susceptance and conductance. The International System of Units' unit of measure for admittance and its constituents is the $m^3/Pa \bullet s$. Some instruments are capable of providing absolute measures of admittance or its components directly in mmho. Other units, especially those that are older, provide only relative measures of compliance. The range of susceptance values measurable varies with probe frequency but usually encompasses 0.2 to 5.0 acoustic mmho. In most current-generation instruments, immittance values are corrected for the immittance of the external auditory meatus, yielding what are called *compensated* values.

In some equipment, the operator may also choose measurements made at the plane of the probe tip that are uncorrected for external canal immittance, the so-called plane tympanometric values. If only compensated measurements at 226 Hz are done, the range of measured admittance values is less than if both plane and compensated measurements are provided and rarely exceeds 2 (cgs) acoustic mmho with normative values ranging from approximately 0.3 to 1.75 acoustic mmho. With the 226 Hz probe, compliance and admittance measures can be used interchangeably with few serious errors since the middle ear is stiffness dominated at this frequency; however, if probes of 678 and 1000 Hz are used, the quantity being measured can no longer be expressed in equivalent volume of air and must be measured either in acoustic mmho of total admittance or in susceptance and conductance via separate metering circuits. As might be expected, instruments that provide both high- and low-frequency probes, compensated admittance measures, and measures of both susceptance and conductance provide the means for the most exacting evaluations and interpretation of the findings. With the reduction of each of these capabilities, then, comes increasing limitations for discriminating between, if not in detecting, various pathologic conditions (Van Camp et al., 1986).

Automatic pump speed in diagnostic units varies from a low of 25 to 600 daPa/second. Screening units uniformly use rapid changes in canal pressure. Values approaching 600 daPa/second are routine although one manufacturer has designed its instrument to slow down to 200 daPa/ second as the tympanometric peak is approached. Because pump speed has a significant effect on tympanogram characteristics, the results may not be interpretable against a common normative database (Margolis and Heller, 1987).

The acoustic reflex–activating system provides pure tone and noise stimuli with adjustable levels and durations that can be directed to a contralateral, supra-aural, or insert earphone or to the probe for ipsilateral measures. The usual pure tone frequencies provided for contralateral activators are the standard octave frequencies from 250 to 4000 Hz as used in audiometry. Noise activators may include broad-band white noise and both low- and high-passed white noise (half-power point typically in the vicinity of 1600 Hz). The range of stimulus levels varies with activator frequency, similar to maximum outputs of audiometers, but for supra-aural earphones, the minimum range is between 50 and 120 dB HL for frequencies 500 to 4000 Hz. Levels higher than this would appear to pose too many risks to be used clinically because of the possibility of temporary threshold shift, permanent threshold shift, and legal action. The ANSI standard (1987) sets calibration values for these activators that roughly correspond to those for audiometers: ± 3 percent for frequency accuracy; ± 3 dB tolerance for SPL for tonal activators; ± 5 dB tolerance for noise activators, and harmonic distortion of no more than 3 percent for supra-aural earphones and no more than 5 percent for insert phones at customary audiometric maximum outputs (e.g., 110 dB HL 500 to 6000 Hz; 90 dB HL at 250 to 8000 Hz), increasing to 5 percent and 10 percent for these respective transducers at higher outputs. Sound evoked immittance changes, presumably the stapedius reflex responses, are displayed visually either via analog or digital devices and can be recorded on printout devices for hard copy. This reflex may be shown as changes from baseline values normalized to preactivator levels or in absolute units.

Ipsilateral activators tend to be fewer in frequency and restricted somewhat in level (typically less than 110 dB SPL). These activators are temporally multiplexed with the probe stimulus and are calibrated, using a 2 cc coupler usually in dB SPL. Standard reference equivalent SPLs may be determined using the procedures that are expected to be included in the revision of ANSI S3.6–1969 (R 1973).

ELECTRIC RESPONSE TESTING

Contrasted with the paucity of information available for psychoacoustic measures and immittance measures, a great deal has been written about the instrumentation needed for measurement of evoked electric responses, particularly the auditory brainstem response (Durrant, 1983; Gorga, Abbas, and Worthington, 1985; Hyde, 1985). This physiologic technique, described in Chapter 7, presents special equipment demands for signal generation and control, for response recording and analysis, and for data storage and presentation.

Stimuli used for auditory brainstem response and middle latency responses always consist of multiple repetitions of impulsive signals. These may be clicks (typically) generated by driving the earphone with 100- μsec pulses of selectable or alternating polarity or brief tone bursts of selectable durations, rise/fall times, and (perhaps) envelope. Signal amplitude may be given in peak values (peak equivalent sound pressure level [$dB_{pe}SPL$] equated to the RMS of a corresponding continuous tone) or normalized for user-assessed samples of listeners ($dB_n HL$). Noise signals of various bandwidths for masking may be available. Transducers may be earphones (supra-aural, circumaural, insert) or a bone vibrator. All the constraints and problems of calibrating these devices for conventional audiometry apply here, too, with the additional complications of using transient stimuli that cannot be measured directly using sound level meters, and the lack of acceptable standards; however, for long-latency auditory evoked potential evaluation using relatively long-duration stimuli, conventional calibration practices are usable or reasonably adaptable. The use of the click, on the other hand, poses the same calibration problems encountered in short-latency evoked responses.

The responses are picked up by electrodes, usually chlorided silver-silver, silver, or gold disks, and relayed to an array of equipment that functions to improve the signal-to-noise ratio of the electric responses and to amplify them via averaging or summing of multiple responses. Most systems provide checks or measurements of electrode impedance. The parameters of many of the steps of response enhancement, for example, filter bandwidth, play a crucial role in the electrical signature called a *response*. These factors are covered comprehensively by Coats (1983) and by Hyde (1985) and are described in Chapter 7. The responses can be visualized on video screens using interactive cursors to identify, label, and quantify various points on the functions. Numeric data quantifying latencies, amplitudes, and derived (calculated) values can be displayed and stored. Printers are used then to provide hard copy of the recorded responses, numeric data, demographic data, and data regarding recording and stimulus parameters.

SOUND-TREATED ROOMS

Testing areas must be maintained at very quiet levels in order to obtain reliable hearing and related measurements. Environments commonly encountered, such as hospitals and professional offices, have ambient noise levels that would elevate thresholds for both earphone and ear-uncovered listening (bone and sound field). Maximum permissible ambient noise levels (ANSI, 1977) for obtaining 0 dB HL thresholds for both of these listening conditions are given in Table 3-4. The amount by which any given noise exceeds these values indicates the lowest hearing level at which reliable thresholds can be measured.

To achieve these conditions, it usually is necessary to install or build a specially designed test room. One of the basic functions of these rooms is to reflect sounds originating from outside the test enclosure to prevent them from being transmitted through the walls and reaching the listener. To accomplish this, outside walls normally are designed from metal to provide low absorption and high reflectivity. To reduce transmission of sounds

through the wall (since not all sound will be reflected by the outside wall), the insides of the walls are lined with highly absorptive material (e.g., glass wool). The interior walls generally are formed of metal mesh to discourage reflection of sound produced inside the test room. The floor is carpeted. The number of reflective surfaces within the test area must be kept to a minimum in order for a free sound field to be approximated. Adequate floor space must be available to allow careful and charted positioning of loudspeakers and comfortable seating for the listener. The orientation of the listener's head to the loudspeakers should be known and standardized. In addition, the listener should be clearly visible from the control room.

Several manufacturers make prefabricated sound-treated rooms of various sizes and configurations. These rooms are rated in terms of their noise reduction characteristics in octave bands. Typical values for one manufacturer for single- and double-walled rooms are given in Table 3-5. The rooms have appropriate ventilation systems, jack panels for interfacing equipment, and windows and doorways designed to preserve the acoustic integrity of the room. Internal electrical wiring and lighting are provided, and specially shielded booths are available for improved electrostatic and electromagnetic artifact reduction, which are of particular application in evoked response testing. Last, an adjacent (typically single-walled) booth is often used as a control room. Although the sound reduction provided by a prefabricated room may not be entirely essential, the control room must be sufficiently quiet so interference is not provided during

TABLE 3-4. MAXIMUM ALLOWABLE SOUND PRESSURE LEVELS FOR TESTING TO 0 dB HL (OVERALL LEVEL IN OCTAVE BANDS)[a]

Condition	125	250	500	1000	2000	3000	4000	6000	8000
Ears not covered	28	18.5	14.5	14	8.5	8.5	9	14	20.5
Ear covered [b]	34.5	23	21.5	29.5	34.5	39	42	41	45

[a] ANSI S3.1–1977.
[b] Ears covered with earphones mounted in MX41/AR cushion.

TABLE 3-5. USUAL NOISE REDUCTION OF PROPERLY ASSEMBLED PREFABRICATED SOUND ROOMS*

Condition	Octave band center frequency							
	63	125	250	500	1000	2000	4000	8000 Hz
Single-wall rooms	33	31	39	50	57	61	68	62 dB
Double-wall rooms	37	52	64	80	93	>93	>93	>93 dB

*Industrial Acoustics Co., Bronx, NY.

any monitored live voice testing that might be used; however, no standards currently exist for examiner rooms, and requirements somewhat depend on the microphone used, the audiometer (i.e., microphone gain), and operator style (i.e., whether one "close-talks" the microphone).

REFERENCES

American National Standards Institute. (1969). *Specifications for audiometers.* ANSI S3.6–1969 (R 1973). New York: Author.

American National Standards Institute. (1972). *Artifical headbone for the calibration of audiometer bone vibrators.* ANSI S3.13–1972 (R 1986). New York: Author.

American National Standards Institute. (1977). *Criteria for permissible ambient noise during audiometric testing.* ANSI S3.1–1977 (R 1986). New York: Author.

American National Standards Institute. (1981). *Reference equivalent threshold force levels for audiometric bone vibrators.* ANSI S3.26–1981. New York: Author.

American National Standards Institute. (1987). *Specifications for instruments to measure aural acoustic impedance and admittance (aural acoustic immittance).* ANSI S3.39–1987. New York: Author.

Coats, A. C. (1983). Instrumentation. In E. J. Moore (Ed.), *Bases of auditory brain-stem evoked responses.* New York: Grune & Stratton.

Dirks, D. D., Lybarger, S. F., Olsen, W. O., & Billings, B. (1979). Bone conduction calibration: Current status. *Journal of Speech and Hearing Disorders, 44,* 143–155.

Durrant, J. D. (1983). Fundamentals of sound generation. In E. J. Moore (Ed.), *Bases of auditory brain-stem evoked responses.* New York: Grune & Stratton.

Durrant, J. D., & Lovrinic, J. H. (1984). *Bases of hearing science.* Baltimore: Williams & Wilkins.

Durrant, J. D., Fung, R., & Ronis, M. L. (1983). *Feasibility study of very low frequency hearing measurements via conventional instrumentation.* Paper presented at the midwinter meeting of the Association for Research in Otolaryngology, St. Petersburg, FL.

Fausti, S. A., Frey, R. H., Erickson, D. A., Rappaport, B. Z.,

Cleary, E. G., & Brummett, R. E. (1979). A system for evaluating auditory function for 8000–20,000 Hz. *Journal of the Acoustical Society of America, 6,* 1713–1718.

Gorga, M. P., Abbas, P. J., & Worthington, D. W. (1985). Stimulus calibration in ABR measurements. In J. Jacobson (Ed.), *The auditory brainstem response.* Boston: College-Hill Press.

Hyde, M. L. (1985). Instrumentation and signal processing. In J. Jacobson (Ed.), *The auditory brainstem response.* Boston: College-Hill Press.

Killion, M. D. (1984). New insert earphones for audiometry. *Hearing Instruments, 35* (7), 28, 46.

Margolis, R. H., & Heller, J. W. (1987). Screening tympanometry: Criteria for medical referral. *Audiology, 26,* 197–208.

Morgan, D. E., Dirks, D. D., & Bower, D. R. (1979). Suggested threshold sound pressure levels for frequency-modulated (warble) tones in the sound field. *Journal of Speech and Hearing Disorders, 44,* 37–54.

Stelmachowicz, P. G., Beauchaine, K. A., Kalberer, A., Langer, T., & Jesteadt, W. (1988). The reliability of auditory thresholds in the 8- to 20-k Hz range using a prototype audiometer. *Journal of the Acoustical Society of America, 83,* 1528–1535.

Stelmachowicz, P. G., Gorga, M. P., & Cullen, J. K. (1982). A calibration procedure for the assessment of thresholds above 8000 Hz. *Journal of Speech and Hearing Research, 25,* 618–623.

Tillman, T., Johnson, R., & Olsen, W. O. (1966). Earphone versus sound-field threshold sound-pressure levels for spondee words. *Journal of the Acoustical Society of America, 39,* 125–133.

Tonndorf, J., & Kurman, B. (1984). A new high-frequency audiometer. *Journal of Laryngology and Otology.* Supplement, 9, 101–105.

Van Camp, K. J., Margolis, R. H., Wilson, R. H., Creten, W. L., & Shanks, J. E. (1986). Principles of tympanometry. *ASHA Monographs, 24.* Rockville, MD: American Speech-Language-Hearing Association.

Wilber, L. A. (1985). Calibration: Puretone, speech and noise signals. In J. Katz (Ed.), *Handbook of clinical audiology.* Baltimore: Williams & Wilkins.

Zwislocki, J., Kruger, B., Miller, J. D., Niemoeller, A. F., Shaw, E. A., & Studebaker, G. (1988). Earphones in audiometry. *Journal of the Acoustical Society of America, 83,* 1688–1689.

CHAPTER 4

Otologic Evaluation

Jerry L. Northern • Gerald M. English

The management of hearing-impaired adults and children requires both medical and nonmedical professional attention. Patients with hearing loss may require medical or surgical treatment, or both, from a physician, as well as individualized counseling, hearing aid amplification, and auditory therapy as provided by audiologists. The association of audiologists with otolaryngologists has been mutually beneficial over the years, much to the benefit of the hearing-handicapped patients (Alford and Jerger, 1977).

According to public health estimates, hearing impairment is among the most common of physical disabilities. It is estimated that 22 million Americans have significant hearing loss including some 2 million profoundly deaf individuals. Each year 3000 to 4000 deaf babies are born in the United States, and an additional 5000 infants are born with significant hearing impairment that requires hearing aid amplification or special speech and language habilitation. The public health impact of hearing loss is extensive in terms of educational and economic implications as well as individual and family psychological and social adjustment problems. The problems of hearing loss and communication handicap will be even more serious as our general population grows older. Recent studies indicate that as many as 8.8 million (40%) of persons over 60 years of age have significant hearing loss, yet fewer than 10 percent of this group uses personal hearing aids (Lichtenstein, Bess, and Logan, 1988). The solitude created by hearing loss often separates the hearing-impaired individual from social activities, work environment, family, and friends.

The role and scope of audiology are well described by Jacobson and Northern in Chapter 1. Otorhinolaryngology is the medical specialty for the study of diseases and disorders affecting the ears, nose, and throat. This title, however, is commonly shortened in the United States to otolaryngology even though the specialty has actually been recently broadened to include diseases of the head and neck. The broad nature of ear, nose, throat/head, and neck diseases and disorders permits some otolaryngologists to limit their practice to specific areas of interest and skills, such as *otology* — the study and treatment of diseases and disorders of the auditory and vestibular systems. Otolaryngologists must have 4 to 5 years of surgical training following completion of medical school. They must also pass extensive oral, practical, and written examinations to become board certified by the American Academy of Otolaryngology — Head and Neck Surgery.

Prior to the advent of the antibiotic era of the early 1940s, diseases of the ear and temporal bone often created life-threatening infections. As these serious problems subsided with aggressive medical treatment, otologists were able to focus attention on innovative surgical procedures to eliminate disease and restore hearing. With the development of the binocular operating microscope during the 1950s, surgical procedures for hearing loss and dizziness problems gave rise to the need for comprehensive hearing tests to provide accurate diagnostic information about the nature of the problem, as well as pre- and postsurgical hearing evaluations. Thus, the fields of audiology and otolaryngology became associates in the evaluation, treatment, and management of hearing-impaired children and adults.

OTOLOGIC EXAMINATION

A wide variety of defects, diseases, and disorders cause hearing losses of varying degrees. The treatment of a specific otologic disease is not always the same among physicians, and in fact, considerable controversy may exist concerning preferred treatment protocols. Many factors influence each physician's decisions about treatment including the patient's age, sex, occupation, social status,

67

general health, presenting symptoms, and other concomitant disorders. Medical and surgical treatment are often integrated during the course of a disease, and one therapy does not necessarily exclude the other. The medical and surgical treatment of most diseases is a continually evolving process, with the formation of new concepts and revision of older ideas changing as new diagnostic information is noted. A thorough description of the medical and surgical treatment of hearing loss has been published by English and Sargent (1988).

During the otologic examination, the subjective complaints of the patient must be evaluated to determine if they form a system complex related to a specific disease process, or if in fact the symptoms are nonrelated problems. It is advantageous to always take the patient history and perform the physical examination in the same standard order with every patient. A summary of common complaints related to hearing loss is presented in Table 4-1 (Wood, 1979).

Several essential questions will help to more accurately define the patient's problem: (1) What is the principal problem? (2) How long have you had this difficulty? (3) Did the problem arise suddenly or slowly? (4) Has the problem become worse? (5) Have you had any medical treatment in the past? (6) Do you have any other illnesses? (7) Has this problem caused you any social or economic difficulties? Patients may give inaccurate answers to some of these questions due to lack of knowledge or to the anxiety of the situation. For example, when patients are asked to identify how long they have had a hearing impairment, the patient almost always underestimates the duration of the problem. It is often helpful to have a close relative, such as the patient's spouse or another family member, present during the history questionnaire. The relative may actually provide more accurate information than the patient. Most hearing impairments develop slowly and insidiously, and the patient may not be aware of the hearing loss until it has become more pro-

---

TABLE 4-1. SUBJECTIVE COMPLAINTS RELATED TO HEARING LOSS

HEARING — NORMAL OR ABNORMAL

Symmetric
If loss, gradual or sudden onset
Better ear?
Ear used with telephone
Hear but not understand
Worse in crowds or noise?
Loss: constant or fluctuating?
Previous use of hearing aid
Associated symptoms: tinnitus (ringing or buzzing), dizziness, drainage from ear, fullness in ear
Past medical history
Head: trauma, unconsciousness
Previous surgery
Ear infections
Noise exposure: occupational, military, gunfire, tractors, airplanes, explosions, heavy equipment
Drugs: aminoglycosides (injections, wound irrigations), diuretics
Family history: hearing loss, ear surgery, hearing aids, dizziness, renal disease, congenital anomalies (von Recklinghausen's disease, low-set ears, Waardenburg's syndrome)

TINNITUS

Bilateral or unilateral
High-pitched ringing or buzzing
Continuous, intermittent, pulsatile
Longstanding or recent onset
Altered by head position
Altered by pressure on neck
Associated symptoms: hearing loss, fullness or pressure in ears, dizziness
Drugs: aspirin, quinine

DISCHARGE

Unilateral, bilateral
Continuous, intermittent
Odorless, foul
Colored (yellow, green), clear, watery, bloody
Painful, painless
Associated symptoms: hearing loss, fever, dizziness, headache, upper respiratory infection, facial weakness
Past medical history: diabetes, head trauma, loss of consciousness, ear surgery, ear trauma

PAIN

Duration
Continuous, intermittent
Location (deep, superficial, circumaural)
Nature (sharp, dull, etc.)
Associated symptoms: drainage, hearing loss, tinnitus, dizziness, odynophagia, dysphagia, sore throat)

PINNA DEFORMITY

Acquired: traumatic, recent, old
No trauma — other cartilaginous structures affected
Congenital: bilateral, unilateral
Other members of family affected
  Hearing loss?
  Renal disease: patient, other family members

Source: From Wood, R. P. (1979). History taking in otolaryngology. In R. P. Wood & J. L. Northern, *Manual of otolaryngology*. Baltimore: Williams & Wilkins. With permission.

nounced. Some patients deny that they have a hearing impairment, even though their relatives and friends may have recognized the existence of the problem and discussed it with them.

A practical method of compiling and organizing the data from a clinical evaluation is the problem-oriented system of record keeping (Weed, 1971). The ultimate goal of this approach is to collect data in an organized, logical manner, which will lead to an accurate diagnosis. The problem-oriented record provides a clear picture of the clinical pattern from chief complaint to diagnosis and treatment. This system is composed of four parts creating the acronym *SOAP:* (1) the *S*ubjective complaint, (2) the *O*bjective findings, (3) the *A*ssessment, and (4) the *P*lan of treatment. The subjective complaint (S) lists the patient's symptoms. It should include the onset (sudden or slow), the duration, and other associated symptoms. The objective findings (O) are the result of the physical examination and any tests that have been performed. The assessment (A) is the diagnosis or differential diagnosis of the patient's disease, which may also include the pathogenesis of the disorder. The plan (P) is the proposed treatment for the particular diagnosed disorder.

The exact time of onset is important, particularly when the symptom occurs suddenly. A sudden hearing loss usually stimulates the patient to seek an examination much earlier than slowly progressive hearing loss. Many problems affect only one ear, and a significant unilateral hearing problem may be more apparent to the patient than a slowly progressive problem that affects both ears.

It is important to question the familial occurrence of the hearing problem since many causes of hearing loss are genetic. The patient may initially state that there is no history of deafness in the family; however, on further questioning, they may recall members of the family who were indeed afflicted with a hearing impairment. On the other hand, it may be true that there is "no deafness in the family" because genetic hearing loss may skip generations in recessive hereditary deafness.

When relating to the patient, every effort must be put forth to make the situation as relaxed as possible so that the patient will be at ease. Patients with hearing problems or otologic disease generally appear to be in good health, although careful evaluation may uncover coexisting symptoms or other associated medical problems.

MAIN COMPLAINT

The patient's chief complaint should be recorded exactly as stated by the patient. The most common complaints are "I'm going deaf"; "I've lost the hearing in my ear"; "There is noise in my ear, ears, or head"; "I have an earache"; "My ear feels plugged"; "My ears don't clear"; "My balance is poor." It is important to determine as accurately as possible the onset of the patient's chief complaint, its duration, severity, and what activity increases or decreases the problem. The chief complaint is what usually makes the patient seek help; however, it may not be an accurate indicator of the ongoing disease process.

PATIENT HISTORY

The patient's past history should be elicited through several lines of questioning. The occurrence of otitis media and the methods used to treat those episodes should be determined. Ototoxic drugs, head trauma, noise exposure, and occupational history are essential items of information in the history. Alcohol and tobacco use may be contributing factors to otologic disease. Previous otologic surgery and the previous or current use of amplification may provide information concerning the patient's disease process.

The duration of hearing impairment is sometimes difficult to determine, and, as stated previously, it may be necessary to discuss this issue with family members or friends. Whether or not the loss is unilateral or bilateral, progressive, stable, or intermittent is important since this information may help to determine the nature of the pathologic process. Patients with a conductive hearing loss frequently have *paracusia Willisii* (the ability to hear better in a noisy environment than a quiet one). Patients with some forms of sensory hearing loss may have recruitment (tolerance problems for loud sounds), causing them to avoid noisy situations. *Diplacusis* is the perception of a single auditory stimulus as two sounds, and it usually indicates pathology within the cochlea. Pain, fullness, and pressure in the ear are symptoms that cause patients to seek prompt medical attention. The severity and duration of those complaints are important. These symptoms may be unilateral, bilateral, and continuous, or intermittent, and they may be associated with tinnitus, crepitus (crackling sounds), or otorrhea (drainage). Drainage from the ear may be clear and watery, mucoid, purulent, or bloody. The duration of this problem and whether or not it is continuous or intermittent are important. Unilateral drainage may indicate a more severe disease than bilateral drainage. Fever, pain, swelling, or tenderness around the ear are important associated complaints.

Itching of one or both ears is a relatively common symptom. The duration, frequency, side of involvement, and any associated symptoms of pain, drainage, hearing loss, tinnitus, and dizziness are important to determine.

PHYSICAL OTOLOGIC EXAMINATION

The physical examination of the ear should be performed in a systematic fashion as described in classic otolaryngologic textbooks such as English's (1976) and Goodhill's (1979). The auricle and postauricular region should be inspected to detect abnormalities such as the scars from previous surgery, swelling, redness, or tenderness. Finger pressure on the mastoid bone may produce pain in the patient with an acute otitis media. Tenderness in this area may indicate bony destruction and an advanced suppurative process.

When the auricle is retracted upward and backward, the ear canal is straightened, a maneuver that will greatly assist the examination of the ear canal and tympanic membrane (Figure 4-1). A suitable ear speculum is then gently introduced into the ear canal. A speculum that is too small will not permit adequate illumination or a large enough field of examination; a speculum that is

Figure 4-1. Normal tympanic membrane landmarks. (From Jafek, B. and Barcz, D. [1984]. The otologic evaluation. In J. Northern [Ed.], *Hearing disorders.* Boston: Little, Brown. With permission.)

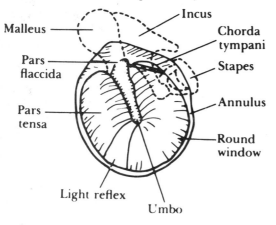

too large causes patient discomfort. The external auditory canal (EAC) may be occluded with wax, debris, or other materials, which should be removed carefully (see Chapter 8, case 1). There may be "sagging" of the posterior-superior EAC wall near the tympanic membrane, indicating bone destruction in patients from acute suppurative otitis media. Deformities of the posterior-superior bony canal wall may indicate a fracture of the temporal bone.

Several tumors, cysts, and bony growths arise in the ear canal. Bony outgrowths in the EAC come in two forms: multiple growths, termed *exostoses;* and single growths, termed *osteomas.* Osteomas are the most common neoplasms of the EAC and appear as smooth, hard, round nodules covered with normal skin. Exostoses do not require removal unless they interfere with cerumen removal, impair hearing, or cause obstruction. Osteomas usually continue to grow and hence require surgical removal.

Occasionally just touching the pinna will cause the patient to wince or react with noticeable discomfort. Conditions most frequently responsible for this phenomenon are (1) external otitis, (2) perichondritis, or (3) furunculosis of the EAC (Baker and Northern, 1976), or a combination of these.

Otitis externa is an inflammation of the skin of the EAC most frequently due to bacterial infection or fungal infection. The skin of the canal in acute external otitis is usually red, quite tender, with some form of drainage present. It is of interest that external otitis is frequently found in hearing aid users. The presence of an occlusive ear mold results in increased moisture in the ear canal, which may stimulate the external otitis condition. Do not be surprised if the otolaryngologist treating the case suggests that the patient either switch the hearing aid to the opposite ear or, in certain instances, go without the aid for awhile until the condition clears. The use of open-type ear molds may help prevent this condition.

Perichondritis is an inflammation of the covering of the cartilage of the pinna or ear canal. It is usually secondary to trauma of the cartilage, either accidental or surgical. The pinna is usually red and tender with generalized swelling. The infection may deprive the cartilage of needed blood supply. The resultant lack of nourishment to the cartilage may cause subsequent deformities of the pinna.

A *furuncle* of the external canal is a boil or pimple. It is exquisitely tender because the skin of the ear canal is tightly applied to the cartilage.

The normal tympanic membrane is a pearly gray color, and its anatomic landmarks, the short and long process of the malleus, the cone of light, and the anterior and posterior malleolar folds, should be easily seen (Figure 4-1). The tympanic membrane appears normal in diseases of the inner ear and the EAC when pathologic processes have not extended to or involved the tympanic membrane. A normal tympanic membrane is also encountered when hearing loss is due to noninflammatory diseases of the middle ear such as otosclerosis and traumatic or congenital ossicular defects (see Chapter 8, cases 10, 14, and 16).

An intact tympanic membrane may have an abnormal color or alterations in its anatomic landmarks. These changes are commonly seen in middle ear effusions and acute otitis before the tympanic membrane perforates (see Chapter 8, cases 7 and 12). An intact tympanic membrane may have an abnormal color when there is a glomus jugular tumor of the middle ear (Brown's sign). A red area noted through the intact tympanic membrane in the regions of the promontory is an indication of active otoclerosis (Schwartze's sign).

Perforations of the tympanic membrane occur most frequently from trauma and infections of the middle ear. The location of the perforation (central, marginal, or attic) in chronic otitis media indicates different disease processes and may help determine the management of the particular disease. Occasionally, polyps and granulation tissue may protrude through a tympanic membrane perforation. A perforation of the tympanic membrane is also encountered when tumors of the middle ear erode through the tympanic membrane (see Chapter 8, case 5).

A pulsatile mass in the middle ear often indicates a glomus jugulare tumor or arteriovenous malformation. Occasionally, an abnormal jugulare bulb may lie in the middle ear, which presents as a bluish mass behind the tympanic membrane. An excellent guide with color photographs of normal and abnormal views of the tympanic membrane has been published by Hawke (1987).

The presence of fluid running from the EAC is obviously of concern. Fluid from the EAC may be divided into three categories: (1) clear; (2) cloudy, whitish, or yellow; and (3) bloody (Baker and Northern, 1976).

Clear fluid may represent spinal fluid leaking from a skull fracture, which offers a ready route for access for infection into the cranial cavity. This condition requires prompt otologic consultation by physical examination, x-ray studies, and perhaps surgical exploration of the ear to confirm and repair the leakage.

Cloudy fluid usually represents inflammation of the EAC, a condition known as *external otitis*. Cloudy discharge may also result from an inflamed middle ear space with existing perforation of the tympanic membrane. External otitis should be treated before performing immittance audiometry as insertion of the probe tip may cause pain. Actually, immittance evaluation is unlikely to provide additional diagnostic information in such an ear.

Blood coming from the EAC frequently results from self-mutilation of the ear canal to relieve itching or remove ear wax. Blood coming from the ear canal may also be the result of a fracture of the temporal bone, which necessitates immediate medical consultation. Obviously, presence of any fluid drainage from the EAC requires immediate referral and investigation by a qualified otolaryngologist.

TUNING FORK TESTS

Tuning fork tests are an important part of the otologic evaluation. They are simple, quick, and give a relatively accurate estimation of the type of hearing impairment, such as conductive or sensory, and in skillful hands may provide a general estimate of the degree of the hearing loss (Girgis and Shambaugh, 1988).

A basic screening assessment of audiologic function and hearing sensitivity can be undertaken with tuning forks. These results *must correlate* with the results of otologic assessment, audiogram, and acoustic immittance measurements. When disagreement exists, either the patient is not fully cooperating with the behavioral tests, or error exists within the responses to the tuning fork tests. In any event, the disagreement must be resolved.

Tuning forks of different frequencies (e.g., 512 Hz and 1024 Hz) may be used to rapidly map the patient's audiogram relative to the audiogram of the audiologist. The 256 Hz fork is not used often because of the tactile sensation it produces by bone conduction, and the tactile vibrations may be mistaken by the patient for sound. In addition, because more sound intensity is required at low frequencies to reach the normal hearing threshold, the 256 Hz tuning fork must be hit sufficiently hard (often creating overtones of higher frequencies) so the patient will perceive the sound. Finally, the pitch of the 256 Hz tuning fork is easily masked by environmental and clinical noises.

The Mueller speaking tube, with Barany noisemaker masking the opposite ear, may be used to supplement tuning fork tests in the otologic examination. The speaking tube is used for loud speech and provides from 120 to 154 dB sound pressure level (SPL), depending on how loudly the examiner speaks into the tube. The Barany noisemaker is an effective masking device because its frequency response is from 500 to 6000 Hz, with a maximum power output of 130 dB SPL at 1000 Hz. With this frequency response, the noisemaker is very good for masking the opposite ear when testing the patient's ability to hear speech. The output of both of these elementary devices is often in excess of signal generated by conventional audiometers so they must be used with caution as to not induce noise trauma hearing loss. The technique can be used to offer qualitative estimates of hearing in patients with severe losses (Jafek and Barcz, 1984).

Varying points of view are often expressed about the value of tuning fork tests. Many argue that the subjective response to tuning forks is too variable to be useful, and that the tuning fork test results are only qualitative and not quantitative (Stankiewicz and Nowry, 1979). The opposing point of view advocates the need to use tuning fork tests to "check" the accuracy of the audiometric evaluation (Sheehy, Gardner, and Hambley, 1971). In fact, since most otolaryngologists use the tuning fork tests in the examination of each patient, it behooves the audiologist to be equally adept at using tuning forks. Some audiologists

recommend the use of tuning fork tests prior to bone conduction threshold testing to evaluate the lateralization of bone-conducted signals and the need for opposite ear masking. In otologic practice, tuning forks are a routine part of the work-up of every patient with impaired hearing, especially if surgery is being considered (Girgis and Shambaugh, 1988).

The most helpful tests in the evaluation process are the Rinne and the Weber, but other tuning fork tests such as the Schwabach and Bing tests are still employed (Figure 4-2). To perform the Weber test, a vibrating tuning fork is placed firmly in the middle of the forehead, over the bridge of the nose, or on the upper incisor teeth. The patient may hear the sound equally in both ears or more loudly in the affected ear. The sound lateralizes to the affected (worse-hearing) ear in a unilateral conductive hearing loss. It is heard in the better-hearing ear of patients with nonsymmetric sensory hearing loss. An audiometric Weber test can also be conducted with a bone vibrator.

To perform the Rinne test, a vibrating tuning fork is placed in front of the meatus (air conduction) and then pressed firmly against the mastoid bone (bone conduction). The patient is asked to indicate which sound from those two positions was the louder. When the air conduction is louder than the bone conduction, the Rinne is defined as "positive." A positive Rinne is found in normal

Figure 4-2. Tuning fork tests. (A) The Weber test. (B) and (C) The two positions for conducting the Rinne test. (From Downs, M., and Northern, J. [1976]. The evaluation of hearing. In G. English, *Otolaryngology: A textbook*. Hagerstown, MD: Harper & Row. With permission.)

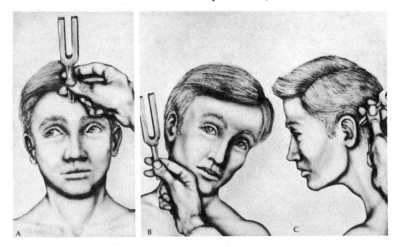

subjects and patients with a sensory hearing loss. When bone conduction is louder than air conduction, the Rinne is defined as "negative" and is associated with conductive hearing loss. When the bone conduction is equal to the air conduction, the Rinne test is "equivalent," but this result may indicate a mild conductive hearing impairment. Although the literature differs, it is estimated that at least a 40 dB air-bone gap must exist before a negative Rinne is considered accurate (Chandler, 1964; Wilson and Woods, 1975).

As a variation of the above Rinne technique, some examiners press the tuning fork on the mastoid bone until the patient no longer hears it. The tuning fork is then placed in front of the meatus, and the patient is asked to indicate whether air conduction is greater than, equal to, or less than the bone-conducted tone.

The Schwabach test is a comparison of the bone conduction of the patient with that of the examiner or a normal subject. The vibrating tuning fork is pressed against the patient's mastoid until the patient no longer hears the sound. The tuning fork is then placed on the examiner's mastoid. When the examiner hears the tuning fork better than the patient, the patient has a sensory hearing loss. This is not a very precise test, and consequently it is not commonly used.

The Bing test may be used to help identify the presence of a conductive component as part of the patient's hearing problem. With the tuning fork in the midline position, the examiner gently occludes the patient's EAC with a finger. When middle ear function is normal, occlusion of the ear canal results in an increase in loudness of the bone-conducted tuning fork tone with a lateralization of the sound toward the occluded ear. Patients with even a small conductive loss component will not notice a change in the loudness of the tone when the ear canal is occluded with the finger tip.

This phenomenon of enhanced bone conduction sensitivity with occlusion of the EAC is only noted when the middle ear is normal; the *occlusion effect* may be as great as 25 dB in the low frequencies but varies greatly from person to person (Keith, 1984). Zwislocki (1953) reported that placement of an earplug in the cartilaginous outer two-thirds of the EAC creates more occlusion effect than when an earplug is placed more deeply into the medial (or bony) third of the EAC. Thus, many clinicians favor the use of insert earphones for audiometric evaluation to eliminate occlusion contamination of bone conduction test results.

TASTE

There may be abnormalities of taste associated with various middle ear diseases when the chorda tympani has been damaged or cut, as in stapes surgery. The patient often describes a unilateral metalliclike taste in the mouth.

FACIAL NERVE

Weakness or paralysis of the facial nerve should be investigated for possible internal auditory canal, middle ear, or mastoid diseases. A variety of studies, including the Hilger Nerve Excitability test, electromyography, or other electrical nerve studies are available. These tests, in conjunction with topographic evaluation, help to determine the location of the disease process and whether or not there are reversible or irreversible changes in the nerve. A surgical procedure (facial nerve decompression) may be indicated in some patients (see Chapter 8, case 8).

RADIOGRAPHY AND LABORATORY TESTS

X-ray examinations of the ear are often used to confirm a suspected diagnosis and to evaluate more completely abnormalities, structural defects, or destruction caused by disease processes. The otolaryngologist requests specific x-ray studies that will be most effective at illuminating the structural area of concern. Requests for radiographic studies must include consideration of which test is least invasive, most cost-effective, and least likely to expose patients to potentially damaging amounts of radiation, and most likely to yield the most accurate view of the potential disease area. These radiologic studies assist the otologist in making a more accurate diagnosis and planning specific medical or surgical treatment. A thorough discussion of the use of radiology in otologic diagnosis has been published by Rose (1984).

The traditional x-ray views that are most useful in evaluating otologic problems include frontal, lateral, and Towne's views of the skull. A Stenver's view of the temporal bone is obtained to show asymmetry of the internal auditory canals, suggesting the presence of an acoustic neuroma. When standard x-rays are insufficient, additional higher-resolution radiologic studies may be ordered.

Petrous bone tomography is important to identify subtle congenital anomalies, detection of inflammatory or neoplastic involvement of the temporal bone, revealing trauma to the auditory canal or middle ear ossicles, and diagnosing the diseases of otosclerosis and Ménière's disease. Tomography has a higher diagnostic yield than standard radiography but involves considerably more expense and higher radiation exposure for the patient.

Computed axial tomography is a technique in which a computerized reconstruction of absorption density is noted. With this technique small tumors of the cerebellopontine angle can be detected, and brain lesions including tumors, strokes, and infection can be identified.

Magnetic resonance imaging is also a technique of picture elements generated by a computer. This radiographic technique has numerous advantages over plain radiography and computed tomography, particularly in the evaluation of head and neck problems. Magnetic resonance imaging is extremely sensitive to soft tissue changes resulting from infection, trauma, ischemia, demyelination, and other degenerative disorders (Hughes, 1985) and is capable of identifying very small acoustic tumors.

The use of laboratory tests as an aid to accurate diagnosis is an important aspect of the medical work-up. In some situations the laboratory test serves as a health-screening procedure; in other patients a quantitative result provides specific numbers; qualitative findings are reported on some physical effect such as a change in color or clamping of particles; a morphologic laboratory study identifies a given entity such as a bacterium, a fungus, a cell, or a parasite. An excellent review of the use of laboratory diagnosis in otologic disease has been published by White (1984).

IMMITTANCE AUDIOMETRY

Immittance audiometry, to include tympanometry and acoustic reflex examination, provides efficient, objective, and often illuminating information to the otologist and audiologist. Immittance audiometry, as described in detail by Stach and Jerger in Chapter 6, can be used as a cross-check technique to confirm audiometric behavioral results, or to provide information to help determine the nature and cause of an otologic problem. Careful interpretation of contralateral and ipsilateral presence of the acoustic reflex can be used to confirm site of lesion of hearing disorder to the middle ear, inner ear, acoustic nerve, or brainstem.

A number of otologic applications routinely use immittance measurements. Acoustic immittance should be included as part of the preoperative and postoperative evaluation of otologic surgical patients. Immittance techniques are well described for use of this technique in eustachian tube evaluation, fistula testing, identification of the glomus tumor, and as a facial nerve test (Northern, 1980). Chapter 8 provides a comprehensive series of case studies using immittance audiometry and audiometric findings.

DISORDERS OF IMBALANCE

Vertigo is defined as an abnormal perception of motion. It is a sensation of a rotary movement that is often related to disorders of the vestibular system of the inner ear. Other symptoms can arise from the inner ear, central nervous system, or neck. The difference between a subjective vertigo (in which the patient is spinning) and objective vertigo (in which the environment is spinning) is of little importance. The symptom of vertigo includes fainting, loss of consciousness, lightheadedness, unsteadiness, and dizziness.

In a few disorders, the patient's symptoms are more important in making a diagnosis. If the diagnosis cannot be formed on the basis of the patient's history, there is little likelihood of ever reaching the correct diagnosis. It is important to avoid descriptive suggestions to the patient of his or her symptoms. The primary objective is to determine whether or not the patient's complaint is vertigo or some other form of imbalance or dizziness. This distinction makes it possible to determine whether the symptom is vestibular in origin. Some diseases affect only the vestibular labyrinth, but there are also disorders that cause central diseases. Other patients' complaints may be psychogenic in origin (Table 4-2).

Whether or not the onset is gradual or sudden is important. The pattern of the attacks, whether continuous or episodic, may be helpful in making the diagnosis. The duration of the attacks and their frequency should be established. The relative intensity (mild, moderate, or severe) is also important. The associated symptoms of nausea

TABLE 4-2. HISTORY OF PATIENTS WITH VERTIGO

History of vertigo	Labyrinthine diseases	Central diseases	Psychogenic disorders
Onset	Sudden	Insidious	Vague
Pattern	Episodic and paroxysmal	Continuous; occasionally paroxysmal	No pattern; associated with anxiety, depression, and crowds
Sensation	Illusion of motion	Unsteadiness	Weakness, fainting, floating, swimming, detached sensation
Severity of symptom	Intense	Mild, sometimes progressive	Variable
Duration	+5 minutes, several hours, days	Days, weeks, months, or years	Instantaneous, continuous
Head position	Alters the vertigo	No change	Vague
Disturbance of consciousness	Rare	More common	Fainting, wooziness, swimming

Source: From English, G. M. (1976). *Otolaryngology: A textbook*. Hagerstown, MD: Harper & Row. With permission.

and vomiting are a good indication of the severity of the symptom. A positional relationship should be established to determine whether the symptom arises when the patient is recumbent, sitting, standing, arising, turning the head to one side, and looking up or down. The vertigo may arise immediately on assuming a certain position or there may be a latency period.

A hearing loss in either or both ears may be associated with vertigo. A hearing loss that fluctuates with the attack is characteristic of Ménière's disease. The speech recognition score may be normal or abnormal, and the patient may have an increased sensitivity to loud sounds. Tinnitus may be associated with vertigo, and the pitch, intensity, and whether or not it is unilateral or bilateral should be determined (see Chapter 9, case 1).

Patients with vertigo may have the associated symptoms of headache, double vision, unconsciousness, a tendency to fall, loss of sensation, and decreased vision. These important symptoms can indicate central nervous system problems. The otologic examination is most often normal.

A full diagnostic audiologic test battery should be conducted in all patients with vertigo. An x-ray examination is indicated when a vascular disease or a cerebellopontine angle tumor (acoustic neuroma) is possible.

A variety of disorders may produce dizziness that is not consistent with true vertigo. Some of the common nonotologic problems that cause dizziness are anxiety neurosis, orthostatic hypotension, hypoglycemia, and hyperventilation syndrome. These patients may require evaluation by a neurologist or internist.

Four common, relatively similar disorders cause vertigo including epidemic vertigo, vestibular neuronitis, benign positional vertigo, and cervical vertigo. These patients often have vertigo without a hearing problem. Epidemic vertigo usually follows an upper respiratory infection (cold) in about 7 to 10 days. These patients have an acute onset of vertigo that is continuous and severe for 48 to 72 hours. The symptom subsides and usually disappears in about 1 week. After the first 2 to 3 days, the patient may experience positional vertigo with nausea and occasional episodes of vomiting. The examination reveals normal hearing and a spontaneous nystagmus. These clinical findings resolve without any residual defect.

A similar disorder is vestibular neuronitis. The onset is acute; however, it resolves more slowly than the other common vertigo disorders. The patient may have vertigo that lasts from 6 to 9 months, and there may be a persistent positional vertigo that is permanent or improves slowly over a longer period. The hearing is normal. Spontaneous nystagmus is present but disappears after a few weeks or months and is replaced by positional nystagmus.

Patients with benign positional vertigo (cupulolithiasis) have vertigo with a direction-fixed nystagmus: It is produced in more or less specific head postions. The most striking feature is its positional character. It may be either sudden or insidious in onset, and there is a latency period between assuming the position and the onset of the vertigo. The severity of the attacks tends to subside with repeated assumption of the triggering position.

Cervical vertigo (postwhiplash) is characterized by the onset of positional vertigo after a neck injury. It may develop immediately or after a period of time. Tinnitus may be associated with the vertigo. The nystagmus is usually horizontal, and there may be mild unsteadiness between the attacks. There may be little visible nystagmus with the eyes open. The audiometric tests are usually normal. The ENG typically reveals nystagmus with neck position changes.

The vertigo caused by vascular diseases is not associated with a hearing loss. The three most common vascular disorders are basilar artery insufficiency, Wallenberg's syndrome, and the subclavian steal syndrome. These disorders cause other neurologic findings, including diplopia, dysphagia, and dysarthria.

Vertigo and hearing problems can result from head injuries that range in severity from a simple concussion to a temporal bone fracture. The symptoms vary from transient vertigo and tinnitus to severe vertigo with a mild to severe sensory hearing loss. The vertigo occurs almost immediately after the head injury. A fracture of the temporal bone rarely occurs without loss of consciousness. The physical examination may reveal a laceration or hematoma of the scalp (Battle's sign) or bleeding from the EAC. The ENG will usually show a spontaneous nystagmus that persists for several weeks after the injury. Later, the nystagmus may become positional. An x-ray examination and other diagnostic techniques may be necessary to make an accurate and complete diagnosis.

The two types of temporal bone fracture are longitudinal and transverse. Longitudinal fractures are less destructive to the cochlea than the transverse fracture. Hearing loss following a longitudinal fracture may be conductive, sensory, or mixed, and the degree of associated loss may range from mild to severe. Transverse temporal bone fractures are less common than the longitudinal type but are more destructive and often bilateral. Most transverse fractures result in "dead" ears with no measurable responses to auditory stimuli (Zarnoch and Northern, 1988).

The vertigo that arises after ear surgery (stapedectomy) may be due to inflammation of the labyrinth (labyrinthitis), or a perilymph fistula. Serous labyrinthitis is a transient disorder consisting of mild vertigo accompanied with a sensory hearing loss and a slight decline in speech recognition. A spontaneous nystagmus is present. There may be complete resolution of the symptom or a persistence of the hearing loss.

Suppurative labyrinthitis may be associated with surgery on the otic capsule, cholesteatoma erosion, or meningitis that produces severe vertigo and profound hearing loss. The inner ear may be completely destroyed. There is a spontaneous nystagmus and no hearing or vestibular response in the affected ear.

Vertigo caused by ototoxic drugs (aminoglycoside antibiotics) may or may not have an associated hearing loss. These drugs have a predilection for either the cochlear or vestibular portion of the inner ear. Although ototoxic symptoms usually arise during the administration of the drug, they may be delayed for variable periods after the drug has been discontinued. The affects are usually, but not always, present in both ears. The patient may have tinnitus that is constant. Difficulty walking in the dark from vestibular damage may be noted. An audiometric evaluation may reveal normal hearing or a sensory hearing loss that ranges from mild to complete.

The treatment of vertigo ranges from none to highly specialized otoneurosurgical resection of an acoustic neuroma. Symptomatic therapy is somewhat unpredictable in terms of response. These patients should always be referred to an otolaryngologist for specific evaluation and treatment. The diagnosis and evaluation of balance disorders are treated in detail in Chapter 13.

TINNITUS

One of the most disturbing otologic symptoms is tinnitus. *Tinnitus* is the perception of an abnormal sound, which is usually localized to one or both ears. *Subjective tinnitus* is heard only by the patient; *objective tinnitus* can be heard by both the patient and the examiner. Objective tinnitus is far less common than subjective tinnitus and is usually heard by the examiner using a stethoscope on the ear, neck, or skull. Tinnitus can be either continuous or intermittent and may be described as a wide variety of internal sounds including ringing, whistling, buzzing, whirring, chirping, roaring, hissing, humming, and clicking. Overall, the character of the tinnitus sound is of little diagnostic value except for pulsatile tinnitus, which may be related to carotid pulsations, jugular bulb tumor, or arteriovenous malformation.

Tinnitus is among the most common of health complaints. The broad scope of the problem is reflected in a U.S. Department of Health, Education, and Welfare National Center on Health Statistics (1968) report that some 36 million adults in the United States experience tinnitus. Of this number, 7.2 million (20%) complain of severe tinnitus. The causes of tinnitus are many and the degree to which the patient suffers covers a wide range of complaints. Tinnitus may also make some patients unable to concentrate or conduct routine daily duties. Tinnitus is often reported to be worse at night and prevent adequate sleep, thereby creating in some persons depression, annoyance, and insecurity. Tyler and Baker (1983) report results of a survey of 97 members of a tinnitus self-help group who reported their difficulties to include effects on lifestyle (93%), emotional content (70%), general health (56%), and hearing difficulties (53%). An excellent textbook concerning the mechanism and management of tinnitus has been published recently by Hazell (1987).

Treatment of the tinnitus patient can be approached in many ways. Obviously otologic evaluation is extremely important to rule out any pathologic condition that might be medically or surgically treatable. Nearly every conceivable scheme has been attempted to reduce the symptoms of tinnitus, but unfortunately no universal treatment has been found. Treatments for tinnitus include surgery, various drug prescriptions, auditory masking devices, reassurance and self-help groups, biofeedback, psychotherapy, and behavioral modification (Sweetow, 1987).

The vast majority of patients with tinnitus also have some degree of sensory hearing loss. All patients with a complaint of tinnitus require thorough audiologic and otologic evaluation to rule out underlying treatable pathology. Additional tests may also be in order including auditory brainstem response audiometry, ENG, and radiographic procedures. Most patients are satisfied to understand that no serious pathology exists, and

an explanation of the problem with appropriate reassurance is all that is necessary. A small group of patients will continue to express problems associated with their tinnitus and experience severe disability. These patients require continued counseling and a full regimen of therapeutic attempts to relieve their symptoms.

The rupture of the round-window membrane (perilymph fistula) may produce dizziness and hearing loss that is sudden in onset, or the symptoms may not occur until weeks, months, or years after the insult. It is sometimes associated with a "popping" sound in the ear. An increase in cerebrospinal fluid pressure that is transmitted to the perilymph of the labyrinth may cause a rupture of the membrane. This occurs most often from the pressure changes associated with scuba diving, heavy physical exertion, or Valsalva maneuvers brought on by coughing or sneezing. Vertigo is sometimes an associated symptom.

A *fistula test* is conducted by directing positive air pressure into the ear canal either with a Siegle otoscope or an acoustic immittance measuring instrument and is reported to be indicative of a leak of perilymph at the oval or round window. A positive fistula test is associated with the sudden onset of whirling vertigo and nystagmus in the patient associated with positive EAC air pressure (English, 1976). The patient's eyes should be covered and observed through Frenzel glasses. Spontaneous nystagmus and gaze nystagmus may be observed (Table 4-3). Positional nystagmus may be detected with the patient seated or supine and the head hanging right or left (Figure 4-3). Additional testing of the vestibular system must be performed with ENG or posturography as described in Chapter 13 (see also Chapter 9, case 6).

OTOTOXICITY

An unfortunate side effect of certain drugs is damage to the auditory or vestibular system, or both, of the patient. Ototoxity causes hearing loss and cellular degeneration of the inner ear, including the end organs and neurons of the cochlear and the vestibular divisions of the eighth nerve. Individual susceptibility to drug-related ototoxicity varies greatly although it is generally believed that infants, elderly persons, and those patients with pretreatment sensory hearing loss may be at higher risk for inner ear involvement (Bergstrom and Thompson, 1984).

TABLE 4-3. SPONTANEOUS NYSTAGMUS

	Peripheral (labyrinth, vestibular nerve)	Central nervous system
Visual fixation	Nystagmus suppressed	Nystagmus not suppressed; may be enhanced by visual fixation
Form	Horizontal or horizontorotary	Occurs in any direction, including vertical, horizontal, rotary, and diagonal
Location	Bilateral	Unilateral. A vertical, unilateral nystagmus indicates brainstem disease
Intensity	Pronounced at onset, decreases after several hours or days	Continuous for several days and weeks; may increase in severity
Auditory	Frequently with auditory symptoms or signs	Rarely associated auditory symptoms or signs, but associated neurologic symptoms
Vertigo	Present	Variable
Past-pointing and falling	In direction of slow phase	In direction of fast phase
Duration	Minutes–weeks	Weeks–months
Direction of fast component	Toward "stimulated" labyrinth; away from "destroyed" labyrinth	Toward the side of the central nervous system lesion

Source: From English, G. M. (1976). *Otolaryngology: A textbook*. Hagerstown, MD: Harper & Row. With permission.

Figure 4-3. Procedure used to elicit positional nystagmus. (A) Subject's head turned to the right. (B) Subject's head turned to the left. (C) Subject's head maintained in midline position. (From English, G. [1976]. Otoneurologic examination. In G. English, *Otolaryngology: A textbook*. Hagerstown, MD: Harper & Row. With permission.)

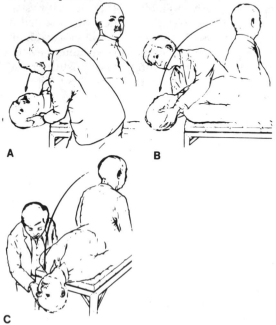

A

B

C

The incidence of ototoxicity, either on an overall basis or for individual specific drugs, has not been accurately determined. Prospective studies over the past few years have emphasized the need for standardized protocols to evaluate potential damage to the cochlear and vestibular portions of the inner ear. Ototoxic drugs are most commonly associated with anti-infectives, analgesic pain relievers, and diuretics that remove excess fluid from the body (Brandell, Brandell, and Hult, 1988). The aminoglycoside antibiotics constitute a family of drugs that have a common chemical structure effective in the treatment of gram-negative and acid-fast bacteria. They are an essential part of treating many life-threatening infections and are often the only drug of choice. Unfortunately, the aminoglycosides are noted for their ototoxic and nephrotoxic potential. Each of the aminoglycosides may create permanent damage to the hair cells of the inner ear and the macula of the utricle and semicircular canals, and in addition, each member of this family of drugs tends to cause specific damage to either area of the otic capsule as shown in Table 4-4.

Thompson and Northern (1981) describe an audiometric monitoring program for patients being treated with potentially ototoxic drugs. These authors discuss the evaluation of auditory

TABLE 4-4. DEGREE OF DAMAGE CAUSED BY OTOTOXIC ANTIBIOTICS ON VESTIBULAR AND COCHLEAR ORGANS

Antibiotic	Vestibular	Cochlear
Streptomycin	+++	+
Dihydrostreptomycin	+	++++
Neomycin	+	++++
Kanamycin	+	+++
Gentamycin	++	+
Viomycin	+++	++
Vancomycin		+++
Polymycin	++	+

+, little damage; ++++, great damage.
Source: From Brandell, M. E., Brandell, R. R., & Hult, R. (1988). Drugs and ototoxicity. *Hearing instruments, 39*(11), 41. With permission.

TABLE 4-5. HIGH-RISK PATIENTS FOR AUDIOMETRIC MONITORING DURING THERAPY WITH OTOTOXIC DRUGS

1. Ototoxic drug administered in the presence of decreased renal function
2. Ototoxic drug administered in increased daily doses or for an extended period
3. Assay showing high-peak or trough level of ototoxic drug
4. Multiple ototoxic drugs administered concurrently or in consecutive courses (within 1 week)
5. Special patient conditions such as preexisting hearing loss or severe visual impairment or blindness
6. Ear symptoms reported by patient: tinnitus, hearing loss, dizziness

Source: From Thompson, P., & Northern, J. L. (1981). Audiometric monitoring of patients treated with ototoxic drugs. In S. A. Lerner, G. I. Matz, J. E. Hawkins, & E. F. Lanze (Eds.), *Aminoglycoside ototoxicity* (p. 239). Boston: Little, Brown. With permission.

TABLE 4-6. AUDIOMETRIC POTENTIAL FOR PATIENTS ON OTOTOXIC DRUG THERAPY

1. Baseline hearing level established as soon as possible
2. Obtain air conduction thresholds bilaterally at 0.5, 1.0, 2.0, 4.0, and 8.0 kHz
3. If hearing loss noted, bone conduction thresholds are obtained, and referral for additional audiologic and otologic work-up considered
4. Patient questioned about ear symptoms: tinnitus, hearing loss, dizziness. Dizzy patients referred for electronystagmography
5. Results are recorded in patient's hospital chart
6. Criterion for change: 15 dB at any test frequency

Source: From Thompson, P., & Northern, J. L. (1981). Audiometric monitoring of patients treated with ototoxic drugs. In S. A. Lerner, G. I. Matz, J. E. Hawkins, & E. F. Lanze (Eds.), *Aminoglycoside ototoxicity* (p. 240). Boston: Little, Brown. With permission.

function in patients who are at increased risk of hearing loss, that is, patients who report otologic symptoms including tinnitus, fullness of the ear, dizziness, or any change in hearing status (Table 4-5). Many of these patients are very sick, and audiometric testing must be conducted at the bedside under conditions of ambient hospital noise. Success in obtaining reliable hearing test results often depends on the skill of the audiologist performing the test. The recommended protocol of audiometric monitoring of patients tested with ototoxic drugs is presented in Table 4-6.

A baseline audiogram should be established as soon as possible, even prior to the initial administration of the potentially damaging drug. Routine audiometric monitoring should be continued weekly throughout the period of drug therapy. Following completion of drug administration, additional audiometric tests should be conducted at 1 week, 1 month, and 3 months to monitor delayed onset of hearing loss. Additional audiologic work-up may be appropriate when ototoxic hearing loss is noted. Audiometric follow-up for infants may be necessary up to age 3 or 4 years. The audiologist must be prepared to offer counseling, rehabilitative assistance with amplification or cochlear implant, or any other aural rehabilitation needed (see Chapter 9, case 7).

EVALUATION OF PERMANENT HEARING HANDICAP

A necessary part of otologic and audiologic services is the definition of permanent hearing impairment for medical-legal purposes and the establishment of compensation awards (AMA, 1971). Considerable debate has been held through the years concerning the question of when does hearing impairment become a hearing handicap and which is the "best" method for determining hearing disability and the appropriate amount of monetary settlement. Many factors influence these decisions including individual differences in susceptibility to injury from noise, normal auditory aging or presbycusis, years on the job, and so forth. The best that these compensation systems can hope to offer is a reasonable approximation in the relationship of compensation to handicap in auditory function (Melnick, 1988).

A task force of the American Speech-Language-Hearing Association (1981) published a thorough review of various definitions of hearing

TABLE 4-7. PERCENTAGE OF
BINAURAL HEARING
IMPAIRMENT AS RELATED
TO WHOLE-PERSON IMPAIRMENT

Impairment of Binaural hearing (%)	Whole person (%)
0–1.7	0
1.0–4.2	1
4.3–7.4	2
7.5–9.9	3
10.--13.1	4
13.2–15.9	5
16.0–18.8	6
18.9–21.4	7
21.5–24.5	8
24.6–27.1	9
27.2–30.0	10
30.1–32.8	11
32.9–35.9	12
36.0–38.5	13
38.6–41.7	14
41.8–44.2	15
44.3–47.4	16
47.5–49.9	17
50.0–53.1	18
53.2–55.7	19
55.8–58.8	20
58.9–61.4	21
61.5–64.5	22
64.6–67.1	23
67.2–70.0	24
70.1–72.8	25
72.9–75.9	26
76.0–78.5	27
78.6–81.7	28
81.8–84.2	29
84.3–87.4	30
87.5–89.9	31
90.0–93.1	32
93.2–95.7	33
95.8–98.8	34
98.9–100.0	35

Note: Impairment of whole person contributed by binaural hearing impairment may be rounded to the nearest 5% *only* when it is the sole impairment involved.

1. The average of the hearing threshold levels at 500, 1000, 2000, and 3000 Hz is calculated for each ear.
2. The percentage impairment for each ear is calculated by multiplying by 1.5 percent the amount by which the aforementioned average hearing threshold level exceeds 25 dB (low fence). A maximum of 100 percent is reached at 92 dB (high fence).
3. The binaural hearing impairment should then be calculated by multiplying the smaller percentage (better ear) by 5, adding this figure to the larger percentage (poorer ear), and dividing the total by 6.

Melnick (1988) points out that the specific formula used for assessing compensatory hearing loss is a major factor but not the only consideration in determining eligibility claimants and the size of the monetary award. Each state makes its own decisions regarding how handicapping a hearing loss is to the percentage of impairment to the whole person. Table 4-7 shows the relation of binaural hearing impairment (as determined with the American Academy of Otolaryngology — Head and Neck Surgery formula) to whole-person impairment.

REFERENCES

Alford, B., & Jerger, J. (1977). Audiology and otolaryngology: A continuing partnership. *Archives of Otolaryngology, 103,* 249–250.
American Academy of Otolaryngology — Head and Neck Surgery, Committee on Hearing and Equilibrium, and the American Council of Otolaryngology, Committee on the Medical Aspects of Noise. (1979). Guide for the evaluation of hearing handicap. *Journal of the American Medical Association, 133,* 396–397.
American Medical Association. Committee on Rating Mental and Physical Impairment. (1971). Ear, nose and throat related structures. In *Guides to the evaluation of permanent impairment* (pp. 103–111). Chicago: American Medical Association.
American Speech-Language-Hearing Association. (1981). Report of the task force on the definition of hearing handicap. *ASHA, 23,* 293–297.
Baker, B., & Northern, J. (1976). Medical conditions of the external ear. *Maico Audiological Library Series,* XIV, Report 7.
Bergstrom, L., & Thompson, P. (1984). Ototoxicity. In J. Northern (Ed.), *Hearing disorders* (2nd ed., pp. 119–134). Boston: Little, Brown.
Brandell, M. E., Brandell, R. R., & Hult, R. (1988). Drugs and ototoxicity. *Hearing Instruments, 39*(11), 41–43.
Chandler, J. R. (1964). Partial occlusion of the external auditory meatus. Its effect upon air and bone conduction hearing acuity. *Laryngoscope, 74,* 22–54.

handicap as well as a summary of numerous schemes devised to assess hearing disability for compensation purposes. Melnick (1988) reports that the most common method used for calculating hearing handicap is that proposed in 1979 by the American Academy of Otolaryngology — Head and Neck Surgery. This procedure for converting hearing threshold levels into percentages of hearing impairment is reproduced below:

English, G. M. (1976). *Otolaryngology: A textbook.* Hagerstown, MD: Harper & Row.

English, G. M., & Sargent, R. S. (1988). Medical and surgical treatment of hearing loss. In N. Lass, L. McReynolds, J. Northern, & D. Yoder (Eds.), *Handbook of speech-language pathology and audiology* (pp. 1237–1264). Toronto: B.C. Decker.

Girgis, T. F., & Schambaugh, G. E., Jr. (1988). Tuning fork tests: Forgotten art. *American Journal of Otology, 9*(1), 64–69.

Goodhill, V. (1979). *Ear diseases, deafness and dizziness.* Hagerstown, MD: Harper & Row.

Hawke, M. (1987). *Clinical pocket guide to ear disease* (p. 136). Philadelphia: Lea & Febiger.

Hazell, J. W. P. (1987). *Tinnitus.* London: Churchill-Livingstone.

Hughes, G. (1985). *Textbook of clinical otology.* New York: Thieme-Stratton.

Keith, R. W. (1984). The basic audiological evaluation. In J. Northern (Ed.), *Hearing disorders* (2nd ed., pp. 13–24). Boston: Little, Brown.

Lichtenstein, M., Bess, F., & Logan, S. (1988). Validation of screening tools for the hearing impaired elderly in primary care. *Journal of the American Medical Association, 259*(19), 2875–2878.

Melnick, W. (1988). Compensation for hearing loss from occupational noise. *Seminars in Hearing, 9*(4), 339–349.

National Center for Health Statistics. (1968). Hearing status and ear examination: Findings among adults, United States, 1960–1962. In *Vital and Health Statistics* (Series 11, No. 32). Washington, DC: U.S. Department of Health, Education, and Welfare.

Northern, J. L. (1980). Clinical measurement procedures in impedance audiometry. In J. Jerger & J. Northern (Eds.), *Clinical impedance audiometry* (2nd ed., pp. 19–39). Acton, MA: American Electromedics.

Rose, J. S. (1984). Radiology in otologic diagnosis. In J. Northern (Ed.), *Hearing disorders* (2nd ed., pp. 85–100). Boston: Little, Brown.

Sheehy, T., Gardner, G., & Hambley, W. (1971). Tuning fork tests in modern otology. *Archives of Otolaryngology, 94,* 132.

Stankiewicz, J. A., & Nowry, H. J. (1979). Clinical accuracy of tuning fork tests. *Laryngoscope, 12,* 1956–1963.

Sweetow, R. W. (Ed.). (1987). Management of the tinnitus patient. *Seminars in Hearing, 8*(1), 1–74.

Thompson, P., & Northern, J. L. (1981). Audiometric monitoring of patients treated with ototoxic drugs. In S. A. Lerner, G. I. Matz, J. E. Hawkins, & E. F. Lanze (Eds.), *Aminoglycoside ototoxicity* (pp. 237–245). Boston: Little, Brown.

Tyler, R. S., & Baker, L. J. (1983). Difficulties experienced by tinnitus sufferers. *Journal of Speech and Hearing Disorders, 48,* 150–154.

Weed, L. L. (1971). *Medical records, medical education and patient care: The problem-oriented record as a basic tool.* Cleveland: Case Western Reserve University Press.

White, J. D. (1984). Laboratory diagnosis of otologic disease. In J. L. Northern (Ed.), *Hearing disorders* (2nd ed., pp. 75–83). Boston: Little, Brown.

Wilson, W. R., & Woods, L. A. (1975). Accuracy of the Bing and Rinne tuning fork tests. *Archives of Otolaryngology, 101,* 81–85.

Wood, R. P. (1979). History taking in otorhinolaryngology. In R. P. Wood & J. L. Northern (Eds.), *Otolaryngology: A symptom-oriented text.* Baltimore: Williams & Wilkins.

Zarnoch, J. M., & Northern, J. L. (1988). Audiological manifestations. In N. Lass, L. McReynolds, J. Northern, & D. Yoder (Eds.), *Handbook of speech-language pathology and audiology* (pp. 1076–1093). Toronto: B.C. Decker.

Zwislocki, J. (1953). Acoustic attenuation between the ears. *Journal of the Acoustical Society of America, 25,* 752–759.

CHAPTER 5

Otoneurologic Diseases and Associated Audiologic Profiles

J. Michael Dennis • J. Gail Neely

The literature in audiology and otorhinolaryngology contains an impressive array of scientific and clinical information describing the deleterious effects of otoneurologic diseases on general health as well as the proclivity of many of these disorders to produce hearing loss and communication compromise. As clinical evaluation techniques have developed and progressed, it has become apparent that a thorough and complete knowledge of these diseases and their associated audiologic profiles precurse accurate diagnosis and successful treatment. This chapter will overview the auditory pathology, pathophysiology, and audiologic findings of common diseases as they affect the external ear, the middle ear, the inner ear, the auditory division of the eighth cranial nerve, and the central auditory pathways. Audiologic descriptions will include basic pure tone, speech, and immittance audiometric results as well as symptomatology. In some cases additional audiologic tests will be included, for example, auditory brainstem responses (ABRs).

TRAUMATIC DISEASES

TEMPORAL BONE FRACTURE

Head injury results in the basic phenomena of concussion, fracture, contusion, and hemorrhage. All may coexist after a single injury. Secondary phenomena such as brain swelling, infection, and scarring add to the severity of the insult. Temporal bone fractures resulting from head injury are categorized as longitudinal or transverse. Longitudinal fractures course posteriolaterally over the mastoid, through the pneumatized spaces lateral to the otic capsule, and extend to the root of the zygoma. These injuries frequently involve the squa-

mous bone contribution to the external auditory meatus (EAM). This creates visible fracture in the external auditory canal (EAC), canal skin laceration, and frequently tympanic membrane perforation. Ossicular chain dislocations are common. The most frequent ossicular involvements are separation of the incudostapedial joint or fracture of the long process of the incus. Dislocation of the incudomalleal joint or luxation of the stapes is less common. Occasionally, a bone fragment from the EAC may impinge on the ossicular chain.

Longitudinal temporal bone fractures typically cause conductive hearing loss because the fracture line transverses the bony tympanic cavity with possible tearing of the tympanic membrane, hemorrhage of the middle ear, and disruption of the ossicular chain (Kinney, 1986); however, high-frequency hearing loss can occur because of the concussive effect to the cochlea (Schuknecht, 1974). The middle ear involvement from longitudinal temporal bone fracture usually produces a 40 to 60 dB unilateral, conductive hearing loss with excellent word recognition ability (Jerger and Jerger, 1981). Immittance audiometry produces a type A_D or type B tympanogram (Jerger, 1970). The crossed stapedius reflexes are often absent with sound presented to either side, and the uncrossed reflexes are present on the unaffected side. Figure 5-1 illustrates the audiometric results from longitudinal temporal bone fracture. Occasionally, the crossed stapedius reflex may be present when the measurement probe is located on the affected side. In these relatively rare instances, there may be a fracture through the stapes crura or a functional connection remaining between the stapes tendon and the tympanic membrane (Dennis, 1983; Jerger and Jerger, 1981).

Transverse fractures account for 20 to 30 percent of temporal bone fractures. These fractures

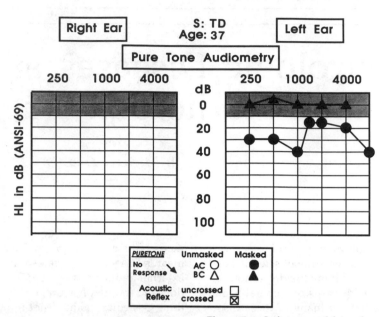

Figure 5-1. Left temporal bone longitudinal fracture with illustration of hearing sensitivity at 5 weeks after motor vehicle accident. Note the conductive hearing loss (25-dB SRT) with normal speech recognition score (98%). The tympanogram was type A_D. Crossed and uncrossed stapedius reflexes were absent with the measurement probe in the left ear canal. With treatment the air-bone gap was closed and the immittance results were normal.

extend from foramen to foramen through the otic capsule, which is the hardest bone in the body. Such a severe injury usually results from an occipital or frontal blow of extreme force. Intercranial damage from these impacts usually has maximum effects along surfaces and tissue changes such as the bone-dura interfaces or venous attachments. Consequently, injuries above the tentorium are much more frequent. Isolated brainstem injuries without diffuse cortical damage are rare if ever present.

Transverse fractures extend horizontally across the petrous pyramid, causing sensory hearing loss because of damage to cochlear structures. The onset of hearing loss is usually acute. Transverse temporal bone fractures generally produce severe to profound sensory loss of hearing sensitivity on the involved side with no residual word recognition ability. In rare cases, the contralateral side may be involved (Podoshin and Fradis, 1975). Immittance findings generally produce a normal tympanogram with the crossed and uncrossed stapedius reflex absent with sound to the involved ear; however, the tympanogram may be abnormal because of middle ear involvement (Jerger and Jerger, 1981).

On some occasions, conductive and sensory hearing loss are transient. Tos (1971) reported that 80 percent of the conductive hearing loss resulting from temporal bone fractures improved spontaneously. Conductive or sensory hearing loss that tends to progress or fluctuate, especially that associated with spontaneous, episodic, or positional vertigo, may be associated with a perilymph fistula through a fractured or subluxed stapes. These cases require middle ear exploration after the resolution of the hemotympanum. Finally, a nonorganic component to the hearing loss may be present in areas of temporal bone fracture. Barber (1969) reported a 7 percent incidence of exaggerated hearing levels in temporal bone fracture patients.

ELECTROCUTION

Very little information is available about the pathology and pathophysiology of auditory injuries from electrocution. A clinical and histologic review of lightning-damaged ears is provided by Bergstrom et al. (1974). These authors documented numerous auditory injuries, including inferior pars tensa tympanic membrane perforation, hemorrhage within the pneumatized spaces of the temporal bone, rupture of Reissner's membrane, degeneration of the stria vascularis and organ of Corti, possible microfractures of the otic capsule, edema of the intracanalicular portion of the facial nerve, and herniation of the cerebellum into the internal auditory meatus (IAM).

Bergstrom et al. (1974) also documented and described hearing loss from lightning injuries to the ear. Initially, the hearing loss can be mixed in nature because this type of injury frequently involves conductive and sensory structures. Unilateral involvement occurs more often than a bilateral configuration. Immittance testing produces abnormal tympanometric and stapedius reflex findings. There appears to be greater residual loss in the higher frequencies after the conductive portion of the loss is cleared. The sensory component of the hearing loss does not recover. The mechanisms to explain the hearing loss are the direct effect of electrocution, the blast effect of the thunderclap, and the traumatic effect of being thrown to the ground. The direct effect of electrocution may affect auditory structures by means of two pathways. The first is conduction of current from external body tissues through the EAC. The second is electrical conduction through intracranial contents and the IAM to the cochlea.

GUNSHOT WOUNDS

Gunshot wounds that affect auditory structures usually result in a whole bullet or bullet fragments impinging on the otic capsule without bone penetration. Consequently, the end result can be conductive, sensory, or mixed hearing loss because of damage to the sound-conducting mechanism, sensory structures, and microvascular anatomy (Jerger and Jerger, 1981; Kinney, 1986).

Generally, the audiologic profile for conductive hearing loss from gunshot wounds can be similar to that described for temporal bone fracture. Sensory hearing loss can range from mild to profound with word recognition scores affected in a manner that parallels the degree of loss and cochlear damage. Stapedius reflexes may be present or absent with sound delivered to the affected side depending on the amount of sensitivity loss.

RADIATION

Therapeutic levels of radiation result in occlusive vasculitis and inflammation of the skin and mucous membranes. Middle ear effusion from mucositis of the mucosa of the pneumatized spaces of the temporal bone is the most common auditory dysfunction seen with radiation of the ear. Avascular necrosis of the long process of the incus can also occur, which may produce a disarticulation of the ossicular chain. Radiation can result in late complication of hearing loss secondary to atrophy of the spiral ligament, rupture of the cochlear duct, and degeneration of the organ of Corti. Atrophy of the annular ligament surrounding the stapes may result in an oval-window fistula. Infection of this devitalized region is a problem. This results in osteitis and osteomyelitis, which frequently bears the name *osteoradionecrosis with infection*. This is a serious infection of the base of the skull. Thus, myringotomy to relieve serous middle ear effusion must be cautiously done if at all.

Conductive and sensory hearing loss from the reaction of the temporal bone and associated structures to radiation injury have been documented (Moretti, 1976; O'Neil, Katz, and Skolnik, 1979; Schuknecht, 1974). Conductive hearing loss results from the effusion of the middle ear space or ossicular necrosis. The loss is usually unilateral and varies in degree. The acoustic immittance profile reflects tympanogram and stapedius reflex abnormality.

Sensory hearing loss from radiation may begin soon after treatment or have a delayed onset up to several years. The degree of loss ranges from mild to profound and is dosage related. The hearing loss may be stable or progressive and usually involves both ears. There is limited information about audiometric profile; however, one report (Moretti, 1976) relates a flat audiometric pattern with mild sensitivity loss and a sloping contour with more severe hearing loss. Word recognition ability varies with the degree of hearing loss.

SURGICAL TRAUMA

Hearing loss is well documented as a possible complication of otologic surgery. A recent publication provides a comprehensive treatment of this topic (Weiet and Causse, 1986). Surgical trauma to the auditory system is also often planned or predicted from the disease requiring surgical intervention. For example, an individual with a cholesteatoma that has partially or completely eroded the incus or stapes will occasionally have normal hearing sensitivity. This results from the cholesteatoma participating with the residual ossicular components as a conductive mechanism. The removal of the cholesteatoma, of course, results in a significant conductive hearing loss prior to reconstruction.

Conductive hearing loss can occur during or subsequent to middle ear surgery. Tympanic membrane injury, unintended ossicular disruption, prosthesis malfunction, persistent tympanic membrane perforation, and development of cholesteatoma are some causal factors that can be involved. The hearing loss is unilateral, mild to moderately severe in range, and the immittance battery can be helpful in determining the nature of the conductive disorder.

Labyrinthine injury from middle ear surgery can produce sensory hearing loss. Inadvertent fistula involving the membranous labyrinth may result in irreversible, severe, or total deafness on the unoperated ear. Touching the intact ossicular chain with a bone-cutting burr can result in permanent high-frequency sensory hearing loss (Crabtree, 1986; Helms, 1976).

Surgical damage to the auditory division of the eighth cranial nerve can occur with middle fossa or posterior fossa resection of the vestibular nerve for vertigo, acoustic tumor resection, and fifth and seventh cranial nerve decompression procedures. This can result in irreversible, unilateral sensory hearing loss ranging from mild to profound in degree. Intraoperative evoked potential monitoring using ABRs is used to detect and avoid auditory nerve injury and hearing loss during the procedures (Dennis, 1987, 1988; Dennis and Early, 1988; Dennis, Early, and Neely, 1987; Schwartz, Blum, and Dennis, 1985).

Sudden sensory hearing loss has been reported as a possible complication of nonotologic surgery (Miller, Toohill, and Lehman, 1982). The hearing loss is often unilateral, moderately severe in degree, with pronounced reduction in word recognition ability. Partial recovery in pure tone sensitivity and word recognition scores can occur. This category of traumatic hearing loss is usually associated with coronary bypass surgery, but other procedures have been implicated. It is assumed the hearing loss has a vascular etiology, encompassing hypofusion of the inner ear and embolic interference with cochlear blood supply.

ACOUSTIC TRAUMA

It is well known that exposure to intense sound can produce temporary and permanent sensory hearing loss (Jerger and Jerger, 1981; Lonsbury-Martin and Martin, 1986; Ward, 1976). The permanent hearing loss is the result of damage to sensory structures by excessive sound stimulation. Hearing deficits resulting from excessive noise are traditionally separated into noise-induced hearing loss and acoustic trauma.

Noise-induced hearing loss is the result of repetitive exposure to damaging sound over a con-siderable period of time, usually years. The pathophysiology of noise-induced hearing loss is still poorly understood. Pathologic correlates include hair cell injury and loss, as well as other structural and metabolic inner ear changes. Noise-induced hearing loss is usually bilateral and begins in the higher-frequency region between 3000 and 6000 Hz (Jerger and Jerger, 1981), with maximum loss of sensitivity often occurring at 4000 Hz. Initially, the hearing loss is very mild and goes unnoticed; however, with repeated exposures, it progresses and encompasses frequency regions critical for understanding of speech. Eventually, noise-induced hearing loss plateaus around 60 to 70 dB HL for the mid and higher frequencies. Generally, the audiometric profile is a sloping configuration. Word recognition scores vary depending on the amount of hearing loss and the frequencies that are involved. Acoustic immittance testing shows normal middle ear function with crossed and uncrossed stapedius reflexes present at hearing levels typically seen for cochlear impairment.

Acoustic trauma is the second category of hearing loss that can result from exposure to intense sound. Acoustic trauma occurs from a single exposure to a very intense, usually percussive type of sound (e.g., explosion or gunshot). The pathology of hearing loss from a single exposure to a very loud sound is mechanical rupture and laceration of tissues and cell membranes in the inner ear and occasionally the middle ear. Another example of sound that can potentially result in acoustic trauma is the screech of a suction tube adjacent to soft tissue during otologic surgery. Care is taken to avoid this type of exposure since the intensities of these sounds can reach 140 dB sound pressure level.

The hearing loss in acoustic trauma is acute in onset and may be unilateral or bilateral. Both middle ear and inner ear structures can be involved. Audiometric patterns for acoustic trauma vary greatly. Conductive and mixed losses of hearing sensitivity are seen because of middle ear involvement. Sensory hearing loss can vary from mild to very severe, and there are instances of partial and complete recovery. Word recognition scores will generally reflect the amount of hearing loss and sensory involvement. Findings from the acoustic immittance battery will vary depending on the site of involvement and degree of hearing loss.

METABOLIC AND OTHER DISEASES

DIABETES MELLITUS

Diabetes mellitus characteristically creates hypertrophy and proliferation of vascular endothelium. These result in vascular occlusion because of the effect on the lumens of arterioles, capillaries, and venules. In addition to these small-vessel anomalies, arteriosclerosis of larger vessels and atherosclerosis of the largest vessels are found with increased incidence in the diabetic patient. Arteriosclerosis may result in hypertension, which increases the probability of cerebrovascular accident, and atherosclerosis further decreases the integrity of cerebral vessels. Thickening capillary walls in the striae vascularis have been documented in diabetics, particularly those with retinopathy and nephropathy.

Diabetes mellitus may predispose the EAC to a condition known as *malignant external otitis,* or more properly, *acute necrotizing external otitis.* This is a potentially deadly external otitis in a diabetic or otherwise immune-compromised individual. The predominant organism is *Pseudomonas aeruginosa.* This condition causes expanding necrotizing vasculitis and osteomyelitis of the base of the skull. Diagnosis is suspected when a refractory, progressive external otitis is present, particularly in a diabetic patient. Vigorous medical and occasionally surgical treatment are necessary to save the patient's life.

Descriptions of structural and functional sequelae of metabolic disturbances resulting from diabetes mellitus include both sensory and vascular elements of the peripheral ear. It is, therefore, compelling to associate sensory hearing loss with diabetes mellitus. Indeed, this association has been present in the literature for years. Generally, the hearing loss is described as sensory, bilateral, and progressive in nature (Taylor and Irwin, 1978). The degree of hearing loss ranges from mild to severe, and higher frequencies are reportedly most affected. Word recognition scores vary with the degree of hearing loss and involvement. Acoustic immittance findings generally show normal tympanograms. The stapedius reflex is described as being present for losses of cochlear origin and elevated or absent with losses of eighth nerve involvement.

Although evidence indicates that cochlear and retrocochlear hearing loss are present in some cases with diabetes mellitus (Jerger and Jerger, 1981; Miller et al., 1983), controversy exists as to whether diabetes mellitus directly causes hearing loss (Harper, 1981; Schuknecht, 1974). Harper (1981) found no evidence of hearing loss in adult-onset diabetes mellitus when he controlled for other causal factors. Jerger and Jerger (1981) reported an interesting case of diabetes mellitus in a patient presenting with an asymmetric hearing loss. The pure tone, speech, and acoustic immittance profile indicated a cochlear, retrocochlear, and facial nerve disorder on the more involved side.

HYPOTHYROIDISM

Hypothyroidism is the constellation of metabolic changes resulting from the deficiency of thyroid hormones (Kaplan and Griep, 1986). Experimentally, hypothyroidism tends to result in thickening of the tympanic membrane and middle ear mucosa. Cochlear hair cell loss from endolymphatic hypertension, and degeneration of the spiral ganglion, tectorial membrane, and organ of Corti also occur. Hypothyroidism can result in eustachian tube edema, leading to middle ear effusion. *Pendred's syndrome* is a simple autosomal recessive genetic disease that includes hypothyroidism. Individuals with Pendred's syndrome tend to develop goiter in their early teens and have a high incidence of Mondini's dysplasia of the inner ears.

Hearing loss accompanying hypothyroidism can be mixed or sensory. Liston and Meyerhoff (1986) report nongenetic cretinism is accompanied by progressive, mixed bilateral hearing loss at a rate of 50 to 100 percent. Perhaps as many as 25 percent of patients with acquired hypothyroidism have hearing loss that is usually sensory or mixed and tends to be reversible when the hypothyroid state is reversed. Bhatia et al. (1977) studied hypothyroidism and found progressive, bilaterally symmetric mild to moderately severe cochlear hearing loss. Although acquired hypothyroidism has been known to reverse with thyroid hormone therapy (Liston and Meyerhoff, 1986), hearing improvement with thyroid hormone therapy remains controversial (Kaplan and Griep, 1986).

HYPERLIPIDEMIA

Evidence that hyperlipidemia may result in hearing loss was presented in a controlled cross-over study (Rosen, Olin, and Rosen, 1970). A low-fat diet was administered to one group of patients and a regular diet to a controlled group. After 5 years the diets were reversed. Those patients first receiving the low-fat diet had significantly better hearing. Interestingly, those in the initial high-fat diet group had improvement in their hearing sensitivity when placed on the lower-fat diet. All who were initially on the low-fat diet experienced diminished auditory sensitivity when placed on the higher-fat diet. Animals receiving a 1 percent cholesterol diet for 6 months showed a significant deterioration in the ABR after 5 months of the high-fat diet.

Pillsbury (1986) in a series of experiments showed significant synergism between hypertension, high-fat diets, and noise exposure. He found that hypertension and high-fat diets alone did not produce significant hearing loss in experimental animals; however, the addition of high noise exposure to this combination created significant effects. Anatomically the lesions were predominately in the outer row of the outer hair cells in the first and second turns of the cochlea. Cochlear blood flow was decreased in the spiral ganglion and lateral portion of the first and second cochlear turns.

STROKE

Ischemic disease of the central nervous system is categorized into major and minor strokes and transient ischemic attacks. Major strokes result from major arterial disruption or occlusion. Minor strokes occur from small tributary artery disruption or obstruction. Transient ischemic attacks result from embolic phenomenon. It is frequently difficult to correlate the anatomic pathology with physiologic dysfunction because of the propensity for more than one vessel to be involved.

Obstructions or emboli within the internal carotid artery system often compromise the middle cerebral artery, which supplies a large portion of the temporal lobes. The occlusion of this cerebral vessel creates brain softening and diffuse, hemorrhagic areas of ischemia. The immediate effect of this vessel occlusion is loss of metabolic processes and function of neural tissue within 5 to 10 minutes following occlusion. Ischemic lesions ultimately lead to coagulative necrosis with hemorrhage in the grey matter and coagulative necrosis without hemorrhage in the white matter. Localized edema and myelin degeneration are com-

mon near the lesion. However, gradual or even complete occlusion of the vessel may not create ischemia if collateral vessels develop abundantly.

Ischemic changes within the vertebral-basilar system are less common than within the carotid system. The usual site of lesion is the subclavian artery. In the event the vertebral-basilar system is involved, the most common site for ischemia is within the paramedian branches of the basilar artery. This does not ordinarily cause auditory dysfunction. Occlusion of the anterior inferior cerebellar artery, which ultimately supplies the tegmen of the pons, medulla oblongata, and the inner ear, is rarely involved. Parenthetically, the most common etiology for occlusion of this vessel is from surgery.

Stroke or cerebrovascular accident principally affects the central auditory pathways and structures. Conventional pure tone and speech audiometric measures are generally insensitive to central auditory damage (Neely, Dennis, and Lippe, 1986). If these measures show deficit, it is frequently related to the patient's age, history of noise exposure, or associated with other otologic manifestations. Generally, the acoustic immittance battery shows normal tympanograms and stapedius reflexes. Some exceptions to the standard audiologic battery are highlighted by Jerger and Jerger (1981). They remind us that stroke accompanied by aphasia may produce depressed word recognition scores because of expressive or receptive disorders.

Central auditory abnormalities resulting from cerebrovascular accident can be detected by specially constructed psychoacoustic and electrophysiologic tests (Neely et al., 1986). Those patients with stroke involving the brainstem auditory pathways typically show depressed scores on monotic degraded speech tasks. Additionally, various parameters of the ABR can be abnormal. Those patients with stroke affecting the auditory pathways and structures of the temporal lobe consistently show depressed function on dichotic degraded speech tasks. Frequently, the performance of the ear contralateral to the side of temporal lobe involvement is most affected. Additionally, the auditory middle latency response can be abnormal with temporal lobe involvement (Kraus et al., 1982).

HYPERTENSION

Hypertension can create a variety of lesions secondary to the hypertrophy of the muscularis layer within arteries. This results in gradual occlusion of the lumen of arteries, elongation, and tortuosity of vessels. These changes cause a diminished sensitivity to oxygen and carbon dioxide tension. Additionally, the tortuosity may create flow inefficiencies into branch vessels. These vessel changes also increase the probability of vasospasms resulting in transient ischemia, focal edema, and local necrosis. Hypertension may also cause the development of microaneurysms, which create flow inefficiencies in tributary vessels.

The vascular complications of hypertension can result in a reduction of the supply of oxygen to the inner ear with developing sensory hearing loss. The loss of hearing sensitivity is usually bilateral and relatively symmetric. Hearing sensitivity may fluctuate but usually stabilizes if the condition persists. Often there is greater involvement of the higher frequencies, although all frequencies may be depressed. Special tests of auditory function delineate a cochlear site of involvement.

MEDICATIONS AND TOXINS

Hearing problems caused by medications and toxins may be permanent, temporary, occur acutely, or have a delayed onset. The hearing loss associated with ototoxicity is sensory in nature and usually begins in the high-frequency regions; however, involvement can progress to middle and lower frequencies and in some cases result in profound deafness. Risk factors associated with development of ototoxic hearing loss include impaired renal function, elevated serum levels of the ototoxic agent, preexisting sensory hearing loss, treatment with more than one ototoxic agent, greater than 14-days treatment with a potentially ototoxic agent, and advanced age. Prudent audiologic monitoring of patients receiving ototoxic medications includes a preadministration test if possible, then serial evaluation during therapy and at intervals up to 1-year postcessation of treatment.

ASPIRIN

Orally administered salicylates are absorbed from the gastrointestinal tract into the vascular system within 15 to 20 minutes. When this occurs salicylates are immediately detectable in the blood vessels of the stria vascularis and spiral ligament. Within 1 hour they are found in the outer tunnel of the organ of Corti, around the outer hair cells, and within Rosenthal's canal surrounding spiral ganglion cells. Within 2 hours the maximum concentration of salicylates is found in the perilymph at approximately one-fourth to one-third blood level concentration.

Some evidence shows that salicylates inhibit several transaminase dehydrogenase systems, which interfere with the transfer of hydrogen in hair cells, cochlear neurons, or both; however, light microscopy and electron microscopy have demonstrated no anatomic defects in the inner ear or hair cells including the stereocilia or in the eighth cranial nerve. No definite evidence to date shows permanent hearing loss with ingestion of salicylates. Generally, tinnitus occurs, and hearing loss, if it exists, is temporary and reverses.

AMINOGLYCOSIDES

Aminoglycosides are antibiotics so named because each contains amino sugars and glycosidic linkage. They are not adequately absorbed after oral administration, do not penetrate the blood-brain barrier, and are rapidly excreted by the kidneys. Antibiotics are administered by intramuscular or intravenous injection to treat gram-negative bacterial infections. It is not clear how these drugs pass from the bloodstream and enter the perilymph and endolymph; however, it is established that they appear in the perilymph, and their clearance from the perilymph is slower than clearance from blood serum. Aminoglycoside ototoxicity may involve two steps. The initial effect is on the phospholipids in the cell membrane, which is reversible and antagonized by calcium. The second effect is noncompetititve and irreversible. This step results in destruction of cochlear hair cells and sensory epithelium of the vestibular system.

Ototoxic effects tend to be either predominately vestibulotoxic or cochleotoxic. Vestibular toxicity creates selective destruction of hair cells in the crista ampullaris. Cochleotoxic effects destroy the outer hair cells beginning with the basal turn and progressing toward the apex. Inner hair cells are also destroyed. Interestingly, the inner hair cell damage tends to begin at the apical end of the cochlea although destruction of these cells can be quite varied in its pattern. Early changes in ototoxicity result in clubbing of the distal end of stereocilia, fusing of stereocilia into giant cilia, and vacuolization of cell bodies (Schacht, 1986). Continued destruction of sensory epithelium can occur after the termination of treatment and may be asymmetric. Secondary degeneration of cochlear neurons can be extensive.

When considered as a group, a 10 percent incidence of some degree of hearing loss is associated with aminoglycoside antibiotics (Quick, 1986). Occurrence and progression of hearing loss after cessation of treatment can occur with dihydro-streptomycin, gentamicin, and tobramycin. A change in hearing sensitivity occurs approximately 10 percent of the time with tobramycin, 16 percent of the time with gentamicin, and 2 percent of the time with netilmycin (Rybak and Matz, 1986). Generally, the initial stage of ototoxicity presents with loss of hearing sensitivity confined to the higher frequencies. If the loss progresses, all frequencies can be involved in a pattern that is usually flat to sloping in nature. Word recognition scores vary with the degree of hearing loss. The immittance battery is consistent with cochlear insult.

DIURETICS

Diuretics known to have significant ototoxic effects include furosemide and ethacrynic acid. These agents are termed *loop diuretics* because they inhibit the transport of chloride and thus sodium absorption from the distal segment of the loop of Henle in the nephron in the kidney. Additionally, ethacrynic acid inhibits glycolytic and respiratory energy in most cells. These loop diuretics influence ion pumps in the cochlear duct by blocking the transport of potassium chloride out of the marginal cells in the striae vascularis. Ethacrynic acid also allows increased penetration of aminoglycosides into the inner ear. Histologic changes from loop diuretic ototoxicity predominately affect the stria vascularis with edema and cystic changes. The dark cell areas of the vestibular system are also affected with the cystic changes. Ototoxic effects of these drugs are frequently temporary and reversible; however, severe tissue destruction produces permanent results and permanent dysfunction.

A 7 percent incidence of hearing loss occurs with furosemide (Tuzel, 1981). The hearing loss can be temporary or permanent and primarily involves the higher frequencies. Word recognition scores are generally good but will reflect the degree of pure tone sensitivity loss. The immittance battery produces findings typically associated with cochlear hearing loss.

CIS-*PLATINUM*

The potential for *cis*-platinum to produce hearing loss is well recognized. The reported incidence of hearing loss with this drug ranges from 9 to 91 percent. The loss of hearing sensitivity is usually bilateral and initially involves higher frequencies. Progression can occur with therapy. Tinnitus occurs in 2 to 26 percent of patients treated with *cis*-platinum and some evidence exists of reversibility for those with very mild hearing loss (Rybak and Matz, 1986). Figure 5-2 depicts progressive audiometric changes that occurred concomitantly with *cis*-platinum therapy.

MIDDLE EAR INFECTIONS AND TOXINS

Pathologic changes in the scala tympani of the inner ear occur in 82 percent of acute purulent and 77 percent of chronic purulent ears (Paparella et al., 1972). This work suggested that one sequelae of otitis media could include the diffusion of small molecules such as bacterial toxins and enzymes through the round-window membrane. This resulted in a serofibrinous precipitation in the scala tympani adjacent to the round-window membrane, which spread longitudinally up the scala tympani through the helicotrema into the scala vestibuli. Acute and chronic inflammatory cells may also enter the round-window membrane. Toxins and inflammatory cells penetrated the basilar membrane from the scala tympani and predominately invaded the endolymphatic system, first at the basal turn and progressed toward the apex. The outer hair cells were most vulnerable to damage; the stria vascularis was reasonably resistant. Endolymphatic hydrops sometimes occurred as a result of this serous labyrinthitis. These cochlear changes were associated with a slowly progressive high-frequency sensory hearing loss and the degree of loss correlated with duration of inflammation.

CARBON MONOXIDE POISONING

Carbon monoxide (CO) couples with hemoglobin to form carboxyhemoglobin. Carboxyhemoglobin prevents oxygen from combining with hemoglobin, which reduces the oxygen-carrying capacity of the blood. This results in acute or chronic ischemia. Autopsies on nonsurvivors of CO poisoning have revealed diffuse small hemorrhages, focal necrosis, edema, and demyelinization predominately within the brainstem and cerebrum, particularly the globus pallidus. It is usually lethal if carboxyhemoglobin reaches the level of 60 percent of available hemoglobin. Car-

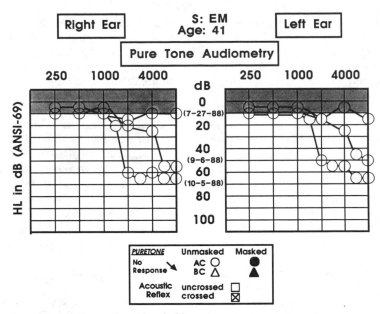

Figure 5-2. Progressive, permanent pure tone threshold changes that occurred during 2-month course of *cis*-platinum chemotherapy. Audiogram is baseline (7-27-88). Initial changes were noted at 1 month (9-6-88) and involved frequencies at 4000 Hz and above. The audiogram at 2 months (10-5-88) showed bilateral, moderately severe sensory involvement at frequencies beyond 1500 Hz. Word recognition ability was below normal when the 2-month audiogram was obtained.

diac and central nervous system symptoms occur at approximately 20 to 30 percent carboxyhemoglobin; however, vision and hearing systems may show decreased function at levels at or below 5 percent.

CO affects the vestibular system more commonly than it does the auditory system; however, symmetric, high-frequency sensory hearing loss resulting from chronic CO poisoning has been reported. Baker and Lilly (1977) described a case of acute CO poisoning that resulted in bilateral sensory hearing loss with a symmetric, trough-shaped audiometric configuration. Human and animal studies have shown hemorrhage and cellular degeneration within the inner ear, eighth nerve, and brainstem. Damage occurs predominately in the cochlear nuclei, vestibular nuclei, and spiral ganglion. The effect within the cochlea involves degeneration of the ganglion cells predominately at the basal turn, congestion of the stria vascularis, and vascularization of the cytoplasm of supporting cells. The hair cells are much more resistant to this type of ischemia than are the supporting cells or the acoustic nerve.

CONGENITAL AND DEVELOPMENTAL DISEASES

AURAL ATRESIA

The term *atresia* derives from the Greek *A*, meaning "none" or "negative" and *tresis* meaning "a hole." Hence, *atresia* denotes a complete absence or closure of a normal body orifice. *Stenosis*, on the other hand, means "narrowing of a stricture, duct, or body orifice without complete obstruction." These are anatomic statements and do not imply cause or time. Aural atresia may be congenital or acquired; however, most atresias occur within the congenital time frame, from fertilization to birth. Technically, *congenital aural atresia*, refers to the EAM; however, the term is used to imply other external and middle ear congenital anomalies.

The pinna, the EAM, the middle ear, and the inner ear must be determined prior to initiation of treatment. The condition of the pinna may be normal or microtic. *Microsia* refers to a pinna that is reduced in size. They are graded into types I, II, and III. The type I closely resembles the normal pinna but is reduced in size. The type II pinna forms the anatomic approximation of a question mark or a capital *I*. The type III does not resemble a pinna and simply exists as a mass of tissue. The most severe of all pinna configurations is its complete absence.

The condition of the EAM may be normal or reduced in diameter (stenotic) or completely closed (atretic). The stenosis of atresia may be from soft tissue or soft tissue and bone. The middle ear may be normal, or present mild to severe anatomic deviation. In like manner, the inner ear may be normal, mildly deformed, or severely deformed. Anatomic dysplasias of the inner ear may exist and these are described in the following section. A direct relationship exists between the severity of the pinna deformity and the middle and inner ear deformities. Distinct exceptions to this are congenitally drug-induced external and middle ear anomalies and certain hereditary conditions such as the trisomies and Treacher Collins syndrome.

The anatomic manifestations of aural atresia prevent efficient transmission of air-conducted sound to the inner ear. With the exception of very mild cases, the functional sequelae of aural atresia is usually conductive hearing loss with maximum air-bone gap. The involvement can be bilateral or unilateral. Associated malformations of the inner ear may introduce a sensory component (Crabtree, 1986). Bone conduction ABR testing is very useful in establishing inner ear function with infants and young children who present with aural atresia. This facilitates intervention by means of a bone conduction hearing aid in those cases of bilateral involvement with adequate cochlear function.

MONDINI'S DYSPLASIA

Mondini's dysplasia is a developmental disorder of the inner ear affecting the bony and membranous labyrinth of the auditory and vestibular systems. The presence of this deformity implies an early insult to inner ear development.

The spectrum of osseous and membranous abnormality is quite broad, ranging from very slight to almost total agenesis. It tends to be bilateral but asymmetric. The osseous abnormalities include a shortened, dilated cochlea, dilated vestibule, and shortened and dilated semicircular canals with decreased angle between the superior and horizontal canals. Within the cochlea there is a scala communis, which is an osseous dehiscence of the interscalar septum between the middle and apical coils.

The membranous abnormalities include dilatation of the saccule and endolymphatic duct, degeneration of the organ of Corti, and stria vascularis. Partial or complete cochlear and vestibular neuron loss may also be seen. In the more severe dysplasias, there may be a congenital dehiscence of the stapes footplate or absence of the round window membrane, or both. This may also be associated with congenital dehiscence of the medial wall of the vestibule, which would allow abnormal communication of cerebrospinal fluid into the dilated vestibule and, ultimately, through the stapes or round window dehiscences into the middle ear. This can result in recurrent meningitis, cerebrospinal fluid middle ear effusion, otorrhea, or rhinorrhea (Neely, 1985). A triad of profound congenital sensory hearing loss, profound vestibular weakness, and recurrent meningitis is associated with this severe Mondini malformation with anomalous cerebrospinal fluid continuity. Therefore, it is advisable that any child with a profound hearing loss, unilateral or bilateral, be screened for Mondini's malformation.

SCHEIBE'S DYSPLASIA

The Scheibe or cochleosacular dysplasia is a congenital malformation of the membranous labyrinth of the saccule and cochlea. Anatomically, the stria vascularis may be dysplastic or aplastic with occasional areas of hyperplasia. Reissner's membrane is frequently collapsed, suggesting a correlation between function of the stria vascularis and production of endolymphatic fluid. The tectorial membrane may be detached from hair cells and retracted to occupy the inner sulcus. Supporting elements of the organ of Corti may be distorted or collapsed and hair cells may be missing. The saccule is usually collapsed. Unlike some of the more severe cases of Mondini's dysplasia, the cochlear neurons remain normal throughout life.

Characteristically, Scheibe's and Mondini's inner ear dysplasia present with profound, bilateral sensory hearing loss (Northern and Downs, 1978); however, residual hearing has been reported. Schuknecht (1974) described a Mondini case that presented with a slowly progressive, bilateral, sensory hearing loss with poor word recognition scores. The final audiometric configuration was flat to 4000 Hz with no measurable hearing sensitivity at higher frequencies. Histologic examination of the temporal bone showed severe loss of basal hair cells and neurons with partial involvement throughout the rest of the cochlea.

TRISOMY DYSPLASIA

Trisomy refers to the individual having one extra chromosome. Ordinarily a normal individual has 46 chromosomes grouped into 23 pairs. An individual with this disorder has 47 chromosomes representing 23 pairs with a third chromosome included in one of the pairs, thus a trisomy. Trisomy can result in severe abnormalities that may or may not include those affecting the ear. *Trisomy 21*, meaning that there are three 21 chromosomes, is the common form of this disorder and type of *Down's syndrome*. Ear abnormalities are not usually part of this syndrome, although hearing loss has been reported (Northern and Downs, 1978). Two syndromes that are quite severe and may be incompatible with life are Pataus' syndrome (trisomy 13) and Edwards' syndrome (trisomy 18). These trisomies have characteristically external, middle, and inner ear abnormalities associated with low-set, poorly formed pinnae, EAC atresia, absence or reduction of the middle ear cleft, and aplasia of the striae vascularis and organ of Corti. The membranous labyrinth is collapsed and the saccular macula is underdeveloped. These syndromes also have eye, palate, and mandibular abnormalities.

DEVELOPMENTAL DELAYS

Developmental delays as well as the inner ear dysplasias are responsible for a significant percentage of congenital hearing loss. Often these conditions are associated with a number of different syndromes. The audiologic pattern is varied because of the range of cochlear developmental abnormalities (Northern and Downs, 1978; Schuknecht, 1974). The hearing loss is generally sensory in nature and spans from mild to profound in degree; however, the majority of losses are in the severe to profound category. The hearing loss may be present at birth or develop postnatally. The involvement is usually bilateral and relatively symmetric, but threshold asymmetry has been documented. There is no characteristic audiometric contour. The profile may be flat, sloping, rising, or parabolic in shape. Word recognition scores correlate with the degree of hearing loss and age of onset. Acoustic immittance testing usually shows type A tympanograms, and stapedius reflexes are often detected if the degree of loss is not severe.

Genetic sensory hearing loss may be present at birth or develop later in life (Jerger and Jerger, 1981). It occurs most often during childhood, and it is estimated that 50 percent of childhood hearing loss is genetic in nature. Genetic hearing loss tends to be stable if present at birth. On the other hand, a delayed onset is more associated with progressive loss.

It is critically important to identify infant and childhood deafness as early as possible (Dennis, 1987; Dennis et al., 1984). This facilitates procurement of suitable hearing aid amplification and initiation of appropriate remediation. The overall management of these patients involves a team of specialists from the disciplines of medicine, communication disorders, and education. Audiologists are specifically involved with the identification and monitoring of the hearing loss, selection of appropriate amplification, and, in some cases, the therapy process to develop or augment auditory and language abilities.

COLLAGEN AND AUTOIMMUNE DISEASES

AUTOIMMUNE INNER EAR DISEASE

At present the definition of *autoimmune inner ear disease* is relatively rapid or suddenly progressive bilateral, sensory hearing loss and concomitant vestibular involvement. The auditory and vestibular symptoms occur over a time frame from weeks to months. There may be fluctuation of symptoms similar to Ménière's disease. Factors that create a suspicion of immunological mediated insult are the presence of coincidental systemic immunologic disorders, increased sedimentation rate or C-reactive protein, presence of cryoglobulins or elevated serum complement levels, and symptomatic improvement with steroid treatment.

Autoimmune inner ear diseases can be localized only to the inner ear or secondary, with involvement of other organs (e.g., Cogan's syndrome). The temporal bone pathology seen in presumed autoimmune inner ear disease shows vasculitis, emptied and somewhat degenerated blood vessels, and a granulomatosis substrate (Hughes et al., 1986). Auditory and vestibular nerve pathology may also be involved with this disease.

Sensory hearing loss associated with autoimmune inner ear disease is usually described as progressive in nature, presenting with bilateral, asymmetric involvement (Hughes, 1984, 1987; McCabe, 1979, 1981). Developmentally, the time course of the hearing loss varies. It usually progresses over several weeks or months, with less frequent presentation of sudden hearing loss or hearing loss developing over a period of years. The loss of hearing sensitivity ranges from mild to profound degree, and word recognition scores vary with severity of the hearing loss. Immittance testing typically produces type A tympanograms with the presence of crossed and uncrossed stapedius reflexes determined by the degree of pure tone involvement; however, immittance testing profiles may reflect conductive disorder in those rare cases where there is occurrence of tissue destruction involving the external or middle ear.

Immunosuppressant medications have been documented to improve or stabilize hearing levels and word recognition ability in some patients with autoimmune otologic involvement. Consequently, hearing loss from autoimmune inner ear disease is one of the few forms of sensory deafness that may respond to treatment. The following case summary is an example from our series on steroid-responsive sensory hearing loss. A 65-year-old man in good health noticed decreased hearing beginning in June of 1986. The audiogram at that time showed a pure tone average of 40 dB HL on the right ear and 10 dB HL on the left ear. A repeat audiogram in October of 1986 revealed a pure tone average of 60 dB HL on the right and 18 dB HL on the left. In February of 1987 audiologic testing showed no change in pure tone hearing levels bilaterally; however, word recognition ability had decreased from 96 to 48 percent on the right ear. Likewise, the left ear score had deteriorated from 86 to 48 percent. Treatment with prednisone was initiated and the patient hospitalized for adjustment of steroid dosage. At discharge, audiometric pure tone averages were 45 dB HL for the right ear and 15 dB HL for the left ear. Word recognition scores were 84 and 90 percent for the right and left ears, respectively. The hearing levels and word recognition ability have remained stable in both ears with continued treatment.

COGAN'S SYNDROME

Cogan's syndrome is defined as nonsyphilitic, interstitial keratitis, acute unilateral or bilateral sensory hearing loss, and reduced vestibular response. This is a systemic disease that may affect other organs and can be fatal. The histopathology associated with this disease is an infiltrate of lymphocytes and plasma cells both in the cornea and the spiral ligament (McDonald, Vollertsen, and Younge, 1985).

ACQUIRED IMMUNODEFICIENCY SYNDROME

Acquired immunodeficiency syndrome (AIDS) interferes with the normal immune responsiveness of the body. This results in an increased susceptibility to infection, a higher incidence of malignancy, and occurrence of other autoimmune diseases, such as rheumatoid arthritis, systemic lupus erythematosus, idiopathic thrombocytopenia purpura, autoimmune hemolytic anemia, and Sjögren's syndrome (Campbell, Montanaro, and Bardana, 1983). The most common sites of infection are the paranasal sinuses, middle ear, and lungs. These infections tend to be chronic and unresponsive to antibiotics.

Information relating hearing loss to AIDS is limited but emerging. Flower and Sooy (1987) reported 14 percent of 54 AIDS patients had significant sensory hearing loss. These authors described a profile of bilateral, moderate to severe hearing loss principally involving the higher frequencies. They also reported a large number of ABR abnormalities. Real, Thomas, and Gerwin (1987) described a case report of unilateral sudden-onset sensory hearing loss in a patient diagnosed with AIDS. Although they speculated direct involvement of sensory auditory structures by the human immunodeficiency virus as a possible cause, the etiology of hearing loss in AIDS is likely multifactorial and awaits further study.

NEOPLASMS AND GROWTH

OSTEOMAS AND EXOSTOSES

Osteomas are single, unilateral pedunculated bony masses that occur at the lateral aspect of the EAM. They become symptomatic when they totally occlude the EAC. Osteomas in the EAC lead to conductive hearing loss if they become large enough to block the passage of air-conducted sound along the ear canal to the middle ear structures. The combination of a relatively large osteoma and accumulated cerumen and squamous debris can have the same effect (Smith, 1986). Although rare, osteomas may occur in the mastoid or about the IAM where they may compress the seventh and eighth cranial nerves.

Exostoses occur at the medial end of the EAC adjacent to the notch of Rivinus on the tympanosquamous and tympanomastoid suture lines. They are usually bilateral, small, and asymptomatic. These fairly common lesions are caused by repeated exposure of the EACs to cold water.

KERATOSIS OBTURANS AND EXTERNAL CANAL CHOLESTEATOMA

Keratosis obturans refers to a rare condition in which the EAC is obliterated by an accumulation of keratin and circumferential sheets of desquamated squamous epithelium. This lesion gradually erodes and enlarges the EAC and partially or completely occludes the EAM. Conductive hearing loss is present with complete occlusion of the canal. Keratosis obturans is sometimes associated with bronchiectasis of the lung.

External canal cholesteatoma is an expanding, bone destructive, squamous epithelial ulcerating lesion located in the floor of the EAC lateral to the osseous tympanic annulus. This type of cholesteatoma creates an accumulation of desquamated squamous epithelium and keratin. It is frequently associated with ulceration of the canal skin and exposure of bone, which may produce osteitis. Unlike keratosis obturans, it rarely produces a conductive hearing loss.

CHOLESTEATOMA

Cholesteatoma is a skin cyst or sac. The term *keratoma* better describes the true characteristic of this lesion. The three principal classifications are congenital, primary acquired, and secondary acquired cholesteatoma. The congenital cholesteatoma originates behind an intact tympanic membrane and is usually not infected unless it perforates the ear drum or bone of the EAM. The sites or origin for primary and secondary acquired cholesteatomas, respectively, include the pars flaccida and pars tensa areas of the tympanic membrane. These acquired cholesteatomas have openings to the external environment through "perforations" in respective areas of the ear drum. These "perforations" are not actual but simply represent the mouth or origin of the sac.

The pathology of cholesteatoma is the epidermal surface of the drum retracted into the middle ear, forming an ever-increasing squamous epithelial cyst. The cholesteatoma is composed of two parts: the matrix and the debris. The *matrix* is the lining of the cyst, and the *debris* is the contents of the cyst, which include desquamated squamous epithelial cells and keratin. This material fills the cyst and assists in its ever-increasing expansion and destructive capabilities. Cholesteatomas create a mass effect and are symptomatic relative to their location and production of bone destruction.

There is usually involvement of the ossicular chain during late development. Cholesteatomas can develop to the point of blocking the eustachian tube, thus producing middle ear effusion. Although rare, cholesteatomas can occur in the posterior fossa as isolated epidermal cysts of the meninges. These may be present as acoustic tumors; however, these lesions are unassociated with the previous description of cholesteatoma.

Cholesteatomas usually involve the middle ear but on rare occasions the site of the disorder may be cochlear or retrocochlear, or both. Typically, the pure tone audiogram shows a unilateral, conductive loss of hearing sensitivity that may have been gradual in onset. Degree of sensitivity loss varies from mild to moderately severe and depends on the encroachment of the lesion on the tympanic membrane and ossicular chain. In some cases the ossicular chain may be disrupted because of erosion that produces significant conductive loss; however, it is possible for the tumor to bridge, thereby functionally connect, the disrupted ossicular chain, producing very little conductive hearing loss (Martin, 1981). Word recognition scores are within normal bounds.

The immittance profile is also variable depending on the effect of the cholesteatoma on middle ear transmission. A type A_D tympanogram can result from ossicular disruption. Complete envelopment of the ossicular chain by the cholesteatoma may produce a type B tympanogram because of a mass effect. Finally, pressure on the ossicular chain by the cholesteatoma can yield a fixation profile or type A_S profile. Crossed and uncrossed stapedius reflexes may be present at normal levels, elevated in threshold, or absent, depending on the degree of hearing loss and the extent of the cholesteatoma involvement on the affected ear.

GLOMUS TUMORS

Glomus tumors are paragangliomas composed of the large polyhedral, neoplastic paraganglia cells and abundant vessels supplying them. These tumors are exceedingly vascular and bleed extensively when manipulated. They originate from paraganglion cell nests, which are scattered along the ninth and tenth cranial nerve sites in the mediastinum, the neck, the jugular bulb, and the middle ear.

There are several types of glomus tumors. An aggregate of paraganglion cells called the carotid body naturally occurs in the bifurcation of the carotid artery. Paragangliomas arising from this area are termed *carotid body tumors*. The paraganglion nests in the jugular bulb or middle ear are referred to as *glomus bodies*. Accordingly, paragangliomas originating from these locations are termed *glomus body tumors*. *Glomus jugulare tumors* arise in the adventitia of the jugular foramen between the jugular bulb and the jugular foramen. *Glomus tympanicum tumors* originate in the middle ear along Jacobson's nerve on the promontory. Glomus jugulare tumors may extend into the middle ear; glomus tympanicum tumors may course down into the jugular bulb.

Glomus tumors expand through available spaces and then ultimately destroy bone. They may extend into the petrous apex, in and around the internal carotid artery, and into the posterior fossa as they migrate medially about the otic capsule. Otic capsule invasion will damage the inner ear, and their expansion intracranially may impinge on the eighth nerve; however, their predominate presentation is conductive hearing loss with a low-pitched pulsatile tinnitus. In this instance they are usually visible as a red mass behind the tympanic membrane. However, they may also present as a low-pitched pulsatile tinnitus only, without conductive hearing loss and visibility behind the eardrum.

The glomus tympanicum tumor almost always produces conductive hearing loss since the primary site of the disorder is within the middle ear. The glomus jugulare tumor may cause conductive hearing loss by means of invasion of the middle ear space or sensory loss by bony erosion of the labyrinth (Graham and Kemink, 1986). The pure tone and acoustic immittance results produce patterns consistent with conductive or sensory involvement. Word recognition scores are usually within normal limits in those cases with conductive hearing loss and vary according to the degree of hearing loss in cases with sensory impairment. Periodic immittance changes that are synchronous with the patient's pulse rate can occur during immittance audiometry. These immittance fluctuations coincide in time with vascular changes within the tumor.

SQUAMOUS CELL CARCINOMAS

A squamous cell carcinoma is a malignant neoplasm of squamous epithelial cells. They usually originate from the ear canal skin, present as a nonhealing ulcer with granulation tissue in the EAC, and simulate an external otitis that tends not to heal. These neoplasms may become exophytic and partially or totally exclude the EAC. Direct extension can occur to the pneumatized spaces of the temporal bone, as well as externally into the temporomandibular joint and other adjacent skin without occluding the canal. They are frequently associated with a preexisting perforation of the tympanic membrane, which may be a chronic otitis media with intermittent or persistent suppurative discharge. Delay in diagnosis of the carcinoma can occur if the chronic otitis media draws attention away from the ulceration that exists in the EAC. These lesions may rapidly extend beyond the confines of the pneumatized spaces of the temporal bone and EAC to extend intracranially. Additionally, they can metastasize to the neck or other distant areas.

ACOUSTIC TUMORS

The term *acoustic tumor* is not a precise histologic description. It infers a neoplasm of whatever origin that affects the eighth cranial nerve. The tumor can arise from the nerve itself, or originate in adjacent tissues and secondarily involve the nerve by means of impingement. The term *acoustic neuroma* is also not a precise histologic description and implies a primary neurogenous tumor of the auditory nerve. The more precise terms that are histologically based and have clinical implication are those that describe the several types of primary neurogenous tumors that may affect the eighth nerve. These categories are the solitary schwannoma or neurilemoma, the multiple schwannoma or neurilemoma, and the neurofibroma associated with von Recklinghausen's neurofibromatosis. The most common is the solitary schwannoma and the second is the neurofibroma. These tumors are almost always benign.

Solitary schwannomas originate within the nerve and expand both within the nerve of origin and can become exophytic. As they expand, they displace remaining nerve fibers to their periphery and, over time, can ultimately consume all nerve fibers. The neurofibroma tends to be bilateral and associated with other neurogenous tumors such as meningiomas, other neurofibromas of the cauda equina in the spinal cord, and optic gliomas. The neurofibroma likewise begins in the nerve of origin, but unlike the solitary schwannoma it expands in a manner that incorporates the nerve fibers within its substance without total fiber destruction. Solitary schwannomas and neurofibromas may result in total loss of auditory function. Conversely, function may be partially or completely maintained even in cases of large tumors.

It is not possible to resect a neurofibroma and spare any nerve fibers. Near total resection of solitary schwannoma with preservation of some nerve fibers can occur in some cases; however, total solitary schwannoma resection with fiber preservation may not be possible (Neely, 1984). The mechanism by which these neurogenous tumors compromise the eighth nerve dysfunction remains unclear. Destruction and reduction of numbers of nerve fibers are obvious means; however, these alone do not account for the dysfunctions seen (Neely, 1981). Another suspected mechanism is change in myelin of the remaining nerve fibers (Neely and Hough, 1986; Neely et al., 1981).

Acoustic tumors produce sensorineural auditory dysfunction primarily through involvement of the eighth cranial nerve and secondarily the cochlea. A myriad of audiometric profiles can result. The hearing loss is usually unilateral in nature, and the degree of pure tone involvement ranges from normal to severe hearing levels. In

some cases, hearing is absent. A characteristic pure tone profile is unilateral sensorineural loss with greater involvement in the high frequencies rather than middle- or low-frequency regions (Jerger and Jerger, 1981). Word recognition scores are affected and can be disproportionately low compared to the amount of pure tone sensitivity loss. Typically, significant roll over is seen on the performance-intensity (PI) function.

The immittance battery generally produces a type A tympanogram. Crossed and uncrossed stapedius reflexes may be present at appropriate hearing levels when testing the involved side but more typically are elevated in threshold or absent. When these thresholds are present, it is relatively common to observe significant stapedius reflex decay when testing the involved ear at 500 and 1000 Hz. Tone decay (per stimulatory threshold adaptation) frequently occurs. The ABR has proved to be the most sensitive and specific audiologic test for detection of acoustic tumors (Jerger, 1983; Josey, Glasscock, and Musiek, 1988). ABR abnormalities in cases with acoustic tumor include significant interaural latency difference, prolonged absolute peak latencies, increased interwave intervals, and absence of the ABR when pure tone hearing levels range from normal to moderately severe. Figures 5-3 and 5-4 present preoperative audiologic and ABR data, respectively, obtained from a case with a 2-cm acoustic tumor confirmed by magnetic resonance imaging and the subsequent surgery.

Figure 5-3. Right acoustic tumor. This patient had noted a slowly progressive unilateral hearing loss with tinnitus for 8 years. The audiogram showed a right-sided sensory loss of hearing sensitivity of moderate degree. Sensitivity in the left ear was normal with the exception of a 4000 Hz notch. Interestingly, word recognition scores were normal on the right without roll over on the PI function. Crossed and uncrossed stapedius reflexes were absent when testing the right ear. This is a significant finding in the presence of a moderate degree of sensitivity loss.

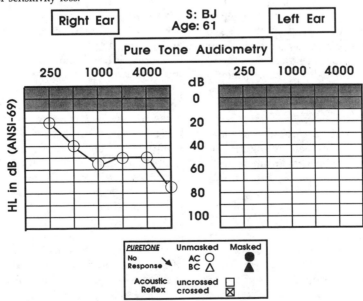

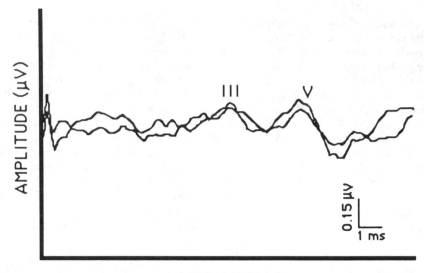

LATENCY (ms)

Figure 5-4. ABR results for right acoustic tumor case described in Figure 5-3. ABR findings were obtained at 95 dB nHL with appropriate contralateral masking. Note the dysmorphic waveforms with relatively poor intertrial repeatability. The absolute peak latency values of wavelets III and V were prolonged beyond the acceptable upper tolerance limits established for our instrumentation.

It should be mentioned that when the magnitude of hearing loss in the affected ear exceeds the moderately severe level, the more contemporary audiologic tests may produce ambiguous results because of the extent of the pure tone involvement. When this ambiguity occurs, the administration of one or more of the classic tests may assist in clarifying eighth nerve disorders.

MENINGIOMAS

Meningiomas are benign tumors that originate from arachnoid villi of the meninges. They affect the temporal bone by expanding from areas that contain arachnoid villi. These locations include the facial hiatus, the porous acousticus, the medial surface of the jugular bulb, and along the inferior or superior petrosal sinus. Lesions that extend into the posterior fossa usually present similarly to acoustic tumors; however, the tumor mass tends not to enter the IAM. Involvement of the seventh and eighth cranial nerves is secondary, thus, it is frequently possible to remove the meningioma and preserve nerves. Meningiomas have also been found to originate in the middle ear around the stapedius muscle and present as a vascular mass.

BRAINSTEM GLIOMAS

Gliomas are neoplasms arising from glial tissue within the brain. These tumors exist predominately above the tentorium in adults, and below the tentorium in children, often locating in the cerebellum or brainstem. Gliomas are classified by cellular origin and include astrocytomas, medulloblastomas, and glioblastomas. Brainstem tumors in children are predominately astrocytomas. Characteristically, astrocytomas are slow growing with wide infiltration of brain tissue. Interestingly, the involved brain areas often continue to function relatively well (Jerger, Neely, and Jerger, 1980).

Exophytic meningiomas and brainstem gliomas may grow into the cerebellopontine angle and produce audiologic signs similar to those observed in patients with acoustic tumors. Since these tumors usually arise outside the IAC, they must become large before producing signs and symptoms of eighth nerve involvement. Consequently, audiologic tests have a slightly lower detection rate because some of these tumors are not large enough to affect auditory function (Brackman and Gherini, 1986).

Brainstem gliomas, as well as other tumors that are intrinsic to the brainstem, produce long-tract auditory signs. Pure tone hearing sensitivity is often within normal limits, although there are occasions where mild, principally higher-frequency bilateral hearing loss can occur (Jerger and

Jerger, 1981). In most instances there is bilateral reduction in performance on degraded monotic word or sentence recognition tests. When the mass is eccentric to one side of the brainstem, there can be a greater degradation of speech recognition performance on the ear contralateral to the side of greater involvement. Crossed and uncrossed stapedius reflexes may be elevated or absent when the caudal brainstem is involved. ABR abnormalities are frequently encountered and are generally characterized by dysmorphic wave forms, delayed peak and interpeak latencies, and absent wavelets of the response complex. Although rare, meningiomas affecting the temporal lobe produce audiologic signs generally similar to those illustrated in the section describing the patterns seen for stroke patients. Serial audiometric measures have been used to measure the effects of tumor growth, exacerbation, and responses to therapy (Jerger, Neely, and Jerger, 1975).

OSSEOUS TUMORS

Lesions that create bone growth within the temporal bone are rare; however, a number of lesions will produce excessive bone. These are fibrous dysplasia, osteopetrosis, meningiomas, ossifying fibromas, metastic carcinomas (particularly from the prostrate or breast), Paget's disease, and osteosarcoma. Benign lesions tend to be painless and not create nerve injury. Malignant lesions are painful and produce early involvement of cranial nerves. These tumors frequently present as osseous obstruction of the EAM and dense bony lesions on x-ray of the temporal bone. Diagnosis is important and derived by clinical history, radiographic appearance, and biopsy (Schrimpf et al., 1982).

INFLAMMATORY DISEASES

RELAPSING POLYCHONDRITIS

Relapsing polychondritis is a rare systemic disease resulting in recurring inflammation of the cartilages of the body, both articular and nonarticular. The cartilages of the ear, nose, larynx, trachea, eustachian tube, and other areas of the body are recurrently involved. This condition causes the cartilage of the pinna to be erythematous, somewhat edematous, and tender. Involvement may be unilateral or bilateral. Sparing of the cartilaginous and osseous external canal clinically

differentiates this process from external otitis. Inflammation of the sclera and middle and inner ears, anemia, and fever are also associated with the disease.

Histologically, the cartilage shows chondrolysis and inflammation. The perichondrium also shows inflammation. Ultimately, the cartilage is destroyed and replaced by granulation tissue, which eventually becomes fibrous. Middle ear symptoms and conductive hearing loss predominately develop from serous effusions secondary to collapse of the eustachian tube. Sensory hearing loss or vestibular symptoms may result from vasculitis associated with the disease.

PERICHONDRITIS

Perichondritis and chondritis are the result of a bacterial infection of the perichondrium and cartilage of the pinna. The offending organism is usually *Pseudomonas aerguinosa*. This condition results from trauma such as an infected hematoma or burn of the pinna. It presents in the pinna only, is not intermittent, and does not have middle or inner ear involvement. Most frequently, it is unilateral. Without vigorous surgical and medical treatment, the cartilage of the pinna will ultimately necrose and the pinna will collapse into an unsightly convoluted mass.

WEGENER'S GRANULOMATOSIS

Wegener's granulomatosis is a presumed autoimmune disease characterized by the development of granulomas and vasculitis in specific target organs such as the upper and lower respiratory tracts and kidneys. Vasculitis resulting from Wegener's granulomatosis may occur anywhere in the body. The most common presentation is that of sinusitis with rhinorrea, fever, and general malaise. Ulcerative granulomatous lesions appear in the nose or sinuses. Involvement of the middle ear may be secondary to the nose and paranasal sinus infection or actual granulomatosis of the eustachian tube, middle ear, or tympanic membrane. Although rare, inner ear involvement can occur from direct extension of the granulomas through the round or oval windows and presumably vasculitis of the labyrinthine arteries.

Inflammatory processes such as Wegener's granulomatosis and relapsing polychondritis may involve the middle ear, mastoid, and eustachian tube, resulting in conductive hearing loss (Hughes, Barna, and Calbrese, 1986; Nadol, 1986). The overall audiologic pattern is similar to that described for otitis media with effusion, which is described in the following section. Invasion of the inner ear may produce severe sensory hearing loss.

MIDDLE EAR INFECTIONS AND EFFUSIONS

The five regions of pneumatization within the temporal bone are the middle ear, the mastoid, the petrous apex, the perilabyrinthine air cells, and the accessory air cells. Bacterial inflammation of the mucosal lining in any one of these spaces usually involves the other regional spaces to varying degrees. Consequently, otitis media, which refers to an inflammation in the middle ear, is also an inflammation of the other pneumatized spaces such as the mastoid and petrous apex; however, it should be mentioned that terms such as *mastoiditis* and *petrositis* are reserved for mastoid and petrous apex infections that have gone beyond the pneumatized spaces to involve surrounding bone or adjacent structures. Effusion or perfusion of fluid is frequently associated with the inflammation within the spaces.

The fluid is characterized as serous, mucinous, and suppurative or purulent. Serous fluid has less viscosity and is somewhat amber in color. Mucinous fluid is much more viscous and sometimes resembles glue. It is frequently hazy and translucent. Purulent or suppurative fluid is distinctly opaque and sometimes white or yellow. The clinical description of the fluid may be recognized by looking through the transparent or translucent tympanic membrane. Any one of these fluids contained behind an intact drum is referred to as an *effusion*. The fluids are termed *discharges* if they extrude from a tympanic membrane perforation. *Acute, subacute,* and *chronic* are terms that relate to duration of involvement. *Acute* refers to otitis media that has existed less than 3 weeks. *Subacute* means 3 weeks, to 3 months, duration, and *chronic* implies greater than three months of involvement. The bacteria causing the infection are usually gram-positive, penicillin, or penicillin-derivative sensitive and are likely to be single organism in nature. Perforations of the tympanic membrane result in involvement of more organisms that are often gram-negative and not penicillin sensitive. Acute bacterial suppurative otitis media will occur in approximately 80 percent of children between age 1 and 6 years.

Frequently, it requires 3 months for an acute infection to stage from suppurative to serous and ultimately dissipate down the eustachian tube. Severe acute or chronic inflammations may gradually occlude the nutrient arteries along the long process of the incus. This can result in avascular necrosis at the junction of the long process and the lenticular process of the incus and create an ossicular discontinuity. Inner ear involvement occurs by direct extension of ototoxic enzymes, chemicals, or, in rare instances, bacteria, through the round-window membrane. This can result in high-frequency sensory hearing loss as well as vestibular symptoms. It is wise, however, not to assume inner ear involvement is necessarily secondary to the middle ear infection. The inner ear dysfunction must be systematically evaluated independent of the middle ear condition, otherwise, concomitant diseases such as acoustic tumors may be missed.

Complications that have the potential to be devastating or fatal can occur from acute or chronic suppurative ear disease. These include meningitis, brain abscess, and hydrocephalus. Signs of potential complications include persistence of the disease despite treatment of acute infection for more than 2 weeks, persistent foul-smelling discharge, retro-orbital pain, lethargy, and headache.

Conductive hearing loss is the most frequent sequela of otitis media with effusion (Bess, 1986). The degree of air conduction hearing loss is variable and ranges from levels within normal bounds to hearing loss as great as 50 dB HL. Bilateral involvement is common. Fria et al. (1984) reported on the variability of air conduction thresholds in cases of middle ear disease with effusion. They concluded that the variability might be related to the presence or absence of air-fluid levels or bubbles in the fluid contained within the middle ear space, or both. Koko (1974) reported audiometric profiles from a cohort of individuals with middle ear effusion. These data included air conduction thresholds from 161 ears and bone conduction thresholds for 122 ears. The typical air conduction audiometric contour was usually flat with a slight rise in the profile peaking at 2000 Hz. The average degree of air conduction hearing loss throughout the speech frequency range was 28 dB HL. The average bone conduction hearing level was 3 dB HL, producing an average air-bone gap of 25 dB HL.

Word recognition scores are typically within normal limits. The immittance battery produces a flat, type B, or rounded tympanometric shape. Tympanometry enjoys a high rate of sensitivity for the detection of middle ear effusion; however, test specificity is low, which means that tympanometry often produces an unacceptably high rate of false-positives when used for detection of middle ear disease with effusion. Uncrossed stapedius reflexes are typically absent when the sound-eliciting stimulus is presented to the involved side. Crossed stapedius reflexes can be absent or elevated. Figure 5-5 shows the audiologic findings for a 5-year-old boy with acute serous otitis media. Persistent cases of otitis media with effusion have been shown to produce a sensory component to the hearing loss. Generally, the audiometric contour is sloping in these patients (Jerger and Jerger, 1981), and word recognition scores may be slightly reduced.

LABYRINTHITIS

Inflammation of the labyrinth usually affects the auditory and vestibular components, which can create sensory hearing loss and vertigo with nystagmus. Agents creating the inflammation are

Figure 5-5. Pure tone and immittance audiometric findings for otitis media with effusion. The hearing loss was conductive in nature, mild in degree, and symmetric. Word recognition scores were within normal limits. The tympanometric profile reflected the commonly encountered type B. The absence of crossed and uncrossed stapedius reflexes supported the presence of bilateral, conductive disorder.

viri, bacteria, or their toxic products. Viri enter the labyrinth by hematogenous dissemination predominately through modialor vessels. Bacteria and bacterial toxic products enter the labyrinth from the middle ear through the round-window membrane, the cerebrospinal fluid, or the IAC. It is important to differentiate viral labyrinthitis from labyrinthitis secondary to middle ear infection because the latter may be life-threatening. Viri known to hematogenously disseminate to the labyrinth in utero or in postnatal life are mumps, measles, rubella, cytomegalic inclusion virus (CMV), and a host of other respiratory organisms. They may create mild to severe auditory and vestibular deficits. Sudden idiopathic sensory hearing loss with or without vertigo is presently presumed to be caused by viral labyrinthitis.

Labyrinthitis from middle ear infection is unilateral and classified into three types. Serous labyrinthitis occurs when toxic products of bacteria enter the perilymphatic space through the round window or secondary defects in the otic capsule. Bacterial labyrinthitis can result from bacterial invasion through the round window or via secondary otic capsule defects from trauma, congenital dehiscences, or infection. Chronic labyrinthitis occurs when soft tissue enters the perilymphatic spaces usually from destruction of the otic capsule over the horizontal semicircular canal from erosive cholesteatoma. The presence of soft tissue alone may be totally asymptomatic unless manipulated mechanically or with air pres-

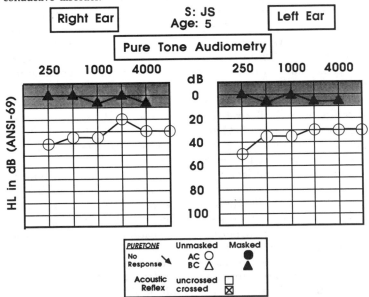

sure. When manipulated, sudden severe vertigo can occur. This secondary defect in the otic capsule creates a path for toxic bacteria products or bacteria to enter the labyrinth.

The imminent danger with labyrinthitis from middle ear infection is the potential for total destruction of the inner ear and rapid development of meningitis from spread of the infection from the labyrinth to the cerebrospinal fluid. Serous or toxic labyrinthitis tends to be less severe in its effects on hearing and vestibular function; however, it may precede bacterial labyrinthitis by minutes to hours or occur concomitantly with the onset of bacterial labyrinthitis. These patients need to be identified immediately and hospitalized for medical and surgical treatment.

Hearing loss associated with mumps occurs rapidly and is unilateral in approximately 80 percent of reported cases (Davis, 1986; Northern and Downs, 1978). The hearing loss is sensory in nature and typically ranges from severe to profound in degree. When there is measurable hearing sensitivity, the high frequencies seem to be more affected than the lower frequencies. Word recognition ability, if existent, is very severely affected. The tympanometric pattern is generally a type A, and crossed as well as uncrossed stapedius reflexes are usually absent when stimulating the affected side because of the degree of hearing loss.

Maternal rubella occurring in the first trimester of pregnancy reportedly produces hearing loss in 50 percent of the infants that survive the pregnancy (Davis, 1986; Northern and Downs, 1978). Hearing loss occurs approximately 10 to 20 percent of the time in those instances where maternal rubella occurred in the second or third trimester of pregnancy (Davis, 1986). Rubella deafness is principally sensory in nature, although conductive overlay can occur. The degree of hearing loss is usually severe to profound and bilateral. The audiometric contour generally reflects a flat hearing loss at all frequencies or one that gently slopes toward the higher-frequency range. One report, however, presented children having parabolic audiograms with the greatest degree of hearing loss occurring between 500 and 2000 Hz (Bordley and Alford, 1970). Word recognition scores are very poor and in some cases there may be progression of hearing loss. Ames et al. (1970) described central auditory disorders in some children with congenital rubella. They presented a clinical picture of delayed speech-language development in the face of normal or near-normal hearing sensitivity.

Hearing loss in children with congenital or prenatally acquired CMV infection is reported as high as 40 percent in those that survive the neonatal period (Davis, 1986). The hearing loss is sensory in nature and frequently involves both ears to a severe or profound degree. The audiometric contour is variable, but usually there is a greater loss for the higher frequencies. Unilateral, sensory hearing loss ranging from moderate to severe has also been reported. In some cases the hearing loss is progressive. Word recognition scores vary with the degree of hearing loss but are usually severely reduced. The immittance profile generally shows a type A tympanogram with absent stapedius reflexes. Harris et al. (1984) reported five cases of hearing loss in a group of fifty children with congenital CMV. Four of these cases had bilateral profound sensory hearing loss, and a fifth case had presumed mild sensory loss. Mild to moderate sensory hearing losses have been reported among children with subclinical CMV. Johnson et al. (1986) concluded, however, that *perinatally* acquired CMV infection is not associated with significant sensory hearing loss in premature or full-term infants through age 3.

MENINGITIS

Meningitis is an inflammation of the meninges. Usually the leptomeninges (pia and arachnoid) are involved. The pachymeninges (dura) may be involved in certain conditions. Viri and bacteria are by far the most common causal organisms; however, hosts of other more esoteric organisms may cause meningitis. Bacteria from meningitis may enter the IAM and ultimately reach the labyrinth by means of the modiolus and perilymphatic canaliculi in the osseous spiral lamina. Bacterial invasion of the labyrinth creates a severe destructive process and frequently incites obliteration of the otic capsule with ultimate generation of fibrous tissue and bone within the inner ear. Auditory brainstem involvement has been documented (Ozdamar, Kraus, and Stein, 1983). Bacterial labyrinthitis from meningitis is typically bilateral and devastating.

Hearing loss associated with meningitis is predominately sensory in nature, presents with bilateral involvement, and is frequently severe to profound in degree (Guiscafre et al., 1984; Martin, 1981). Infrequently, unilateral sensory hearing loss may occur (Ruben, 1983). Word recognition scores vary but are usually markedly depressed. Immittance audiometry typically illustrates a type A tympanogram unless there is an associated middle ear involvement. Crossed and uncrossed stapedius reflexes are usually absent with sound delivered to the involved ear.

Mild to moderate hearing losses following meningitis have been reported (Rosenhall and Kankkunen, 1980). These authors also reported complete or partial recovery of hearing in some patients with hearing loss following meningitis. Keane et al. (1983) reviewed 100 cases of meningitis in which audiologic assessment had been obtained. They found six cases of sensory hearing loss, which ranged in degree from mild to profound. There were five cases of bilateral and one case of unilateral hearing loss. The audiometric profile was typically bilateral and symmetric with a flat or gradually sloping audiogram. One of the cases reported by these authors initially presented with a severe sensory loss with no word recognition ability. The hearing deficit recovered to a mild loss with good word recognition ability. Fluctuating hearing loss following meningitis has been described (Rosenhall and Kankkunen, 1981). This has been associated with a presumed endolymphatic hydrops as well as overlying middle ear effusion.

Lebel et al. (1988) recently concluded that administration of dexamethasone significantly reduced the incidence of moderate to profound sensory hearing loss in 102 patients with bacterial meningitis. Although this report is encouraging, there has been some criticism of the methodology used (Smith, 1988).

SYPHILIS

Histopathologically, syphilis affects the eighth nerve and labyrinth directly or affects the bone by osteitis and secondarily involves the membranous labyrinth. Histologically, the bone involvement is an inflammatory osteitis with areas of rarification, round-cell infiltration, giant cells, and endarteritis. Histologic involvement of the inner ear shows early mononuclear leukocytic infiltration and obliterative arteritis with ultimate endolymphatic hydrops, perilymphatic fibrous tissue proliferation, and destruction of the organ of Corti and cochlear neurons (Schuknecht, 1974).

Sudden, progressive, or fluctuating, bilateral, nearly symmetric sensory hearing loss may be caused by syphilitic infection of the labyrinth or eighth nerve, or both. Both acquired and congenital syphilis may be involved. Late, or tardive, congenital syphilis is most frequently involved as a cause of sensory loss of obscure origin meeting this criteria. Neural syphilis, particularly symptomatic neural syphilis, has a much higher incidence of sensory hearing impairment; however, the incidence of neural syphilis is exceedingly small.

Early acquired syphilitic hearing loss occurs during secondary syphilis (Saltiel, Melmed, and Portnoy, 1983) and is usually sudden, rapidly progressive, and affects both ears. Late acquired luetic hearing loss generally occurs during the tertiary stage of syphilis. The audiologic pattern is similar to that of late congenital syphilitic deafness.

Acoustic immittance results in congenital and acquired syphilitic hearing loss generally produces normal middle ear mobility. Crossed and uncrossed stapedius reflexes are frequently present at hearing levels consistent with cochlear hearing loss; however, stapedius reflexes are absent in cases of severe to profound impairment and may be elevated or absent when there is neural involvement. Although relatively infrequent, presentation of secondary middle ear involvement will produce a conductive signature to the immittance findings. Finally, pure tone hearing sensitivity and word recognition ability have been shown to improve or fluctuate during drug therapy.

Diagnosis of syphilis is best done by the fluorescent treponemal antibody absorption serologic test (Zoller et al., 1978). Some luetic hearing losses are reversible or are partially reversible with early detection and immediate treatment with high doses of intravenous penicillin and oral steroids (Pillsbury and Shea, 1979; Wong et al., 1977). Unfortunately, the treponemes pallida, the spirochetes resulting in syphilis, have been demonstrated in body fluids and tissues after tremendous doses of penicillin (Schuknecht, 1974).

DEGENERATIVE AND IDIOPATHIC DISEASES

MENIERE'S DISEASE

Ménière's disease is a clinical diagnosis characterized by fluctuating cochlear hearing loss and episodic vertigo that is ultimately discovered to be idiopathic. These symptoms coincide or one may precede in time. Remission of symptoms often occurs and frequency of attacks is variable. Histologic evidence has shown endolymphatic system distention with displacement of membranous structures and possible rupture (Schuknecht, 1974). Patients with similar symptoms, that is, Ménière's disease in which a probable cause is identified, are said to have the disease most associated with that cause (e.g., perilymphatic fistula) and are not diagnosed as Ménière's disease. Patients with Ménière's disease may show little or no endolymphatic hydrops; however, hydrops of the pars inferior still remains the most significant correlate of Ménière's disease (Paparella, 1984).

The classic audiologic description of early Ménière's disease is fluctuating unilateral sensory hearing loss, tinnitus, and vertigo. At this stage of the disease, there is generally greater loss of hearing sensitivity for the lower test frequencies. The onset of vertigo may be preceded by feelings of pressure or fullness in the ear (Jerger and Jerger, 1981). During the early stages of the disease, these symptoms may exhibit a complete remission. As the disease continues, the hearing loss typically progresses to a moderate or moderately severe sensory impairment. The configuration changes to a relatively flat profile. Word recognition scores are reduced from normal and are consistent with the degree of hearing loss and shape of the pure tone audiometric profile. Immittance findings show a type A tympanogram. Crossed and uncrossed stapedius reflexes are generally present at hearing levels below 100-dB HL. Stapedius reflex decay results and ABR are usually consistent with a cochlear site of involvement. The hearing loss is unilateral in approximately 80 percent of patients (Pulec, 1976). Electrocochleography has shown an enlarged summating potential amplitude in patients with symptoms of Ménière's disease (Coats, 1981).

SUDDEN IDIOPATHIC SENSORY HEARING LOSS

Sudden sensory hearing losses can result from numerous etiologies that may be potentially harmful or correctable. Possible causes must be thoroughly investigated before assuming the hearing loss is idiopathic in nature. Theories of etiology for idiopathic sudden sensory hearing loss include labyrinthine membrane ruptures, viral infections, vascular insults, and autoimmune inner ear diseases. Specific support for the viral autoimmune etiologies is increasing (Cole and Jarhsdoerfer, 1988).

Sudden idiopathic sensory hearing loss is usually unilateral, severe to profound in degree, with poor word recognition ability. Byl (1978) reported an incidence of approximately 11 cases per 100,000 individuals. In some instances, the degree of loss can be mild to moderate (Jerger and Jerger, 1981). When hearing sensitivity can be measured, the audiometric contour is more often flat, but sloping and rising audiograms have been reported (Sheehy, 1960). In unilateral cases the Stenger test is negative. Immittance findings show a type A tympanogram. Tone decay testing, PI functions, stapedius reflex testing, and ABR results may be consistent with cochlear or eighth nerve site of involvement.

Serial audiometric measurements are important in cases of idiopathic sensory hearing loss since partial to full recovery has been documented (Mattox and Simmons, 1977). Snow (1973) reported that one-third of patients with sudden idiopathic sensory hearing loss stabilized with permanent impairment across the frequency range. One-third recovered thresholds within the mild to severe range, and one-third recovered to normal. If recovery occurs, findings on specialized tests that reflected cochlear or eighth nerve site may produce normal findings (Jerger and Jerger, 1981). Byl's data (1978) indicated that spontaneous recovery occurs in about 25 to 50 percent of cases. Additionally, recovery appeared to occur a greater number of times in those cases that were medically treated within 10 days of the onset of symptoms.

MULTIPLE SCLEROSIS

Multiple sclerosis (MS) is a static or progressive demyelinating disease within the central neural axis that creates areas of demyelinization and gliosis called plaques. Symptoms occur when these plaques are active and changing. Signs and symptoms of the lesion may be silent when the anatomy of these plaques is static, even though demyelinization still exists. Occasionally, MS will affect the auditory system. Histopathology has verified involvement of the auditory tracts within the brainstem (Arnold and Bender, 1983).

Basic pure tone and speech audiometric tests do not provide predictable characteristic audiologic data that can be generally associated with MS. The seminal work of Nofsinger et al. (1972) provided comprehensive audiologic data on 66 MS patients. These authors reported that 88 percent of the ears studied had pure tone sensitivity within normal bounds through the speech frequencies. When pure tone hearing loss was present, it tended to be bilateral, sensory in nature, with a maximum loss confined to the higher-frequency regions. However, greater loss of sensitivity in the lower frequency regions has been reported (Cohen and Rudge, 1984).

Word recognition scores on the average are high, but the variation is considerable, and in some instances these scores may be substantially lower than one would expect on the basis of the pure tone levels. Roll over on the PI function can be seen with MS patients. Although crossed and uncrossed stapedius reflexes may be present at expected hearing levels, it is fairly common for these reflexes to be elevated, absent, or present with significant reflex decay (Keith et al., 1987). A high percentage of MS patients show abnormalities on the ABR (Robinson and Rudge, 1977; Starr and Achor, 1975; Stockard and Sharbrough, 1977). These abnormalities include lack of ABR in the presence of relatively good pure tone hearing sensitivity, absence of later wavelets of the ABR complex, delayed absolute peak latencies, prolonged interwave latencies, and significant degredation of the ABR at fast click rate presentation (Jacobson, Murray, and Deppe, 1987). The ABR is an extremely useful audiologic test with the MS population.

Generally, audiologic tests indicate eighth nerve or brainstem involvement, or both. Audiologic abnormalities noted when a patient is symptomatic may fully or partially return to normal during periods of remission (Jerger and Jerger, 1981).

PRESBYCUSIS

Presbycusis is a term reserved for hearing loss that is caused only by advancing age. Many individuals labeled as presbycusic may be identified as having a familial- or genetic-related hearing loss (Lowell and Paparella, 1977). Schuknecht (1974) has described four types of presbycusis by audiometric profile and light microscopic temporal bone studies. Sensory presbycusis is characterized by atrophy of the organ of Corti in the basal turn, creating an abrupt high-frequency sensory hearing loss. There is concomitant light microscopic evidence of atrophy of the hair cells and their supporting cells to a degree consistent with the hearing loss. Neural presbycusis is described by loss of cochlear neurons with preservation of hair cells and supporting structures. This is ac-

companied by a high-frequency sensory loss with disproportionately low speech recognition scores. Strial presbycusis is characterized by atrophy of the stria vascularis, with flat sensory hearing loss and excellent word recognition. Finally, Schuknecht described cochlear conductive presbycusis, a condition in which light microscopy fails to identify sensory or neural degeneration sufficient to explain a sloping sensory hearing loss.

Recently, electronmicroscopy of the ear and careful light microscopic studies of the central nervous system have confirmed and expanded these earlier observations. Electronmicroscopy has shown primary hair cell and supporting cell degeneration in the basal turn of the cochlea with secondary neural degeneration consistent with sensory presbycusis (Nadol, 1988). Electronmicroscopy has been particularly important in identifying neuron loss in patients with descending audiometric profiles. These changes included reduced numbers of synapses at the base of the hair cells, degenerative changes and abnormalities in the arborizing dendrites to the hair cells, and degeneration of the fibers in the osseous spiral lamina and spiral ganglion cells. These findings further explain neural presbycusis and may be somewhat supportive of the existence of cochlear conductive loss (Nadol, 1979, 1988). Electronmicroscopy has also identified marked thickening of the basilar membrane, particularly in the basal turn due to increased numbers of fibrils and accumulation of amorphous osmiophilic material. This adds morphologic support to the concept of cochlear conductive presbycusis (Nadol, 1979). Light microscopy studies of the cochlear nuclei have identified neuron loss as high as 50 percent in presbycusic patients compared to normal (Arnesen, 1982).

The typical audiologic pattern seen for presbycusis is a slowly progressive, bilateral, sloping sensory loss of hearing sensitivity that is usually symmetric in nature. Presbycusic patients frequently complain of a high-pitched tinnitus. Jerger and Jerger (1981) noted greater high-frequency loss due to presbycusis in males than in females. Conversely, they described greater hearing loss in females in the low-frequency range. Word recognition scores may be typical or greater than might be expected on the basis of the hearing loss. There may be significant roll over on the PI function. The immittance battery shows a normal tympanogram. Stapedius reflexes are usually present at expected hearing levels but may show abnormality in terms of elevation, absence, or reflex decay. Abnormalities may be noted on the ABR (Jerger and Hall, 1980). In general, the audiologic pattern may show cochlear or retrocochlear disorder. Central speech audiometric deficits have been widely reported (Jerger, 1973; Jerger and Hayes, 1977; Orchik and Burgess, 1977; Welsh, Welsh, and Healy, 1985).

OTOSCLEROSIS

Otosclerosis is an autosomal dominant inherited disease of the otic capsule characterized by localized, abundant hypervascular bone with reduced density. This condition eventually ankyloses or subluxes the stapes footplate. The penetrance of this inherited disease is approximately 40 percent (Causse and Causse, 1984).

The oval window at the fistula antefenestra is the most frequent site of lesion. Other less frequent sites include the margins of the round window and the apical medial wall of the cochlea (Schuknecht and Barber, 1985). Pathologic progression of the lesions occurs, but it is variable between lesions and individuals. An early age of onset is correlated with greater involvement of the stapes footplate and obliteration of the oval-window niche. A later age of onset is associated with reduced involvement of the stapes footplate, predominately at the anterior pole (Gristwood and Venables, 1982).

Some patients with otosclerosis have concomitant progressive mixed hearing loss with a significant sensory component. Approximately 84 percent of these patients will demonstrate low-density lesions in the otic capsule adjacent to the cochlea and semicircular canals. Virtually all of these cases can be found to demonstrate decreased absorption in the otic capsule (Valvassori and Dobben, 1985), and the presence of a labyrinthine otosclerosis is irrefutable, both radiographically and histologically (Schuknecht and Barber, 1985); however, the term *cochlear otosclerosis* is often used to denote a controversial and unproved assumption of cause and effect. The assumption is that the sensory hearing loss in patients with otosclerosis is caused by the otosclerotic lesion or cochlear otosclerosis. This is an erroneous use of the term because to this date, the size, the cellular activity, and the location of the otosclerotic lesions within the otic capsule are not correlated with the magnitude of the sensory hearing loss (Schuknecht and Barber, 1985).

A slowly progressive, conductive hearing loss is characteristic of otosclerosis. A ringing or hissing tinnitus may accompany later stages of the hearing loss (Wofford, 1981). Initially, the pure tone sensitivity loss is principally confined to the lower frequencies. This audiometric pattern reflects a stiffness-dominated middle ear transmission system. The hearing loss is usually bilateral, and as stapes fixation progresses, the audiometric contour obtains a relatively flat profile. Very late in the disease there may be some downward slope to the higher frequencies (Houck and Harker, 1986). The hearing loss stabilizes at moderate to moderately severe hearing level. Word recognition scores are within normal limits. The tympanometric profile usually shows a normal pressure compliance function; however, the peak compliance may be somewhat diminished, as characterized by the type A_s tympanogram. Crossed and uncrossed stapedius reflexes are usually absent. During the initial stages of the disease, a diphasic acoustic reflex may be seen, which is characterized by a brief impedance or compliance change that coincides in time with the onset and offset of the reflex-eliciting stimulus.

The bone conduction line on the audiogram often forms a characteristic shape with maximum threshold depression occurring at 2000 Hz. This is termed the *Carhart notch* and was originally described by Carhart in a report that is now considered one of the classics of the audiologic literature (Carhart, 1950). Specifically, bone conduction threshold elevation averages 5, 10, 15 and 5 dB at 500, 1000, 2000, and 4000 Hz, respectively. These "thresholds" represent mechanical artifact introduced by the disease and do not reflect actual organic hearing sensitivity. The notch is likely due to the disease altering the overall contributions of middle ear and ossicular chain resonance to the total bone conduction response. The reader is referred to the work of Tondorff (1971) for further study.

REFERENCES

Ames, M. D., Plotkin, S. A., Winchester, R. A., and Atkins, T. E. (1970). Central auditory imperception: A significant factor in congenital rubella deafness. *Journal of the American Medical Association, 213,* 419.

Arnesen, A. R. (1982). Presbycusis — loss of neurons in the human cochlear nuclei. *Journal of Laryngology and Otology, 96*(6), 503–511.

Arnold, J. E., & Bender, D. R. (1983). BSER abnormalities in a multiple sclerosis patient with normal peripheral hearing acuity. *American Journal of Otology, 4*(3), 235–237.

Baker, S. R., & Lilly, D. J. (1977). Hearing loss from acute carbon monoxide intoxication. *Annals of Otology, 86,* 323–328.

Barber, H. (1969). Head injury: Audiological and vestibular findings. *Annals of Otology, Rhinology, and Laryngology, 78,* 239–252.

Bergstrom, L., Neblett, L. M., Sando, I., Hemenway, W. G., & Harrison, G. D. (1974). *Archives of Otolarygology, 100,* 117–121.

Bess, F. B. (1986). Audiometric approaches used in the identification of middle ear diseases in children. In J. E. Kavanaugh (Ed.), *Otitis media and child development.* Parkton, MD: York Press.

Bhatia, P. L., Gupta, O. P., Agarwal, M. K., & Mishr, S. K. (1977). Audiological and vestibular tests in hypothyroidism. *Laryngoscope, 87,* 2082–2089.

Bordley, J. E., & Alford, B. R. (1970). The pathology of rubella deafness. *International Audiology, 9,* 58.

Brackman, D. E., & Gherini, S. G. (1986). Differential diagnosis of skull base neoplasms involving the posterior fossa. In C. W. Cummings et al. (Eds.), *Otolaryngology — Head and neck surgery* (pp. 3421–3426). St. Louis: C.V. Mosby.

Byl, F. (1978). Sudden Hearing Loss Research Clinic. *Otolaryngology Clinics of North America, 11,* 71.

Campbell, S. M., Montanaro, A., & Bardana, E. J. (1983). Head and neck manifestations of autoimmune disease. *American Journal of Otolaryngology, 4,* 187–216.

Carhart, R. (1950). Clinical application of bone conduction audiometry. *Archives of Otolaryngology, 51,* 798.

Causse, J. R., and Causse, J. B. (1984). Otospongiosis as a genetic disease. Early detection, medical management, and prevention. *American Journal of Otology, 5*(3), 211–223.

Coats, A. C. (1981). The summating potential in Ménière's disease. 1. Summating potential amplitude in Ménière and non-Ménière ears. *Archives of Otolaryngology, 107,* 199–208.

Cohen, M., & Rudge, P. (1984). The effect of multiple sclerosis on pure tone thresholds. *Acta Oto-laryngologica (Stockholm), 97*(3–4), 291–295.

Cole, R. R., & Jahrsdoerfer, R. A. (1988). Sudden hearing loss: An update. *American Journal of Otology, 9*(3), 211–215.

Crabtree, J. A. (1986). Surgery for congenital atresia. In R. J. Wiet & J. B. Causse (Eds.), *Complications in otolaryngology-head and neck surgery: Vol. 1. Ear and skullbase* (pp. 91–96). Toronto: B.C. Decker.

Davis, L. E. (1986). Infections of the labyrinthe. In C. W. Cummings et al. (Eds.), *Otolaryngology — head and neck surgery* (pp. 3137–3147). St. Louis: C.V. Mosby.

Dennis, J. M. (1983). Atypical acoustic reflex results in ossicular chain discontinuity. *Audiology, 8*(12), 114–117.

Dennis, J. M. (1987). Using the auditory brainstem response in the operating room as a means of detection and prevention of hearing loss in infants and children. In K. P. Gerkin & A. Amochaev (Eds.), Hearing in infants: Proceedings from the National Symposium. *Seminars in Hearing, 8,* 115–123.

Dennis, J. M. (1988). Intraoperative monitoring with evoked responses. *Seminars in Hearing, 9.*

Dennis, J. M., & Earley, D. A. (1988). Monitoring surgical procedures with the auditory brainstem response. In J. M. Dennis (Ed.), Intraoperative monitoring with evoked responses. *Seminars in Hearing, 9,* 113–125.

Dennis, J. M., Earley, D. A., & Neely, J. G. (1987). *Predictive value of intraoperative evoked potential monitoring.* Paper presented at the annual meeting of the American Speech-Language-Hearing Association.

Dennis, J. M., Sheldon, R., Toubas, P., & McCaffree, M. A. (1984). Identification of hearing loss in the neonatal intensive care unit population. *American Journal of Otology, 5,* 201–205.

Flower, W. M., & Sooy, C. D. (1987). AIDS: An introduction for speech language pathologists and audiologists. *ASHA, 11,* 25–30.

Fria, T. J., Cantekin, E. I., Eichler, J. A., Mandel, E. M., & Bluestone, C. D. (1984). The effect of otitis media with effusion ("secretory otitis media") on hearing sensitivity in children. In D. J. Limb, C. D. Bluestone, J. O. Klein, & J. D. Nelson (Eds.), *Recent advances in otitis media with effusion.* Philadelphia: B.C. Decker.

Graham, M. D., & Kemink, J. L. (1986). Neoplasms. In C. W. Cummings et al. (Eds.), *Otolaryngology — head and neck surgery* (pp. 351–352). St. Louis: C.V. Mosby.

Gristwood, R. E., & Venables, W. N. (1982). A note on progression of the otosclerotic focus. *Clinical Otolaryngology, 7*(4), 257–260.

Guiscafre, H., Benitez-Diaz, L., Martinez, M. C., & Munoz, O. (1984). Reversible hearing loss after meningitis. Prospective assessment using auditory evoked responses. *Annals of Otology, Rhinology, and Laryngology, 93*(3, Pt. 1), 229–232.

Harper, J. G. (1981). Hearing and adult onset diabetes mellitus. *Otolaryngology — Head and Neck Surgery, 89,* 322–327.

Harris, S., Ahlfors, K., Ivarsson, S., Lernmark, B., & Svanberg, L. (1984). Congenital cytomegalovirus infection and sensorineural hearing loss. *Ear & Hearing, 5,* 352–355.

Helms, J. (1976). Acoustic trauma from the bone cutting burr. *Journal of Laryngology and Otology, 90,* 1143–1149.

Houck, J. R., & Harker, L. A. (1986). Otosclerosis. In C. W. Cummings et al. (Eds.), *Otolaryngology — head and neck surgery* (pp. 3095–3112). St. Louis: C.V. Mosby.

Hughes, G. B. (1987). Current controversies in autoimmune inner ear disease. *Insights in Otolaryngology, 2*(6). St. Louis: C.V. Mosby.

Hughes, G. B., Barna, B. T., & Calabrese, L. H. (1986). Manifestations of systemic disease. In C. W. Cummings et al. (Eds.), *Otolaryngology — head and neck surgery* (pp. 3149–3172). St. Louis: C.V. Mosby.

Hughes, G. B., Kinney, S. E., Barna, B. P., & Calabrese, L. H. (1986). Autoimmunity in otology. *American Journal of Otolaryngology, 7*(3), 197–199.

Hughes, G. B., Kinney, S. E. Calabrese, L. H., & Barana, B. P. (1984). Practical vs theoretical management of autoimmune inner ear disease. *Laryngoscope, 94,* 758.

Jacobson, J., Murray, J., & Deppe, U. (1987). The effects of ABR rate presentation in multiple sclerosis. *Ear & Hearing, 8,* 115–120.

Jerger, J. (1970). Clinical experience with impedance audiometry. *Archives of Otolaryngology, 92,* 311–324.

Jerger, J. (1973). Audiological findings in aging. *Advances in Otorhinolaryngology, 20,* 115–124.

Jerger, J., & Hall, J. (1980). Effect of age and sex on the auditory brainstem response. *Archives of Otolaryngology, 106–*387.

Jerger, J., & Hayes, D. (1977). Diagnostic speech audiometry. *Archives of Otorhinolaryngology, 103,* 216–223.

Jerger, J., Neely, J. G., & Jerger, S. (1980). Speech, impedance, and auditory brainstem response audiometry in brainstem tumors. Importance of a multiple test strategy. *Archives of Otolaryngology, 106,* 218–223.

Jerger, S. (1983). Decision matrix and information theory analyses in the evaluation of neuroaudiologic tests. *Semi-*

nars in Hearing, 4 (2), 121–132.

Jerger, S., & Jerger, J. (1981). Auditory disorders: A manual for clinical evaluation. Boston: Little, Brown.

Jerger, S., Neely, J. G., & Jerger, J. (1975). Recovery of crossed acoustic reflexes in brainstem auditory disorder. Archives of Otolaryngology, 101, 329–332.

Johnson, S., Hosford-Dunn, H., Paryani, S., Younger, A., & Malachowski, N. (1986). Prevalence of sensorineural hearing loss in premature and sick term infants with perinatally acquired cytomegalovirus infection. Ear & Hearing, 7, 325–327.

Josey, A. F., Glasscock, M. E., & Musiek, F. E. (1988). Correlation of ABR and medical imaging in patients with cerebellopontine angle tumors. American Journal of Otology, 9, 12–16.

Kaplan, J. N., & Griep, R. J. (1986). Disorders of the thyroid gland. In C. W. Cummings et al. (Eds.), Otolaryngology — head and neck surgery (pp. 2499–2509). St. Louis: C.V. Mosby.

Keane, W. M., Potsic, W. P., Rowe, L. D., Konkle, D. F., & Eve, I. L. (1983). Meningitis and hearing loss in children. Hearing Journal, 36, 24–27.

Keith, R. W., Garza-Holquin, Y., Smolak, L., & Pensak, M. L. (1987). Acoustic reflex dynamics and auditory brainstem responses in multiple sclerosis. American Journal of Otology, 8, 406–413.

Kinney, S. P. (1986). Trauma. In C. W. Cummings et al. (Eds.), Otolaryngology — head and neck surgery (pp. 3033–3046). St. Louis: C.V. Mosby.

Koko, E. (1974). Chronic secretory otitis media in children. Acta Oto-laryngologica (Stockholm), 372 (Suppl.), 7–44.

Kraus, N., Ozdamar, O., Hier, D., & Stein, L. (1982). Auditory middle latency responses (MLRs) in patients with cortical lesions. Electroencephalography and Clinical Neurophysiology, 54, 275–287.

Lebel, M. H., Freij, B. J., Syrogiannopoulos, G. A., Chrane, D. F., Hoyt, M. J., Stewart, S. M., Kennard, E. D., Olsen, K. D., & McCracken, G. H. (1988). Dexamethasone therapy for bacterial meningitis. Results of two double blind, placebo-controlled trials. New England Journal of Medicine, 319, 964–971.

Liston, S., & Meyerhoff, W. L. (1986). Metabolic hearing loss. In G. M. English (Ed.), Otolaryngology: Diseases of the ear (Vol. 1, chap. 33). Philadelphia: Harper & Row.

Lonsbury-Martin, B. C., & Martin, G. K. (1986). Auditory dysfunction from excessive sound stimulation. In C. W. Cummings et al. (Eds.), Otolaryngology — head and neck surgery (pp. 3173–3187). St. Louis: C.V. Mosby.

Lowell, S. H., & Paparella, M. M. (1977). Presbycusis: What is it? Laryngoscope, 87 (10, Pt. 1), 1710–1717.

Martin, F. K. (1981). Medical audiology: Disorders of hearing. Englewood Cliffs, NJ: Prentice-Hall.

Mattox, D. E., & Simmons, F. B. (1977). Natural history of sudden sensorineural hearing loss. Annals of Otology, Rhinology, and Laryngology, 86 (4, Pt. 1), 463–480.

McCabe, B. F. (1979). Autoimmune sensorineural hearing loss. Annals of Otology, Rhinology, and Laryngology, 88, 585.

McCabe, B. F. (1981). Treatment of autoimmune inner ear disease. In G. E. Shambaugh & J. J. Shea (Eds.), Proceedings of the Sixth Shambaugh International Workshop on Otomicrosurgery and the Third Shea Fluctuant Hearing Loss Symposium. Huntsville, AL: Strode Publishers.

McDonald, T. J., Vollertsen, R. S., & Younge, B. R. (1985). Cogan's syndrome: Audiovestibular involvement and prognosis in 18 patients. Laryngoscope, 95, 650–654.

Miller, J. J., Beck, L., Davis, B., Jones, D. E., & Thomas, A. B. (1983). Hearing loss in patients with diabetic retinopathy. American Journal of Otolaryngology, 4, 342–346.

Miller, S. J., Toohill, R. J., & Lehman, R. H. (1982). Sudden sensorineural hearing loss: Operative complications in non-otologic surgery. Laryngoscope, 92, 613–617.

Morretti, J. A. (1976). Sensorineural hearing loss following radiotherapy to the nasal pharynx. Laryngoscope, 85 (4), 598–602.

Nadol, J. B., Jr. (1979). Electron microscopic findings in presbycusic degeneration of the basal turn of the human cochlea. Otolaryngology — Head and Neck Surgery, 87 (6), 818–836.

Nadol, J. B., Jr. (1986). Manifestations of systemic disease. In C. W. Cummings et al. (Eds.), Otolaryngology — head and neck surgery (pp. 3017–3032). St. Louis: C.V. Mosby.

Nadol, J. B., Jr. (1988). Application of electron microscopy to human otopathology. Ultrastructural findings in neural presbycusis, Ménière's disease and Usher's syndrome. Acta Oto-laryngologica (Stockholm), 105 (5–6), 411–419.

Neely, J. G. (1981). Gross and microscopic anatomy of the eighth cranial nerve in relationship to the solitary schwannoma. Laryngoscope, 91, 1512–1531.

Neely, J. G. (1984). Is it possible to totally resect an acoustic tumor and conserve hearing? Otolaryngology — Head and Neck Surgery, 92, 162–167.

Neely, J. G. (1985). Classification of spontaneous cerebrospinal fluid middle ear effusion: Review of forty-nine cases. Otolaryngology — Head and Neck Surgery, 93 (5), 625–634.

Neely, J. G., & Hough, J. V. (1986). Histologic findings in two very small intracanalicular solitary schwannomas. Annals of Otology, Rhinology, and Laryngology, 95 (5), 460–465.

Neely, J. G., Armstrong, D., Benson, J., & Neblett, C. (1981). "Onion bulb" formation associated with a solitary neoplasm of the eighth nerve sheath. American Journal of Otolaryngology, 2, 307–313.

Neely, J. G., Dennis, J. M., & Lippe, W. R. (1986). Anatomy of the auditory end organ and neuropathways. In C. W. Cummings et al. (Eds.), Otolaryngology — head and neck surgery (pp. 2571–2608). St. Louis: C.V. Mosby.

Nofsinger, D., Olsen, W., Carhart, R., Hart, C., & Sahgal, V. (1972). Auditory and vestibular aberration in multiple sclerosis. Acta Oto-laryngologica Supplement. (Stockholm), 303, 1.

Northern, J. L., & Downs, M. P. (1978). Hearing in children. Baltimore: Williams & Wilkins.

O'Neil, J. V., Katz, A. H., & Skolnik, E. M. (1979). Otologic complications of radiation therapy. Otolaryngology — Head and Neck Surgery, 87 (3), 359–363.

Orchik, D., & Burgess, J. (1977). Synthetic sentence identification as a function of the age of the listener. Journal of the American Audiology Society, 3, 42–46.

Ozdamar, O., Kraus, N., & Stein, L. (1983). Auditory brainstem responses in infants recovering from bacterial meningitis. Audiologic evaluation. Archives of Otolaryngology, 109 (1), 13–18.

Paparella, M. D. (1984). Pathology of Ménière's disease. Annals of Otology, Rhinology, and Laryngology, 112, 31–35.

Paparella, M. M., Oda, M., Hiraide, F., & Brady, O. (1972). Pathology of sensorineural hearing loss in otitis media. Annals of Otology, Rhinology, and Laryngology, 81 (5), 632–647.

Pillsbury, H. C. (1986). Hypertension, hyperlipoproteinemia, chronic noise exposure: Is there synergism in cochlear pathology? *Laryngoscope, 96,* 1112–1138.

Pillsbury, H. C., & Shea, J. J. (1979). Luetic hydrops — diagnosis and therapy. *Laryngoscope, 89* (7, Pt. 1), 1135–1144.

Podoshin, L., & Fradis, M. (1975). Hearing loss after head injury. *Archives of Otolaryngology, 101,* 15–18.

Pulec, J. L. (1976). Ménière's disease. In J. L. Northern (Ed.), *Hearing disorders* (pp. 153–160). Boston: Little, Brown.

Quick, C. A. (1986). Ototoxicity. In G. N. English (Ed.), *Otolaryngology.* New York: Harper & Row.

Real, R., Thomas, M., & Gerwin, J. M. (1987). Sudden hearing loss in acquired immunodeficiency syndrome. *Otolaryngology — Head and Neck Surgery, 97,* 409–412.

Robinson, K., & Rudge, P. (1977). Abnormalities of the auditory evoked potentials in patients with multiple sclerosis. *Brain, 100,* 19.

Rosen, S., Olin, P., & Rosen, H. V. (1970). Dietary prevention of hearing loss. *Acta Oto-laryngologica* (Stockholm), *70,* 242–247.

Rosenhall, U., & Kankkunen, A. (1980). Hearing alterations following meningitis: Hearing improvement. *Ear & Hearing, 1,* 185–190.

Rosenhall, U., & Kankkunen, A. (1981). Hearing alterations following meningitis, II — variable hearing. *Ear & Hearing, 2,* 170–176.

Ruben, R. J. (1983). Diseases of the inner ear and sensorineural deafness. In C. V. Bluestone & S. E. Stool (Eds.), *Pediatric otolaryngology* (pp. 577–604). Philadelphia: W.B. Saunders.

Rybak, L. P., & Matz, G. J. (1986). Auditory and vestibular effects of toxins. In C. W. Cummings et al. (Eds.), *Otolaryngology — head and neck surgery* (pp. 3161–3172). St. Louis: C.V. Mosby.

Saltiel, T., Melmed, C. A., & Portnoy, D. (1983). Sensorineural deafness in early acquired syphilis. *Canadian Journal of Neurological Science, 10,* 114.

Schacht, J. (1986). Molecular mechanisms of drug-induced hearing loss. *Hearing Research, 22,* 297–304.

Schrimpf, R., Karmody, C. S., Chasin, W. D., & Carter, B. (1982). Sclerosing lesions of the temporal bone. *Laryngoscope, 92,* 1116–1119.

Schuknecht, H. F. (1974). *Pathology of the ear.* Cambridge: Harvard University Press.

Schuknecht, H. F., & Barber, W. (1985). Histologic varients in otosclerosis. *Laryngoscope, 95* (11), 1307–1317.

Schwartz, D. M., Blum, M. J., & Dennis, J. M. (1985). Perioperative monitoring of auditory brainstem responses. *Hearing Journal, 38,* 9–14.

Sheehy, J. (1960). Vasodilator therapy in sensorineural hearing loss. *Laryngoscope, 70,* 885.

Smith, A. L. (1988). Neurologic sequelae of meningitis. *New England Journal of Medicine, 319,* 1012–1013.

Smith, R. J. H. (1986). *Medical diagnosis and treatment of hearing loss in children* (pp. 3225–3246). St. Louis: C.V. Mosby.

Snow, J. (1973). Sudden deafness. In M. Paparella & D. Shumrick (Eds.), *Otolaryngology* (pp. 357–364). Philadelphia: Saunders.

Starr, A., & Achor, J. (1975). Auditory brainstem responses in neurological disease. *Archives of Neurology, 32,* 761–768.

Stockard, J., & Sharbrough, F. (1977). Detection and localization of occult lesions with brainstem auditory responses. *Mayo Clinic Proceedings, 52,* 761–769.

Taylor, I., & Irwin, J. (1978). Some audiological aspects of diabetes mellitus. *Journal of Laryngology and Otology, 92,* 99–113.

Tondorf, J. (1971). Animal experiments in bone conduction: Clinical conclusions. In I. M. Ventry, J. B. Chaiklin, & R. F. Dixon (Eds.), *Hearing measurement: A book of readings* (pp. 130–141). New York: Appleton-Century-Crofts.

Tos, M. (1971). Prognosis of hearing loss in temporal bone fracture. *Journal of Laryngology and Otology, 85* (2), 1147–1159.

Tuzel, I. J. (1981). Comparison of adverse reactons to bumetanide and furosemide. *Journal of Clinical Pharmacology, 21,* 615.

Valvassori, G. E., & Dobben, G. D. (1985). CT densitometry of the cochlear capsule in otosclerosis. *American Journal of Neurology, 6* (5), 661–667.

Ward, W. D. (1976). Noise-induced hearing loss. In J. L. Northern (Ed.), *Hearing disorders* (pp. 161–170). Boston: Little, Brown.

Welsh, L. W., Welsh, J. J., & Healy, M. P. (1985). Central presbycusis. *Laryngoscope, 95* (2), 128–136.

Wiet, R. J., & Causse, J. B. (1986). *Complications in otolaryngology — head and neck surgery: Vol. 1 Ear and skullbase.* Philadelphia: B.C. Decker.

Wofford, M. (1981). Audiological evaluation and management of hearing disorders. In F. N. Martin (Ed.), *Medical audiology: Disorders of hearing* (pp. 145–173). Englewood Cliffs, NJ: Prentice-Hall.

Wong, R. T., Lepore, M. L., Burch, G. R., & Henderson, R. L. (1977). Luetic hearing loss. *Laryngoscope, 87* (10, Pt. 1), 1765–1769.

Zoller, M., Wilson, W. R., Nadol, J. B., Jr., & Girard, K. F. (1978). Detection of syphilitic hearing loss. *Archives of Otolaryngology, 104* (2), 63–65.

PART II

Auditory Assessment

CHAPTER 6

Immittance Measures in Auditory Disorders

Brad A. Stach • James F. Jerger

Immittance audiometry is one of the most powerful individual tools available for the diagnosis of auditory disorder. It is simultaneously sensitive in detecting middle ear disorder, accurate in differentiating cochlear from retrocochlear pathology, and useful in predicting degree of peripheral hearing sensitivity as a cross check to pure tone audiometry. As a reflection of its value to audiologic diagnosis, immittance audiometry is now used clinically on a routine basis in most audiologic settings.

This chapter will cover the many aspects of analysis and interpretation of immittance measures as they relate to the diagnosis of auditory disorder. Although increasingly sophisticated analyses of the various aspects of immittance audiometry are being made, this chapter will focus on those measures that are currently used clinically. Throughout, two major points will be emphasized: (1) in isolation, results from a specific immittance measure are almost always ambiguous; and (2) in combination, immittance measures represent an indispensible component of the audiologic evaluation.

BASIC IMMITTANCE MEASURES AND THEIR CLINICAL RELEVANCE

Three immittance measures are commonly used in the clinical assessment of middle ear function: tympanometry, static immittance, and the acoustic reflex.

TYMPANOMETRY

Tympanometry is simply the measure of how acoustic immittance in the plane of the tympanic membrane changes as a function of varying degrees of air pressure in the external auditory meatus. The fundamental concept of tympanometric measurement relies on the fact that transmission of sound through the middle ear mechanism is maximum when air pressure is equal on both sides of the tympanic membrane. For a normal ear, maximum transmission occurs at, or near, atmospheric pressure. Early studies, by Thomsen (1958) and Terkildsen and Thomsen (1959), showed that middle ear pressure could be assessed by varying pressure in the sealed ear until the sound pressure level (SPL) of the probe tone was at its minimum, reflecting maximum transmission of sound through the middle ear mechanism. As the pressure was varied above or below this point of maximum transmission, the SPL of the probe tone in the external auditory meatus increased, reflecting a reduction in sound transmission through the middle ear. These same principles were applied to clinical problems (Alberti and Kristensen, 1970; Brooks, 1969; Lidén, Peterson, and Bjorkman, 1970), and the use of tympanometry as a measure of the condition of the middle ear began.

Investigations by Lidén et al. (1970) and Jerger (1970) represented the germinal descriptions of the clinical efficacy of tympanometric measures. These authors described patterns of tympanometric shapes that were related to various auditory disorders. Lidén (1969) first described the classification system of three tympanogram types that is

113

still in widespread use today. As a relatively objective measure of middle ear function, tympanometry rapidly gained widespread use and still holds its position today as an almost indispensable diagnostic tool.

Since this early work, many efforts have been directed toward enhancing the diagnostic sensitivity of tympanometric measures by either (1) the use of multiple probe-tone frequencies, (2) the use of more sophisticated analyses of tympanometric shape, or (3) the use of the three immittance measures as an interpretive battery.

Early investigations of probe-tone frequency (Alberti and Jerger, 1974; Lidén, Harford, and Hallen, 1974) suggested that additional, multipeaked tympanometric shapes could be delineated by use of a higher-frequency probe tone. These studies, along with many subsequent investigations, concluded that higher-frequency probe tones were of limited diagnostic value. In general, they were too sensitive to minor tympanic membrane aberrations that did not reflect an active pathologic condition. In addition, it was found that multipeaked tympanograms could be measured in normal as well as pathologic ears, thereby limiting their diagnostic value. Nevertheless, the search has continued for a technique that will render these frequency-dependent differences useful. For example, Colletti (1977) and Funasaka, Funai, and Kumakawa (1984) described systems for the measurement of multifrequency tympanometry, and current commercial instrumentation typically includes high-frequency probe-tone capabilities. This search is encouraged by the contention that middle ear pathology will have a greater effect on high-frequency tympanometric shape (e.g., Shanks, 1984). Although of important academic interest, enthusiasm has not developed for clinical applications, presumably because of a lack of knowledge of the sensitivity and, especially, the specificity of such measures to treatable middle ear disorder.

Tympanometric shape has also been scrutinized as a means for enhancing the sensitivity of tympanometry. Although conventional classification of shape is into one of three types, some investigators, such as Paradise, Smith, and Bluestone (1976), suggested that tympanograms be classified into more specific types. Others, such as Brooks (1969), suggested a more precise quantification of the shape, by measuring the so-called gradient of the tympanogram. Still others suggest that two-component, multiple-frequency measurements be made and tympanograms be plotted in the form of admittance and phase angle, susceptance and conductance, impedance and phase angle, reactance and resistance, phasor diagram, and three-dimensional (Shanks et al., 1988).

The final approach to tympanometric enhancement concedes that tympanometry, regardless of the sophistication with which it is analyzed, is not an altogether useful technique in the clinic because of its lack of sensitivity to some pathologic conditions and its excessive sensitivity to some nonpathologic conditions. Rather, tympanometry gains its diagnostic power when interpreted in combination with the other two components of the total battery — static immittance and the acoustic reflex.

STATIC IMMITTANCE

Static acoustic immittance is a measure of the absolute immittance of the middle ear vibratory system. The conventional procedure for obtaining static immittance involves measurement of probe-tone SPL in the external ear canal with a pressure of +200 decaPascal (daPa). At that pressure, the middle ear is thought of as being effectively excluded, and the subsequent measurement reflects the volume of air in the external ear canal. Air pressure is then adjusted to the point of maximum immittance, and probe-tone SPL is again measured. The difference in SPL or its equivalent volume of air between the two measurements is considered the equivalent volume or static acoustic immittance of the middle ear system. Thus, a middle ear system with substantial stiffness due to some pathologic condition would have a relatively small static immittance, and a middle ear system that lacked appropriate stiffness would have a relatively large static immittance.

Static immittance measurement is useful because tympanogram types can be similar in very different types of auditory disorder. For example, tympanometric measurement of both a normal middle ear and a middle ear with excessive stiffness due to otosclerosis will result in type A tympanograms. Similarly, a middle ear that has effusion and a tympanic membrane that has a perforation can both result in type B tympanograms. The nature of these disorders can often be clarified by the measurement of static immittance.

Static immittance, however, is much too variable to be used as an isolated metric of middle ear function. It has been found to differ as a function of sex (Zwislocki and Feldman, 1970), as a function of age (Jerger, Jerger, and Mauldin, 1972), and, perhaps most important, as a function of the pressure used to estimate the immittance of the external ear canal (Margolis and Smith, 1977). These factors limit the usefulness of static immittance to such an extent that, in isolation, it can be used to differentiate only between normal and extreme pathologic conditions.

ACOUSTIC REFLEX

When a sound is of sufficient intensity, it will elicit a consensual reflex of the middle ear musculature, primarily the stapedius muscle in humans. When the stapedius muscle contracts in a normally functioning middle ear, it exerts tension on the stapes and stiffens the ossicular chain. The result of this additional stiffness is an increase in probe-tone SPL in the external auditory meatus as a result of a reduction of low-frequency energy transmission through the middle ear. Thus, when the stapedius muscle contracts in response to high-intensity sounds, it can be measured quite easily with conventional immittance techniques. In addition, since both middle ear muscles contract in response to sound delivered to either ear, both an ipsilateral (uncrossed) and a contralateral (crossed) reflex can be recorded with sound presented to each ear.

Although the acoustic reflex had been studied for many years, its first clinical implementation can be attributed to the work of Otto Metz (1946). Metz described a system for clinical measurement of the reflex and later showed that reflex thresholds could be recorded at reduced sensation levels in patients with Ménière's disease. At the time, it appeared that the real importance of these results was in the discovery both of an objective measure of recruitment and of a means to differentiate between a conductive and sensory hearing loss. This changed, however, when, more than 20 years later, Anderson, Barr, and Wedenberg (1969) described the effectiveness of acoustic reflex measurement in the diagnosis of eighth nerve tumors. By 1970, instrumentation for acoustic reflex measurement was widely available commercially, and large diagnostic strides followed with corroboration of the Anderson et al. findings (Jerger and Jerger, 1974, 1975; Jerger, Harford, Clemis, and Alford, 1974; Jerger, Neely, and Jerger, 1975; Olsen, Noffsinger, and Kurdziel, 1975; Sanders, Josey, and Glasscock, 1974; Thomsen and Terkildsen, 1975), the implementation of uncrossed reflex measurement (Griesen and Rasmussen, 1970), and the understanding of the substantial diagnostic power of crossed versus uncrossed reflex patterns (Jerger, 1975; Jerger and Jerger, 1977). Assessment of the suprathreshold characteristics of decay, latency, amplitude, amplitude relationships, and sequential variability followed (e.g., Borg, 1982; Bosatra, Russolo, and Poli, 1975; Bruschini et al., 1984; Jerger and Hayes, 1983; Jerger et al., 1978; Jerger, Oliver, and Jenkins, 1987; Jerger, Oliver, Rivera, and Stach, 1986; Mangham and Miller, 1979; Yamane and Nomura, 1984) and are still being pursued for their excellent sensitivity to disorder of the neural auditory system.

Threshold Measures

The *threshold* is the most common measure of the acoustic stapedial reflex and can be defined as the lowest intensity level at which a middle ear immittance change can be detected in response to sound. Detection of this threshold, of course, is confounded by numerous variables, including sensitivity of the instrumentation used to record the reflex (Karlsson and Hagerman, 1984; Mangham and Lindeman, 1980; Stach and Jerger, 1984) and the intensity and frequency of the probe tone (Peterson and Lidén, 1972; Terkildsen, Osterhammel, and Scott–Nielsen, 1970). With commerically available equipment, normal crossed reflex thresholds can be detected from 70 to 100 dB HL. Uncrossed stimulation will result in slightly lower thresholds, as will binaural stimulation (Moller, 1962; Zakrisson, Borg, and Blom, 1974). Threshold measures are useful for at least two purposes: differential diagnosis of auditory disorder and prediction of peripheral hearing sensitivity.

Reflex threshold measurement has been valuable in both the assessment of middle ear function (Jerger, Anthony, Jerger, and Mauldin, 1974) and in the differentiation of cochlear from retrocochlear disorder (Anderson et al., 1969; Antonelli, Bellotto, and Grandori, 1987; Cohen and Prasher, 1988; Hirsch and Anderson, 1980b; Jerger, Anthony, Jerger, and Mauldin, 1974; Johnson, 1977; Olsen et al., 1975; Sanders et al., 1974, 1981; Sheehy and Inzer, 1976; Thomsen and Terkildsen, 1975). In terms of the latter, whereas reflex thresholds occur at reduced sensation levels in ears with cochlear hearing loss, they are typically elevated or absent in ears with eighth nerve disorder. Similarly, reflex thresholds are often abnormal in patients with brainstem disorder (Antonelli et al., 1987; Bosatra, Russolo, and Poli, 1976; Cohen and Prasher, 1988; Colletti, 1975; Greisen and Rasmussen, 1970; Grenman et al., 1984; Hannley, Jerger, and Rivera, 1983; Jerger and Jerger, 1974, 1975; Jerger et al., 1975; Jerger, Neely, and Jerger, 1980; Jerger, Oliver, Chmiel, and Rivera, 1986; Jerger, Oliver, Rivera, and Stach, 1986; Kofler, Oberascher, and Pommer, 1984; Stephens and Thornton, 1976). Comparison of crossed and uncrossed thresholds has also been found to be helpful in differentiating eighth nerve from brainstem disorder (Jerger, 1975; Jerger and Jerger, 1977; Stach, 1987).

Although threshold measures are valuable, interpretation of absence or abnormal elevation of an acoustic reflex threshold can be difficult because the same abnormality can result from a number of pathologic conditions. For example, the absence of a right crossed acoustic reflex can result from (1) a severe sensory hearing loss on the right ear; (2) a substantial conductive loss on the right ear; (3) right eighth nerve tumor; (4) a lesion of the crossing fibers of the central portion of the reflex arc; (5) left facial nerve disorder; or (6) left middle ear disorder. For this reason the addition of uncrossed reflex measurement, tympanometry, and static immittance is important in reflex threshold interpretation.

Acoustic reflex thresholds have also been used for the prediction of peripheral auditory sensitivity. In 1972, Niemeyer and Sesterhenn reported that they could exploit cochlear bandwidth effects on the acoustic reflex to predict degree of hearing loss (Niemeyer and Sesterhenn, 1972, 1974). The procedure was simplified in 1974 (Jerger, Burney, Mauldin, and Crump, 1974) and was applied successfully for clinical purposes. Although numerous encouraging reports followed, many others amplified the weaknesses of this technique. Despite criticism of the use of acoustic reflex thresholds in the prediction of hearing sensitivity because of its lack of precision (see Silman et al., 1984 for a summary), it continues to be clinically viable as a powerful cross check to behavioral audiometry, especially in children.

Suprathreshold Measures

Suprathreshold analysis of the acoustic reflex includes such measures as decay, latency, amplitude, amplitude relationships, and sequential variability.

Decay

Acoustic reflex decay is often a component of routine immittance measurement used to differentiate cochlear from eighth nerve disorder. Al-

though various measurement techniques and criteria for abnormality have been developed (Fowler and Wilson, 1984), reflex decay testing is typically carried out by presenting a 10-second signal at 10 dB above the reflex threshold. Results are considered abnormal if amplitude of the resultant reflex decreases to less than half of its initial maximum value. Reflex decay has been shown to be a sensitive measure of eighth nerve disorder (Anderson et al., 1969; Hirsch and Anderson, 1980a, 1980b; Jerger et al., 1974; Mangham, Lindeman, and Dawson, 1980; Olsen et al., 1975; Olsen, Stach, and Kurdziel, 1981, 1983; Sanders et al., 1974, 1981; Sheehy and Inzer, 1976; Thomsen and Terkildsen, 1975), brainstem pathology (Jerger and Jerger, 1977; Stephens and Thornton, 1976), and neuromuscular disease (Blom and Zakrisson, 1974; Kramer et al., 1981; Warren et al., 1977). One of the problems associated with reflex decay testing, however, is a high false-positive rate in patients with cochlear hearing loss. Positive reflex decay has been reported in as many as 27 percent of patients with Ménière's disease (Olsen et al., 1981). Although this false-positive rate can be lowered by altering the definition of normalcy, the increase in specificity is inexorably accompanied by a decrease in sensitivity (Jerger and Jerger, 1983).

Latency

Acoustic reflex latency and rise time have also been used as diagnostic measures and have been shown to be abnormal in ears with eighth nerve disorder (Clemis and Sarno, 1980; Mangham and Miller, 1979; Mangham et al., 1980), multiple sclerosis (Bosatra et al., 1975, 1976; Hess, 1979; Jerger, Oliver, Chmiel, and Rivera, 1986; Jerger, Oliver, Rivera, and Stach, 1986), and other brainstem disorders (Bosatra et al., 1975, 1976). Despite these encouraging findings, at least two problems have been encountered in the clinical measurement of latency. First, evidence suggests that latency is not delayed due to an acoustic tumor, rather the apparent delays reported were simply artifacts of amplitude reduction (Borg, 1982; Jerger and Hayes, 1983; Jerger, Oliver, and Stach, 1986; Jerger et al., 1987). That is, the presence of an acoustic tumor will reduce the amplitude of a reflex, but if it is compared to a reflex of comparable amplitude obtained from the other ear, no latency differences will exist. Although this finding holds for abnormality resulting from acoustic tumors, true latency delays have been reported as a result of brainstem disorder (Jerger,

Oliver, Rivera, and Stach, 1986). The second problem in the measurement of latency results from limitations of instrumentation (Lilly, 1984). Response times of commercial instrumentation may be too slow to accurately reproduce temporal characteristics of the acoustic reflex. Indeed, data have suggested that average acoustic reflex rise times in neurologically normal subjects can actually be faster than the rise time of a commercial immittance instrument (Jerger, Oliver, and Stach, 1986). Despite these measurement difficulties, reflex temporal characteristics have been found to be sensitive to brainstem disorder.

Amplitude

Acoustic reflex amplitude is a suprathreshold measurement that is often ignored because of excessive subject and measurement variability (Silman, 1984). Parameters contributing to this variability include signal characteristics, patient age, previous middle ear disorder, and difficulty of direct comparison of crossed to uncrossed reflexes due to differences in transducers. Despite these problems, depressed reflex amplitudes have been reported in patients with eighth nerve tumors (Hayes and Jerger, 1983; Jerger and Hayes, 1983; Mangham et al., 1980; Stach and Jerger, 1984), multiple sclerosis (Bosatra et al., 1975, 1976; Hayes and Jerger, 1983; Hess, 1979; Jerger, Oliver, Chmiel, and Rivera, 1986; Jerger Oliver, Rivera, and Stach, 1986; Stach and Jerger, 1984), and other brainstem disorders (Bosatra et al., 1975, 1976).

Amplitude Relationships

One technique for reducing amplitude variability, first described by Möller (1961) and later exploited by Jerger et al. (1978), is the use of a dual-probe assembly for simultaneous measurement of crossed and uncrossed reflexes. Such a system permits analysis of relationships among reflex amplitudes within a single subject. To carry out such a measurement, the ipsilateral transducer of one probe is used to deliver the eliciting signal, and both crossed and uncrossed reflexes resulting from the signal are recorded simultaneously. A signal is then delivered to the other ear, and the process is repeated. Amplitude measurements of the resultant four reflexes are cast into formulae for intrasubject comparison. Three indices are used to express amplitude relationships. The *afferent index* (AI) represents the difference between reflex amplitudes with sound presented to one ear and those with sound to the other ear. The *efferent index* (EI) represents the difference

between reflex amplitudes recorded from one probe and those recorded from the other probe. The *central pathway index* (CPI) represents the difference between uncrossed and crossed amplitudes. These indices have been helpful in reducing much of the problem associated with the variability of amplitude measurement (Hayes and Jerger, 1983; Stach and Jerger, 1984, 1987b). With this procedure, patterns of reflex amplitude abnormalities have been found in patients with various types of neuropathology (Hall, 1982b; Hayes and Jerger, 1983; Jerger, Oliver, Rivera, and Stach, 1986; Stach, 1987; Stach and Jerger, 1984; Stach, Jerger, and Jenkins, 1984).

Sequential Variability

Sequential variability is measured as the standard deviation of amplitude or latency values over successive samples of the acoustic reflex waveform. Jerger et al. (1987) reported recently on increased sequential variability of reflex latency in a patient with an acoustic neuroma. Sixteen signals were presented, and variability was computed for both amplitude and latency. Results showed that onset latency of the crossed acoustic reflex was substantially more variable when sound was presented to the ear with an acoustic neuroma than when sound was presented to the opposite ear. Sequential variability may prove to be a dimension of reflex analysis that further enhances sensitivity of the acoustic reflex measurement.

BASIC PRINCIPLES OF INTERPRETATION

PARADOX

It is an interesting paradox that a group of diagnostic tests may sometimes be relatively ineffective when interpreted individually but quite powerful when viewed as a whole. In diagnostic audiometry the best example of this paradox is the immittance test battery. Viewed separately, the individual components of the immittance battery — tympanometry, static immittance, and acoustic reflex thresholds — are relatively ambiguous.

To be sure, certain tympanometric shapes are diagnostically useful. The type C tympanogram, for example, clearly signals reduced air pressure in the middle ear space. Similarly the type B tympanogram suggests mass loading of the vibratory mechanism. But the type A tympanogram may be ambiguous to interpret. Fixation of the chain should produce an abnormally shallow type A tympanogram, and ossicular discontinuity should produce an abnormally deep tympanogram, but the distributions of tympanometric amplitudes in these two clinical entities overlap the distribution of normal tympanometric amplitudes to such an extent that it is hazardous to ascribe diagnostic significance to what appears to be either a shallow or deep type A tympanogram.

Static immittance is also subject to ambiguous interpretation. Certain pathologies of the middle ear act to render the static immittance abnormally low; others should have the opposite effect. But the distribution of static immittance in normal ears is so broad (95% interval from 0.3–1.6 cc) that only very extreme changes in immittance are sufficient to drive the static immittance outside the normal boundaries.

Similarly, acoustic reflex thresholds are difficult to interpret in isolation. Elevation of the reflex threshold, or its disappearance entirely, may be related to a number of clinical entities, including middle ear disease, retrocochlear loss, facial nerve disorder, and even severe cochlear loss. Thus the fact that an ipsilateral or contralateral reflex threshold is elevated, or that the reflex cannot be observed at all, is, when viewed in isolation, an observation with little diagnostic value. But when immittance data are combined with information about the pure tone audiogram, the combination of these two pieces of information can lead to extremely precise prediction. Suppose, for example, that tympanograms are type A, but no reflexes, crossed or uncrossed, can be elicited with sound in either ear. This observation alone is consistent with any of three possibilities: (1) a moderate bilateral conductive loss, (2) a severe bilateral cochlear loss, or (3) a brainstem disorder.

If the immittance data are now combined with the observation of a normal pure tone audiogram, then there is strong evidence for a brainstem disorder, since each of the other possibilities would be characterized by a uniquely different audiometric contour. Table 6-1 summarizes these three possibilities. It illustrates how the combination of just two pieces of information, the audiogram and the immittance pattern, can lead to relatively specific prediction of site of disorder.

Consider another example. Suppose that an active 3-year-old child is being tested. Air conduction thresholds are established to be within normal limits on the right ear but at about a 40 dB level on the left ear. Bone conduction thresholds would establish whether the loss on the left ear is

TABLE 6-1. ILLUSTRATION OF HOW THE COMBINATION OF ACOUSTIC REFLEX DATA AND PURE TONE AUDIOMETRIC DATA CAN LEAD TO A SITE-SPECIFIC PREDICTION

Reflex pattern	Audiogram	Predicted site
Neither crossed nor uncrossed can be elicited from either ear	Bilateral air-bone gap	Middle ear
Neither crossed nor uncrossed can be elicited from either ear	Bilateral severe sensory loss	Cochlea
Neither crossed nor uncrossed can be elicited from either ear	Normal	Brainstem

conductive or sensory, but the child's cooperation is waning, and the possibility of obtaining valid bone conduction thresholds for the left ear while appropriately masking the right ear is poor. Very often in such a situation, the immittance data will be sufficient to make the distinction between conductive and sensory without the need for bone conduction thresholds. If both tympanograms are type A, and all reflex thresholds are within normal bounds, it may be safely assumed that the loss is sensory. If, on the other hand, the tympanogram is type A on the right ear but type B on the left ear, and reflex thresholds are beyond equipment limits for both the left uncrossed reflex and the right-to-left crossed reflex (i.e., whenever the probe is in the left ear), then the loss on the left ear is most likely conductive.

Thus the key to the successful interpretation of immittance data lies not in the examination of individual results, but in the examination of the pattern of results characterizing the entire audiometric assessment. Within this frame of reference, the following observations are relevant:

1. The acoustic reflex is exceedingly sensitive to middle ear disorder. Only a 5 to 10 dB air-bone gap is usually sufficient to eliminate the reflex when the immittance probe is in the ear with conductive loss. As a corollary, it is well to keep in mind that the most common reason for an abnormality of the acoustic reflex is middle ear disorder. Thus the possibility of middle ear disorder, as an explanation for any observed reflex abnormality, must always be ruled out.

2. Reflex threshold testing should be carried out at frequencies of 500, 1000, 2000, and 4000

Hz. But the tester must keep in mind that, even in normal ears, results are unstable at 4000 Hz. Apparent abnormality of the reflex threshold at this test frequency may not be diagnostically relevant.

3. Reflex-eliciting stimuli should not exceed 110 dB HL for any signal, unless clear evidence exists of a substantial air-bone gap in the ear to which sound is being delivered. Unless duration of presentation is carefully controlled and kept quite short (i.e., less than 1 second), there is the ever-present danger that stimulation at these exceedingly high levels will be upsetting to the patient. Indeed, several case reports (Elonka, 1986; Lenarz and Gulzow, 1983; Miller, Hoffman, and Smallberg, 1984; Portman, 1980) have documented temporary or permanent auditory changes in patients following reflex testing. For this reason we advise the abandonment, or very judicious use, of the reflex decay test, in which stimulation is continuous for 5 to 10 seconds. Because of the high false-positive rate associated with this test procedure and the danger of excessive acoustic exposure, the cost-benefit ratio seems rather unfavorable.

UNIQUE PATTERNS

The diagnostic value of the immittance battery lies in the fact that the overall pattern of results is uniquely different depending on whether the problem is in the middle ear, the cochlea, or the retrocochlear system. The following sections summarize these unique patterns.

Middle Ear Disorder

The typical overall immittance pattern associated with middle ear disorder is as follows:

1. Some abnormality of the normal tympanometric shape
2. Some abnormality of the static immittance
3. No observable acoustic reflex to either crossed or uncrossed stimulation when the probe is in the affected ear

Cochlear Disorder

The typical overall immittance pattern associated with cochlear disorder is as follows:

1. Normal tympanogram
2. Normal static immittance
3. Normal reflex thresholds so long as the sensitivity loss by air conduction does not exceed 50 dB HL. Above this level, however,

the reflex threshold is elevated in proportion to degree of loss

Retrocochlear Disorder

The typical overall immittance pattern associated with retrocochlear disorder is as follows:

1. Normal tympanogram
2. Normal static immittance
3. Abnormal elevation of reflex threshold, or absence of reflex response, whenever the reflex-eliciting signal is delivered to the suspect ear in either the crossed or the uncrossed mode

Thus, in the case of a right-sided acoustic tumor, the abnormality would be observed for the right uncrossed and the right-to-left crossed reflex responses. The key factor differentiating retrocochlear from cochlear elevated reflex thresholds is the audiometric level at the test frequency. In the case of cochlear loss, reflex thresholds are not elevated at all until the audiometric loss exceeds 50 dB HL. And even above this level, the degree of elevation is proportional to the audiometric level. In the case of retrocochlear disorder, however, the elevation is much more than would be predicted from the audiometric level. One might, for example, see the reflex threshold elevated by 20 to 25 dB even though the audiometric level shows no more than a 5 to 10 dB loss. It is certainly the case, however, that if the audiometric loss exceeds 70 to 75 dB, then the absence of the acoustic reflex is ambiguous. The abnormality could be attributed either to retrocochlear disorder or to severe cochlear loss.

POTENTIAL SOURCES OF CONTAMINATION

Two factors — age and previous middle ear disease — can create problems in the interpretation of acoustic reflex data.

Age

Since age impacts virtually every aspect of audition, it is not surprising that it may contaminate the interpretation of reflex data as well. The primary effect of age is to widen the dispersion of absolute amplitude and latency measures, that is, to increase the distance between the upper and lower boundaries of normalcy (Jerger, Oliver, Rivera, and Stach, 1986). In the case of amplitude, the lower boundary changes little after age 30, but in the case of onset and offset latencies, there is a systematic increase in the upper boundary over the entire age range from 10 to 80 years. It is important, therefore, that age be taken into account when absolute measures of amplitude and latency are being evaluated. Fortuitously, however, there is no significant age effect on any of the three relative indices used to describe amplitude relationships. Thus age may be disregarded when evaluating any of these indices.

Previous Middle Ear Disorder

Previous middle ear disease may have a profound effect on reflex characteristics. Hall (1982a), for example, showed dramatic differences in suprathreshold reflex amplitude when he compared two groups matched for age and degree of hearing loss but differing in immittance characteristics. In the control group, all tympanograms and static immittance scores were within normal limits. In the experimental group, however, there was some abnormality of either or both of these measures. Interestingly, only 5 of the 17 subjects in the experimental group reported a previous history of middle ear disease. But amplitude of both the crossed and the uncrossed reflex at 1000 Hz was as much as 4 times greater (measured in equivalent volume) in the control group than in the experimental group at high signal levels (105–110 dB).

These results illustrate the vulnerability of the acoustic reflex to even seemingly minor episodes of middle ear disease. The prudent clinician, therefore, learns to look carefully at the basic tympanometric and static immittance measures and to take into account in the interpretation of reflex data any evidence of even minor deviation from normalcy.

CLINICAL APPLICATIONS

MIDDLE EAR FUNCTION

Principles of Clinical Application

Middle ear function is assessed by scrutiny of the unique patterns of measurement of static immittance, tympanometry, and acoustic reflexes. Each measure is evaluated in isolation against normative data and then in combination to discern the necessary pattern. Interpretation of the pattern may fall into one of five categories, which are described in Table 6-2: (1) results consistent with normal middle ear function; (2) results consistent with an increase in the mass of the middle ear mechanism; (3) results consistent with an increase in the stiffness of the middle ear mechanism; (4) results consistent with excessive immittance of the middle ear system; and (5) results consistent with significant negative pressure in the middle ear space.

Illustrative Cases

Increased Mass

Figure 6-1A shows immittance results on an 8-year-old girl. The right ear results are characterized by a type B tympanogram, excessively low static compliance, and absent right uncrossed and left crossed acoustic reflexes. These results are consistent with increased mass of the right middle ear mechanism. The left ear immittance results are normal. The tympanogram is a type A, static immittance is within normal limits, and left uncrossed reflexes are present. The absence of right crossed reflexes in the presence of left uncrossed reflexes suggests that the right middle-ear disorder has produced a substantial conductive hearing loss on the right ear. Figure 6-1B shows a

TABLE 6-2. TYPICAL PATTERNS OF IMMITTANCE MEASUREMENT RESULTS IN THE ASSESSMENT OF MIDDLE EAR DISORDER

Middle ear condition	*Tympanogram*	*Static immittance*	*Acoustic reflex*
Normal	A	Normal	Normal
Increased mass	B	Low	Absent
Increased stiffness	A	Low	Absent
Excessive immittance	A	High	Absent
Negative pressure	C	Normal	Abnormal

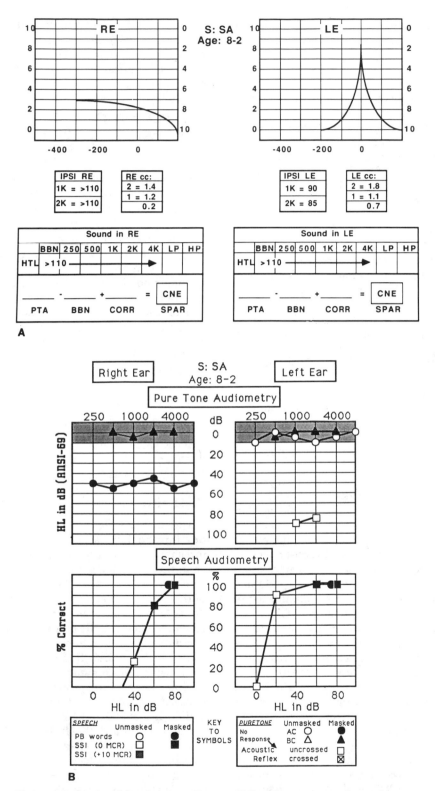

Figure 6-1. Results of immittance audiometry (A) and pure tone and speech audiometry (B) on an 8-year-old girl with a diagnosis of otitis media with effusion.

moderate conductive hearing loss and confirms this suspicion. The diagnosis was otitis media with effusion.

Increased Stiffness

Immittance results on a 34-year-old woman are shown in Figure 6-2A. Both the right and left ears are characterized by type A tympanograms, relatively low static immittance, and absent acoustic reflexes. These results are consistent with an increase in stiffness of both middle ear mechanisms. Figure 6-2B shows bilateral mild conductive hearing loss. The diagnosis was otosclerosis.

Excessive Immittance

Figure 6-3A shows immittance results on a 24-year-old man who was evaluated following mild head trauma. The left ear results are characterized by a type A tympanogram, excessively high static immittance, and absent acoustic reflexes, probe left (left uncrossed and right crossed). The right ear immittance results are normal. The tympanogram is a type A, static immittance is within normal limits, and right uncrossed reflexes are present. The absence of left crossed reflexes in the presence of right uncrossed reflexes suggests that the left middle ear disorder is causing a substantial conductive hearing loss on the left ear. Figure 6-3B shows a moderate conductive hearing loss and confirms this suspicion. The diagnosis was ossicular discontinuity.

Tympanic Membrane Perforation

Immittance results on a 14-year-old boy are shown in Figure 6-4A. The right ear results are characterized by a flat tympanogram, unmeasurable static immittance, and absent acoustic reflexes, probe right (right uncrossed and left crossed). These results are consistent with a perforated tympanic membrane. The left ear immittance results are normal. The tympanogram is type A, static immittance is within normal limits, and left uncrossed reflexes are present. The slight elevation of right crossed reflexes in the presence of normal left uncrossed reflexes suggests that the right middle ear disorder is causing a mild conductive hearing loss on the right ear. Audiometric results shown in Figure 6-4B confirm both the degree and type of loss.

Negative Middle Ear Pressure

Figure 6-5 shows immittance results on a 2-year-old boy. Results are identical on both ears and are characterized by type C tympanograms (peak at −200 and −250 daPa in the right and left ear, respectively), normal static immittance, and absent acoustic reflexes. These results are consistent with significant negative pressure in the middle ear space.

PREDICTION OF HEARING SENSITIVITY

Principles of Clinical Application

For purposes of illustration, the sensitivity prediction by the acoustic reflex (SPAR) will be the technique used to estimate hearing sensitivity. The concept for this technique was first described by Niemeyer and Sesterhenn (1974) and later adapted for clinical use by Jerger, Burney, Mauldin, and Crump (1974). It is based on the well-documented difference between acoustic reflex thresholds to pure tones versus broad-band noise and on the change in broad-band noise thresholds, but not pure tone thresholds, as a result of sensory hearing loss. To compute the SPAR value, the broad-band noise threshold is subtracted from the average reflex threshold to pure tones of 500, 1000, and 2000 Hz in normal-hearing subjects. The magnitude of this difference will vary according to the specific equipment used to carry out the measures. A correction is applied to yield a SPAR value of 20. If a patient's SPAR value is less than 15, there is a high probability of a sensory hearing loss.

Illustrative Cases

The first case illustrates the use of acoustic reflex thresholds in a child on whom behavioral threshold measures could not be carried out. The child was evaluated at the age of 2 years 1 month. Her mother suspected a hearing loss. Regardless of the nature or intensity of our efforts, we were not able to carry out behavioral audiometry and could not elicit a startle reflex at equipment intensity limits. Results of immittance audiometry are shown in Figure 6-6. Tympanograms are type A, with maximum immittance at 0 daPa. Static immittance was symmetric and within normal limits. Crossed acoustic reflex thresholds were present and normal at 500 and 1000 Hz, elevated at 2000 Hz, and absent at 4000 Hz, bilaterally. SPAR was only 4 dB bilaterally, suggesting a significant sensory hearing loss. Based on the SPAR and on the configuration of the crossed threshold pattern, these immittance measures predicted a sensory hearing loss, greater in the high-frequency region

123

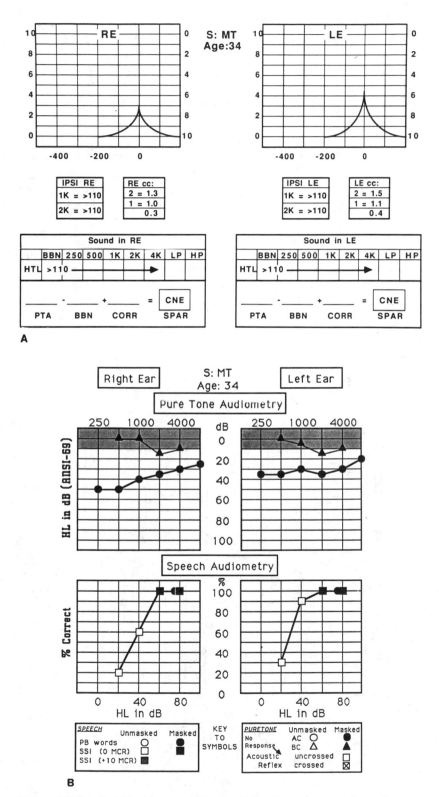

Figure 6-2. Results of immittance audiometry (A) and pure tone and speech audiometry (B) on a 34-year-old woman with a diagnosis of otosclerosis.

124

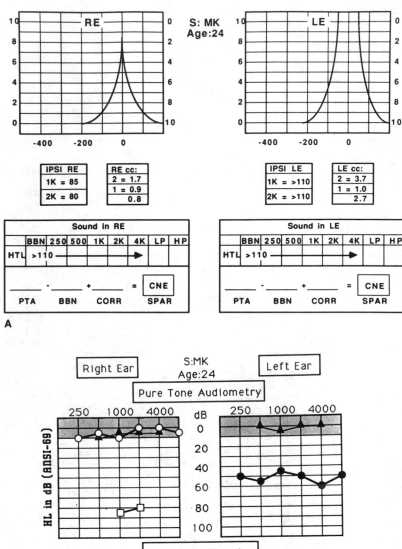

A

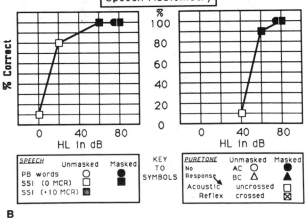

B

Figure 6-3. Results of immittance audiometry (A) and pure tone and speech audiometry (B) on a 24-year-old man with a diagnosis of ossicular discontinuity.

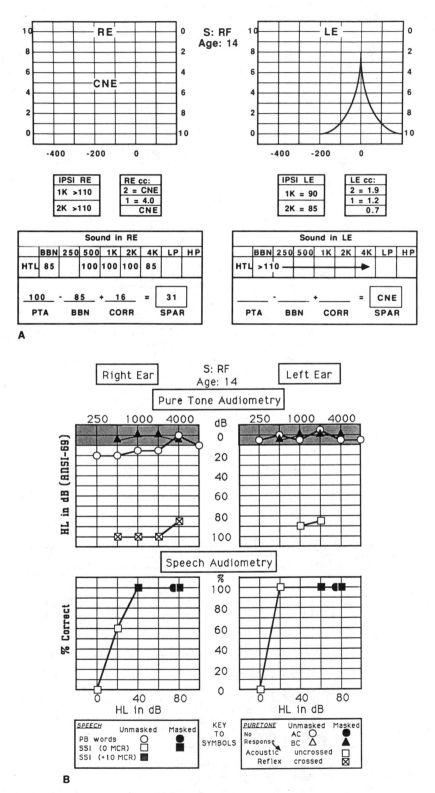

Figure 6-4. Results of immittance audiometry (A) and pure tone and speech audiometry (B) on a 14-year-old boy with a tympanic membrane perforation.

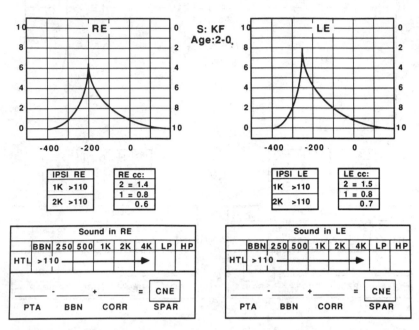

Figure 6-5. Results of immittance audiometry on a 2-year-old boy with significant negative pressure in the middle ear space.

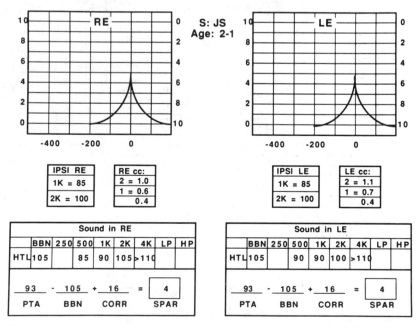

Figure 6-6. Results of immittance audiometry on a 2-year, 1-month-old boy with a moderate, bilateral sensory hearing loss.

of the audiogram than in the low. Auditory brainstem response audiometry later confirmed these suspicions. Click thresholds were 90 dB, and thresholds to 500 Hz tone bursts predicted a 50 dB hearing loss in the lower-frequency region of the audiogram.

The second case illustrates the use of reflex measurement for sensitivity prediction in a patient with a nonorganic hearing loss. This 34-year-old male patient was evaluated for a right ear hearing loss, secondary to an industrial accident when he was exposed to high-intensity noise as a result of steam release from a broken pipe at an oil refinery. Results of immittance audiometry are shown in Figure 6-7A. The tympanogram, static immittance, and acoustic reflex thresholds are all within normal limits. SPARs of 20 and 22 dB and a flat reflex threshold configuration predict normal peripheral sensitivity bilaterally. Results of behavioral testing are shown in Figure 6-7B. Right ear pure tone thresholds interweaved with reflex thresholds, strongly supporting the suspicion of functional hearing loss. Subsequent auditory evoked potential testing showed auditory brainstem response click thresholds of 10 dB and late vertex response thresholds of 10 dB for pure tone signals of 500 and 2000 Hz. The overall pattern of results predicted normal peripheral sensitivity bilaterally.

RETROCOCHLEAR DISORDER

Threshold Measures

Principles of Clincal Application

Differentiating cochlear from retrocochlear disorder is based exclusively on the acoustic reflex threshold or suprathreshold patterns, assuming either that the tympanogram and static immittance are normal and suggest normal middle ear function, or that the nature of any middle ear disorder and its effect on the reflex measures are well understood. For diagnostic interpretation, acoustic reflex measures are probably best understood if viewed in the context of a three-part reflex arc, the sensory or input portion (afferent), the central nervous system portion that transmits neural information (central), and the motor or output portion (efferent) (see, for example, Stach and Jerger, 1987a). An afferent abnormality occurs as the result of a disordered sensory system on one ear. An example of a pure afferent effect would result from a profound unilateral sensory hearing loss on the right ear. Both reflexes with

the signal presented to the right ear (right uncrossed and right crossed) would be absent. An efferent abnormality occurs as the result of a disordered motor system or middle ear mechanism on one ear. A pure efferent effect would result from unilateral right facial nerve paralysis. Both reflexes measured by the probe in the right ear (right uncrossed and left crossed) would be absent. A central pathway abnormality occurs as the result of brainstem pathway disorder and is manifested by the elevation or absence of one or both of the crossed acoustic reflexes in the presence of relatively normal uncrossed reflex thresholds.

Illustrative Cases

The first case illustrates normal immittance results in a patient with a sensory hearing loss. Figure 6-8A shows the immittance results on a 54-year-old female patient who was diagnosed as having acute labyrinthitis resulting in a unilateral hearing loss and dizziness. Tympanograms, static immittance, and acoustic reflex thresholds are within normal limits. Figure 6-8B shows the audiometric results. Even with the substantial sensory hearing loss in the right ear, reflex thresholds remain within normal limits.

The second case illustrates an afferent acoustic reflex abnormality resulting from retrocochlear disorder. Immittance results on a 48-year-old male patient who was diagnosed as having a right acoustic neuroma are shown in Figure 6-9A. Although tympanograms, static compliance, and acoustic reflexes, with sound to the left ear, are normal, reflexes with sound presented to the right ear (right uncrossed and right crossed) are absent. This pattern of abnormality suggests an afferent disorder that, in the absence of a severe degree of hearing loss, is consistent with retrocochlear disorder. Figure 6-9B shows a mild hearing loss in the right ear that is of an insufficient magnitude to account for the absence of acoustic reflexes when sound is presented to that ear.

The third case illustrates an efferent acoustic reflex abnormality resulting from brainstem disorder. Figure 6-10 shows immittance results on a 40-year-old woman with a confirmed diagnosis of multiple sclerosis. Among other symptoms, she had left-side facial weakness. In addition, she had no history of previous middle-ear disorder and no auditory complaints. Although the tympanogram and static immittance are normal on both ears, no reflexes could be measured from the left ear, regardless of which ear was being stimulated.

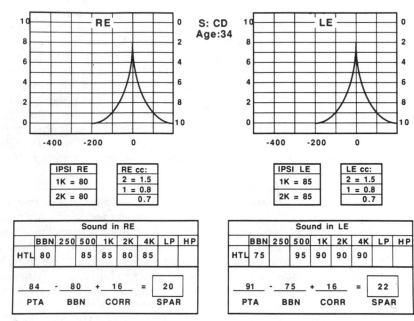

A

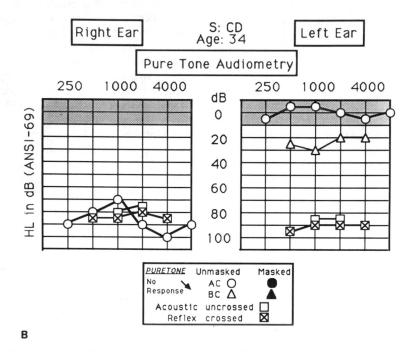

B

Figure 6-7. Results of immittance audiometry (A) and pure tone and speech audiometry (B) on a 34-year-old man with a suspected functional hearing loss.

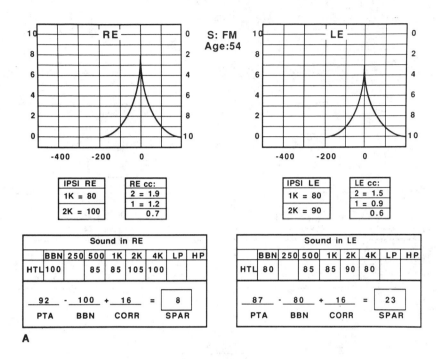

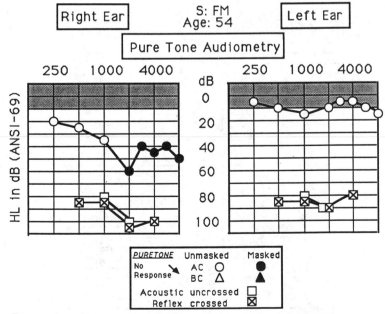

Figure 6-8. Results of immittance audiometry (A) and pure tone audiometry (B) on a 54-year-old woman with a diagnosis of sensory hearing loss.

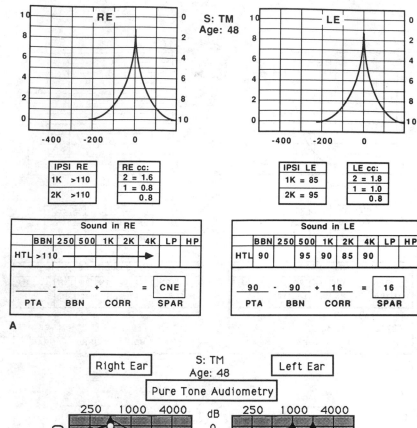

A

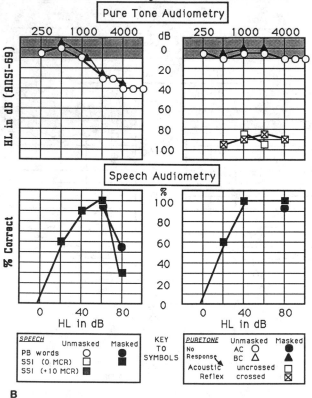

B

Figure 6-9. Results of immittance audiometry (A) and pure tone and speech audiometry (B) on a 48-year-old man with a right acoustic neuroma.

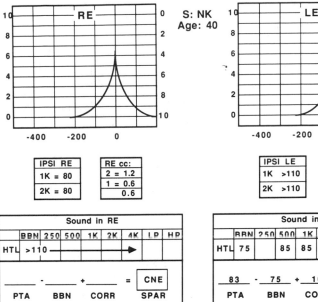

Figure 6-10. Results of immittance audiometry on a 40-year-old woman with a confirmed diagnosis of multiple sclerosis.

This pattern of abnormality suggests an efferent disorder, which, in the absence of any middle ear dysfunction is consistent with a neurologic disorder, probably affecting the motor nucleus of the seventh cranial nerve.

The fourth case illustrates a central pathway abnormality resulting from brainstem disorder. Immittance results on a 61-year-old man with a brainstem infarct are shown in Figure 6-11. Static immittance and tympanograms are normal bilaterally. In addition, uncrossed reflexes are normal for both ears, right crossed reflexes are present at normal levels, and left crossed reflexes are absent. The presence of a left uncrossed reflex rules out the possibility of either a substantial hearing loss or an acoustic tumor on the left side. The presence of a right uncrossed reflex rules out the possibility of middle ear disorder on the right side. The absence of a left crossed reflex, then, can only be explained as the result of a brainstem disorder.

Suprathreshold Measures

Principles of Clinical Application

Examination of the waveform of the suprathreshold reflex provides additional diagnostic information not necessarily evident in the pattern of reflex threshold abnormalities. From the suprathreshold waveform morphology, one may compute the amplitude of the reflex, as well as its onset and offset latencies. In our clinical work we have found that comparison of the amplitudes of the four suprathreshold waveforms, right uncrossed, left uncrossed, right-to-left crossed, and left-to-right crossed, can be extremely sensitive to site of disorder. In the past, the amplitude of the acoustic reflex has not been regarded as particularly promising from the diagnostic standpoint because of its considerable intersubject variability. As noted earier, however, the computation of the three amplitude indices — afferent, efferent, and central pathway — effectively attenuates the problem of variability by averaging across the two ears. The pattern of results based on all four reflexes, the two uncrossed and the two crossed, offer a powerful technique for differentiating among the various possible reasons for reflex abnormality.

Illustrative Cases

If the basis for the reflex abnormality is insufficient loudness in the ear receiving the reflex-eliciting signal (a disorder of the afferent portion of the reflex arc), then the abnormality will be observed on the two reflexes involving presentation of sound to the suspect ear, but the other two reflexes will be spared. In the case of a left acoustic tumor, for example, the crossed left-to-right reflex and the uncrossed left reflex will be abnormal, but the other two will typically be spared. This pattern is illustrated in Figure 6-12. The pa-

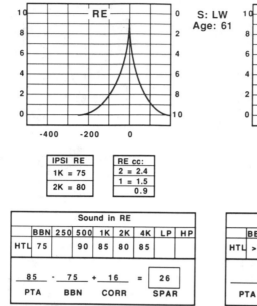
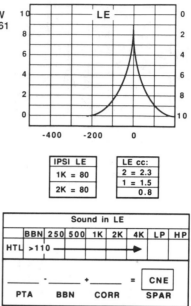

S: LW
Age: 61

		Sound in RE						
	BBN	250	500	1K	2K	4K	LP	HP
HTL	75		90	85	80	85		

$$\underline{85} - \underline{75} + \underline{16} = \boxed{26}$$

PTA	BBN	CORR	SPAR

		Sound in LE						
	BBN	250	500	1K	2K	4K	LP	HP
HTL	>110							

$$\underline{} - \underline{} + \underline{} = \boxed{CNE}$$

PTA	BBN	CORR	SPAR

Figure 6-11. Results of immittance audiometry on a 61-year-old man with a brainstem infarct.

tient was a 27-year-old man with a left acoustic tumor. The audiogram (Figure 6-12A) showed a mild sensory loss in the left ear (pure tone audiometry = 28 dB), and speech audiometry showed "rollover" of both the performance-intensity–phonetically balanced and performance-intensity–synthetic sentence identification functions. Note that in spite of the relatively mild loss on the left ear, left-to-right crossed thresholds were elevated to 110 dB HL at 500 and 1000 Hz and were absent at 2000 and 4000 Hz. Yet, in comparison with the thresholds on the right ear, the abnormality in reflex thresholds was not striking. Figure 6-12B shows the four suprathreshold reflex waveforms for a reflex-eliciting signal at 1000 Hz and 110 dB SPL. Note the relatively well-formed reflex morphology for both the crossed and uncrossed reflexes with sound to the right ear, but the greatly attenuated amplitudes for both crossed and uncrossed reflexes with sound to the left ear. Calculation of the AI yielded a value of 1.48, well beyond the normal limit of 0.7. The commonality in the two abnormal reflexes is that both represent presentation of sound to the left ear. It does not matter which ear the probe is in because the problem is in the afferent branch of the reflex arc. When sound is delivered to the left ear, the resulting sensation of loudness is not sufficient to elicit the reflex.

If, on the other hand, the basis for the reflex abnormality is a problem in the ear housing the

acoustic probe, either because of middle ear or facial nerve disorder (a problem in the efferent portion of the reflex arc), then the two reflexes measured with the probe in the suspect ear will be involved, but the other two will be spared. Suppose for example, that the left facial nerve is paralyzed. Then the left uncrossed and the right-to-left crossed reflexes will be abnormal, but the other two will be spared. The commonality in the two abnormal reflexes is that both represent a condition in which the probe is in the left ear. It does not matter to which ear the sound is delivered because the problem is in the efferent branch of the reflex arc. When the probe is in the left ear, the reflex does not appear, even though the sensation of loudness evoked by the reflex-eliciting signal in either ear is sufficient. Figure 6-13 illustrates these principles in a 44-year-old woman with a left Bell's palsy. The audiogram (Figure 6-13A) shows a mild sensory loss in the affected ear (unusual in Bell's palsy). All speech audiometric results were within normal limits. Conventional reflex thresholds were present in the right uncrossed mode, and in the left-to-right crossed mode but were absent in the left uncrossed and the right-to-left crossed modes. Figure 6-13B shows the four suprathreshold waveforms for a 1000 Hz tone at 110 dB SPL. Calculation from the four amplitudes

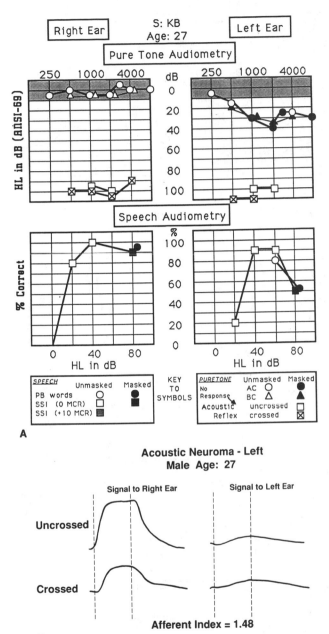

Figure 6-12. Results of pure tone and speech audiometry (A) and averaged acoustic reflexes (B) on a 27-year-old man with a left acoustic tumor. The reflex-eliciting signal was a 1000 Hz tone presented at 110 dB SPL.

of the EI yielded a value of 1.93, far beyond the normal limit of 1.00.

If the problem is in the brainstem portion of the reflex arc, then one or both of the crossed reflexes will be abnormal, but the two uncrossed reflexes will typically be spared. The commonality in the two abnormal reflexes is that both represent a condition in which the sound is delivered to one ear and the probe is sealed in the opposite ear. Here the problem is in neither the afferent nor the efferent portions of the reflex arc but in the neural pathways linking the cochlear nucleus on one side of the brainstem with the motor nucleus of the facial nerve on the opposite side. Lesions at this site will typically spare both uncrossed reflexes since the neural pathways sub-

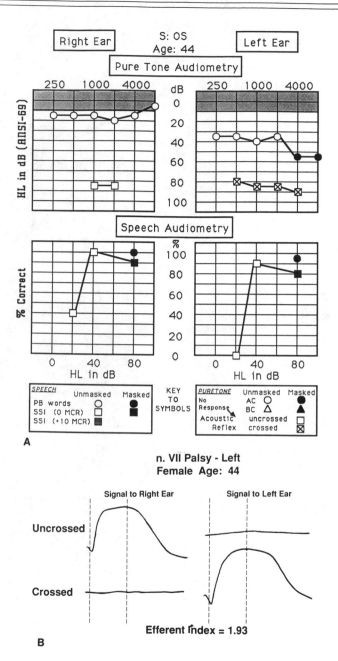

Figure 6-13. Results of pure tone and speech audiometry (A) and averaged acoustic reflexes (B) on a 44-year-old woman with a left Bell's palsy. The reflex-eliciting signal was a 1000 Hz tone presented at 110 dB SPL.

serving these two reflexes do not cross the brainstem. These principles are illustrated in Figure 6-14 in the case of a 34-year-old woman with multiple sclerosis. Note the relatively normal pure tone and speech audiometric results (Figure 6-14A). The four waveforms in Figure 6-14B show well-formed uncrossed reflex responses but greatly attenuated amplitudes for the two crossed reflex responses. The resultant CPI was 1.08, well beyond the normal limit of 0.8.

The final case illustrates the sensitivity of both the amplitude index measure and the onset latency variability measure. The patient is a 54-year-old man with a right acoustic neuroma. The audiogram (Figure 6-15A) shows a mild high-frequency sensory hearing loss on the left ear and a

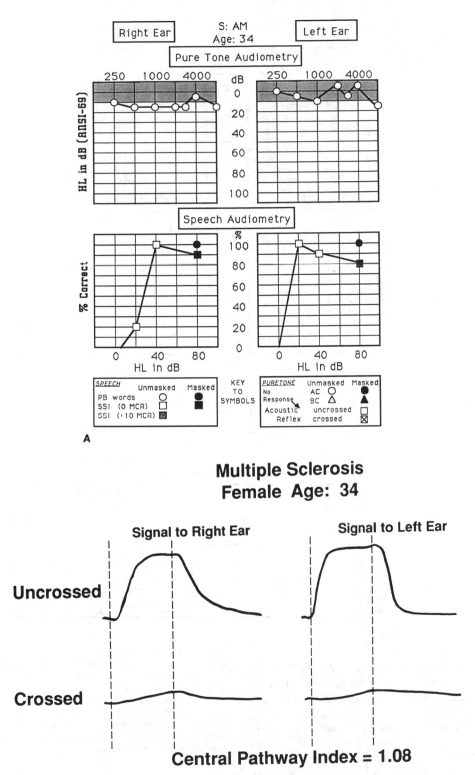

Figure 6-14. Results of pure tone and speech audiometry (A) and averaged acoustic reflexes (B) on a 34-year-old woman with multiple sclerosis. The reflex-eliciting signal was a 1000 Hz tone presented at 110 dB SPL.

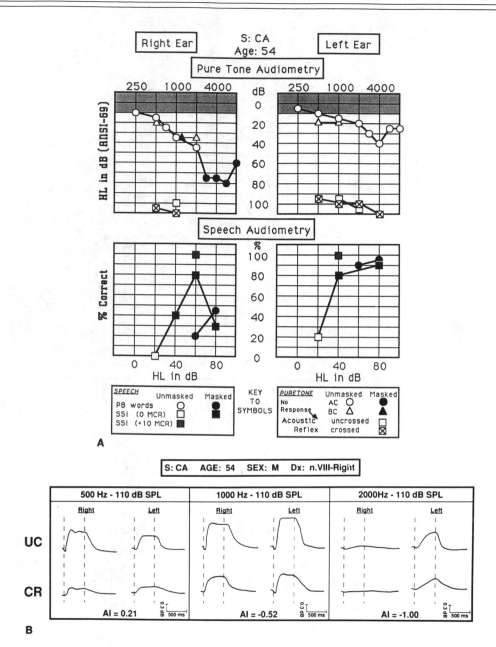

Figure 6-15. Results of pure tone and speech audiometry (A) on a 54-year-old man with a right acoustic tumor. B. Representative averaged reflex waveforms at 500, 1000, 2000 Hz to a signal at an intensity level of 110 dB SPL. C. Reflex waveforms at 1000 Hz (top panel) and standard deviations of onset latency, amplitude, and offset latency, calculated over 16 successive waveforms. Shaded area represents the 95 percent normal confidence interval.

moderate high-frequency sensory loss on the right ear. Conventional crossed reflex thresholds were present at 500 and 1000 Hz on the right ear at levels of 105 and 110 dB HL, respectively. At 2000 and 4000 Hz, however, responses were not obtained at 110 dB HL. Figure 6-15B shows representative suprathreshold-averaged reflex waveforms (n = 8) at 500, 1000, and 2000 Hz. In all cases, the intensity level of the reflex-eliciting signal was 110 dB SPL. Note that at 500 and 1000 Hz, responses were well defined in both the

crossed and uncrossed modes. Additionally, the AI was within normal limits (less than 0.70) at both frequencies. At 2000 Hz, however, the con-

S: CA Age: 54 Sex: M Dx: n. VIII-Right

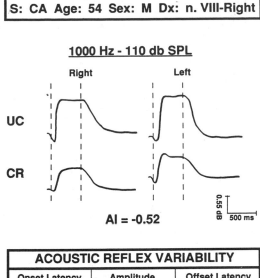

1000 Hz - 110 db SPL

Right　　　　Left

UC

CR

AI = -0.52

0.55 dB | 500 ms

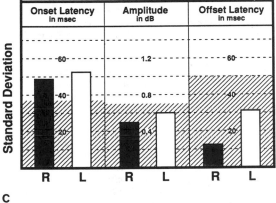

ACOUSTIC REFLEX VARIABILITY

Onset Latency in msec	Amplitude in dB	Offset Latency in msec

Standard Deviation

C

sizes that the abnormality in sequential variability was confined to the onset dimension of the reflex waveform.

These four cases illustrate the important point that suprathreshold waveform morphology of the acoustic reflex may yield more sensitive diagnostic information than conventional reflex thresholds.

SUMMARY

Immittance audiometry is a powerful tool for the evaluation of auditory disorder. Careful examination of the three components of the immittance battery — the tympanogram, the static immittance, and the acoustic reflex, both crossed and uncrossed — provides information about middle ear, cochlear, and retrocochlear disorder. The key to successful use of the immittance battery in clinical evaluation is to view the results in combination with the totality of the audiometric examination rather than in isolation. As the immittance battery becomes an integral part of basic audiometric assessment, the clinician will come to appreciate the unique patterns characterizing each distinct clinical entity. When immittance results are viewed within this framework, rather than in isolation, the clinician will learn more quickly to appreciate their importance to the total audiometric evaluation.

siderably attenuated amplitudes of the right uncrossed and right-to-left crossed waveforms led to a significant AI of 1.00. Figure 6-15C repeats the four reflex waveforms at 1000 Hz, showing the nonsignificant AI (AI = −0.52). In the lower panel of this figure is plotted the standard deviation of onset, amplitude, and offset latencies, calculated over 16 successive individual waveforms. The shaded areas along the lower boundary represent the range of normal expectation (95 percent confidence interval) for these variability measures. Note that the onset variability scores exceed the norm on both ears. This abnormality is particularly striking in view of the fact that all other threshold and suprathreshold measures of individual or averaged waveforms were within normal limits at this test frequency. In addition, the fact that neither amplitude nor offset latency variability exceeded the normal range empha-

REFERENCES

Alberti, P., & Jerger, J. (1974). Probe-tone frequency and the diagnostic value of tympanometry. *Archives of Otolaryngology, 99,* 206.

Alberti, P., & Kristensen, R. (1970). The clinical application of impedance audiometry. *Laryngoscope, 80,* 735–746.

Anderson, H., Barr, B., & Wedenberg, E. (1969). Intra-aural reflexes in retrocochlear lesions. In C. Hamberger & J. Wersall (Eds.), *Nobel Symposium 10: Disorders of the skull base region* (pp. 49–55). Stockholm: Almquist & Wiskell.

Antonelli, A. R., Bellotto, R., & Grandori, F. (1987). Audiologic diagnosis of central versus eighth nerve and cochlear auditory impairment. *Audiology, 26,* 209–226.

Blom, S., & Zakrisson, J. E. (1974). The stapedius reflex in the diagnosis of myasthenia gravis. *Journal of Neurological Sciences, 21,* 71–76.

Borg, E. (1982). Dynamic properties of the intra-aural reflex in lesions of the lower auditory pathway. *Acta Oto-laryngologica* (Stockholm), *93,* 19–29.

Bosatra, A., Russolo, M., & Poli, P. (1975). Modifications of the stapedius muscle reflex under spontaneous and experimental brain-stem impairment. *Acta Oto-laryngologica* (Stockholm), *80,* 61–66.

Bosatra, A., Russolo, M., & Poli, P. (1976). Oscilloscopic

analysis of the stapedius muscle reflex in brain stem lesions. *Archives of Otolaryngology, 102,* 284–285.

Brooks, D. (1969). The use of the electro-acoustic impedance bridge in the assessment of middle ear function. *International Audiology, 8,* 563–569.

Bruschini, P., Sellari–Franceschini, S., Bartalena, L., Aghini-Lombardi, F., Mazzeo, S., & Martino, E. (1984). Acoustic reflex characteristics in hypo- and hyperthyroid patients. *Audiology, 23,* 38–45.

Clemis, J. D., & Sarno, C. N. (1980). The acoustic reflex latency test: Clinical applications. *Laryngoscope, 90,* 601–611.

Cohen, M., & Prasher, D. (1988). The value of combining auditory brainstem responses and acoustic reflex threshold measurements in neuro-otological diagnosis. *Scandinavian Audiology, 17,* 153–162.

Colletti, V. (1975). Stapedius reflex abnormalities in multiple sclerosis. *Audiology, 14,* 63–71.

Colletti, V. (1977). Multifrequency tympanometry. *Audiology, 16,* 278–287.

Elonka, D. R. (1986). Letter to the editor. *American Journal of Otology, 7,* 164–165.

Fowler, C. G., & Wilson, R. H. (1984). Adaptation of the acoustic reflex. *Ear & Hearing, 5,* 281–288.

Funasaka, S., Funai, H., & Kumakawa, K. (1984). Sweep-frequency tympanometry: Its development and diagnostic value. *Audiology, 23,* 366–379.

Greisen, O., & Rasmussen, P. E. (1970). Stapedius muscle reflexes and oto-neurological examinations in brain-stem tumors. *Acta Oto-laryngologica* (Stockholm), *70,* 366–370.

Grenman, R., Lang, H., Panelius, M., Salmivalli, A., Laine, H., & Rintamaki, J. (1984). Stapedius reflex and brainstem auditory evoked responses in multiple sclerosis patients. *Scandinavian Audiology, 13,* 109–113.

Hall, J. W. (1982a). Acoustic reflex amplitude. II. Effect of age-related auditory dysfunction. *Audiology, 21,* 386–399.

Hall, J. W. (1982b). Quantification of the relationship between crossed and uncrossed acoustic reflex amplitudes. *Ear & Hearing, 3,* 296–300.

Hannley, M., Jerger, J. F., & Rivera, V. M. (1983). Relationships among auditory brainstem response, masking level difference and the acoustic reflex in multiple sclerosis. *Audiology, 22,* 20–33.

Hayes, D., & Jerger, J. (1983). Signal-averaging of the acoustic reflex: Diagnostic applications of amplitude characteristics. *Scandinavian Audiology.* Supplementum, *17,* 31–36.

Hess, K. (1979). Stapedius reflex in multiple sclerosis. *Journal of Neurology, Neurosurgery and Psychiatry, 42,* 331–337.

Hirsch, A., & Anderson, H. (1980a). Audiologic test results in 96 patients with tumours affecting the eighth nerve. *Acta Oto-laryngologica.* Supplement (Stockholm), *369,* 1–26.

Hirsch, A., & Anderson, H. (1980b). Elevated stapedius reflex threshold and pathologic reflex decay. *Acta Oto-laryngologica.* Supplement (Stockholm), *368,* 1–28.

Jerger, J. (1970). Clinical experience with impedance audiometry. *Archives of Otolaryngology, 92,* 331–324.

Jerger, J. (1975). Diagnostic use of impedance measures. In J. Jerger (Ed.), *Handbook of clinical impedance audiometry.* New York: American Electromedics Co.

Jerger, J., & Hayes, D. (1983). Latency of the acoustic reflex in eighth-nerve tumors. *Archives of Otolaryngology, 109,* 1–5.

Jerger, J., & Jerger, S. (1974). Auditory findings in brainstem disorder. *Archives of Otolaryngology, 99,* 342–350.

Jerger, J., & Jerger, S. (1983). Acoustic reflex decay: 10-second or 5-second criterion? *Ear & Hearing, 4,* 70–71.

Jerger, J., Anthony, L., Jerger, S., & Mauldin, L. (1974). Studies in impedance audiometry III. Middle ear disorders.

Archives of Otolaryngology, 99, 165–171.

Jerger, J., Burney, P., Mauldin, L., & Crump, B. (1974). Predicting hearing loss from the acoustic reflex. *Journal of Speech and Hearing Disorders, 39,* 11–22.

Jerger, J., Harford, E., Clemis, J., & Alford, B. (1974). The acoustic reflex in eighth nerve disorder. *Archives of Otolaryngology, 99,* 409–413.

Jerger, J., Hayes, D., Anthony, L., & Mauldin, L. (1978). Factors influencing prediction of hearing level from the acoustic reflex. *Monographs in Contemporary Audiology, 1,* 1–20.

Jerger, J., Jerger, S., & Mauldin, L. (1972). Studies in impedance audiometry: I. Normal and sensorineural ears. *Archives of Otolaryngology, 96,* 513–523.

Jerger, J., Neely, J. G., & Jerger, S. (1980). Speech, impedance, and auditory brainstem response audiometry in brainstem tumors. *Archives of Otolaryngology, 106,* 218–223.

Jerger, J., Oliver, T. A., & Jenkins, H. (1987). Suprathreshold abnormalities of the stapedius reflex in acoustic tumor: A series of case reports. *Ear & Hearing , 8,* 131–139.

Jerger, J. F., Oliver, T. A., Chmiel, R. A., & Rivera, V. M. (1986). Patterns of auditory abnormality in multiple sclerosis. *Audiology, 25,* 193–209.

Jerger, J., Oliver, T. A., Rivera, V., & Stach, B. A. (1986). Abnormalities of the acoustic reflex in multiple sclerosis. *American Journal of Otolaryngology, 7,* 163–176.

Jerger, J., Oliver, T. A., & Stach, B. A. (1986). Problems in the clinical measurement of acoustic reflex latency. *Scandinavian Audiology, 15,* 31–40.

Jerger, S., & Jerger, J. (1975). Extra- and intra-axial brain stem auditory disorders. *Audiology, 14,* 93–117.

Jerger, S., & Jerger, J. (1977). Diagnostic value of crossed vs uncrossed acoustic reflexes. Eighth nerve and brainstem disorders. *Archives of Otolaryngology, 103,* 445–453.

Jerger, S., Neely, J. G., & Jerger, J. (1975). Recovery of crossed acoustic reflexes in brain stem auditory disorders. *Acta Oto-laryngologica* (Stockholm), *101,* 329–332.

Johnson, E. W. (1977). Auditory test results in 500 cases of acoustic neuroma. *Archives of Otolaryngology, 103,* 152–158.

Karlsson, K., & Hagerman, B. (1984). A clinical comparison between a laboratory and a commercial impedance audiometer. *Scandinavian Audiology, 13,* 199–203.

Kofler, B., Oberascher, G., & Pommer, B. (1984). Brain-stem involvement in multiple sclerosis: A comparison between brain-stem auditory evoked potentials and the acoustic stapedius reflex. *Journal of Neurology, 231,* 145–147.

Kramer, L. D., Ruth, R. A., Johns, M. E., & Sanders, D. B. (1981). A comparison of stapedial reflex fatigue with repetitive stimulation and single fiber EMG in myasthenia gravis. *Annals of Neurology, 9,* 531–536.

Lenarz, T., & Gulzow, J. (1983). Acoustic inner ear trauma by impedance measurement. Acute acoustic trauma? *Laryngologie, Rhinologie, and Otologie, 62,* 58–61.

Lidén, G. (1969). The scope and application of current audiometric tests. *Journal of Laryngology and Otology, 83,* 507–520.

Lidén, G., Harford, E., & Hallen, O. (1974). Tympanometry for the diagnosis of ossicular disruption. *Archives of Otolaryngology, 99,* 23–29.

Lidén, G., Peterson, J., & Björkman, G. (1970). Tympanometry. *Archives of Otolaryngology, 92,* 248–257.

Lilly, D. J. (1984). Evaluation of the response time of acoustic-immittance instruments. In S. Silman (Ed.), *The acoustic reflex.* New York: Academic Press.

Mangham, C. A., & Lindeman, R. C. (1980). The negative acoustic reflex in retrocochlear disorders. *Laryngoscope, 90,* 1753–1761.

Mangham, C. A., & Miller, J. M. (1979). A case for further quantification of the stapedius reflex. *Archives of Otolaryngology, 105,* 593–596.

Mangham, C. A., Lindeman, R. C., & Dawson, W. R. (1980). Stapedius reflex quantification in acoustic tumor patients. *Laryngology, 90,* 242–250.

Margolis, R., & Smith, P. (1977). Tympanometric asymmetry. *Journal of Speech and Hearing Research, 20,* 437–446.

Metz, O. (1946). The acoustic impedance measured on normal and pathological ears. *Acta Oto-laryngologica.* Supplement (Stockholm), *63,* 1–254.

Miller, M. H., Hoffman, R. A., & Smallberg, G. (1984). Stapedial reflex testing and partially reversible acoustic trauma. *Hearing Instruments, 35,* 15, 49.

Moller, A. R. (1961). Bilateral contraction of the tympanic membrane in man examined by measuring acoustic impedance change. *Annals of Otology, Rhinology, and Laryngology, 70,* 735–753.

Moller, A. (1962). The sensitivity of contraction of the tympanic muscle in man. *Annals of Otology, 77,* 86.

Niemeyer, W., & Sesterhenn, G. (1972). Calculating the hearing threshold from the stapedius reflex threshold for different sound stimuli. Presented at the Eleventh International Congress of Audiology, Budapest.

Niemeyer, W., & Sesterhenn, G. (1974). Calculating the hearing threshold from the stapedius reflex threshold for different sound stimuli. *Audiology, 13,* 421–427.

Olsen, W. O., Noffsinger, D., & Kurdziel, S. (1975). Acoustic reflex and reflex decay. Occurrence in patients with cochlear and eighth nerve lesions. *Archives of Otolaryngology, 101,* 622–625.

Olsen, W. O., Stach, B. A., & Kurdziel, S. A. (1981). Acoustic reflex decay in 10 seconds and in 5 seconds for Ménière's disease patients and for VIIIth nerve patients. *Ear & Hearing, 2,* 180–181.

Olsen, W. O., Stach, B. A., & Kurdziel, S. A. (1983). Reply to Jerger and Jerger. *Ear & Hearing, 4,* 71.

Paradise, J., Smith, C., & Bluestone, C. (1976). Tympanometric detection of middle ear effusion in infants and young children. *Pediatrics, 58,* 198–210.

Peterson, J. L., & Lidén, G. (1972). Some static characteristics of the stapedial muscle reflex. *Audiology, 11,* 97.

Portman, M. (1980). Impedance audiometry is not always without risk. *Revue de Laryngologie, Otolologie, Rhinolologie* (Bordeaux), *101,* 181–182.

Sanders, J. W., Josey, A. F., & Glasscock, M. E. (1974). Audiologic evaluation in cochlear and eighth nerve disorders. *Archives of Otolaryngology, 100,* 283–289.

Sanders, J. W., Josey, A. F., Glasscock, M. E., & Jackson, C. G. (1981). The acoustic reflex test in cochlear and eighth nerve pathology ears. *Laryngoscope, 91,* 787–793.

Shanks, J. E. (1984). Tympanometry. *Ear & Hearing, 5,* 268–280.

Shanks, J. E., Lilly, D. J., Margolis, R. H., Wiley, T. L., & Wilson, R. H. (1988). Tympanometry. *Journal of Speech and Hearing Disorders, 53,* 354–377.

Sheehy, J. L., & Inzer, B. E. (1976). Acoustic reflex test in neurotologic diagnosis. *Archives of Otolaryngology, 102,* 647–653.

Silman, S. (1984). Magnitude and growth of the acoustic reflex. In S. Silman (Ed.), *The acoustic reflex.* New York: Academic Press.

Silman, S., Gelfand, S. A., Piper, N., Silverman, C. A., & Van Frank, L. (1984). Prediction of hearing loss from the acoustic-reflex threshold. In S. Silman (Ed.), *The acoustic reflex.* New York: Academic Press.

Stach, B. A. (1987). The acoustic reflex in diagnostic audiology: From Metz to present. *Ear & Hearing.* Supplement, *8,* 36–42.

Stach, B. A., & Jerger, J. F. (1984). Acoustic reflex averaging. *Ear & Hearing, 5,* 289–296.

Stach, B. A., & Jerger, J. F. (1987a). Acoustic reflex patterns in peripheral and central auditory system disease. *Seminars in Hearing, 8,* 369–377.

Stach, B. A., & Jerger, J. F. (1987b). Techniques for acoustic reflex measurement and analysis. *Seminars in Hearing, 8,* 359–367.

Stach, B. A., Jerger, J. F., & Jenkins, H. A. (1984). The human acoustic tensor tympani reflex. A case report. *Scandinavian Audiology, 13,* 93–99.

Stephens, S. D. G., & Thornton, A. R. D. (1976). Subjective and electrophysiologic tests in brain-stem lesions. *Archives of Otolaryngology, 102,* 608–613.

Terkildsen, K., & Thomsen, K. A. (1959). The influence of pressure variations on the impedance of the human ear drum. *Journal of Laryngology and Otology, 73,* 409.

Terkildsen, K., Osterhammel, P., & Scott–Nielsen, S. (1970). Impedance measurements. Probe-tone intensity and middle ear reflexes. *Acta Oto-laryngologica* (Stockholm), *263,* 205.

Thomsen, K. A. (1958). Investigation on the tubal function and measurement of the middle-ear pressure in pressure chamber. *Acta Oto-laryngologica.* Supplement (Stockholm), *140,* 269.

Thomsen, K., & Terkildsen, K. (1975). Audiological findings in 125 cases of acoustic neuromas. *Acta Oto-laryngologica* (Stockholm), *280,* 353–361.

Warren, W. R., Gutmann, L., Cody, R. C., Flower, P., & Segal, A. T. (1977). Stapedius reflex decay in myasthenia gravis. *Archives of Neurology, 34,* 496–497.

Yamane, M., & Nomura, Y. (1984). Analysis of stapedial reflex in neuromuscular diseases. *Archives of Otology, Rhinology, and Laryngology, 46,* 84–96.

Zakrisson, J. E., Borg, E., & Blom, S. (1974). The acoustic impedance change as a measure of stapedius muscle activity in man. A methodological study with electromyography. *Acta Oto-laryngologica* (Stockholm), *78,* 357.

Zwislocki, J., & Feldman, A. (1970). Acoustic impedance of pathological ears. *ASHA Monographs, 15.*

CHAPTER 7

Strategies for Optimizing the Detection of Neuropathology from the Auditory Brainstem Response

Daniel M. Schwartz • Michele D. Morris

Since its initial description by Jewett, Romano, and Williston (1970), the auditory brainstem response (ABR) has been used extensively to evaluate the functional integrity of the peripheral and central auditory pathways. Audiologically, the ABR has enjoyed widespread popularity in the evaluation of hearing whenever behavioral audiometric techniques are precluded, such as with infants, uncooperative children, and adults. In neurodiagnostics it has been used to verify demyelinating, compressive, vascular, or metabolic disease in patients who present with neurologic signs and symptoms. When clinical signs and symptoms are ambiguous, the ABR has helped define an abnormality or it has detected insidious or occult lesion in the otherwise asymptomatic patient. In an adjacent neurologic role, the ABR also has proved valuable in neural monitoring of central nervous system status during operative procedures that place the peripheral or central auditory pathway, or both, at risk for neurologic compromise and for the serial assessment of brainstem integrity in the comatose head-injured patient. Without question, therefore, the ABR has become an essential part of audiologic, otologic, and neurologic medicine.

During the past decade a sundry of book chapters have been written on each of the aforementioned ABR applications. In general, these have represented introductory overviews of fundamental principles and assumptions that underlie ABR measurement and interpretation, descriptions of clinical methodology based on early historical works in ABR, or concentrated uncritical literature reviews on some specific application often augmented by case studies. Much less often have such chapters focused on clinical testing

protocols and strategies actually adopted by the author(s) and justification for their use.

This chapter on neurodiagnostic applications of the ABR concentrates on testing strategies that are used in the authors' own clinical neurophysiology practice to optimize information that will identify electrical abnormality along the auditory pathway. A unique aspect of this chapter is a *What If?* section that provides a troubleshooting guide to sometimes perplexing clinical situations. Throughout, limitations in conventional methodology or specific research studies are addressed based on many years of specialized clinical practice in multimodality evoked potentials. The aim is not to judge what is right or wrong, rather to present a philosophy predicated on optimizing the ABR from which to base a rational, defensible diagnostic impression regarding the presence, type, and perhaps the anatomic distribution of a disease process.

This chapter is not meant to serve as a primer for the inexperienced reader. Rather, the authors assume fundamental knowledge of the neurophysiologic bases of the ABR, the normal ABR and its variants, and the effects of parametric changes in recording parameters and subject variables that can affect waveform latency, amplitude, and morphology. Indeed a long roster of existing textbooks and book chapters deal quite adequately with the elementary aspects of auditory evoked potentials.

The objective was not to write "yet another chapter" on neurologic applications of the ABR but to relate clinical knowledge that has been gained from an evoked potential practice that transcends the more traditional otolaryngic referral base. This goal will have been achieved if readers can transfer these insights into their own clinical practice.

141

TOWARD MAXIMIZING THE ABR FOR DIAGNOSTIC INTERPRETATION

Originating from the antecedent works of Jewett and Williston (1971), Hecox and Galambos (1974), and Starr and Achor (1975), the methodology most commonly employed to record the ABR has been governed by historical convention based on early pioneering literature. Although this approach serves to maintain consistency across laboratories, it does not necessarily reflect optimal stimulating and recording parameters for high-quality response detection. Clinicians often seem to be "locked" into one set procedure regardless of the patient or the quality of the response. Perhaps this "inflexibility" is a byproduct of clinical comfort based on what has been taught at a workshop, by a supervisor, or what has appeared in literature review–type book chapters. Unfortunately failure to explore alternatives to traditional structure or to deviate from a conventional protocol is guaranteed to increase the false-negative or -positive rates for disease detection. Moreover, it limits new insights into the power of the ABR in neurodiagostics.

OPTIMIZING THE RECORDING MONTAGE

Based on historical precedent, the most common electrode montage for neurodiagnostic testing has been a single channel with the noninverting electrode at the vertex (Cz) or high forehead (Fpz), the inverting one usually at the ipsilateral mastoid (M1-M2) or earlobe (A1-A2) and ground on the contralateral mastoid or earlobe.

The goal of clinical practice is to solicit maximum information as to the electrical integrity of the auditory system from which to form the bases of an accurate diagnostic impression. Consequently, a four-channel recording derivation similar to that described by Hall et al. (1984) is advocated in an effort to achieve voltage maxima of specific peaks by aligning the recording electrodes in the direction of the presumed electrical dipole. No single electrode montage can reliably detect all far-field generators. Thus, in addition to the conventional orthogonal arrangement from ipsilateral earlobe to vertex (Cz-A1-A2), the authors always record simultaneously from the contralateral earlobe (channel 2), between ears (A1-A2) representing a horizontal montage (channel 3), and from vertex to a noncephalic reference (channel 4) on the second cervical vertebra (Cz-C2). The common or ground electrode is typically placed at Fpz.

Figure 7-1 depicts a four-channel recording obtained from an audiologic and neurologic normal patient. Observe the relative size and latencies of different peak components between electrode derivations.

Figure 7-1. Example of a four-channel ABR recording from a neurologically normal patient. *SP* refers to the summating potential.

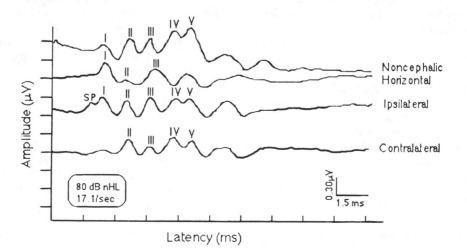

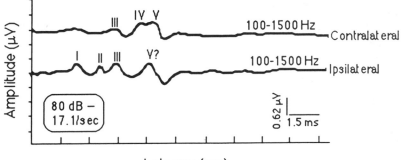

Figure 7-2. Example of how the contralateral ABR recording channel helps unfuse a IV/V complex for correct peak identification.

On the contralateral recording, the important feature is that wave IV appears slightly earlier and wave V later in time than on the ipsilateral recording. This is attributed to the notion that in normal ears, the dipole vector for wave V turns toward the stimulated ear. Hence, this robust ABR component will reach its peak amplitude sooner than it would along the line from vertex to contralateral ear. Wave IV, on the other hand, would actually achieve maximum amplitude earlier on the contralateral side since it rotates in the opposite direction to wave V. The clinical value of this is seen when wave IV and V become fused, thus confounding peak identification, as shown in Figure 7-2. It is easily seen how the contralateral channel serves to separate the fused rostral wave complex owing to the differences in their respective dipole orientations.

The horizontal channel is used to enhance wave I amplitude and definition when it is poorly

Figure 7-3. Example of how the horizontal recording channel helps define an ambiguous or poorly resolved wave I.

resolved on the ipsilateral channel response as illustrated in Figure 7-3. The reason for this improvement in wave I is that the ear-to-ear configuration lies along the general line of action potential propagation and has horizontal dipole equivalents (Starr and Squires, 1982). When information from this third channel is viewed with that from the second contralateral channel, which typically has no wave I but a more prominent wave II, identification of these distal and proximal eighth nerve responses is clarified greatly.

The value of the fourth noncephalic reference channel, shown in Figure 7-4, lies in the improved definition and increased voltage of wave V, particularly when a broad-filter passband (30–1500 Hz) is used. The orientation of vertex to cervical vertebra appears to follow the axis of the brainstem. In their studies of the 3-channel Lissajous' trajectory of the ABR in humans, Sininger et al. (1987) also indicated that on the basis of vector amplitude plots, the maximum voltage for wave V is obtained from a vertex to high cervical vertebra electrode montage. Borrowing from the somatosensory works of Cracco and Cracco (1976) and Desmedt and Cheron (1980), a noncephalic refer-

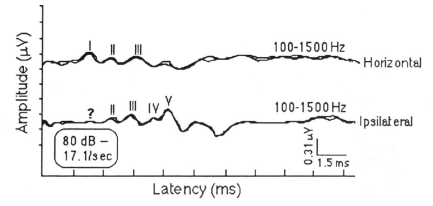

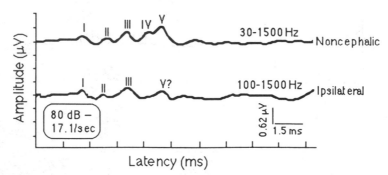

Figure 7-4. Advantage of a noncephalic reference recording channel clarifying wave V definition and amplitude.

ence seems to permit better correspondence between electrical potentials derived from a near field and those from a distant far field relative for subcortical neural-generating sources.

This multiple-channel recording montage has been invaluable in unveiling the "true" peak component(s) in perplexing clinical situations where wave identification often would be left to "guesswork." This not only influences greatly clinical decision making but certainly reduces false-negative and -positive rates. It is also comforting to know that ABR mapping studies (Sininger et al., 1987; Starr and Squires, 1982) support these clinical observations.

OPTIMIZING THE BANDPASS FILTER SETTING

The selection of an optimal analog filter passband should be governed by the frequency content of the potential of interest and the signal-to-noise ratio. Perhaps the most popular filter settings are a high pass of 150 Hz and low pass of 3000 Hz. The advantage of setting the high-pass cutoff above 100 Hz is that it reduces electrical (60 Hz) and myogenic interference that will contaminate the average waveform while permitting clear observation of the ABR fast components. The disadvantage to such extreme filtering, however, is suppression of the low-frequency slow component, which contributes heavily to wave V amplitude (Kavanagh et al., 1988; Kevanishvili and Aponchenko, 1979; Laukli and Mair, 1981; Mason, 1984).

Since the amplitude of wave V is significantly greater than that of the faster, earlier waves for most patients, minor voltage reductions and waveform distortions due to low-frequency filtering (150 Hz) usually have little influence on wave identification. Yet, as discussed previously, many patients display a poorly resolved wave V, thereby making accurate peak identification difficult, at best.

Recall that both contralateral and noncephalic electrode derivations are used to facilitate wave V identification. If the high-pass filter cutoff of the noncephalic channel is lowered to 30 Hz, it will optimize wave V identification still further since the waveform will represent the algebraic sum of the slow and fast components of the ABR (Figure 7-5). The result can be as much as a 20 percent voltage gain (Kavanagh et al., 1988). This is particularly critical in pediatric work when attempting to estimate the degree of hearing loss from wave V threshold or in neurodiagnostics when wave V is ambiguous. (See Schwartz and Schwartz (1989) for a more detailed discussion of filter selection in brainstem evoked response audiometry.)

Clinically, the high-pass setting for individual channels should be selected according to the major frequency content of the peak component(s) of interest. Since the majority of the spectral energy of the early waves I–III is above 100 Hz, the high-pass cutoff from the ipsilateral, contralateral, and horizontal channels is 100 or 150 Hz, depending on the instrumentation used. For the noncephalic channel, used primarily for wave V identification, the high cutoff frequency is set at 30 or 50 Hz.

There appears to be no obvious advantage to the conventional low-pass cutoff of 3000 Hz since no appreciable ABR spectral energy is above 1000 Hz. Rather, a 1500 Hz setting, which eliminates the overriding high-frequency noise commonly seen and provides a better waveform clarity overall, is recommended.

OPTIMIZING STIMULUS REPETITION RATES

Since the ABR represents the summation of synchronously locked neural discharges within

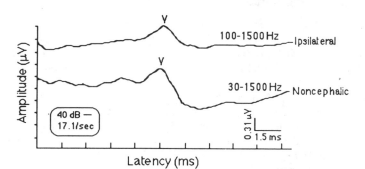

Figure 7-5. Example of how a noncephalic recording site (Cz-C2) combined with a broad-filter passband serve to enhance wave V amplitude, particularly for low-intensity ABR recordings.

the auditory nervous system, successful recording depends on the temporal characteristics of the stimulus. Accordingly, a transient signal and a relatively slow rate of stimulus presentation are required for defining the early, faster peak components (I through III).

Most clinicians present click stimuli at odd integers near 10 per second (usually 11.1/second). One important reason for selecting an odd integer is to avoid harmonic interaction with 60 Hz line noise. The rationale for selecting a nominal 10 per second, however, is unclear. Perhaps it stems from the seminal work of Jewett and Williston (1971) who stated that "we frequently found that at click rates higher than about 10 stimuli/sec the baseline preceding the click artifact was not as flat as at slower rates" (p. 689). Given that they found the best waveform clarity at a rate of 2 per second, subsequent more clinically minded individuals may have considered 10 per second to represent a suitable compromise between the slow rate needed to maximize neural synchrony and the number of averages necessary to present a clinically interpretable waveform series. Regardless of its origin, the advantage of a slow rate is to ensure synchronous neural discharge.

Although the choice of an 11.1 per second stimulus repetition rate is certainly defensible, the authors have deviated from this standard and use a rate of 17.1 per second. The rationale for this comes from finding essentially no difference in wave I morphology and amplitude at 17.1 per second versus 11.1 per second for the broad spectrum of patients that are evaluated. The advantage of a 17.1 per second rate is that it saves valuable testing time that can be used for additional routine ABR measures, or for acquiring more averages when the patient is "noisy." Of course, when

faced with an unusual patient who presents with a poorly resolved wave I, even on the horizontal channel, the rate is slowed, as will be discussed later in the *What If?* section of this chapter.

Note: Rates more than 20 per second often will reduce wave I amplitude by 20 percent or more in ears with high-frequency sensory hearing loss; therefore, repetition rate should be held below 20 per second in neurodiagnostics.

In addition to using a relatively slow rate to ensure adequate neural synchrony, the authors are also great proponents of the routine use of a rapid rate of stimulus presentation as a means of affecting central synaptic efficiency. Although several studies have suggested faster rates of presentation (greater than or equal to 50/second) result in abnormal latency prolongation and waveform distortion in selected patients with neuropathology (Fowler and Noffsinger, 1983; Gerling and Finitzo-Hieber, 1983; Jacobson, Murray, and Deppe, 1987; Pratt et al., 1981; Robinson and Rudge, 1977; Shanon, Gold, and Himmelfarb, 1981; Stockard, Stockard, and Sharbrough, 1977; Yagi and Kaga, 1979), few centers have followed the recommendation for a dual-rate ABR protocol. This dual-rate strategy is not more popular for several reasons. First might be the notion that in the majority of neuropathologic patients, particularly those with acoustic tumor, the ABR abnormality will be apparent on the slow-rate recording. This is exactly the conclusion drawn most recently by Campbell and Abbas (1987). In a comparison of wave V latency shift as a function of stimulus rate (9.7, 39.7, 49.7, and 59.7/second) among 20 subjects with asymmetric cochlear hearing loss and 8 with confirmed acoustic tumor, they reported that although the shift was significantly greater in the poorer ear of the tumor group at the 59.7 per second rate, sufficient overlap between groups negated the benefits of using an increased rate. Moreover, in all tumor patients the ABR was already abnormal at a slow rate (9.7/second). This statement implies that the only neuro-pathology of interest in ABR diagnosis is acoustic tumor, or at best, space-occupying neoplasm.

Although it certainly is true that the addition of a rapid repetition rate in the presence of an already abnormal slow-rate ABR adds nothing to disease detection rate, it is equally true that a sufficient number of patients with insidious brainstem pathology show ABR abnormality only when the repetition rate is sufficiently fast to alter the synaptic efficiency (e.g., multiple sclerosis).

Consider, for example, the patient whose audiogram is shown in Figure 7-6. This 45-year-old man presented with a 6-month history of progressive hearing loss accompanied by ringing tinnitus in the left ear and episodes of imbalance. His physical examination was essentially unremarkable. Audiologic findings revealed unilateral mild to severe sloping cochlear hearing loss characterized by a 3000 Hz notch. Diagnostic speech audiometry showed no evidence of pathologic roll over. The tympanograms supported the otoscopic findings, and no acoustic reflex threshold or decay abnormalities were found other than some crossed/uncrossed threshold asymmetries that were attributable to the high-frequency hearing loss.

In addition to the negative audiometric data, electronystagmography with caloric irrigation was also within normal limits, bilaterally. There was no

spontaneous, gaze, or positional nystagmus, and ocular fixation was present.

Represented in Figure 7-7 is the slow rate (17.1/second) ABR recorded to rarefaction clicks (the ABR to condensation clicks also was recorded but is not shown since it did not add to the diagnosis) at 90 dB HL (125.0 dB pSPL) for the right and left ears, respectively. Results for the right ear (left panel) are clearly normal with regard to absolute and interpeak latency, absolute and relative (V/I) amplitude, and waveform morphology. Equally normal is the left ear ABR, despite the high-frequency sensitivity loss. On the basis of these results to a slow stimulation rate, therefore, one would report no evidence of auditory brainstem electrical abnormality.

The ABR in Figure 7-8 was recorded to a rapid rate (65.1/second), which is a routine part of the authors' diagnostic protocol. The latency and amplitude of wave V only are marked since interest is primarily in the shift and morphologic organization of this rostral component imposed by the increase in rate. For the right ear, wave V remains clearly visible with no dramatic distortions in wave shape and the latency shift of only 0.3 msec relative to the 17.1 per second condition is within normal tolerance. For the left ear, however, there

Figure 7-6. Audiologic results of a 45-year-old man with a 6-month history of progressive left ear hearing loss, ringing tinnitus, and imbalance.

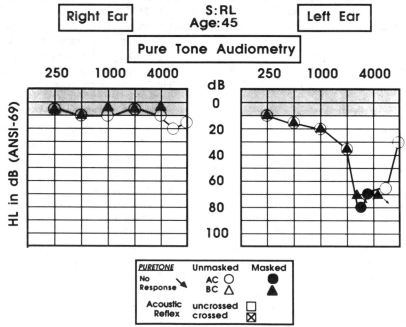

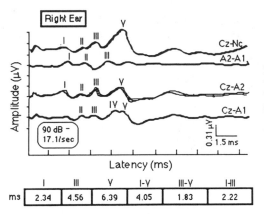

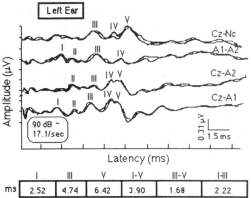

ms	I	III	V	I–V	III–V	I–III
	2.34	4.56	6.39	4.05	1.83	2.22

ms	I	III	V	I–V	III–V	I–III
	2.52	4.74	6.42	3.90	1.68	2.22

Figure 7-7. Slow rate (17.1/sec) ABR to rarefaction clicks for the patient whose audiogram is shown in Figure 7-6.

was a dramatic increase in wave V amplitude on the ipsilateral channel and twice the latency shift (0.6 msec) as that in the right ear despite only a 0.03 msec interaural wave V latency difference at 17.1 per second. Interestingly, this difference was magnified still further for rapid condensation clicks (ABR not shown) where the shift was 0.36 msec in the right ear and a startling 4.2 msec in the left ear. On the basis of these results to a fast repetition rate, an abnormal ABR most likely secondary to rostral brainstem involvement was reported.

Subsequent magnetic resonance imaging with Gadolinium contrast revealed elongated cerebellar tonsils extending to the level of the foramen magnum. Follow-up neurosurgical consultation resulted in the diagnosis of Arnold-Chiari malformation (type I). If the rapid-rate condition was not included, as is commonly practiced, this would have been a false-negative ABR finding.

Figure 7-8. Rapid rate (65.1/sec) ABR to rarefaction clicks for the patient whose slow rate (17.1/sec) recording is displayed in Figure 7-7. Only wave V is labeled since the salient diagnostic indicator is the wave V latency difference between the two rate conditions.

Although this represents only a single case report, similar results have been experienced on a sufficient sample of patients with apparently silent lesions both to justify and recommend routine inclusion of a rapid repetition rate in the neurodiagnostic ABR protocol whenever results to a slow rate of stimulation are normal. Although others such as Jacobson et al. (1987) also have supported use of such fast rates, their recommendation for its use was disease specific as in the evaluation of demyelinating diseases. This a posteriori approach is founded on the assumption that the patient has been referred for ABR to verify an existing clinical suspicion or impression for a specific disease.

A suggested alternative is to opt for an a priori strategy designed to optimize the magnitude of diagnostic information available from the ABR or other sensory evoked potential tests (e.g., somatosensory or visual). Consequently, all patients are evaluated with both a slow (17.1/second) and rapid (65.1/second) rate of stimulation, in search of occult electrical abnormality.

A second argument often presented for not using a dual-rate protocol is that it prolongs clinical testing time. Considering that it takes only 1 minute to acquire a conservative 2000 averages at

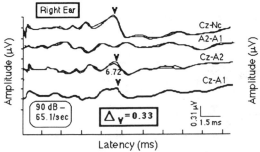

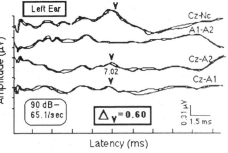

65.1 clicks per second for each run per ear, the diagnostic information gained far outweighs the extra testing time.

OPTIMIZING STIMULUS PHASE (S)

Without question the majority of audiologists performing ABR tests do so using an alternative polarity stimulus. The original rationale for alternating the rarefaction and condensation phases of a stimulus was to reduce the magnitude of stimulus artifact created by magnetic radiation from an electrodynamic earphone. Yet, a plethora of studies has long discouraged continued use of this practice because of the possibility of phase cancellations obscuring the "true" ABR (Borg and Lofqvist, 1982; Chiappa, 1983; Coutin, Balmaseda, and Miranda, 1987; Hughes, Fino, and Gangon, 1981; Kevanishvili and Aphonchenko, 1981; Ornitz and Walter, 1975; Ruth, Hildenbrand, and Cantrell, 1982; Schwartz, Pratt, and Schwartz, 1989; Stockard, Stockard, and Sharbrough, 1978).

The authors routinely record the ABR separately to rarefaction and condensation clicks for several reasons. In concert with the observations of Emerson et al. (1982) and Maurer (1985), a series of select patients have been seen who present either with ABR abnormality to one polarity (usually rarefaction) but not the other, or on both polarities but with different types of deviance.

The ABRs shown in Figure 7-9 depict the rarefaction and condensation recordings from the right ipsilateral channel only (Cz-A2) from a patient with mild-low/mid-frequency (500–1000 Hz) cochlear hearing loss in the right ear and moderate, essentially flat, loss in the left ear. There were no other audiologic abnormalities. His otologic history was remarkable for mild disequilibrium, headaches, and episodes of blurred vision.

The rarefaction results show prolonged brainstem transmission times (I–V = 4.63 msec) owing to the absolute latency delay of wave V. Wave amplitudes were normal, and wave morphology was characterized by a dominant wave IV followed by a reduced amplitude wave V appearing as an entirely separate peak. On the condensation recording, however, wave I latency remained normal and decreased by 0.41 msec while that of wave V decreased by 0.61 msec, which is within normal limits for the instrumentation used. Consequently, interpretation based on the rarefaction stimuli was in favor of rostral brainstem abnormality whereas that for condensation events supported normal brainstem function. Subsequent neuroimaging studies revealed a "pea"-size cerebellar mass.

The results displayed in Figure 7-10 are from the left ear of a 54-year-old man with mild bilateral high-frequency (presumably noise-induced) cochlear hearing loss, tinnitus, and vertigo. His otologic exam was entirely normal, and he was otherwise in good health.

Figure 7-9. Example of an abnormal rarefaction and normal condensation recording in a patient with a "pea"-size cerebellar mass.

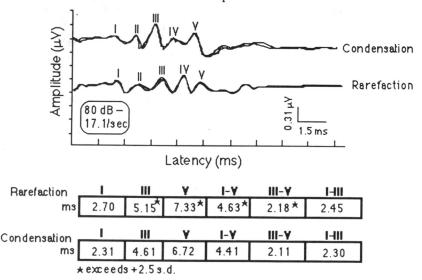

Rarefaction ms	I	III	V	I-V	III-V	I-III
	2.70	5.15*	7.33*	4.63*	2.18*	2.45

Condensation ms	I	III	V	I-V	III-V	I-III
	2.31	4.61	6.72	4.41	2.11	2.30

★ exceeds +2.5 s.d.

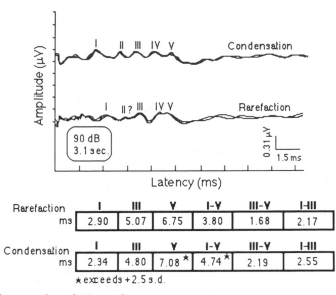

Rarefaction ms	I	III	V	I-V	III-V	I-III
	2.90	5.07	6.75	3.80	1.68	2.17

Condensation ms	I	III	V	I-V	III-V	I-III
	2.34	4.80	7.08 ★	4.74 ★	2.19	2.55

★ exceeds + 2.5 s.d.

Figure 7-10. Example of a normal rarefaction and abnormal condensation ABR in a patient with previous pontine infarct.

Here, the ABR to rarefaction stimuli shows normal absolute and interpeak latencies, although wave II is ambiguous. For the condensation events, wave I appeared earlier as was seen in Figure 7-9; however wave V latency and thus the I–V interval were abnormally prolonged. Although not shown, results for the right ear were entirely normal.

Opposite to the conclusions reached for the patient described in Figure 7-9, the normal rarefaction with abnormal condensation recordings for this patient led us to suspect the possibility of left brainstem vascular disorder rather than mass lesion. (The authors have never seen a brainstem mass cause abnormality only for condensation clicks.) Subsequent T_1- and T_2-weighted magnetic resonance images revealed two punctate foci of abnormal signal intensity involving both the right side of the upper pons as well as the tail of the left caudate nucleus. These were attributed to areas of brainstem infarct with no evidence of neoplastic disease.

Although these two case studies demonstrate the value of a dual-polarity ABR protocol for uncovering occult lesion, one must be cautious when interpreting such paradoxical findings in patients with precipitous high-frequency hearing loss. In such patients, it is sometimes possible to see a wave V distortion and latency delay on condensation recording but not to rarefaction clicks. Given that condensation clicks will yield wave I

amplitudes up to 30 percent less than that with rarefaction events (Coutin et al., 1987; Emerson et al., 1982; Kevanishvili and Aphonchenko, 1981; Schwartz et al., 1989; Stockard et al., 1978; Tietze and Pantev, 1986), it is not surprising that wave V would not also be sensitive to polarity reversal. As a consequence, steeply sloping cochlear hearing loss can confound interpretation of an ABR recorded solely to condensation polarity stimuli. Using positive polarity stimuli alone is not advocated since it will increase the false-positive yield.

In contrast to condensation recordings, experience has shown that the use of an alternating stimulus can lead to a higher false-negative rate. Here, an ABR abnormality that may have surfaced with monopolarity stimulation might be offset with an alternating polarity due to phase cancellation effects.

Clinical experience favors a dual-polarity protocol. If, however, one must choose from among a single monopolarity polarity or alternating phase due to time constraint, a rarefaction click is a better alternative given the amplitude advantage for wave I, the effect of precipitous sensory hearing loss on wave V with condensation events, and the possibility of phase cancellation with alternating polarity signals. However, neither is considered a suitable substitute for the dual-polarity protocol.

Caveat: The importance of ensuring that the polarity of the acoustic stimulus at the earphone is the same as the electrical pulse generated by the evoked potential system is underscored. Unfortunately, most clinicians assume that the manufacturer has calibrated correctly. During a trial period of four systems by one manufac-

turer, stimulus polarity was found to be reversed on every system; that is, when rarefaction was selected on the ABR parameters menu, the stimulus phase at the earphone actually was positive.

OPTIMIZING STIMULUS INTENSITY

In comparison to each of the other recording parameters, there does not appear to be any convention regarding level of stimulation. Most of the neurologic community stimulate at 60 to 70 dB sensation level (SL) relative to the patient's behavioral click threshold in each ear, consistent with the original work of Jewett and Williston (1971) and guided by the recommendations of Chiappa (1983). In contrast, most audiologists stimulate at 70 to 80 dB HL referenced to the average behavioral click threshold of a jury of normal-hearing adult listeners (so-called normalized hearing level [nHL]).

The disadvantage of the sensation level reference is that the signal SPL is different at the two ears, which has an obvious effect on wave latency and amplitude. Consider, for example, a patient whose click threshold on the right ear was 20 dB (re: attenuator setting), whereas that in the left was 0 dB. Interpretation of the right ear will be based on an ABR recorded to a 90 dB stimulus versus a 70 dB click for the left ear. If it is assumed that wave V latency increases approximately 40 μsec per dB decrease in stimulus level, the interaural wave V latency difference will be a significant 0.8 msec. One might conclude erroneously, therefore, that this ABR was abnormal, creating a false-positive result.

There have been a number of case presentations in which a false-negative conclusion was reached for acoustic tumor detection because absolute wave V and interpeak I–V latencies in the hearing loss ear were similar to those of the normal ear despite a 25 dB difference in signal presentation level. Had the ABR for each ear been recorded at equivalent SPLs in both of these examples, however, the interpretation would have been correct in favor of normal and abnormal brainstem function, respectively.

The message here is that click intensity should be sufficiently high (e.g., 115 dB pSPL) to maximize neural discharge so that the ABR reflects optimal auditory system capability. This same level should be delivered to both ears even in the presence of unilateral or asymmetric hearing loss. Many times the degree of high-frequency sensitivity loss in one ear is severe enough to warrant a higher-stimulus intensity level (e.g., 125–130 dB pSPL) for maximum neural discharge. This is particularly important for optimizing wave I amplitude and clarity. In such cases the signal presented to the better-hearing ear should be at the same intensity level so that interpretation will be based on results obtained from equivalent SPLs at the two cochleae. Failure to equate signal SPL ultimately will lead either to a false-positive or -negative error.

Caveat: When collecting normative data for neurodiagnostics, it is important to include those higher (90–95 dB nHL) intensities that are used to compensate for more severe hearing losses.

OPTIMIZING STIMULUS DELIVERY

Without question, the most time-honored method of stimulus delivery in ABR testing is the unshielded electrodynamic earphone (TDH-39/49/50) adopted from pure tone audiometry. The obvious limitation of this transducer is a rather large stimulus artifact, which can smear wave I at high intensities. Such artifact occurs when a magnetic-type earphone, driven by an electrical pulse, generates a magnetic field causing current to spread to the recording electrodes. To reduce stimulus artifact, most clinicians have chosen to use an alternating polarity stimulus without recognizing the diagnostic consequences discussed previously. Two additional problems surrounding the use of an electrodynamic earphone more common to pediatric ABR evaluation are ear canal collapse and SPL variability due to minor displacement of the transducer during testing. (For a detailed discussion of transducer effects in pediatric auditory evoked potentials, see Schwartz and Schwartz, 1989.)

To negate the complications derived from an electrodynamic earphone, routine use of an insert transducer such as the Etymotic Tubephone or the Nicolet Enhancer I is recommended. Each of these insert receivers incorporates a calculated length of tubing that separates the actual transducer from the point of stimulus delivery. The result is a transmission delay (e.g., 0.9 msec for the ER-3 Tubephone) imposed on the ABR waveform such that the stimulus artifact cannot smear any portion of the response, regardless of intensity level.

Note: When substituting an insert receiver for a standard earphone, new normative data should be collected. It is inappropriate simply to subtract a constant 0.9 msec to equate back to earphone norms since the transmission delay is governed by the exact length of tubing.

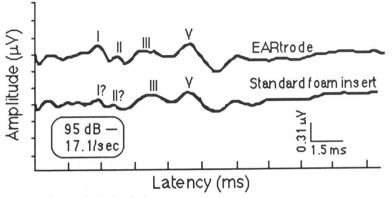

Figure 7-11. Comparison of wave I amplitude between ABR recordings obtained with a standard Etymotic Tubephone insert and with an Etymotic EARtrode.

Moreover, greater amplitudes and less variability have been found with the insert receivers, thus warranting separate norms.

An additional advantage to each of these insert transducers is that a recording ear canal electrode is (Nicolet Enhancer I) or can be (Etymotic Tubephone) part of the stimulus delivery system for optimizing wave I amplitude and definition in troublesome patients. The Nicolet Enhancer I uses a foam earplug separated by a reticulated foam center that is sodden with gel electrolyte. The compressible foam tip used as the earpiece in the Etymotic Tubephone can be replaced by one that is wrapped in a delicate piece of gold foil to which an electrode lead is attached via an alligator clip. Spreading a fine layer of gel electrolyte over the foil to serve as a contact medium is advised.

The benefit of the Etymotic EARtrode is evident from the ABR tracings in Figure 7-11. The bottom recording was obtained with a standard compressible foam tip on an Etymotic Tubephone. The top trace represents the ABR when a gold foil EARtrode was substituted. Note that wave I amplitude increased from 0.7 μV to 0.15 μV, whereas that for wave V improved by 0.16 μV with the EARtrode. In general, both clinical experience and research data support the efficacy of both the EARtrode and Enhancer ear canal electrode-stimulus delivery systems for improving wave I identification and resolution, particularly for patients with steep, severe high-frequency sensitivity loss (Bach, 1988; Ruth et al., 1982).

OPTIMIZING THE ANALYSIS EPOCH

7 Since the normal adult ABR is observed within 5.8 to 6.8 msec (depending on transducer type)

poststimulus onset, it is commonplace to limit the analysis epoch (time base, sweep time to 10 msec; the authors, however, recommend that the epoch should be lengthened to 15 msec for all ABR recordings. The principal advantage to a longer sweep time is that it provides a visual representation of the residual background noise averaged into the response as depicted in Figure 7-12. Note that the peaks and valleys following a presumed wave V in the top tracing indicate myogenic and movement contamination. Since this unwanted noise is undifferentiated from the evoked potential, it too will be averaged into the waveform, producing spurious amplitudes, extra peaks that might confuse interpretation, and poor test-retest consistency. In contrast the bottom recording is characterized by a flat line that returns to baseline following the marked negativity of wave V, supporting an acceptably low residual noise level. In both examples, this information would not have been evident with a 10 msec epoch. This same estimate of background noise can be visualized on the initial portion of the response by introducing a 5 msec stimulus delay.

Another recommended technique incorporates plus/minus averaging that permits an additional on-line measure of residual noise level. During the process of averaging to resolve the ABR, a simultaneous averaged waveform is obtained by alternately adding and subtracting the incoming data; that is, 50 percent of the trials are averaged positive up and 50 percent positive down. Such alternation cancels the constant signal (the reproducible evoked potential) to a flat line and leaves only the background noise, which remains random regardless of its polarity. To the best of our knowledge, however, the only commercial instruments that have sufficient computer memory and

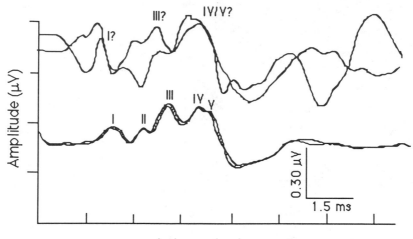

Latency (ms)

Figure 7-12. Comparison of poor waveform reproducibility (top trace) and excellent test-retest reproduction (bottom trace). Note the undulations in the tracing over the last 5 milliseconds of the recording epoch, denoting a poor signal-to-noise ratio.

software routines for plus/minus averaging are the Nicolet Pathfinder and Viking series.

Any of these three clinically applicable approaches to on-line residual noise estimation is far superior to the standard no-stimulus input trial. In the latter case, the patient might be excessively noisy during testing and perfectly quiet at the time of the no-stimulus run, thus leading to the false conclusion that the ABR is uncontaminated by residual noise. Use of a longer epoch either in the form of a 5 msec prestimulus baseline or the same postactivity baseline, or a plus/minus averaging technique reflects background activity at the same time that the evoked potential is being averaged. *Remember the clinical goal is to show little or no residual noise either in the initial or final 5 msec of the response.* When accomplished, the test-retest overlap will be similar to that in the bottom trace of Figure 7-12. Failure to achieve or at least approach that goal should lead the clinician either to reschedule testing to a later time with a request for mild sedation or to take additional steps toward minimizing the consequences of excessive background noise as will be discussed later in the *What If?* section.

OPTIMIZING THE AVERAGING PROCESS

Like so many other aspects of ABR testing, the number of samples averaged to complete the recording derives from the classic works of Jewett and Williston (1971) who averaged 2048 stimuli to resolve the ABR. For some reason, however, many professionals involved in auditory clinical

electrophysiology consider this number to be "cast in stone."

Indeed many individuals will watch the averaged data build (with little or no concern for the "raw" electroencephalogram) only to stop when the "magic" number hits 2000 or 2048, regardless of what the waveform looks like. Perhaps this relates to an inadequate understanding of time domain averaging. (For excellent tutorials on the fundamentals of computer averaging for evoked potentials, the reader is referred to Hyde, 1985; Picton et al., 1983.)

Since the purpose of averaging is to reduce interfering background noise by selectively attenuating random cerebral and nonneural electrical activity, the number of trials acquired should be based on waveform clarity and the estimated residual noise level. When a patient is myogenically quiet, a well-resolved ABR with a flat postanalysis baseline may be seen within 800 to 1000 averages. If, however, there is excessive movement, it may be necessary to pause from averaging manually numerous times and to average 4000 or more trials. Again, one should strive for the best waveform resolution and excellent repeatability exhibited by almost exact overlap among all components of the waveform within a reasonable length of time. Anything less is unacceptable in the majority of situations.

If this cannot be accomplished within an appropriate period of testing time (1.5 hours is a suitable time allotment for a comprehensive neuro-electrodiagnostic evaluation) because the patient is excessively noisy, one should cease averaging and reschedule the patient with sedation. Continuing to average unacceptably high levels of residual noise serves no purpose since a reliable ABR cannot be recorded, regardless of how many samples are acquired. Use of diazepam (10 mg) for adults or chloral hydrate (50 mg/kg) for children and some elderly patients helps relieve tension from anxiety and produces a mild sedation/hypnosis with only minimal chance of respiratory depression. A protocol for administering these sedative/hypnotic agents should be a developed facet of every neurodiagnostic program.

WHAT IF?

Regardless of how much care is taken to optimize all of the recording parameters outlined in the preceding sections, those situations remain where the ABR is confounded by intrinsic (i.e., patient related) or extrinsic (i.e., environmental) variables, or both. All too often clinicians are willing to accept less than "clean" electrophysiologic data for use in the diagnosis of neuropathology. Whether this relates to an unwillingness to take the extra time needed to clarify the response, or to a lack of appreciation of how best to resolve the problem or to identify and correct the complicating source is irrelevant. Since the negative effects of these factors can influence greatly the ultimate interpretation of the data, it is imperative that every attempt be made to solve these often perplexing clinical problems, regardless of time. *Failure to do so will lead to serious decision-making errors.*

To this end, a series of potentially frustrating and confusing clinical situations are presented along with possible solutions. These select examples hopefully will facilitate the acquisition of well-resolved and highly reproducible ABR recordings from which to base a rational defensible diagnostic impression.

WHAT IF WAVE I IS AMBIGUOUS?

Since the latency and amplitude of wave I are used in essentially every aspect of test interpretation, they are indeed the ABR hallmarks of neurodiagnosis. Failure to record a peripheral eighth nerve action potential will most definitely complicate ABR interpretation since it becomes difficult to determine whether latency prolongation of a later wave (e.g., V) was the result of a peripheral hearing loss or a lesion in the auditory nerve or lateral pons.

A variety of manipulations can be taken to optimize wave I resolution. Recall that in our routine neurodiagnostic paradigm a simultaneous horizontal (A1-A2) recording helps to clarify wave I when it is poorly defined on the ipsilateral channel (Cz-A1,A2) as depicted in Figure 7-3. If, however, the presence and location of wave I remain unclear and a monopolarity stimulus is used (preferably rarefaction), then it is best to slow the click rate down considerably (e.g., 3.1, 5.1, 7.1/second) and to raise the stimulus intensity 10 dB or to the attenuator limits. Both of these maneuvers should enhance the amplitude of the compound eighth nerve action potential by increasing the number of eighth nerve fibers activated and by improving neural synchrony.

If these changes in recording parameters are not corrective, the next approach is to couple a slow-rate and high-intensity stimulus presentation with a noninvasive ear canal electrode array such as the Etymotic EARtrode or the Nicolet Enhancer I. Ironically, reversing stimulus polarity to condensation is also helpful at times since the ABR of a minority of patients is characterized by slightly better waveform definition on condensation versus rarefaction for reasons that are not clear. For the most part, however, rarefaction will elicit a more robust wave I response.

The obvious advantage of an ear canal electrode is that it lies closer to the "near field" of the neural generator. This recording montage results in a combined compound action potential recording as in electrocochleography, and the far-field ABR. With the exception of some patients with severe to profound broad-spectrum hearing loss, these approaches to wave I enhancement have been remarkably successful. In these latter instances, it is sometimes possible to extract wave I via a seminoninvasive tympanic membrane electrode made either from multistranded Teflon-insulated silver wire or one similar to that described by Stypulkowski and Staller (1987). (See Ruth, Lambert, and Ferraro (1988) for further discussion of noninvasive ear canal electrodes.)

WHAT IF WAVE V IS AMBIGUOUS?

Ambiguity of wave V appears in many forms, the most common of which is a fused IV/V complex as discussed earlier. Here again, use of a multiple recording montage will most often alleviate this problem since wave V should be identifiable both from the contralateral and noncephalic channels as illustrated in Figures 7-2 and 7-4, respectively.

An unusual, often perplexing situation is a double wave V seen at times in patients with precipitous high-frequency cochlear hearing loss as exemplified in Figure 7-13. The characteristic of this response to high-intensity stimulation is an initial sharp peak occurring within the expected latency range of wave V followed by a broader-shaped component having a deeper negative downstroke. This configuration could lead one to become easily confused as to which of the two peaks should be used to calculate the I–V interpeak interval. If the first component is chosen, brainstem transmission time is normal. Selection of the second peak results in an interpretation that favors abnormality.

Picton and Stapells (1985) explained this enigma of multiple wave Vs on the basis of cochlear mechanics. They hypothesized that at high intensities, the broad-spectrum click stimulates the entire basilar membrane. Since the high-frequency sensitive basal region is synchronized more easily than its low-frequency apical counterpart, and since the traveling wave moves from base to apex, high-intensity stimulation will evoke a sharp potential appearing within the same time domain as the normal wave V. They speculated further that the second peak originates within the low-frequency apical region where there is poorer neural discharge synchrony but, in these patients, better hearing sensitivity. This supposed low-frequency component is manifested as a broader-shaped wave that occurs later in time owing to the traveling wave delay from base to apex.

The latency-intensity series shown in Figure 7-13 illustrates how the first component is abolished as stimulus intensity approaches hearing threshold in the high frequencies. As described by Picton and Stapells (1985), the second later component's threshold occurs at a lower intensity owing to the better low- and mid-frequency hearing. The importance of this phenomenon is that despite the observation that the shape and slope of the second peak appear more like that of the usual wave V, neurodiagnostic interpretation should be based on the latency of the first component. For audiologic purposes, however, threshold estimation can be based on the visual detection levels for each component separately since it will be affected by hearing sensitivity at adjacent frequencies.

In addition to wave V distortions, its amplitude also can be so highly attenuated that peak identification seems open to "guesswork." As with wave I enhancement, a host of parametric manipulations will help unveil wave V. We cannot overstate the value of a contralateral and noncephalic recording montage in these situations. It is much more efficient to record from these derivations simultaneously with every patient than having to interrupt the testing session to affix new electrodes on the patient. In the latter case you may arouse an already quiet, relaxed patient and thus chance contaminating a poorly defined response with unwanted noise. Surely this will result in a "no win" outcome.

This strategy is easily appreciated in Figure 7-14. The ipsilateral channel recording shows a clear wave I and possibly a small wave II (unlabeled) followed by a broad slow wave with an

Figure 7-13. Example of a wave V doublet sometimes seen in patients with steeply sloping high-frequency sensory hearing loss.

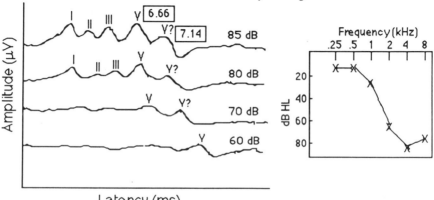

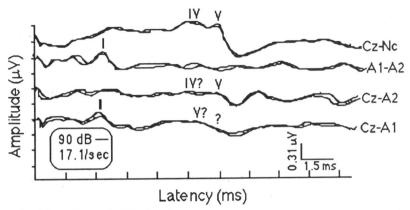

Figure 7-14. Example of how the contralateral and noncephalic recording montages can be used to clarify wave V when it is poorly resolved or ambiguous on the ipsilateral channel response.

abnormal slope assumed to be wave V. Had this been the only recording channel available, confident identification of wave V would not be possible. Owing to the combination of a broad-filter passband (30–1500 Hz) and a vertex to cervical vertebra electrode orientation, wave V is easily recognized.

For other difficult cases, of course, it may be necessary to modify the recording protocol to enhance wave V recognition still further. The combination of a broad-filter passband, a moderately rapid rate (e.g., 37.1/second), and reductions in stimulus intensity are all tactics that can be applied to identify the "real" wave V. It is critical, therefore, that the clinician be a flexible thinker and understand how best to manipulate the testing strategy to resolve a given waveform component, if at all possible. Those who are bound by a set protocol and do not appreciate the power of the many parametric changes available to resolve a given problem will undoubtedly find themselves either accepting less than high-quality recordings or interpreting the ABR via guesswork.

Hearing Loss Correction Factors

One often confusing and frustrating circumstance in neurodiagnostic ABR testing is wave V latency delay in patients with high-frequency cochlear hearing loss. The reason for wave V prolongation in these patients is similar to that for the double-peaked wave V discussed previously. At high stimulus levels, wave V latency is dominated by the high-frequency regions of the cochlea. Given that this basal region is damaged, the apical end becomes more dominant, and wave

V latency is prolonged owing to traveling wave time delay.

The consequences of this wave V latency delay are best appreciated when evaluating a patient with asymmetric or unilateral high-frequency hearing loss; the audiometric "red flag" for eighth nerve lesion. If, in this case, the interaural wave V latency was greater than or equal to 0.4 msec, a false-positive interpretation of conduction blockage secondary to acoustic tumor could result.

To compensate for the confounding influence of high-frequency cochlear hearing loss on wave V latency, several investigators (Hyde and Blair, 1981; Jerger and Johnson, 1988; Jerger and Mauldin, 1978; Rosenhamer, 1981; Selters and Brackmann, 1977) have advocated some type of mathematical correction factor based on degree of sensitivity loss at 4000 Hz. Recent studies by Prosser and Arslan (1987) and Jerger and Johnson (1988) have also indicated that an equivalent sensation level paradigm for the selection of signal intensity will obviate the need for a correction factor.

Each of these two approaches for hearing loss compensation assumes that the salient criterion in diagnostic ABR interpretation is wave V latency. The principal flaw with a constant correction factor is that not all ears with high-frequency sensory hearing loss behave alike. In two patients with similar high-frequency audiometric contour and degree of hearing loss, wave V latency might be normal in one and delayed in the other. Application of a correction factor would move the prolonged wave V into the normal range while forcing the already normal wave V to a latency below the lower cutoff limit for that peak component; that is, it represents overcompensation. Although some clinicians solve this dilemma simply by correcting only when wave V is delayed, this is antithetic to the rules of mathematical constants. *A wave V latency correction factor cannot and should not be used on a selective basis.* One might inadvertently normalize a wave V latency delay in a patient with neuropathology. There is no way to predict wave V latency for any given patient since the interactions between age, gender, and degree and shape of hearing loss simply are too complex.

The best alternative to hearing loss correction factors is to base interpretation on interpeak latencies, since these represent the electrophysiologic hallmark of auditory brainstem pathology. Indeed, the available evidence indicates that interpeak latencies are not significantly affected by peripheral sensitivity loss. In a scatterplot comparison of ABR absolute and interpeak latencies of 220 patients with high-frequency cochlear hearing loss and 30 acoustic tumor ears, Schwartz and Sanders (1983) found that brainstem transmission time (I–V interval) was always normal or shortened among the cochlear hearing loss patients and abnormal for all tumor cases. Similar findings have been reported by Parker, Chiappa, and Brooks (1980) and Zupulla, Karmel, and Greenblat (1981).

The single complicating variable in this approach is the ability to record an interpretable wave I in the presence of high-frequency cochlear hearing loss. If sufficient care is taken to enhance wave I resolution by incorporating the many techniques outlined herein, then it should be possible to clarify this important peak component in the majority of patients. Admittedly this is not possible in some patients. Such cases warrant cautious interpretation in light of an inability to assess peripheral function. Yet, with careful thought and "old-fashioned" clinical insight, it is possible to develop a rational, defensible statement regarding the presence of brainstem electrical abnormality.

If, for example, the patient has broad-spectrum severe to profound cochlear hearing loss and the ABR is characterized by a wave V only, then interpretation can be based solely on the presence of a response. The possibility of a space-occupying neoplasm creating such a severe hearing loss without obliterating the ABR in total would probably be remote. The mere presence of a response argues cautiously against mass lesion. This is exactly why one should always attempt to record the ABR regardless of hearing loss severity.

Likewise, comparison with responses obtained from the contralateral ear also can prove enlightening. Large cerebellopontine angle tumors often will result in anatomic compression and distortion of the brainstem, which will be manifested by an ABR abnormality such as prolonged wave V and III–V interval on the side opposite the tumor. Even if there is no measurable hearing in one ear, never assume that valuable diagnostic information is unavailable from recording an ABR in the unaffected ear.

The recent reports of Prosser and Arslan (1987) and Jerger and Johnson (1988) advocate an equivalent sensation-level stimulus-intensity paradigm based on the average of the pure tone thresholds at 2000 and 4000 Hz in the suspected ear. Prosser and Arslan (1987) recommend basing the interpretation on a ΔV index, which is calculated from the difference between wave V latency of the affected ear and that predicted from a normal latency-intensity function at the same sensation level. In other words, wave V latency to a 90 dB nHL click for an impaired ear having a 75 dB average hearing loss at 2000 and 4000 Hz is compared to that at 15 dB (equal sensation levels) from the normal function. The arguments favoring this technique over an equivalent SPL approach (Jerger and Johnson, 1988) appear to make the invalid assumption that ABR interpretation is based solely on wave V latency in the suspected ear without concern for any other criterion for abnormality (e.g., interpeak latency, amplitude, or morphology) or the results from the contralateral ear. They also state that "a click intensity appropriate for a subject with a substantial high-frequency hearing loss would be too high for a subject with only a mild loss." This has not been our experience. In fact, our normative data were collected at 80, 90, and 95 dB HL in order to accommodate equal SPL when evaluating those with severe sensitivity losses.

If interpretation is based on equal SPL, then interear differences across all ABR parameters become obvious. Using the equivalent sensation level method, however, interpretation is limited to wave V latency between the suspected ear and a predicted normal value. In concert with the theme of this chapter, the authors prefer to optimize the informational database.

WHAT IF THE PATIENT IS NOISY?

When the initial ABR recording is contaminated by electrical interference, it is best to cease testing and eliminate the source rather than to control the artifact by decreasing amplifier sensitivity, averaging more samples, changing the analog filter setting, using a quadratic smoothing algorithm, or simply ignoring it and accepting the response as is.

Perhaps the most obvious and common noise source relates to myogenic and movement activity emanating from the patient. This large random activity will be obvious when monitoring the "raw" input. When seen it is best to ensure that the patient is comfortable. All attempts should be made to have the patient relax and not be anxious. Careful and complete explanation of the test procedures and the importance of having them relaxed and quiet is often all that is needed. Anxiety is a byproduct of the unknown. It is good practice to ask patients (e.g., the elderly) already on anti-anxiety medication (e.g., Valium, Ativan) to take one 30 minutes prior to the ABR, unless otherwise contraindicated. It also is best to have the patient go to the bathroom and to get a drink of water immediately prior to testing. Controlling the temperature in the test room, ensuring that there is sufficient air return, and having blankets available are important aspects of patient comfort. Use of a cervical pillow will assist in relieving neck muscle tension. If, despite all effort, the problem persists, a mild hypnotic/sedative (Valium, 10 mg) *should* be administered. It is inexcusable practice to accept poorly defined and unrepeatable waveforms simply because that is what appeared after two trials of 2000 repetitions.

Caveat. The principal reason for poorly defined and irreproducible evoked potentials is waveform contamination from muscle and other movement artifacts. Even if the evoked potential system has automatic artifact reject capability, transient bursts of residual noise either fall just below the artifact cutoff level or enter the recording before the system can detect it. The importance of being constantly vigilant to the ongoing electroencephalogram to detect interfering artifact cannot be overemphasized. Whenever such noise is apparent on the monitor, even if it does not trigger the reject mechanism, simply pause the averaging manually. When a quiet state is reestablished, resume averaging. Although this simple maneuver might delay testing, the end product is well worth the effort as exhibited by a much more highly resolved waveform and excellent test-retest consistency free from excessive contamination.

In addition to patient-related noise, environmental electrical interference can radiate from fluorescent lights, power cords, other nearby electrical equipment, and the like. Normally this noise will be in the form of a 60 Hz sinusoid. When this is seen in a recording, calculate the reciprocal of the interpeak latency interval (1/msec) to esti-mate the frequency of the interference. If this is 16.6 msec, then it reflects 60 Hz interference.

The easiest method of controlling 60 Hz noise is to offset the repetition rate by an integer not evenly divisible into 60. Other techniques include turning off all lights and unplugging external electrical equipment. Braided short (e.g., 30 in.) electrode sets are preferable to loose, long (60 in.) ones for reducing electrical interference. The latter serve as broadcast antennae. Another approach is to maintain electrode impedance between 1000 and 2000 ohms and to ensure that interelectrode impedance is well balanced. Too often clinicians work under the principle that as long as electrode impedance is less than 5000 ohms, they are safe. If, however, one electrode is set at 1000 ohms and another is at 4500 ohms, then there is much greater opportunity for noise to contaminate the recording. Finally, it is best not to use a 60 Hz notch filter in routine neurodiagnostics. In addition to the possibility of phase shifting, a 60 Hz artifact can occur due to ringing of the notch filter, which will emerge as part of the averaged response, only to confound interpretation.

WHAT IF THE ABR IS NOT REPRODUCIBLE?

Recall from the sections on *Optimizing the Analysis Epoch* (Figure 7-12) and *Optimizing the Averaging Process* that the clinical goal is to eliminate residual noise from the recording to the best extent possible. Since even totally random noise can be manifested as peaks with latencies and polarities similar to those of an actual evoked potential, it is critical to maintain strict criteria for signal-to-noise ratio and reproducibility. Extending the analysis epoch to 15 msec, incorporating a 5.0 msec prestimulus baseline, or recording with a plus/minus averaging paradigm are all techniques for visualizing and estimating the signal-to-noise ratio. If the prestimulus or postanalysis activity returns to baseline and is essentially flat, as illustrated in Figure 7-12, or if the plus/minus average shows little residual noise, then a favorable signal-to-noise ratio is implied and the recording may be considered highly reliable.

From here the goal is to achieve an exact reproduction of that low-noise trace. If there is any deviation from overlap, the background noise represents the irreproducible portion(s) of the response as exemplified in Figure 7-15. In such circumstances it is best to calculate the amplitude ratio between the actual evoked potential and the

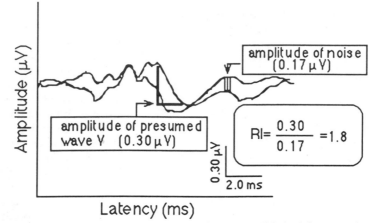

Figure 7-15. Method for quantifying the reproducibility index (RI) of the evoked potential response. The noise is considered the irreproducible portion of the response.

noise as shown in Figure 7-15. If this value is less than or equal to 3.0, reproducibility is clinically unacceptable for diagnostic interpretation. In such instances it is best to quiet the patient and obtain a new averaged response either until there is acceptable overlap or until it is apparent that a reliable recording is unattainable. Judgments based on one well-defined, low-residual noise recording rather than two that demonstrate poor repeatabiity is recommended.

CLOSING COMMENTS

When formulating the structure of this chapter, previous chapters on this topic were reviewed in an effort to determine underlying commonalities and obvious voids. Invariably, a recurrent theme of previous work was the uncritical review of the literature approach. Although some authors may have, at times, espoused a particular preference for a specific protocol, rarely if ever did they explain the philosophic underpinnings of their biases. Overall, clinicians involved in ABR seem to use a recording paradigm based solely on historical precedent. Although this time-honored approach to clinical testing may serve to offer security, it does not necessarily reflect the optimum. Techniques used by the early pioneers often are not the most appropriate given a growing fund of knowledge in clinical neurophysiology and diagnostic testing.

As stated in the introduction, the objective here was not to write "yet another chapter" on neurologic applications of the ABR, but to couple the clinical knowledge that has been gained from a busy evoked potential practice with what has been learned through critical scrutiny of the con-

temporary research literature. Throughout this chapter our biases and concerns have been expressed. At times the conclusions reached by certain investigators relative to formulating a rational clinical decision have been questioned, not as a means of judging right from wrong but to place interpretation of the ABR data in a broader clinical perspective.

Interpretation of an electrodiagnostic test is only as good as the quality of the recording. The concept of optimizing recording parameters is foremost to improve disease detection accuracy. The need to look "beyond" the acoustic neuroma has been highlighted since a host of demyelinating, neurovascular, and metabolic disorders also can compromise auditory brainstem function and thus result in an abnormal ABR. Some of these present obviously with routine recording techniques; others require electrophysiologic "teasing."

Hopefully, students and clinicians who read this chapter will appreciate better the possible power and accuracy of the ABR in neurodiagnostics when sufficient care is given to optimizing response clarity and, hence, response interpretation.

REFERENCES

Bauch, C. (1988). Clinical applications of auditory evoked potentials. In M. S. Robinette & C. Bauch (Eds.), *Proceedings of a Symposium in Audiology*. Rochester, MN: Mayo Clinic.

Borg, E., & Lofqvist, L. (1982). Auditory brainstem response (ABR) to rarefaction and condensation clicks in normal and abnormal ears. *Scandinavian Audiology, 11,* 227–235.

Campbell, K. C. M., & Abbas, P. (1987). The effect of stimulus repetition rate on the auditory brainstem response in tumor and nontumor patients. *Journal of Speech and Hearing Research, 30,* 494–502.

Chiappa, K. H. (1983). *Evoked potentials in clinical medicine* (pp. 129–133). New York: Raven Press.

Coutin, B., Balmaseda, A., & Miranda, J. (1987). Further differences between brain-stem auditory potentials evoked by rarefaction and condensation clicks as revealed by vector analysis. *Electroencephalography and Clinical Neurophysiology, 66,* 420–426.

Cracco, R. Q., & Cracco, J. B. (1976). Somatosensory evoked potentials in man: Farfield potentials. *Electroencephalography and Clinical Neurophysiology, 41,* 460–466.

Desmedt, J. E., & Cheron, G. (1980). Central somatosensory conduction in man: Neural generators and interpeak latencies of the far-field components recorded from the neck and right or left scalp and earlobes. *Electroencephalography and Clinical Neurophysiology, 50,* 382–403.

Emerson, R. G., Brooks, E. B., Parker, S. W., & Chiappa, K. H. (1982). Effects of click polarity on brainstem auditory evoked potentials in normal subjects and patients: Unexpected sensitivity of wave V. *Annals of the New York Academy of Sciences, 388,* 710–721.

Fowler, C. F., & Noffsinger, D. (1983). Effects of stimulus repetition rate and frequency on the auditory brainstem response in normal and VIII nerve/brainstem-impaired subjects. *Journal of Speech and Hearing Research, 26,* 560–567.

Gerling, I. J., & Finitzo-Hieber, T. F. (1983). Auditory brainstem response with high stimulus rates in normal and patient populations. *Annals of Otology, Rhinology, and Laryngology, 92,* 119–123.

Hall, J. W., Morgan, S. H., Mackey-Hargadine, J., Aguilar, E. A., & Jahrsdoerfer, R. A. (1984). Neuro-otologic applications of simultaneous multi-channel auditory evoked response recordings. *Laryngoscope, 94,* 883–889.

Hecox, K., & Galambos, R. (1974). Brainstem auditory evoked response in human infants and adults. *Archives of Otolaryngology, 99,* 30–33.

Hughes, J. R., Fino, J., & Gagnon, L. (1981). The importance of phase of stimulus and the reference recording electrode in brainstem auditory evoked potentials. *Electroencephalography and Clinical Neurophysiology, 51,* 611–623.

Hyde, M. (1985). Instrumentation and signal processing. In J. T. Jacobson (Ed.), *The auditory brainstem response* (pp. 33–62). Boston: College-Hill Press.

Hyde, M. L., & Blair, R. L. (1981). The auditory brainstem response in neuro-otology: Perspectives and problems. *Journal of Otolaryngology, 10,* 117–125.

Jacobson, J. T., Murray, T. J., & Deppe, U. (1987). The effects of ABR stimulus repetition rate in multiple sclerosis. *Ear & Hearing, 8,* 115–120.

Jerger, J., & Johnson, K. (1988). Interactions of age, gender and sensorineural hearing loss on ABR latency. *Ear & Hearing, 9,* 169–175.

Jerger, J., & Mauldin, L. (1978). Prediction of sensorineural hearing loss from the brainstem evoked response. *Archives of Otolaryngology, 104,* 456–461.

Jewett, D. L., & Williston, J. S. (1971). Auditory-evoked far fields averaged from the scalp of humans. *Brain, 95,* 681–696.

Jewett, D. L., Romano, M. N., & Williston, J. S. (1970). Human auditory evoked potentials: Possible brain stem components detected on scalp. *Science, 167,* 1517–1518.

Kavanagh, K. T., Domico, W. D., Franks, R., & Jin-Cheng, H. (1988). Digital filtering and spectral analysis of the low

intensity auditory brainstem response. *Ear & Hearing, 9,* 43–47.

Kevanishvili, Z., & Aponchenko, V. (1979). Frequency composition of the brain stem auditory evoked potentials. *Scandinavian Audiology, 8,* 51–55.

Kevanishvili, Z., & Aponchenko, V. (1981). Click polarity inversion effect upon the human brainstem auditory evoked potential. *Scandinavian Audiology, 10,* 141–147.

Laukli, E., & Mair, I. W. S. (1981). Early auditory-evoked responses: Filter effects. *Audiology, 20,* 300–312.

Mason, S. M. (1984). Effects of high-pass filtering on the detection of the auditory brainstem response. *British Journal of Audiology, 18,* 155–161.

Maurer, K. (1985). Uncertainties of topodiagnosis of auditory nerve and brain-stem auditory evoked potentials due to rarefaction and condensation stimuli. *Electroencephalography and Clinical Neurophysiology, 62,* 135–140.

Maurer, K., Schafer, E., & Leitner, H. (1980). The effect of varying stimulus polarity (rarefaction versus condensation) on early auditory evoked potentials. *Electroencephalography and Clinical Neurophysiology, 50,* 332–334.

Ornitz, E. M., & Walter, D. O. (1975). The effect of sound pressure on human brainstem evoked responses. *Brain Research, 92,* 490–498.

Parker, S. W., Chiappa, K. H., & Brooks, E. B. (1980). Brainstem auditory evoked responses in patients with acoustic neuromas and cerebello-pontine angle meningiomas. *Neurology, 30,* 413–414.

Picton, T. W., & Stapells, D. R. (1985). ABR case study: A "Frank's Run" latency-intensity function. In J. T. Jacobson (Ed.), *The auditory brainstem response* (pp. 410–413). Boston: College-Hill Press.

Picton, T. W., Linden, R. D., Gilles, Hamel, G., & Maru, J. T. (1983). Aspects of averaging. *Seminars in Hearing, 4,* 327–339.

Pratt, H., Ben-David, Y., Peled, R., Podoshin, L., & Scharf, B. (1981). Auditory brainstem evoked potentials: Clinical promise of increased stimulus rate. *Electroencephalography and Clinical Neurophysiology, 51,* 80–90.

Prosser, S., & Arslan, E. (1987). Prediction of auditory brainstem response wave V latency as a diagnostic tool of sensorineural hearing loss. *Audiology, 26,* 179–187.

Robinson, K., & Rudge, P. (1977). Abnormalities of the auditory evoked potentials in patients with multiple sclerosis. *Brain, 100,* 19–40.

Rosenhamer, H. (1981). Auditory evoked brainstem electric response (ABR) in cochlear hearing loss. In T. Lundborg (Ed.), *Scandinavian Audiology. Supplementum, 13.*

Ruth, R. A., Hildenbrand, D. L., & Cantrell, R. W. (1982). A study of methods used to enhance wave I in the auditory brainstem response. *Otolaryngology — Head and Neck Surgery, 90,* 635–640.

Ruth, R. A., Lambert, P. R., & Ferraro, J. A. (1988). Electrocochleography: Methods and clinical applications. *American Journal of Otology, 9*(Suppl.), 1–11.

Schwartz, D. M., & Sanders, J. W. (1983). The effect of audiometric contour on the auditory brainstem response. Unpublished report.

Schwartz, D. M., & Schwartz, J. A. (1989). Auditory evoked potentials in clinical pediatrics. In W. F. Rintelmann (Ed.), *Hearing assessment* (2nd ed.). Austin: Pro-Ed.

Schwartz, D. M., Pratt, R. E., & Schwartz, J. A. (1989). Auditory brainstem responses in preterm infants: Evidence of peripheral maturity. *Ear & Hearing, 10,* 14–22.

Selters, W. A., & Brackmann, D. E. (1977). Acoustic tumor detection with brainstem electric response audiometry.

Archives of Otolaryngology, 103, 181–187.

Shanon, E., Gold, S., & Himmelfarb, M. (1981). Assessment of the functional integrity of brainstem auditory pathways of stimulus stress. *Audiology, 20,* 65–71.

Sininger, Y. S., Gardi, J. N., Morris, J. H., Martin, W. H., & Jewett, D. L. (1987). The 3-channel Lissajous' trajectory of the auditory brain-stem response. VII. Planar segments in humans. *Electroencephalography and Clinical Neurophysiology, 68,* 368–379.

Starr, A., & Achor, L. J. (1975). Auditory brainstem responses in neurological disease. *Archives of Neurology, 32,* 761–768.

Starr, A., & Squires, K. (1982). Distribution of auditory brainstem potentials over the scalp and nasopharynx in humans. *Annals of the New York Academy of Sciences, 388,* 427–442.

Stockard, J. J., Stockard, J. E., & Sharbrough, F. W. (1977). Detection and localization of occult lesions with brainstem auditory responses. *Mayo Clinic Proceedings, 52,* 761–770.

Stockard, J. J., Stockard, J. E., & Sharbrough, F. W. (1978). Nonpathologic factors influencing brainstem auditory evoked potentials. *American Journal of EEG Technology, 18,* 177–209.

Stypulkowski, P., & Staller, S. (1987). Clinical evaluation of a new EcoG recording electrode. *Ear & Hearing, 8,* 304–310.

Tietze, G., & Pantev, Ch. (1986). Comparison between auditory brainstem responses evoked by rarefaction and condensation step functions and clicks. *Audiology, 25,* 44–53.

Yagi, T., & Kaga, K. (1979). The effect of click repetition rate on the latency of the auditory evoked brainstem response and its clinical use for neurological diagnosis. *Archives of Otology, Rhinology, and Laryngology, 222,* 91–96.

Zupulla, R. A., Karmel, B. A., & Greenblatt, E. (1981). Prediction of cerebellopontine angle tumors based on discriminant analysis of brainstem auditory evoked responses. *Neurosurgery, 9,* 542–547.

CHAPTER 8

Diagnosis of Middle Ear Pathology and Evaluation of Conductive Hearing Loss

James W. Hall III • Bechara Y. Ghorayeb

For the majority of patients, otologic pathology producing conductive hearing impairment (external and middle ear abnormalities) can be conclusively diagnosed with a good history and careful physical examination. Audiometry in these cases, in particular the comparison of air versus bone conduction pure tone thresholds, quantifies degree of suspected hearing impairment. Other procedures, such as immittance audiometry, serve to confirm the otologic diagnosis but do not provide new or essential clinical information. This application of audiometry is by no means unimportant and still may contribute to decisions regarding surgical or medical management, especially when the physical examination reveals no obvious abnormality. Probably the most important example of this latter application is differentiation of stapes fixation (as in otosclerosis) versus disruption of the ossicular chain, and quantification of the resulting conductive hearing impairment, by the pattern of findings for pure tone and immittance audiometry (illustrated in cases to follow).

Clinical experience suggests six other, somewhat unique, contributions of audiometry in patients with external/middle ear pathology. These are (1) screening for middle ear dysfunction in children by nonphysicians (Harford, Bess, Bluestone, and Klein, 1978; Holte & Margolis, 1987), (2) detection of middle ear dysfunction in newborn infants or uncooperative, difficult-to-examine children by nonotologists (Paradise, Smith, and Bluestone, 1976), (3) documenting pre- versus posttherapy (surgical or medical) changes in auditory status (Wehrs, 1976), (4) describing the mechanical dysfunction caused by middle ear pathology (Jerger, 1970; Jerger, Anthony, Jerger,

and Mauldin, 1974), (5) evaluation of auditory function in comatose patients who cannot provide a history or respond behaviorally for clinical techniques such as tuning fork tests (Hall, 1989; Hall et al., 1982), and (6) providing otherwise unavailable ear-specific information on sensory integrity in persons with severe bilateral apparently conductive hearing impairment, such as congenital aural atresia (Hall et al., 1986; Jahrsdoerfer and Hall, 1986; Jahrsdoerfer, Yeakley, Hall, Robbins, and Gray, 1985). The first four of these contributions rely almost entirely on a comprehensive battery of immittance measures (tympanometry for low and high probe-tone frequencies, ipsilateral and contralateral acoustic reflexes). The final two contributions require assessment with auditory evoked responses in addition, perhaps, to immittance measures. Both confirmatory and diagnostic applications of audiometry will be discussed here, but the emphasis will be on the latter.

Three general areas of knowledge are fundamental to consistently successful evaluation of conductive hearing impairment but are beyond the scope of this chapter. The first is an understanding of external/middle ear anatomy and physiology. This topic is addressed in greater detail in Chapters 4 and 5; however, a brief description of the salient features of external/middle ear function is presented before reviewing the auditory effects of dysfunction of this important portion of the hearing mechanism. The pinna, by virtue of its orientation (facing forward) and morphology (folds and depressions), modulates sounds, mostly in the high-frequency region, and thereby creates acoustic cues that facilitate localization.

161

The external ear canal protects the ear (by its length and cerumen), offers a channel for passage of sound to the middle ear, and also amplifies, via resonance effects, acoustic energy at approximately 3000 Hz.

The two major and related functions of the middle ear (tympanic membrane and ossicles) are to match low impedance of the vibrations in the air of the external ear canal to the relative high impedance of movement of cochlear fluids. Impedance matching and resultant amplification are accomplished in three well-known ways: (1) an intricate buckling movement of the tympanic membrane (amplification × 4), (2) a lever action created by greater length of the manubrium of the malleus than the incus (amplification × 1.3), and (3) most important, the ratio of area of the relatively large tympanic membrane to the relatively small stapes footplate (amplification × 35). By means of these three properties, the middle ear functions as an acoustic impedance transformer and increases the amount of force transmitted from the external ear canal to the middle ear/inner ear junction (stapes footplate). This amplification is most pronounced in the auditory frequency region from 800 to 2000 Hz. Conductive hearing impairment resulting from external/middle ear pathology, therefore, may be practically defined as failure to collect or transmit sound energy from the environment to the organ of Corti. It is primarily a breakdown in the impedance matching mechanism somewhere between airborn sound arriving at the head and sound-related movement of cochlear fluid. Etiologies for this breakdown, however, are extremely varied, ranging from complete absence of the external ear and ear canal to the more subtle pathology of otosclerosis.

Second, a firm grasp of the acoustic immittance principles and practices is vital for maximum efficiency and effectiveness of audiometry in evaluation of conductive hearing impairment. Current concepts of immittance measurement are reviewed in Chapter 6 and also in several recent publications (Hall, 1985, 1987; Shanks, 1984; Van Camp, Margolis, Wilson, Creten, and Shanks, 1986).

Finally, the clinician must fully appreciate the complexities of air versus bone conduction pure tone audiometry in patients with suspected conductive hearing impairment. In the development of the audiology profession from about 1950 to 1965, pure tone techniques were essentially the only means available for audiometric evaluation of conductive hearing impairment. Immittance measurement was not yet clinically feasible or commercially available, and measurement of auditory evoked responses, namely electrocochleography (ECochG), was invasive and extremely limited in clinical application. It is, therefore, not surprising that this period produced a host of classic reports of air versus bone conduction audiometric findings in conductive hearing impairment. Among the important issues studied were the effect of procedural factors (Dirks, 1964; Hood, 1960; Jerger and Wertz, 1959; Studebaker, 1967; Ventry, Chaiklin, and Boyle, 1961), interaural attenuation (Zwislocki, 1953), masking (Dirks and Malmquist, 1964; Sanders and Rintelmann, 1964; Studebaker, 1962), the masking dilemma (Naunton, 1960), mechanical effects of middle ear pathology on cochlear function (Bekesy, 1960; Carhart, 1950; Huizing, 1960; Tonndorf, 1964), the occlusion effect (Goldstein and Hayes, 1965), and the sensory acuity level (SAL) test. Contemporary clinicians will find the information provided in these publications to be as useful today as their predecessors did over 20 years ago when they were published.

This chapter continues with a discussion of the differential diagnosis of external/middle ear pathology from the otologist's perspective. Then essential clinical procedures for comprehensive audiometric evaluation of external/middle ear dysfunction and conductive hearing impairment are summarized. This is followed by a review of typical patterns of audiometric findings in varied pathologies, along with brief reports of more challenging cases illustrating application of pure tone, immittance, and auditory brainstem response (ABR) audiometry in evaluation of middle ear pathology. The chapter concludes with guidelines for efficient and effective audiometric evaluation of conductive hearing impairment using the wide array of behavioral and electrophysiologic auditory procedures currently available. A glossary of audiologic and medical terminology is appended.

CLINICAL EXAMINATION

A diagnosis is based on the patient's history, symptoms, and clinical signs, and the results of laboratory tests and special diagnostic procedures (including audiometric data). Differential diagnosis is a comparison of this information among diseases that the patient *might* have in order to determine which disease the patient *does* have. The purpose for establishing a diagnosis is to provide a rational basis for selecting appropriate treatment and to estimate prognosis.

HISTORY

When a patient presents with the complaint of hearing loss or fullness in the ear, he or she should be questioned about other pertinent symptoms that may be valuable in reaching a diagnosis. For example, if there is a sensation of fullness, is it unilateral or in both ears? When did it start? Was it preceded by a common cold? Was it first noticed after flying, swimming, diving, or taking a shower? Did the patient "clean" the ear with a cotton swab just before the fullness became apparent? Are there other symptoms, such as earache, itching, tinnitus, discharge (of fluid from the ear), or fever? Did the symptoms start during pregnancy? Has the patient had previous surgery on the ear? Was there exposure to loud sounds or blasts, or any use of firearms? Has the patient taken any potentially ototoxic drugs? In order to consistently obtain an adequate history, the clinician must take the necessary time to put the patient at ease, and ask the appropriate questions. A good history is the first major step toward an accurate diagnosis of external/middle ear disease.

PHYSICAL DIAGNOSIS

Inspection of the External (Outer) Ear

The diagnosis can sometimes be made simply by closely viewing the external ear. Diseases involving the external ear are summarized in Table 8-1. An *absent auricle* (anotia) or a small, malformed auricle (microtia) often leads to the diagnosis of congenital disease of the ear. The presence of other associated maxillofacial deformities may allow the clinician to identify a syndrome. Likewise, obvious bleeding, lacerations, contusions, hematomas, or burns of the auricle and surrounding structures are evidence of *trauma*. More specifically, Battle's sign (bluish postauricular discoloration or ecchymosis) indicates a temporal bone fracture. Temporal bone fracture, as we will demonstrate, may be associated with varied types and degrees of hearing impairment. Facial nerve paresis or paralysis, a possible component of temporal bone fracture, is easily recognized when the patient is conscious but is frequently overlooked in comatose or paralyzed patients.

Redness, swelling, loss of auricular convolutions, weeping auricular skin, and sometimes dis-

TABLE 8-1. DISEASES OF THE EXTERNAL AUDITORY CANAL IN DIFFERENTIAL DIAGNOSIS

Congenital	Acquired
Atresia	Cerumen impaction
Collapsing external canal	Foreign body
	Infections
	Bacterial otitis externa
	Fungal (otomycosis)
	Parasitic
	Granulomas or polyps, or both
	Osteomas or exostoses
	Benign tumors
	Traumatic lesions
	Burns
	Hematomas
	Lacerations
	Fractures
	Scarring

charge or residual crusting are signs of a *diffuse external otitis or perichondritis* of the auricle, which may in turn cause collapse of the external ear canal. Diffuse redness and lateral displacement of the auricle, with or without purulent discharge from the meatus, with obliteration of the postauricular sulcus and generalized postauricular edema, are signs of acute mastoiditis. Swelling and redness over the sternocleidomastoid region indicate a Bezold's abscess. *Tumors of the auricle* that produce hearing impairment are generally large enough to be easily detected by physical inspection. Finally, the clinician should inspect visually for postauricular and endaural (within the meatus of the ear canal) incision scars that would suggest the nature of previous surgery.

Otoscopy of the Outer Ear

Atresia of the external auditory canal (EAC) is easily recognized. It may be associated with auricular deformities, preauricular skin tags, or a perfectly normal auricle. EAC *stenosis* with normal skin lining the canal is a congenital deformity that should be distinguished from a collapsing meatus. The latter consists of a slitlike meatus that opens on gentle posterosuperior retraction of the auricle and allows the examiner to insert the otoscope speculum. The remainder of the ear is usually normal. This condition is fairly common in elderly patients or in those who have undergone surgery via a postauricular incision. An unusually large meatus leading to a posterior cavity is evidence of previous surgery (radical or modified radical mastoidectomy).

Impacted cerumen (ear wax) is probably the most common cause of conductive hearing impairment

It is also the most annoying physical finding encountered by the otologist or audiologist because its removal is time consuming and requires a great deal of dexterity, particularly when it is found in children. Freshly secreted cerumen is soft and yellow. Cerumen becomes harder and turns a dark brown or black color if allowed to remain in the ear canal over time. It may appear dry and flaky and become covered with hair and dandruff, particulary in elderly men. On the other hand, cerumen may appear soft and creamy after swimming or bathing. Cerumen is only secreted in the cartilaginous (outer, hair-bearing) portion of the ear canal and normally tends to migrate and fall out of the canal spontaneously. Any cerumen accumulation in the bony (innermost) portion of the ear canal usually is due to the patient "cleaning" the ear with a cotton swab or some other equally inappropriate object. Patients often ask what they should do about earwax when they are advised not to clean their ears with, for example, a Q-tip. For these patients, it is safe to recommend insertion of a few drops of baby oil.

Foreign bodies in the EAC are common in children but are also observed in adults. Children are notorious for inserting beads, pebbles, milk teeth, and parts of toys in their ears. With adults, however, the object is most often left in the ear canal following insertion of a softer foreign body (cotton tip of a swab, paper tissue, detached pencil eraser) or the plastic cap of a ball point pen, as the patient attempts to scratch or clean the ear canal.

Osteomas or exostoses are occasionally seen in the ear canal during otoscopy. They are covered with thin, shiny, smooth skin and are located deep inside the body portion of the canal. In some cases, an exostosis is large enough to occlude the ear canal lumen (opening). *Acute otitis externa* presents in the form of a boil or abscess in the hair-bearing skin of the outer portion of the EAC. When it is diffuse, the entire canal is swollen, red, wet, and extremely tender on moving the auricle or pressing on the tragus. Insertion of the otoscope into the meatus causes the patient severe pain. The tympanic membrane, when it can be visualized, usually appears normal. *Otomycosis* is diagnosed when a mold is found in the ear canal. Filaments and spores may also be present. Discharge is scanty.

Otoscopy of the Middle Ear

Middle ear pathologies are listed in Table 8-2. In *acute bacterial otitis media*, the EAC is normal

TABLE 8-2. DISEASES OF THE MIDDLE EAR IN DIFFERENTIAL DIAGNOSIS

CONGENITAL

Absence or malformation of the ossicular chain

ACQUIRED

Infections and their sequelae
  Serous otitis media (acute or chronic)
  Purulent otitis media (acute or chronic)
  Tympanic membrane perforation
  Erosion or necrosis of lenticular process of incus
  Polyps
  Cholesteatoma
  Tympanosclerosis
  Atelectasis of middle ear space
Barotrauma
Trauma
  Insertion of foreign object or manipulation resulting in ossicular chain disruption or tympanic membrane perforation, or both
  Iatrogenic
  Blast injuries
  Temporal bone fractures resulting in hemotympanum, ossicular disruption, cerebrospinal fluid otorrhea
  Burns
Tumors
  Benign (adenomas, glomus tympanicum)
  Malignant
Granulomas

DISEASES OF THE OTIC CAPSULE

Otosclerosis

---

with no tenderness when the auricle is manipulated or when the speculum is inserted. With otoscopic inspection, the eardrum appears red and is sometimes bulging. Blood vessels are seen coursing over the manubrium. At a later stage, blood vessels become prominent over the entire tympanic membrane. The usual landmarks of the eardrum (the umbo and the light reflex) are lost. If untreated, the tympanic membrane may rupture, allowing pus to flow out. The tear in the eardrum is usually small and the purulent discharge is occasionally pulsatile. As the disease progresses, there is less discharge, and within days after the spontaneous rupture, the tear in the eardrum closes. At this stage, the eardrum is thinner and there may still be an air-fluid level in the middle ear.

The onset in *acute nonsuppurative otitis media* is sudden, and the tympanic membrane is thin, bluish, and retracted. Bubbles or air-fluid levels are readily visible through the eardrum. *Barotrauma*, caused by sudden changes in ambient pressure (associated with decompression, diving, and flying), is almost identical to this condition. *Chronic serous otitis media (glue ear)* is characterized by a bluish-grey or yellowish tympanic membrane, which is thick, opaque, and, in some cases, retracted.

Chronic purulent otitis media (chronic ear) is an infected middle ear space that drains through a tympanic membrane perforation. The perforation is usually large but could be as small as a pin point. The perforation edges are well defined, smooth, and occasionally slightly thickened. The layer of tympanic membrane skin curls inward along the perforation edge to blend with the medial mucosal lining of the tympanic membrane. Middle ear mucosa is hyperemic, thickened, and wet. Pus may be observed in the most dependent area of the middle ear. Red fleshy polyps occasionally emerge from the perforation. At times, they are so large as to occlude the entire external canal. These polyps are wet, foul smelling, and bleed easily. Removing the polyps by simply pulling on them is ill advised since they may be attached to the ossicles.

A *dry tympanic membrane perforation* is easily recognized. It almost always occurs in isolation and in the pars tensa portion of the tympanic membrane. The perforation may be central, marginal, or total. The round window niche is frequently observed, and in some cases the stapes, stapedius tendon, and incudostapedial joint are visible. The manubrium of the malleus may also be adherent to the promontory. The perforation edges are well defined and smooth. *Tuberculous otitis media* should be suspected if multiple perforations are present.

Perforations of the pars flaccida suggest the possibility of *cholesteatomas*, particularly if shiny skin appears to grow into the middle ear space. This ingrowth may appear as a simple pocket or at times as a tract leading medially and superiorly toward the attic. This invagination or tract could be lined with shiny, pearly white flakes and may be filled with keratin debris and foul-smelling necrotic material and pus. In a large cholesteatoma, the normal anatomy of the eardrum may be completely replaced by these white pearly flakes and keratin debris. Polyps and pus are often present, and the foul smell is overbearing.

Tympanosclerosis (adhesive otitis media) is the result of long-standing middle ear infection. It is characterized by hyaline degeneration of the tympanic membrane and middle ear space, which leads to calcification and sometimes new bone formation. Such calcium deposits may be seen as white plaques in the substance of the eardrum. The eardrum may be extremely thin, transparent, and so severely retracted that it is wrapped around the ossicles. The retraction could easily be mis-

taken for a large perforation when it is plastered to the promontory. This is referred to as *atelectasis of the middle ear.*

Trauma to the middle ear can cause the eardrum to rupture, resulting in an irregular or stellate perforation and fresh blood in the ear canal and middle ear space *(hemotympanum)*. This pattern of findings is usually the result of insertion of a foreign body accidentally into the ear (cotton swab or bobby pin), or it may be iatrogenic, secondary to attempted removal of cerumen or foreign bodies from the EAC. Blasts can produce the same clinical picture and associated inner ear symptomatology. A slap to the ear can trap air under pressure in the ear canal and cause the tympanic membrane to rupture. Occasionally, the tympanic membrane remains intact but the ossicular chain becomes disrupted.

Longitudinal *fractures of the temporal bone* produce a laceration of the EAC skin with fresh bleeding, exposure of bony fragments, tears in the tympanic membrane, and occasionally cerebrospinal fluid leak. When the eardrum is intact, or after it heals, hemotympanum is manifested by a blue, opaque discoloration of the tympanic membrane. Other signs that may be present are facial nerve paralysis, nystagmus, and ataxia. Many of these patients may be comatose and may have other severe brain injuries. Evidence of dysfunction in longitudinal fractures may be first discovered by the otologist or audiologist during an auditory evoked response assessment. It is imperative to remember that such ear injuries are potential ports of contamination to the brain and can lead to meningitis. Therefore, extreme care should be taken in cleaning blood and debris from the EAC, and sterile instruments and technique must be used during the procedure. Some otologists prefer to defer the cleaning procedure for a week or two so that healing of the tympanic membrane and lacerations can occur first. Under no circumstances should the ear be irrigated or a caloric test (ice water calorics or electronystagmography) be performed until the lacerations and tympanic membrane have completely healed. Also, conductive hearing impairment in these patients should be evaluated audiometrically only after resorption of the hemotympanum.

Tumors of the EAC are occasionally mistaken for polyps. They are fleshy, red, bleed easily, and may be associated with chronic otitis media and purulent discharge. Pulsating red masses observed behind the eardrum are usually *glomus tympanicum tumors.*

Finally, *otosclerosis,* a disease of the otic capsule, may produce a physical sign that can be observed with the otoscope. *Schwartze's sign* is a reddish discoloration of the eardrum secondary to an active otosclerotic focus that causes the blood vessels of the promontory to dilate and engorge with blood.

Additional Diagnostic Procedures

For the majority of patients, a diagnosis is made from the history and physical examination. Diseases of the external ear are obvious and easily diagnosed. Difficulties arise when the differential diagnosis narrows down to certain conditions that require additional clinical information. An example of this difficulty is diffuse otitis externa with a tender postauricular lymph node versus swollen purulent ear versus an acute mastoiditis. In such conditions, radiograms of the mastoids and possibly audiologic evaluation, when feasible, help the clinician in reaching a diagnosis.

Other clinical entities exist for which information from the history and physical examination does not consistently lead to a diagnosis. For example, the eardrum may appear normal, even for an experienced clinician, yet tympanometry may indicate middle ear effusion. Cholesteatoma may bridge the ossicular chain and mask a disruption in the ossicular chain by conducting sound waves from the tympanic membrane to the inner ear. Such patients may have little or no conductive hearing impairment with the cholesteatoma in place, but with its removal there may be a conductive hearing impairment of up to 50 dB HL. The same difficulty in correctly diagnosing middle ear disease may be present for the patient with a normal eardrum and an ossicular chain disruption. The most frequent lesion causing this finding is necrosis of the lenticular process of the incus following chronic middle ear disease. A serious (50–60 dB HL) conductive hearing impairment accompanies the disease. When the eardrum is ruptured, the clinician may be able to visualize the pathology.

High-resolution computed tomography is useful in the description of otologic pathology in temporal bone fracture, including definition of ossicular chain disruption. Finally, with chronic adhesive otitis media, the eardrum is so thin and retracted that the contour of the eroded incus or incudostapedial joint may be perceived through the membrane. Occasionally, the long process of the incus is completely eroded and the eardrum wraps around the capitulum of the stapes in what

appears to be a natural tympanoplasty type III effect. Such patients may have normal hearing.

AUDIOLOGIC ASSESSMENT

AURAL IMMITTANCE

Immittance measurement at the outset of an audiometric assessment is the most effective means of differentiating conductive versus sensory hearing impairment, as shown schematically in Figure 8-1. In 1970, Jerger observed that "impedance audiometry represents an invaluable diagnostic tool in clinical audiology. It has become, in our clinic, a routine part of the audiologic assessment of every patient. We frankly wonder how we ever got along without it" (Jerger, 1970, p. 322). Almost 20 years later, immittance measures remain invaluable and a routine component of audiologic assessment.

Rigorous definition of normal immittance findings is crucial for successful application of immittance measures in ruling out middle ear pathology. These normal immittance criteria that must be rigidly adhered to are (1) ear canal volume within normal limits, (2) normal type A tympanograms (not A_s or A_d) bilaterally, and (3) acoustic reflexes clearly and consistently present at expected stimulus levels (95 dB HL or better) bilaterally for both ipsilateral (uncrossed) and contralateral (crossed) conditions. With these immittance findings and pure tone audiometry evidence of hearing impairment, the deficit is almost always considered to be sensory and subsequent audiometric assessment directed toward differentiation of cochlear versus retrocochlear dysfunction, and complete definition of auditory status for one or the other site of lesion (see Chapters 9, 10, and 11). Measurement of acoustic reflex decay is a standard component of the immittance battery and, therefore, the first procedure administered for differentiation of sensory versus neural auditory dysfunction. *Bone conduction pure tone measurement in patients with unequivocally normal immittance findings (with the exception of abnormal acoustic reflex decay) is generally superfluous, that is, noncontributory toward the diagnosis or description of the hearing impairment, and a waste of valuable clinical time.*

Of course, this normal acoustic immittance pattern occurring in combination with normal pure tone hearing sensitivity does not necessarily imply normal function of the peripheral *and* cen-

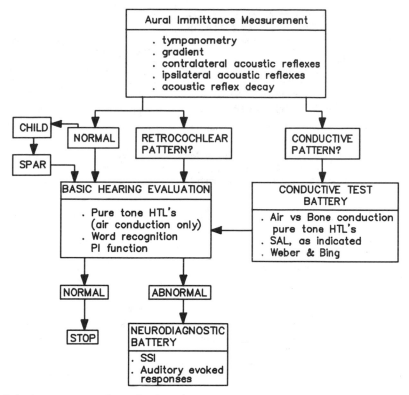

Figure 8-1. Audiologic test strategy for evaluation of conductive hearing impairment.

tral auditory system. With this combination of results, especially for patients with auditory complaints (e.g., difficulty understanding speech under adverse listening conditions), a history of central nervous system disease or insult (e.g., head injury, stroke, multiple sclerosis), or neurologic and neurotologic signs or symptoms (e.g., dizziness, tinnitus), there is a high index of suspicion for central auditory nervous dysfunction. More extensive analysis of acoustic reflex activity (Hall, 1983; Stach and Jerger, 1987) plus diagnostic speech audiometry (Hall, 1984) and assessment of auditory evoked responses (Hall, 1990) are the procedures of choice in these patients. The following general remarks will be limited to clinical evaluation of patients with suspected external/middle ear pathology and associated conductive or mixed hearing impairment. Specific patterns of audiometric findings for patients with various middle ear pathologies will be presented and discussed in a subsequent section.

Since Jerger published his classic paper in 1970 on clinical immittance audiometry experiences with over 400 patients, the unique diagnostic

value of immittance audiometry has been repeatedly reported in the literature and demonstrated clinically (Jerger, 1970; Jerger and Hayes, 1976; Jerger et al., 1974; Jerger, Jerger, and Mauldin, 1972). Analysis of acoustic immittance patterns is the most sensitive audiometric means of identifying middle ear dysfunction and, in addition, of differentiating among mechanical bases of this dysfunction. "Individually . . . each measure has serious limitations. In combination, however, they yield patterns of great diagnostic value" (Jerger, 1970, p. 322). There are numerous detailed descriptions of correlations among immittance patterns and types of underlying middle ear pathology. What follows herein is a summary of the salient immittance findings for types of pathology encountered most often clinically. In Table 8-3, characteristic audiometric patterns are summarized for commonly encountered types of otologic pathology.

Tympanometry

Major tympanogram types according to the Jerger (1970) classification system are illustrated in Figure 8-2. Other approaches for tympanogram analysis have been proposed (Bluestone, Berry,

TABLE 8-3. SUMMARY OF GENERAL PATTERNS OF AUDIOLOGIC
FINDINGS ASSOCIATED WITH MIDDLE EAR PATHOLOGIES

Pathology	Audiologic procedure		
	Pure tone audiometry (db HL)	Tympanometry*	Acoustic stapedial reflexes
Serous otitis media	20–30 dB rising CHL	Type C or B	Absent
Acute otitis media	30–50 dB flat CHL	Type B	Absent
Early otosclerosis	Normal hearing to <20 dB CHL	Type A$_s$	Reverse direction
Otosclerosis	25–60 dB rising CHL or MHL; Carhart's notch	Type A$_s$	Absent
Complete ossicular chain discontinuity	60 dB flat or sloping CHL	Type A$_d$	Absent
Ossicular chain discontinuity with functional connection	30–40 dB flat or sloping CHL	Type A$_d$	May be present
Tympanic membrane perforation: peripheral	Within normal limits	Abnormally large EAC volume	CNE
Tympanic membrane perforation: central	Normal to 25 dB rising CHL	Abnormally large EAC volume	CNE
Tympanic membrane ventilation tube (patent)	Within normal limits	Abnormally large EAC volume	CNE
Cholesteatoma	25–60 dB CHL	Variable	Usually absent
Aural atresia	>60 dB flat or rising MHL or CHL	CNE	CNE

CHL, conductive hearing loss; MHL, mixed hearing loss; EAC, external auditory canal; CNE, cannot evaluate.
* Tympanogram types are described in text and Figure 8-2.

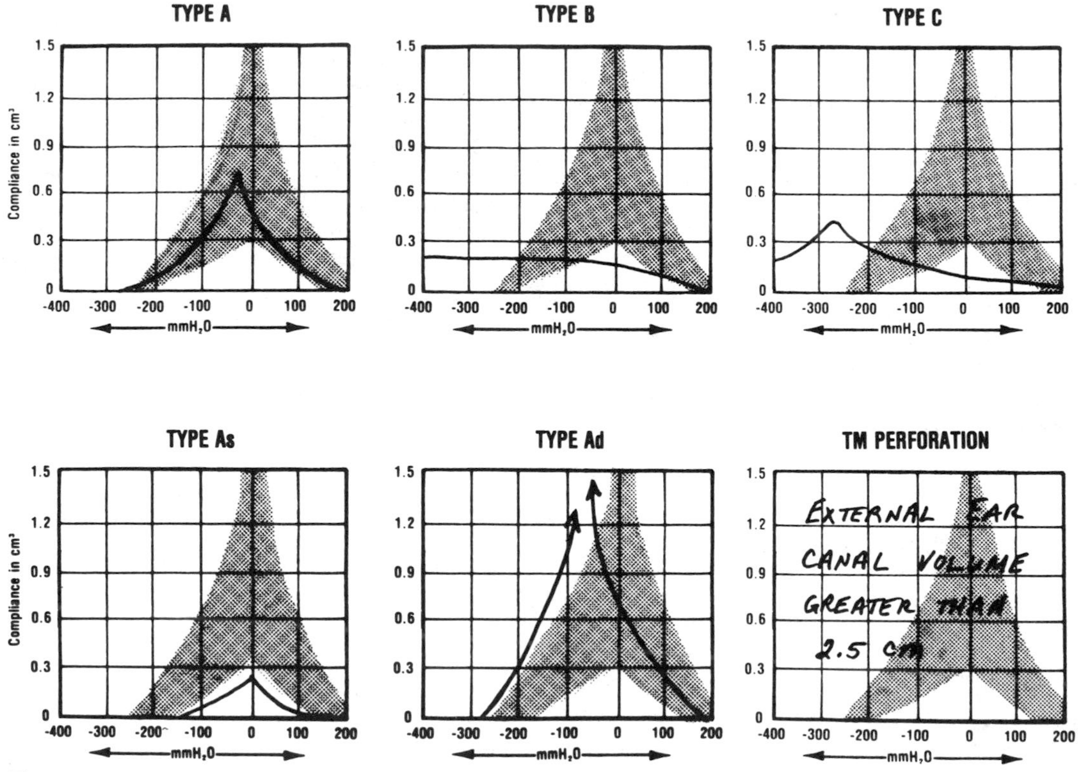

Figure 8-2. Clinically popular tympanogram classification system proposed by Jerger (1970).

and Paradise, 1973; Cooper, Hearne, and Gates, 1982; Feldman, 1976; Van Camp et al., 1986). Among these, the clinical use of multifrequency (e.g., 660 versus 220 Hz probe tone) and multicomponent (e.g., susceptance and conductance versus admittance) tympanometry has been consistently endorsed in the United States and Europe. Some evidence exists that multiple-frequency, multicomponent, and phase-angle tympanometry offer diagnostically useful information in a rather selective category of patients with low-impedance (high-admittance or -compliance) middle ear pathology, such as ossicular chain disruption (Van Camp et al., 1986); however, findings from the combination of a complete medical history, otologic examination, routine immittance measurement, and pure tone audiometry rarely fail to confirm accurate diagnosis of this pathology, as will be demonstrated soon with actual cases. Probably as a consequence, Jerger's relatively simple tympanogram classification schema continues to be the most widely accepted clinically.

The clinician applying this system is advised to follow the test protocol originally described by Jerger, specifically plotting the tympanogram for an approximately 220 Hz probe-tone frequency as air pressure in the EAC is varied in a positive-to-negative direction. It is possible for tympanogram interpretation by the Jerger criteria to be invalidated if the other protocols are used. Probe-tone frequency, the rate and direction of ear canal pressure change, and, of course, the property measured (admittance, susceptance, or conductance) exert clinically important influences on tympanogram measurement (Shanks and Wilson, 1986; Van Camp et al., 1986; Wilson, Shanks, and Kaplan, 1984). It would, therefore, be unwise to routinely record tympanograms with a test parameter not employed by Jerger et al., such as a negative-to-positive versus positive-to-negative ear canal pressure change, and then to interpret the results with their classification system.

Acoustic Reflexes

Acoustic reflexes are usually not observed when recorded with the measuring probe in an ear with middle ear pathology because ossicular chain or tympanic membrane abnormalities obscure detection at the eardrum of the relatively small alterations in middle ear immittance that occur with stapedial muscle contraction. (See Hall, 1984, for a review of acoustic reflex anatomy and physiology.) Acoustic reflexes are almost invariably abnormal for the cases in which they are present. These include minor middle ear pathology, early fixation of the ossicular chain, and, rarely, disruption of the ossicular chain with some type of functional connection between tympanic membrane and stapes. With even subtle middle ear dysfunction in the probe ear, such as the negative pressure associated with eustachian tube obstruction and early serous otitis media, acoustic reflex thresholds are markedly elevated (intensity levels of 95 dB HL or greater are required to elicit reflex activity). Early fixation of the ossicular chain characteristically produces an unusual acoustic reflex waveform. With stimulus presentation, a curious decrease occurs in middle ear impedance (referred to as *negative deflection* of the meter and X-Y plotter pen), rather than the usual increase in impedance (or stiffness). In these cases, hearing sensitivity may still be normal and there may be little or no air-bone gap. If the gap between the stapes and a more lateral portion of the middle ear system (e.g., tympanic membrane or malleus) is bridged in some atypical way, patients with ossicular chain disruption may show acoustic reflex activity. The fortuitous ossicular connection can be made with fibrous adhesions or other material, which serve to transmit stapedius muscle–related changes in middle ear immittance from the stapes to the tympanic membrane. Despite this functional connection, there is usually a maximum (60 dB HL) conductive component to the hearing impairment. As an aside, patients with ossicular chain disruption and other concomitant middle ear pathology, such as cholesteatoma or fluid, may have less hearing impairment because there is a means for mechanical transmission from eardrum to stapes footplate.

PURE TONE AUDIOMETRY

Comparison of hearing threshold levels for air- versus bone-conducted pure tone signals — measurement of the air-bone gap — is the traditional approach for audiometric description of conductive hearing loss associated with middle ear pathology. As noted earlier, the many technical issues of air versus bone conduction pure tone audiometry, among them placement of the bone vibrator, masking criteria and methods, and calibration, are fully addressed in hundreds of articles and scores of basic audiology textbook chapters and will not be reviewed here.

Acoustic Impedance Versus Audiogram Configuration

One aspect of pure tone audiometry in conductive hearing loss that is rarely noted, but diagnostically useful, is the relationship between middle ear pathology and audiogram configuration. Over 40 years ago, long before impedance measurement became incorporated into the basic audiometric test, Johansen (1948) described the hearing loss configurations that were correlated with different components of middle ear impedance. The acoustic impedance components, namely resistance (friction), reactance (mass and stiffness, or its reciprocal compliance), and their dependence on frequency of sound, are now familiar to audiologists. The audiometric correlates are illustrated in Figure 8-3. Resistance abnormalities, which are not common, affect a wide range of mid frequencies in the audiogram. The effect of a mass abnormality is decreased high-frequency hearing sensitivity, whereas abnormally increased stiffness, most commonly found clinically, produces a low-frequency hearing deficit. Thus, a simple inspection of air conduction pure tone audiometry configurations can provide some indica-

Figure 8-3. Relationship of aural acoustic impedance and audiogram configuration. (From Johansen, H. [1948]. Relation of audiograms to the impedance formula. *Acta Oto-laryngologica* [Stockholm] *Suppl. 74.)*

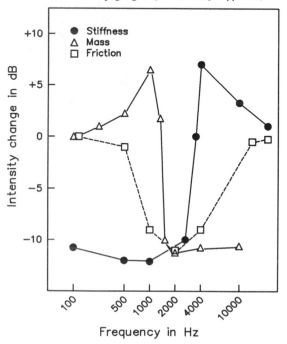

tion of underlying middle ear pathology and confirm otologic and immittance findings.

Masking Dilemma

One of the most challenging problems in clinical audiology is the *masking dilemma* (Jerger and Wertz, 1959; Naunton, 1960), which is presented most often by a person with a moderate to severe bilateral, apparently conductive hearing loss. This audiometric pattern is illustrated with a forthcoming case report of congenital atresia (case 17). The dilemma is that the intensity level of masking noise necessary to effectively mask the non-test ear (e.g., overcome the conductive component on the non-test ear and reach the cochlea at an intensity level about 10 dB higher than any crossed-over test signal) exceeds interaural attenuation (minimally 40–50 dB) and can cross over (via bone conduction) to mask hearing on the test ear. The most vivid demonstration of this potential problem is provided by unmasked air versus bone conduction findings for patients with a total unilateral sensory hearing impairment (a "dead ear"). Unmasked air conduction thresholds are usually in the 50 to 60 dB range, and bone conduction thresholds (obtained with the bone vibrator on the mastoid of the ear in question) may be in the 10 to 20 dB range (Chaiklin, 1967). Both air and bone conduction thresholds in the dead ear are due to cross over to the normal non-test ear.

Three simple techniques can help to resolve this dilemma in some cases. The first two are the audiometric Weber and Bing tests. If a patient with bilaterally symmetric and apparently conductive hearing impairment consistently lateralizes low-frequency pure tone signals to one ear (the Weber test) or shows no occlusion effect (Goldstein and Hayes, 1965) for these signals on one ear (the Bing test), it is likely that this ear has a greater conductive component, and unmasked bone conduction thresholds originate from this ear. Admittedly, these tests generally do not unequivocally resolve the masking dilemma, but the information can be very valuable clinically. A third simple approach to dealing with the masking dilemma is the use of insert earphone cushions (ER-3A) for both air conduction pure tone stimulation and masking during bone conduction stimulation. If these cushions are inserted to maximum recommended depth within the ear canal, they do contribute to increased interaural attenuation for lower frequency (below 1000 Hz) tones. This may reduce the likelihood of stimulus cross over to the non-test ear as well as cross over of the masking noise at high-intensity levels to the test ear. However, minimal interaural attenuation benefit comes from so-called tubephones for higher frequencies, particularly at more typical insertion depths. Also, insert cushions cannot, of course, be used in patients with aural atresia (anotia). This discussion of the masking dilemma presumes that immittance audiometry was consistent with bilateral conductive hearing impairment. If immittance audiometry shows normal tympanometry and acoustic reflex activity on one ear, a sensory hearing impairment can be presumed and there will be no masking dilemma. Two additional approaches for solving the masking dilemma — the SAL test and ABR — will now be presented.

Sensory Acuity Level

The SAL test is perhaps the most underused and underappreciated of clinical audiometric procedures. Rainville introduced in 1955 a new, but rather complicated, technique for assessing sensory function that did not rely on conventional bone conduction audiometry. Several years later, Jerger and Tillman (1960) and then others (Burke, Creston, Marsh, and Shutts, 1965; Jerger and Jerger, 1965; Jerger and Tillman, 1960; Keys and Milburn, 1961; Michael, 1963; Tillman, 1963) provided comprehensive investigations of a clinically feasible modification of the Rainville technique. The two major limitations of conventional bone conduction audiometry motivating the SAL test were the problem with calibration of bone conduction stimuli and difficulties associated with adequately masking the non-test ear, that is, the masking dilemma.

In 1963, Jerger and Jerger described the SAL test protocol, systematically studying the possible effects of certain procedural variables on SAL outcome, including occlusion effect, force of bone vibrator application, effect of noise duration, linearity of masking, effect of correlated noise in non-test ear (i.e., masking level difference phenomena), and the acoustic reflex. Importantly, they found that SAL and conventional bone conduction audiometry hearing threshold levels were equivalent.

In brief, the SAL procedure is as follows: Air conduction pure tone hearing threshold levels for signals of 500, 1000, 2000, and 4000 Hz are first measured for each ear without any masking. Then a masking noise is presented via a bone vibrator placed on the forehead. The intensity level of the noise is 2 volts root-mean-square. Clinically, this level can be approximated by presenting masking noise by bone conduction at the output limit for the audiometer, usually about 55 dB HL for 500 Hz and 60 or 65 dB HL for 1000, 2000, and 4000 Hz. The average shift in air conduction thresholds produced by this noise level at each of the four pure tone stimulus frequencies is determined for a group of normal-hearing subjects, prior to application of SAL testing in a clinical facility. The SAL test cannot, unfortunately, be performed on audiometers that do not permit presentation of a masking noise via the bone vibrator.

The fundamental calculation in SAL testing is comparison of the air conduction hearing threshold level (HTL) shift from the quiet test condition to the bone conduction masking condition in a patient versus the normal expected shift, derived as noted above. If the patient's hearing loss is entirely conductive, his or her shift will equal the normal shift, since the masking noise will have full effect on sensory hearing. Normal bone conduction is presumed. On the other hand, if the hearing loss is sensory, masking noise will not affect hearing until it exceeds the patient's HTL. An approach that facilitates an understanding of SAL is to consider the difference between the patient's noise-produced HTL versus the normal noise-produced HTL as an estimation of air-bone gap, not bone conduction hearing level. If subtraction of the normal air conduction threshold in noise (e.g., 55 dB) from a patient's threshold in noise, for example 65 dB, produces a difference of only 10 dB, then there is a 10 dB air-bone gap. The remainder of the hearing loss is sensory. That is, bone conduction hearing is 10 dB better than air conduction hearing. SAL threshold symbols (diamonds) are plotted at an intensity level 10 dB better than those for air conduction as initially measured in quiet. If the difference for patient versus normal threshold is 60 dB, on the other hand, the air-bone gap is 60 dB (i.e., SAL symbols are plotted at the dB HTL 60 dB better than the air conduction HTL in quiet). A useful form for calculating SAL outcome clinically is shown in Figure 8-4.

Concerns about validity and clinical accuracy of the SAL test expressed in the early 1960s (Goldstein, Hayes, and Peterson, 1962; Martin and Bailey, 1964; Tillman, 1963) were essentially allayed by the findings of Jerger and Jerger in 1965; however, two practical limitations are sometimes encountered in clinical application of SAL in pa-

Patient: _____ Age: ____ Sex: ___

Date of test: _____ Tester: _____

_____
_____

		Test Frequency (Hz)				
Ear	Condition (HTLs in dB)	500	1000	2000	4000	SRT
Right	Quiet					
Right	Noise					
	SAL shift norm					
	Noise - SAL norm (air bone gap)					
Left	Quiet					
Left	Noise					
	SAL shift norm					
	Noise - SAL norm (air bone gap)					

Figure 8-4. Worksheet for computing SAL.

tients with moderate to severe hearing impairment. For patients with severe conductive loss, air conduction threshold levels may be shifted beyond the output limits of the audiometer by the bone conduction noise. An air-bone gap of as much as 60 dB can be confirmed, but the actual sensory hearing level cannot be determined. Also, if a patient showing no shift in air conduction threshold levels with noise has HTLs worse than the intensity level of the noise (e.g., 55–60 dB), one cannot be certain that a pure sensory loss exists, that is, no air-bone gap. Nonetheless, the authors have found SAL testing to be a very effective approach for differentiating between largely conductive versus sensory types of deficits in patients with severe bilateral hearing impairment. Clinical application of SAL testing is illustrated by case reports in the following section.

AUDITORY BRAINSTEM RESPONSE

With infants or young children, and patients of all ages who are uncooperative or for whatever reason untestable with traditional audiometry, it may be impossible to use earphones or bone vi-

brators in behavioral assessment of auditory sensitivity. The SAL test cannot be used in these patients and, furthermore, does not always provide an estimate of air conduction HTL. According to prevailing opinion, ABR by air conduction and bone conduction is similarly limited by masking problems. Acoustic cross-over levels of 50 to 75 dB have been reported for click stimuli (Humes and Ochs, 1982; Reid and Thornton, 1983). Bone conduction ABR is additionally constrained by maximum stimulus output levels of 50 to 60 dB HL.

Numerous clinical reports describe the use of ABR in defining conductive hearing loss (Arlinger and Kylen, 1977; Cornacchia, Martini, and Morra, 1983; Finitzo-Hieber, Hecox, and Cone, 1979; Fria and Sabo, 1980; Hall, 1984; Hall, Morgan, Mackey-Hargadine, Aguilar, and Jahrsdoerfer, 1984; Hooks and Weber, 1984; Jahrsdoerfer et al., 1985; Mauldin and Jerger, 1979; McGee and Clemis, 1982; Weber, 1983) and several attempts to assess sensory function with an ABR SAL-type procedure (Hicks, 1980; Webb and

Greenberg, 1983). To date, the major emphasis seems to have been on applying ABR in accordance with the principles and constraints of behavioral audiometry rather than exploiting the unique advantages of auditory evoked response methodology. For instance, Weber (1983) states that with air conduction ABR, "as with any audiometric procedure, a masking noise must be administered to the non-test ear when the poorer ear is being evaluated" (p. 344), and "because a bone-conducted signal reaches each cochlea with about the same intensity, masking of the non-test ear is essential if information about the individual ear is desired. . . . This masking dilemma in patients with a marked conductive hearing loss is not unique to ABR testing" (p. 348). A similar theme is reiterated by others (Finitzo-Hieber, Hecox, and Cone, 1979).

Although ABR permits assessment of monaural auditory sensitivity with earphone and bone vibrator transducers, even in infants and young children with middle ear pathology, this advantage would appear quite markedly reduced in patients with a serious conductive component to the hearing impairment. That is, if effective masking were necessary and yet could not be applied without the likelihood of overmasking, then ear-specific information would be impossible with air and bone conduction ABR, just as it is with traditional threshold audiometry. The recent commercial availability of insert transducers may, as noted before, offer a partial practical solution to the overmasking problem in behavioral and ABR assessment in some patients. Insert transducers are not useful for patients with complete aural atresia or stenotic ear canals. Furthermore, with the limitation in maximum stimulus output, bone conduction ABR provides little information for patients with a mild to moderate sensory component.

Masking is not invariably necessary in ABR assessment of serious bilateral conductive hearing impairment, or ABR measurement in general. In the authors' experience, ABR assessment can often define the extent of the conductive loss and residual sensory function for each ear (Hall, 1989; Hall et al., 1984; Jahrsdoerfer et al., 1985). A clear wave I in the ipsilateral recording, usually at a high-stimulus intensity level, by air or bone conduction ensures an ear-specific ABR. A delayed wave V component at a high-stimulus intensity level, with no evidence of a wave I, indicates the need for contralateral masking to rule out a cross-over response. Success in obtaining ear-specific information is highest for infants and young children but can be

enhanced in all patients by following a test protocol that includes four major components: (1) an earlobe or, whenever possible, ear canal or promontory inverting electrode (versus mastoid placement) serves to augment wave I amplitude. In fact one of the first clinical applications of ECochG was evaluation of conductive hearing impairment (Lempert, Wever, and Lawrence, 1947); (2) a high-pass filter setting (low-frequency cutoff) of 30 Hz (versus 150 or 300 Hz) encompasses the substantial low-frequency energy that characterizes the ABR. Low-frequency spectral content may be greater, in fact, for the bone conduction ABR, since the frequency response of the transducer is predominately below 1500 Hz; (3) stimulus (click) rate of no greater than 21 per second and occasionally 11.1 per second or even slower; (4) a quiet (natural sleep or sedated) patient, and (5) simultaneous multichannel recordings for air and bone conduction stimulation.

The initial overall objective of these technical maneuvers is to produce a clear wave I for the ipsilateral recording channel (versus no wave I for the contralateral channel), which confirms that the response is arising from the ear stimulated. Masking the non-test ear is superfluous if a wave I is identified in the stimulus ipsilateral waveform. The response cannot, in this case, be due exclusively to stimulation of the non-test ear. A secondary objective is to record a distinct and reliable wave V component that can then be followed as stimulus intensity is decreased in estimation of ABR threshold. With a reliable wave I for at least one intensity level, it is then safe to conclude that waveforms for lower-intensity stimuli are also ear specific, even if a wave I cannot be confidently identified. Guidelines for application of bone conduction ABR are presented in a recently published textbook (Hall, 1990). The application of these ABR techniques in eliciting clinically useful bone conduction responses is illustrated (case 17) in a section that follows.

PATTERNS OF AUDIOMETRIC FINDINGS IN EXTERNAL AND MIDDLE EAR PATHOLOGY

The following illustrative cases highlight findings for a basic audiometric test battery that typify common types of external or middle ear disorders or pathology. The emphasis is on audiometric patterns that permit differentiation of one disorder from the next and contribute to accurate interpretation of findings. As noted at the outset of this chapter, a careful history and thorough physical examination often lead to the correct diagnosis. Certainly, this would be true for most of the following cases; however, the patients first presented to audiology. It is often the audiologist's responsibility to conduct the initial assessment and ensure that the patient receives proper hearing health care. Atypical patterns of findings for middle ear pathology are discussed in the next section.

CASE 1: IMPACTED CERUMEN

A 76-year-old woman presents with the chief complaint of long-standing difficulty in hearing, especially understanding speech in the presence of background noise, but recent onset of increased difficulty in all listening conditions. As shown in Figure 8-5, she had a moderate to severe, sloping mixed hearing impairment bilaterally. Speech audiometry performance was fair for word recognition and synthetic sentence identification (SSI) at a high-intensity level (80 dB HL) but very poor at even a loud conversation level (60 dB HL). Immittance audiometry showed flat type B tympanograms in each ear.

Initial review of audiometry might suggest otitis media. The important audiometric finding for this patient was abnormally small EAC volumes, as estimated from immittance audiometry (Shanks and Lilly, 1981). This prompted otoscopic inspection, which confirmed that cerumen occluded each external auditory meatus. Removal of the cerumen by an otolaryngologist produced a mild to moderate sloping sensory hearing impairment suggested by the bone conduction HTLs in Figure 8-5. The finding of a medically treatable external ear disorder influenced the alternatives for audiologic management of this elderly patient. Otoscopy before immittance audiometry is advisable.

CASE 2: COLLAPSING EAR CANALS

A 69-year-old woman noted a slight decrease in hearing for the left versus right ear. Pure tone audiometry (Figure 8-6) showed a mild high-frequency conductive component bilaterally. Speech audiometry was good for phonetically balanced (PB) word recognition and SSI. SSI scores were higher than PB word scores for low to moderate (40–60 dB) intensity levels. Tympanometry was normal. At this juncture, the presence of a slight conductive component and normal tympanograms would suggest stapes fixation, although this pathology produces a hearing impairment with a rising configuration.

The presence of normal ipsilateral acoustic reflex threshold levels and elevated contralateral acoustic reflexes, especially for higher-stimulus frequencies, led to the suspicion of collapsing ear canals. The immittance probe prevented ear canal collapse, whereas the standard audiometric earphone cushion used for contralateral reflex assessment caused ear canal collapse just as it did during pure tone audiometry. The relative poorer performance for PB word recognition, which depends most on hearing sensitivity in the 2000 Hz region versus SSI materials, which reflect hearing in the 750 Hz region, was consistent with the high-frequency deficit. Elevated contralateral versus ipsilateral acoustic reflexes, a horizontal pattern, are also a sign of brainstem pathology (Hall, 1985). The air-bone gap would not be consistent with this pathology. In addition,

repeat air conduction audiometry following insertion of an otoscope speculum produced HTLs equivalent to those for bone conduction shown in Figure 8-6. A collapsing ear canal produces an apparent hearing deficit of 10 to 15 dB, which is greatest at 2000 Hz (Ventry et al., 1961). It is more often encountered in newborn infants and the elderly than other patient age groups. The possibility of collapsing ear canals should be considered in patients of any age with large "lop" ears.

CASE 3: PATENT VENTILATION TUBES

Ventilation (aeration or pressure equalization) tubes were inserted bilaterally into the tympanic membranes of a 5-year-old boy with recurrent otitis media. Audiometric findings obtained 1 year later (shown in Figure 8-7) confirmed that the ventilation tube for the right ear remained in the tympanic membrane and was patent. EAC volume of 2.3 cc, as estimated by immittance measures (Hall, 1987), greatly exceeded normal expectations for a child (no more than 1.0 cc) and the value for the other canal (0.60 cc). Positive ear canal pressure (+200 decaPascal [daPA]) was relieved by swallowing. *A finding of patent ventilation tube (or tympanic membrane perforation) precludes tympanometry and acoustic reflex measurement (Hall, 1987).* It is improper to perform tympanometry and report a type B tympanogram, since pressure against the eardrum is, in effect, not being varied. Air conduction pure tone HTLs were well within the normal range, although bone conduction testing showed a consistent air-bone gap. Word recognition (PB-K lists) was excellent.

For the left ear, the pattern of immittance findings (normal EAC volume, negative pressure of −300 daPA, and absent acoustic reflexes with probe left) and a mild conductive hearing impairment, with only fair word recognition at a conversational intensity level, indicated extrusion or occlusion of the ventilation tube and apparent recurrence of serous otitis media. The tube was found lying deep within the ear canal on otoscopic inspection with an operating room microscope. The presence of the ventilation tube in the right tympanic membrane was verified otoscopically.

By tympanometric measurement, no distinction exists between a patent ventilation tube and tympanic membrane perforation. History and otoscopic inspection can differentiate between the two. Also, a patent ventilation tube typically causes little or no deficit in hearing sensitivity, although an air-bone gap, as in this case, may be present whereas a very mild conductive hearing component (e.g., 20 dB) at the least is usually found in tympanic membrane perforation.

CASE 4: SCARRED TYMPANIC MEMBRANE

A 55-year-old Spanish-speaking woman complained of recent difficulty understanding what her grandchildren said to her. She reported a history of repeated ear infections and tympanic perforations as a child, but no problems with her ears since then. Tympanometry with a 226 Hz probe tone showed abnormally high compliance (>1.60 cc) bilaterally (Figure 8-8).

Because of the sharp tympanogram peak, it was difficult to remain at maximum compliance and maintain a steady compliance meter during acoustic reflex measurement bilaterally. An attempt to measure acoustic reflexes was abandoned for this reason with probe left. Pure tone audiometry showed a mild, gently sloping sensory hearing impairment bilaterally. Bone conduction threshold assessment was mandated by the abnormal immittance findings. There

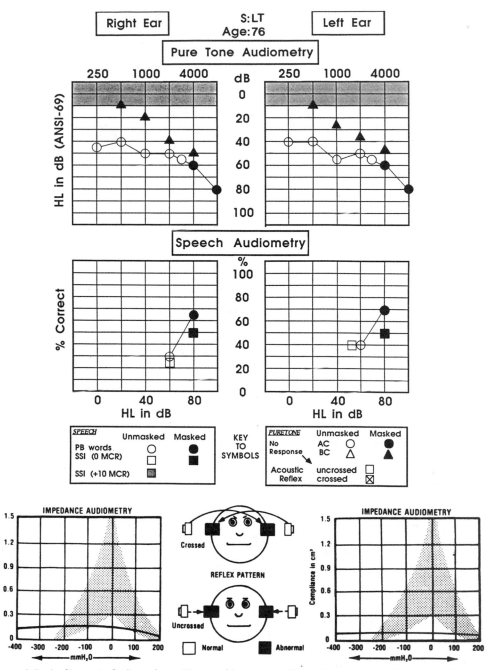

Figure 8-5. Audiometric findings for a 75-year-old woman with presbycusis in combination with impacted cerumen within external auditory canal (case 1).

176

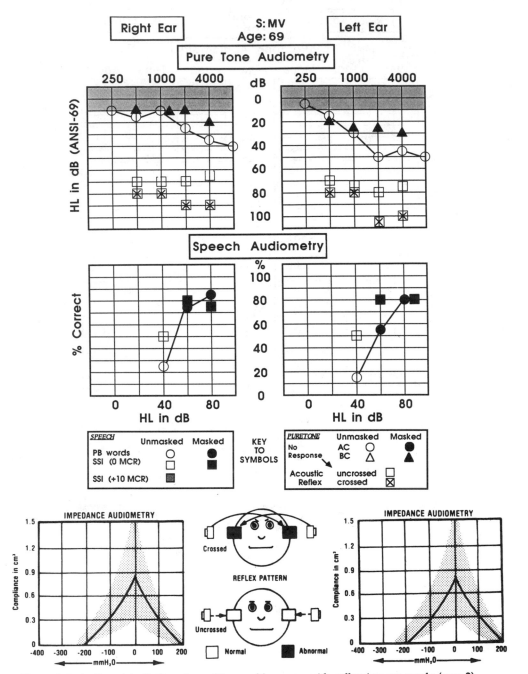

Figure 8-6. Audiometric findings for a 69-year-old woman with collapsing ear canals (case 2).

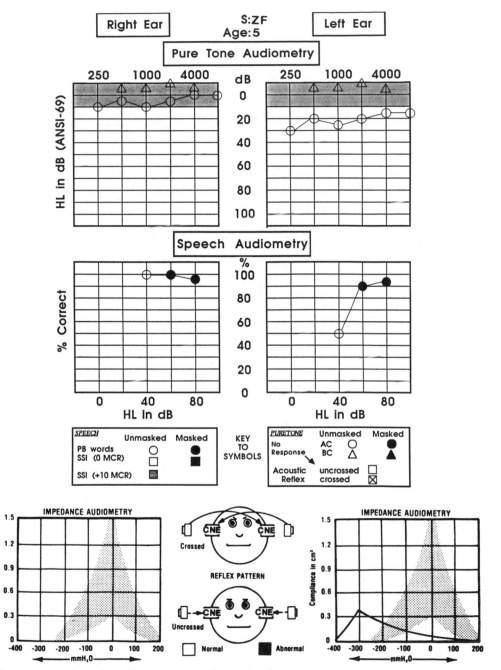

Figure 8-7. Audiometric findings for a 5-year-old boy with patent ventilation tubes (case 3).

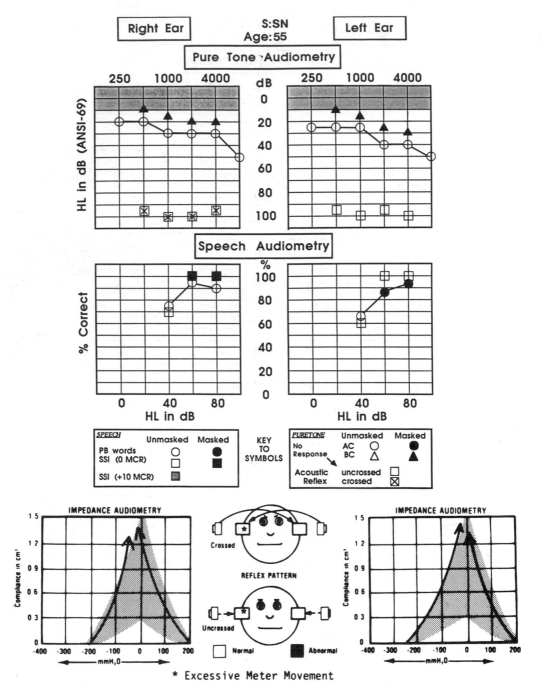

Figure 8-8. Audiometric findings for a 55-year-old woman with scarred tympanic membrane (case 4).

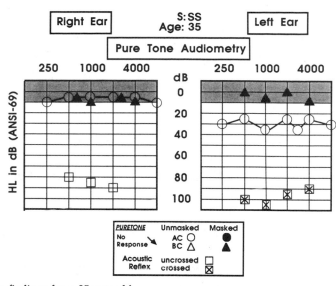

Figure 8-9. Audiometric findings for a 35-year-old woman with perforation of tympanic membrane (case 5).

was no air-bone gap. Selected Spanish word recognition (not standardized) and Spanish language SSI performance were excellent for higher-intensity levels but slightly reduced at conversational level (40 dB HL).

Highly compliant tympanograms suggest the possibility of ossicular chain discontinuity; however, in this case the history and pure tone audiometry are consistent with tympanic membrane dysfunction instead. The pattern of sensory impairment may have been related to presbycusis. Otoscopic examination revealed monomeric membranes and scarring of tympanic membranes bilaterally. The patient was not interested in evaluation for possible amplification at the time of the evaluation.

CASE 5: TYMPANIC MEMBRANE PERFORATION
A 35-year-old woman reported bleeding and slight difficulty hearing on the left ear after she was slapped in the ear during an altercation. Auditory function was normal on the right ear (Figure 8-9). Despite repeated efforts, a seal could not be maintained for tympanometry on the left ear, although an ear canal volume of greater than 2.5 cc was temporarily recorded before pressure was relieved spontaneously. Pure tone audiometry revealed a mild conductive hearing impairment. Acoustic reflexes were present with probe in the normal right ear, although the crossed reflexes were elevated by the degree of conductive component with stimulus left. Audiometric Weber lateralized to the left ear at 500 and 1000 Hz. Otologic examination of the left ear showed a large perforation in the posterior-superior portion of the tympanic membrane.

CASE 6: EUSTACHIAN TUBE DYSFUNCTION
The patient was a 3-year-old child with nasal congestion. Type C tympanograms were evident bilaterally when pressure was varied in a positive-to-negative direction (Figure 8-10). Note, however, that with a negative-to-positive change in ear canal pressure, there was a positive pressure shift in the tympanogram peak that altered interpretation according to the Jerger system. Acoustic reflexes were pres-

ent but at elevated stimulus intensity levels under all conditions (right and left ears, crossed and uncrossed). Hearing sensitivity was borderline normal in each ear. The child was referred for medical management of serous otitis media.

CASE 7: PURULENT OTITIS MEDIA
The patient was an 8-year-old child with a history of chronic ear infections and drainage from both ears, which were managed medically by his pediatrician. Parents and teachers noted reduced attention and poorer school performance. Immittance audiometry (Figure 8-11) showed ear canal volumes within normal limits and flat type B tympanograms bilaterally with absent acoustic reflexes. There was a moderate conductive hearing impairment by pure tone audiometry. SAL testing confirmed normal sensory function bilaterally. Word recognition was good at a high-intensity level but very poor (30–40%) at a quiet conversational level. Otologic management was strongly urged. The child's teachers were informed of the audiometric findings and the need for preferential classroom seating.

CASE 8: FACIAL (SEVENTH CRANIAL) NERVE PALSY
A 46-year-old male oil rig worker reported a recent onset of facial weakness on the left side. The diagnosis was Bell's palsy. He also acknowledged some difficulty in understanding conversational speech. Immittance measurement showed normal tympanometry. Acoustic reflexes, however, were not observed with probe in the left ear. With probe in the right ear, reflexes were at expected intensity levels. Pure tone audiometry (Figure 8-12) indicated a bilateral hearing deficit in the 3000 to 4000 Hz frequency region. There was no air-bone gap and the audiometric Weber was referred to midline. Maximum speech audiometry performance was excellent for words and SSI materials, but roll over was noted on the left ear.

This pattern of findings is consistent with facial nerve palsy on the left side involving the branch to the stapedius muscle. The vertical acoustic reflex pattern on the left is typical of a peripheral disorder, usually middle ear dysfunction. In this case, the normal tympanogram, midline Weber, lack of air-bone gap, and crossed acoustic reflexes at a reduced sensation level with sound left all argument con-

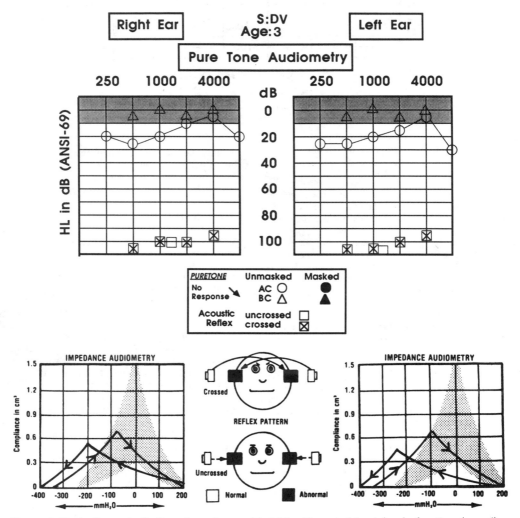

Figure 8-10. Audiometric findings for a 3-year-old child with eustachian tube dysfunction (case 6).

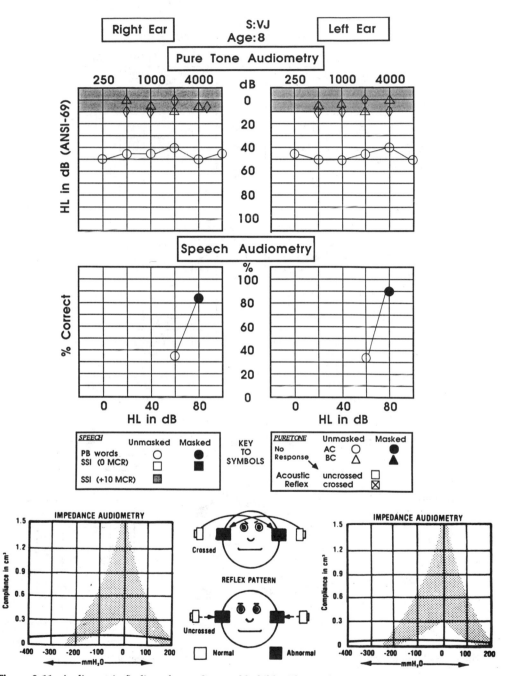

Figure 8-11. Audiometric findings for an 8-year-old child with purulent otitis media (case 7).

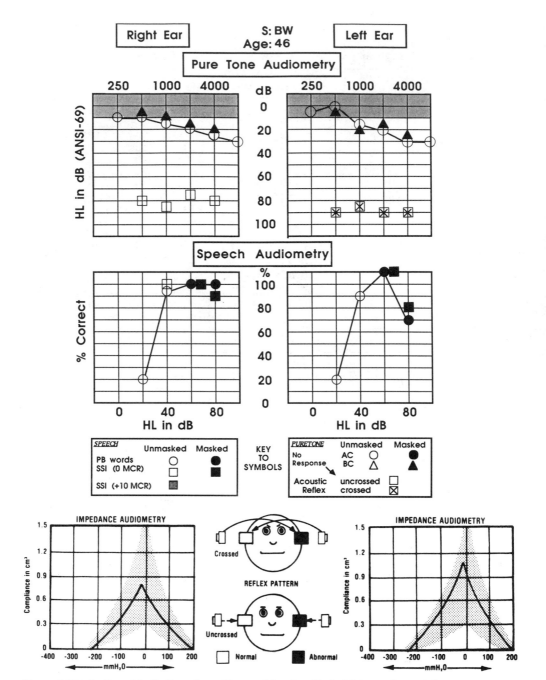

Figure 8-12. Audiometric findings for a 46-year-old male with facial (seventh cranial) nerve palsy (case 8).

vincingly for a seventh nerve etiology versus conductive hearing component. The patient's reported difficulty hearing the relatively high-pitch voices of his wife and children was a reflection of the high-frequency hearing loss. Roll over in speech understanding in ears with no acoustic stapedial reflex activity and normal middle ear function is sometimes found in facial nerve palsy (Hall, 1985).

CASE 9: DISCONTINUITY OF THE OSSICULAR CHAIN

A 26-year-old man was involved in an automobile accident that resulted in head trauma and bilateral hearing impairment. Audiometric findings are illustrated in Figure 8-13. Tympanograms were type A_d bilaterally, and acoustic reflex activity was not observed for maximum (110 dB HL) stimulus intensity levels. Pure tone audiometry showed a severe, slightly sloping, apparently conductive hearing impairment bilaterally. At these air conduction HTLs, there was a masking dilemma. Masking levels needed to overcome the air conduction impairment (greater than 70 dB HL) also exceeded interaural attenuation and could cross over to the test ear. SAL testing (refer back to data displayed in Figure 8-4) confirmed that the loss was entirely conductive bilaterally. Speech audiometry at a high-intensity level was necessarily unmasked, although insert earphones were used to reduce the likelihood of cross over (i.e., to increase interaural attenuation). Surgical otologic management was planned.

CASE 10: OTOSCLEROSIS

A 48-year-old woman reported a gradual, progressive hearing impairment bilaterally, which she first noticed during her college years. Her mother had experienced a similar decrease of hearing. Tympanograms were type A_s bilaterally (Figure 8-14). Acoustic reflexes were not present. Pure tone audiometry showed a primarily conductive hearing impairment bilaterally, with a notch for bone conduction thresholds at 2000 Hz. Speech audiometry performance was excellent at high-intensity levels. The audiometric Weber test produced a midline response. SAL test results generally confirmed the conductive component, but thresholds were better than for conventional bone conduction at 2000 Hz (Tillman, 1963). This case provides a classic illustration of otosclerosis producing stapes footplate fixation and a conductive component. Two other otosclerotic patterns of pure tone audiometry are essentially no air-bone gap (early otosclerosis) and a serious mixed or largely sensory impairment (partially or primarily cochlear focus for otosclerosis).

CASE 11: "CORNER AUDIOGRAM" WITH AIR-BONE GAP

A 3-year-old boy reportedly had normal hearing sensitivity until he contracted meningitis. Within the following month, he had experienced recurrent upper respiratory infections. Audiometric assessment (Figure 8-15) at 1 month after the onset of meningitis showed a "corner audiogram" configuration. There was an apparent air-bone gap for low-frequency stimuli (250 and 500 Hz), suggesting a conductive component to the hearing impairment. Immittance measurement, however, yielded normal tympanograms and evidence of acoustic reflex activity for low-frequency pure tone stimuli. Sensitivity prediction by acoustic reflex was consistent with a severe sensory hearing impairment bilaterally (Hall, 1987). The bone conduction audiometric responses were vibrotactile rather than auditory (Nober, 1964).

AUDIOLOGIC FINDINGS IN ATYPICAL CONDUCTIVE HEARING IMPAIRMENT

CASE 12: OTITIS MEDIA
DIAGNOSED BY SCHOOL NURSE

A 14-year old girl was referred to the audiology service by the school nurse with the diagnosis of right middle ear effusion and approximately 60 dB conductive hearing impairment. Audiometric findings are illustrated in Figure 8-16. Immittance audiometry immediately cast doubt on the suspicion of middle ear effusion. Tympanograms were normal (type A), and the diagonal acoustic reflex pattern was consistent with a severe sensory impairment on the right ear, rather than a conductive component. Hearing sensitivity was normal on the left. For the right ear, air and bone conduction audiometry confirmed the presence of a severe, high-frequency sensory hearing impairment (the patient's shadow curve is also indicated). Audiometric Weber was lateralized to the left ear. Word recognition performance on the right was nil, due to the high-frequency deficit, and the SSI score was 50 percent (reflecting the 60 dB loss at 750 Hz). Without using masking in pure tone testing, the school nurse inferred a conductive hearing impairment on the right ear. Our findings indicated a sensory deficit, and a subsequent ABR confirmed cochlear site of lesion. The patient deferred amplification.

CASE 13: COCHLEAR OTOSCLEROSIS
IN A POSTSTROKE PATIENT

A 64-year-old woman recovering from a stroke was referred for audiologic assessment by a physical medicine and rehabilitation specialist because she was experiencing difficulty understanding speech. Since the stroke, she experienced left-sided paresis of upper and lower extremities. She reported a long-standing hearing impairment for which she had taken fluoride 15 years previously in order to prevent further loss of hearing.

Audiometric findings are shown in Figure 8-17. Immittance audiometry (not shown) yielded shallow type A (A_s) tympanograms bilaterally. Acoustic reflexes were observed at abnormally elevated levels in each ear but were characterized by negative deflections (i.e., an increase versus decrease in compliance with stimulus presentation). There was a severe, flat, primarily sensory hearing loss on the right and a mild to moderate deficit on the left. Audiometric Weber lateralized to the ear with greater conductive component (right). Speech audiometry showed good word recognition but only fair performance for the SSI materials. Speech understanding was relatively poorer on the ear (left) with better hearing sensitivity.

This is an example of otosclerosis with a primarily cochlear focus (Paparella and Shumrick, 1980), although the negative deflection acoustic reflexes are evidence of stapes footplate involvement. Audiologic management was not straightforward. There was central auditory system involvement. Speech understanding was poorer for the ear with better auditory sensitivity (right), presumably because it was contralateral to the cerebral hemisphere involved in the stroke (left). The patient relocated to another city and was referred for amplification.

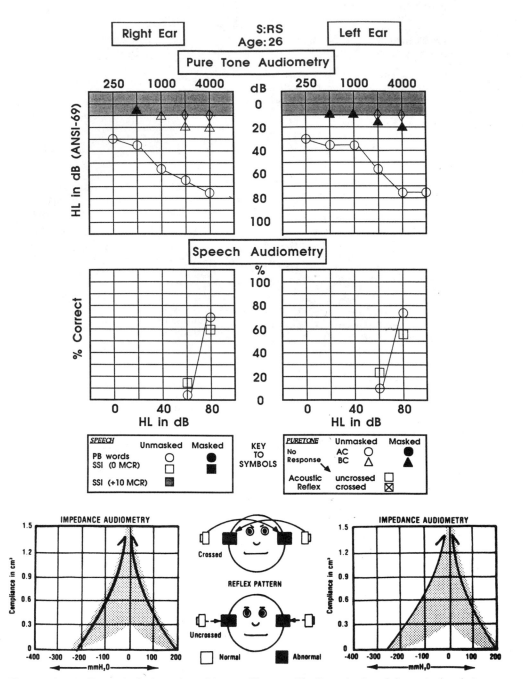

Figure 8-13. Audiometric findings for a 26-year-old man with discontinuity of the ossicular chain (case 9).

185

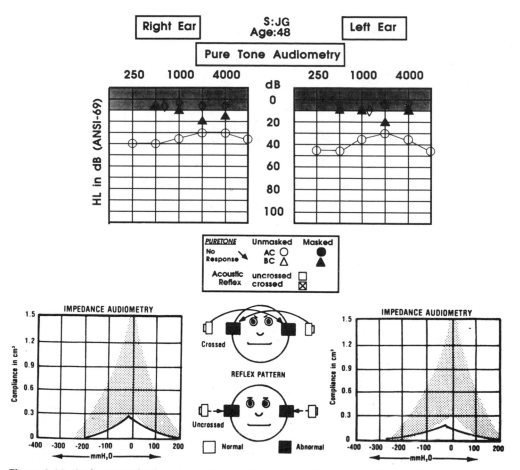

Figure 8-14. Audiometric findings for a 48-year-old woman with otosclerosis (case 10).

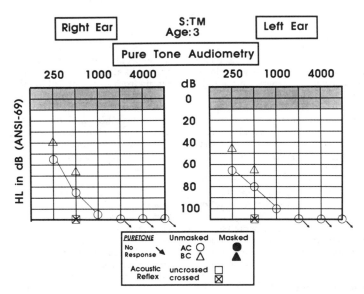

Figure 8-15. Audiometric findings for a 3-year-old boy with corner audiogram (case 11).

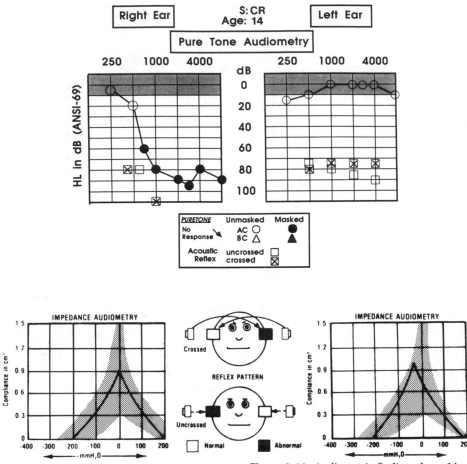

Figure 8-16. Audiometric findings for a 14-year-old girl with suspected middle ear effusion on the right ear (case 12).

CASE 14: POSTSTAPEDECTOMY CHANGES IN SENSORY STATUS

The patient was a 55-year-old woman employed by the local school district. Twenty years previously she had a right ear stapedectomy with a revision five years later. Since then, hearing has reportedly fluctuated in the right ear. She noted mild dizziness and unsteadiness, particularly when getting up from a sitting or supine position. Physical examination of the right ear showed evidence of the previous surgery (chorda tympani nerve adherent to the under surface of the tympanic membrane and curettage of the posterior bony ear canal wall). The left ear examination was normal. The patient underwent a left stapedectomy with oval window drill out, fracture of the crura, disarticulation of the incudostapedial joint, incision of the stapes tendon, and insertion of a platinum Teflon Fisch prosthesis.

Pre- and postoperative audiograms are presented in Figure 8-18. Before surgery, there was a severe, primarily conductive hearing impairment on the left ear and a mild high-frequency sensory loss on the right ear. Three weeks after surgery, audiometric assessment showed a high-frequency, apparently sensory deficit on the left. By 4 months post-operative, however, hearing was bilaterally symmetric.

As this case illustrates, poststapedectomy improvement in hearing loss does not necessarily occur within the initial weeks after surgery. The audiologist would be wise to refrain from any comment to the patient about postoperative changes in hearing until it is clear that hearing has stabilized. In addition, the dynamic interaction of the middle ear and cochlea and the possibility of surgery-related changes in cochlear function (e.g., fistulas, noise-induced damage) can produce temporary or permanent bone conduction deficits that may or may not reflect long-term sensory status.

CASE 15: SUSPECTED MALINGERER

A 9-year-old boy was referred from another audiologist because of inconsistent audiometric findings on two previous test sessions. Hearing sensitivity was described as normal on the left. For the right ear, however, one test showed normal hearing whereas the next showed inconsistent evidence of sensory hearing impairment (Figure 8-19). Immittance measurement was consistent with normal middle ear function on the left (type A tympanogram with uncrossed acoustic reflexes at expected intensity levels).

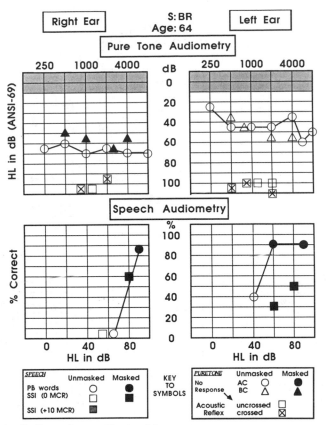

Figure 8-17. Audiometric findings for a 64-year-old poststroke patient with cochlear otosclerosis (case 13).

There was a type A_s tympanogram and no acoustic reflex activity with probe in the right ear, and no acoustic reflex activity for the contralateral mode with sound right. This pattern is consistent with at least a moderate conductive hearing impairment on the right.

Pure tone audiometry confirmed this expectation (Figure 8-19). Pure tone audiometry and speech threshold measures were in close agreement. SAL results were similar to bone conduction thresholds but slightly better at 2000 Hz. The audiometric Weber lateralized to the right ear at 500 and 1000 Hz. Speech audiometry performance was excellent by word recognition bilaterally but slightly depressed for SSI materials on the right ear because of the greater low-frequency hearing deficit.

On questioning, we determined that the first audiologist had done tympanometry but no reflex testing and concluded that the middle ear function was normal. On the first test, she had found normal masked right bone conduction thresholds and rejected the possibility of decreased air conduction thresholds. As the test session wore on, patient and tester became frustrated. The patient was asked to return and on this occasion provided inconsistent evidence of a possible sensory impairment. The mother became disenchanted with the test process and sought a second opinion. The patient was referred for otologic management of an apparent ossicular chain fixation following our audiometric assessment.

CASE 16: OSSICULAR DISCONTINUITY WITH FUNCTIONAL CONNECTON

A 30-year-old man noticed decreased hearing on the left after head trauma. Audiometric assessment (Figure 8-20) showed a normal tympanogram on the right and a type A_d tympanogram on the left ear. Acoustic reflexes were present in each test condition but consistently elevated in the contralateral mode with sound left (probe right) and not observed for several stimulus frequencies with the probe in each ear. Hearing sensitivity was essentially normal on the right ear. There was a moderate to severe sloping conductive hearing impairment on the left ear. Audiometric Weber was referred to the left.

Otologic diagnosis was ossicular chain discontinuity on the left, but with a functional connection along the chain. The audiometric pattern is consistent with discontinuity, except for the presence of acoustic reflexes with probe left. This case illustrates the importance of bone conduction pure tone assessment when any immittance aberration exists (e.g., A_d tympanogram or elevated acoustic reflex thresholds). Presumption of a sensory impairment on the right ear on the basis of an A-type tympanogram and the presence of acoustic reflexes, along with a sloping high-frequency configuration, would have led to a serious error in audiometric interpretation.

CASE 17: CONGENITAL AURAL ATRESIA BILATERALLY

The patient was a 6-year-old girl with congenital aural atresia. A resident of a Middle East country, she was in the

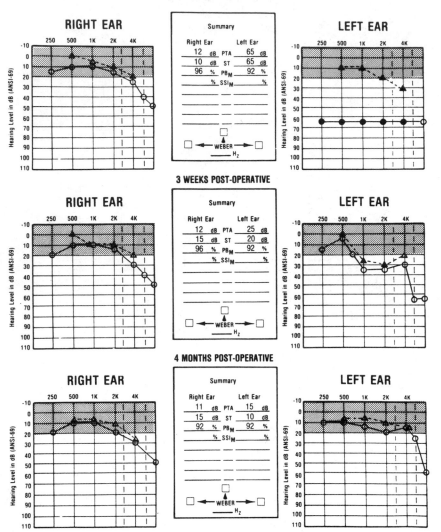

Figure 8-18. Serial pre- and poststapedectomy audiograms (case 14).

United States for evaluation and possible surgical repair of the otologic defect. Pure tone audiometry is illustrated in Figure 8-21. There was a moderate to severe, apparently bilateral and conductive sensitivity loss. The results of SAL audiometry suggested normal bone conduction thresholds in each ear. Unmasked word recognition performance with selected Arabic vocabulary presented by live voice was 100 percent at 90 dB HL but only 20 to 30 percent at 50 dB HL.

ABR assessment was carried out in the operating room under general anesthesia, immediately before high-resolution, thin-slice computed tomography of the temporal bone (Jahrsdoerfer and Hall, 1986). As shown in Figure 8-22, with air conduction stimulation at maximum intensity level (95 dB HL), there was a reliable ABR wave I and V component for the right and left ears with the vertex to

ipsilateral mastoid array. Simultaneous recording with a contralateral mastoid electrode pair, however, revealed no wave I component for either stimulus ear. An ABR wave V was observed for air conduction stimulation at intensity levels down to 75 dB on the right and 85 dB on the left. Bone conduction ABR waveforms for this patient are shown in Figure 8-23. Again, a clear and reliable wave I component was observed with the ipsilateral mastoid electrode array, but the contralateral array failed to yield a wave I. An ABR was recorded for bone conduction stimulation levels down to 10 dB on the right and 20 dB on the left.

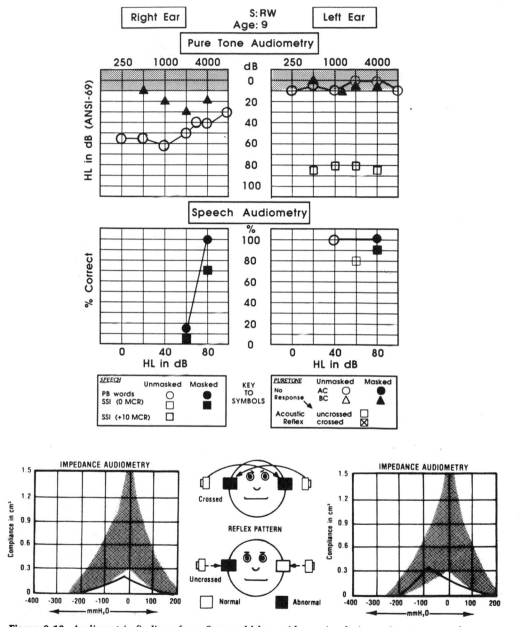

Figure 8-19. Audiometric findings for a 9-year-old boy with previously inconsistent test results classified as a malingerer (case 15).

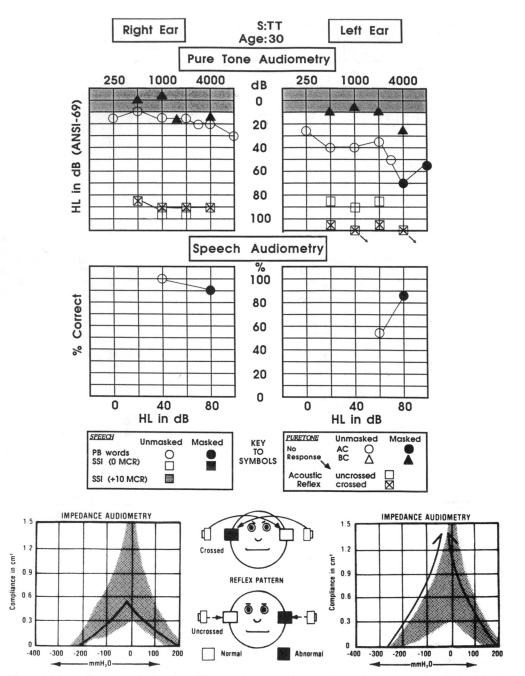

Figure 8-20. Audiometric findings for a 30-year-old man with ossicular chain discontinuity and functional connection (case 16).

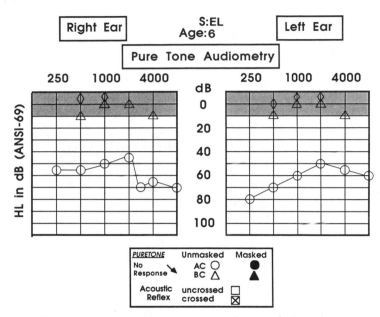

Figure 8-21. Preoperative pure tone audiometry findings for a 6-year-old girl with bilateral aural atresia (case 17).

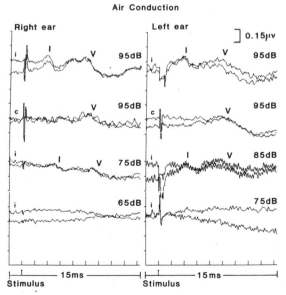

Figure 8-22. ABR waveforms for air conduction stimulation (case 17). Note presence of wave I component in ipsilateral but not contralateral electrode array.

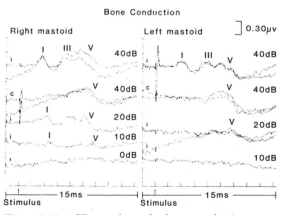

Figure 8-23. ABR waveforms for bone conduction stimulation (case 17). Note presence of wave I component in ipsilateral but not contralateral electrode array.

On the basis of these ABR results and computed tomography scanning, the otologist chose to operate on the right ear. That is, auditory sensitivity for air and bone conduction by ABR appeared to be better for the right than left ear; sensory sensitivity was within normal limits; and the computed tomographic scan showed less anatomic aberration for the right temporal bone. Postoperative pure tone average on the right ear at 3 months was 30 dB HL and speech awareness threshold was 15 dB HL.

CASE 18: SUSPECTED CONGENITAL CHOLESTEATOMA

A 7-year-old boy was referred to the audiology service by the child development center for evaluation of hearing with reported speech-language delay and academic difficulties in school. He had a 4- to 5-year history of otitis media. He had failed a hearing screening in the center. With immittance measurement (Figure 8-24), tympanograms were normal bilaterally, but the acoustic reflex pattern was consistent with middle ear dysfunction on the left ear. Pure tone audiometry showed normal hearing sensitivity on the right and a mild to moderate sloping mixed hearing loss on the left ear. Audiometric Weber at 1000 and 2000 Hz was lateralized to the poorer left ear. Word recognition was good on the right and excellent on the left ear. Otologic consultation was initiated.

Physical examination of the ears revealed retraction pocket enclosing debris. An attic cholesteatoma in the left middle ear was suspected and surgery was scheduled. Exploratory tympanotomy showed that the retraction pocket did not extend into the epitympanum. Adhesions found around the lenticular process of the incus were removed. Hearing sensitivity was normal on postoperative audiologic evaluation.

CASE 19: CHRONIC EAR

The patient was a 6-year-old boy with extensive history of middle ear pathology. Tympanostomy (ventilation) tubes were first placed bilaterally at 6 months of age. Six other sets of tubes were placed since then. At age 2 years, a mastoidectomy and tympanoplasty were peformed on the right side. The patient had been hospitalized 22 times for ear infections that resisted medical treatment. On audiologic assessment (Figure 8-25), each ear was free of tubes. Immittance measurement showed type B tympanograms and reflexes were not detected. There was a conductive component for frequencies through 4000 Hz. Hearing was best at 2000 Hz. Hearing sensitivity was decreased bilaterally above 4000 Hz. In the absence of bone conduction thresh-

Figure 8-24. Audiometric findings for a 7-year-old boy with congenital cholesteatoma (case 18).

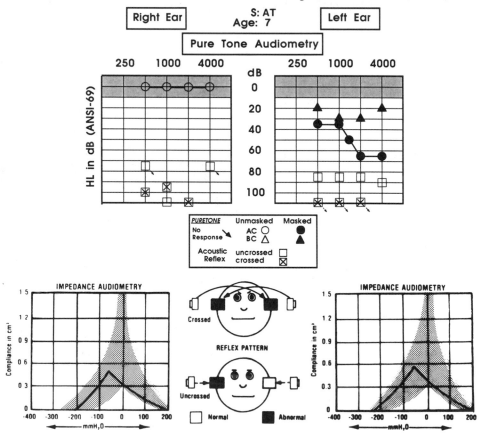

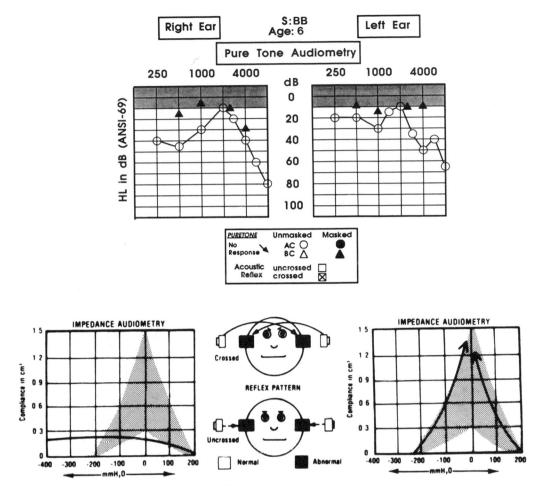

Figure 8-25. Audiometric findings for a 6-year-old boy with chronic middle ear disease (case 19).

olds, it was not clear whether it was conductive or sensory in nature.

Some investigators suggest that a mixed or sensory deficit at 4000 Hz or for higher frequencies may be a component of chronic otitis media (Dommerby and Tos, 1986); others theorize that bone conduction sensitivity is depressed by mechanical changes in middle ear functioning (Walby, Barrera, and Schuknecht, 1983). In any event, bone conduction thresholds may not always represent permanent sensory status. Furthermore, as this case illustrates, chronic otitis media may produce an unusual audiogram configuration.

AUDIOLOGIC MANAGEMENT OF PATIENTS WITH MIDDLE EAR PATHOLOGY

Patients with middle ear pathology constitute an important interface between audiologists and phy-

sicians, usually otolaryngologists or pediatricians. The audiologist may contribute to management of patients with middle ear pathology in four ways. The first is *detection of middle ear pathology* in patients entering the health care system through the audiologist, whether the setting is a school, a hearing center, a hearing aid dispensary, a nursing home, a hospital audiology clinic, or a newborn intensive care unit. Audiologists must have technical skills necessary for evaluating middle ear function and the clinical skills necessary for recognizing and describing varied types of middle ear pathology. *It is imperative that audiologists refer such patients for appropriate medical management before initiating audiologic management.* With most hearing-impaired patients with middle ear dysfunction, immediate audiologic management is at the very least inappropriate and, in many cases, contraindicated. Among them are patients with excessive cerumen, otitis media, tympanic membrane perforations and draining ears, and audiometric evidence of otosclerosis. These conditions are potentially medically and surgically treatable. The audiologist who fails to make a proper medical referral is not only doing the patient a disservice, but also risking medicolegal action and jeopardizing the credibility and reputation of audiologists in general as competent hearing health care professionals. Proper medical referral following detection of middle ear pathology should be viewed with the same seriousness as medical referral of patients with audiologic signs of retrocochlear pathology. Likewise, unexplained and, particularly progressive, sensory hearing loss warrant medical referral. Medical or surgical treatment, or both, may be effective for various etiologies causing sensory deficits (e.g., Ménière's disease or autoimmune pathology).

The second contribution is accurate *description of middle ear function* based on audiometric findings. Even the most complete and well-administered hearing evaluation is of little clinical value if findings are not promptly and accurately reported to the appropriate persons or acted on by the managing audiologist. Pure tone audiometry often permits classification of hearing impairments as conductive, sensory, or mixed. With the inclusion of immittance audiometry to the basic test battery, however, further and more precise description of auditory status is possible. Often, immittance measurements are carried out only to confirm the presence of middle ear dysfunction in patients with air-bone discrepancies by pure tone audiometry. This practice grossly underuses the diagnostic power of aural immittance. As indicated at the outset of this chapter, if the hearing evaluation begins with immittance measurement, it is usually possible to determine quickly and confidently whether hearing impairment has or does not have a conductive component. Bone conduction pure tone audiometry may not be necessary. If evidence of middle ear dysfunction by aural immittance exists, the pattern of tympanometry and acoustic reflex findings often leads to a precise description of the nature of the middle ear dysfunction and narrows down the possible underlying diseases. Then, suspicion of a conductive component by abnormal immittance is confirmed by careful comparison of air versus bone conduction pure tone audiometry.

A key factor in fully exploiting assessment of auditory status with this test battery approach is the precision with which results are described.

Unfortunately, precision is in fact discouraged with the somewhat more traditional approach for assessing audiologic status and reporting audiologic findings.

It is generally accepted that one cannot diagnose ear disease with audiometric findings. As noted in the beginning of this chapter, the results of a hearing evaluation may contribute, but the medical diagnosis is based also on the history, physical examination, and sometimes other information (e.g., laboratory or radiologic procedures). According to the traditional test report philosophy, therefore, the audiologist should carefully avoid any semblance of "making a diagnosis." Terminology used in reports is purposefully vague to accomplish this goal. Rather than endorsing this philosophy, the authors strongly submit that audiologists should take full advantage of the diagnostic power offered by certain procedures, such as immittance measurement, and report findings with as much precision and detail as possible. The principle that "a diagnosis is not made by audiologic tests" is not discarded with this more aggressive reporting style. Terminology and phrases are, in fact, specifically selected to avoid this inference.

Numerous examples of report writing "buzz words" and audiologic descriptors were provided among the case reports presented here. A brief review of audiologic data for an additional patient may serve to illustrate the unfortunate consequences of inadequate audiologic assessment and vague description of hearing status, followed by immediate audiologic management without proper medical referral. A self-referred young female adult was evaluated at a hearing center. She noted a gradual decrease in hearing over the previous 5 or 6 years. Pure tone audiometry showed a mild, flat hearing loss bilaterally. There was a slight air-bone gap in each ear, but the hearing loss was described as "sensorineural." Aural immittance was not done and there was no medical referral. The patient then underwent evaluation for hearing aid use and was fitted with amplification. She recently came to the first author's attention when she was referred for audiologic evaluation on a routine postoperative visit to an otolaryngologist following laryngeal surgery. The hearing impairment had progressed to the moderate to severe range. Immittance findings of type A tympanograms and absent acoustic reflexes, in combination with an air-bone gap and evidence of Carhart's notch, suggested otosclerosis. In contrast to the initial audiologic report, findings for the second evaluation were described directly. Unfortunately, without the potential benefit from medical/surgical intervention over the preceding unknown number of years, the patient's hearing sensitivity had decreased markedly. An otologic referral was made. Pending any medical treatment, a hearing aid reevaluation was essential.

The third contribution of audiologists in patients with middle ear pathology is *pre- versus postoperative evaluation* of hearing status. The audiologic evaluation unequivocally and rather dramatically affects medical management and communicative or medical outcome in several types of patients. Among these are newborn infants with hearing impairment and patients with retrocochlear pathology. In persons with middle ear pathology, audiometric findings often are the most important factor in determination of surgical candidacy. The implication here is quite clear. Inaccurate or incomplete audiometric data may potentially rule out surgery for a patient who could in fact benefit. This outcome would result, for example, from incorrectly describing poor bone conduction thresholds or failing to report any valid bone conduction thresholds because of technical limitations (e.g., masking dilemma). Perhaps worse, audiometry may lead to surgery for a patient with little or no chance for benefit, and furthermore put the patient at risk for total loss of hearing on the operated ear. This outcome, of course, results from overestimation of the air-bone gap and, particularly, the assumption of relatively good bone conduction sensitivity (often because of inadequate contralateral masking) in an ear with a significant sensory component. Clearly, the most important single factor in preoperative evaluation is accurate and valid description of air versus bone conduction thresholds. In cases posing masking problems, the audiologist is obligated to first use all procedures at his or her disposal to obtain accurate and complete air and bone conduction pure tone audiometry results and then to employ a conservative approach to interpreting these results.

In addition to this concern about preoperative test accuracy, the audiologist must be cautious in commenting on postoperative audiologic findings. Some clinical audiologists probably do not devote an appropriate amount of time to patient counseling. For many patients, hearing test results are not adequately explained, and little or no guidance on dealing with their hearing impairment is provided. For patients who have undergone middle ear surgery, however, less explanation of hearing status by the audiologist is often better. The potential for long-term postoperative improvement in bone conduction hearing was vividly illustrated above by case 14. Remarks on the audiologic effects of surgery are certainly premature until repeated postoperative tests have demonstrated stable hearing status. Even then, the audiologist is advised to leave detailed explanations of audiometric test findings to the surgeon who is in a position to interpret audiometric findings in the context of intraoperative and postoperative physical findings. As a general rule, the audiologist who anticipates working closely with otolaryngology colleagues is advised to initiate an open discussion on policies for audiologic management of mutual patients, including counseling of patients after hearing testing.

The fourth, and final, contribution of the audiologist is *management of patients* with middle ear pathology that is not amenable to medical or surgical management. Although such patients are traditionally considered good candidates for amplification, multiple factors add to the challenge of audiologic management, including audiogram configuration, a draining ear, and fluctuations in hearing sensitivity. The patient with a serious conductive component often requires a creative and flexible management approach.

ACKNOWLEDGMENTS

Susan M. Tompkins, M.Ed., Charlotte H. Prentice, M.S., Deborah S. Wilson, M.S., and Lisa Sells contributed to selection of cases.

REFERENCES

Arlinger, S., & Kylen, P. (1977). Bone-conducted stimulation in electrocochleography. *Acta Oto-laryngologica* (Stockholm), *84*, 377–384.

Bekesy, G. von (1960). *Experiments in hearing.* New York: McGraw-Hill.

Bluestone, C. D., Berry, Q. C., & Paradise, J. L. (1973). Audiometry and tympanometry in relation to middle ear effusions in children. *Laryngoscope, 83*, 594–604.

Burke, K. S., Creston, J. E., Marsh, A. J., & Shutts, R. E. (1964). Variability of threshold shift in SAL technique. *Archives of Otolaryngology, 80*, 155–159.

Carhart, R. (1950). Clinical application of bone conduction audiometry. *Archives of Otolaryngology, 51*, 798.

Chaiklin, J. B. (1967). Interaural attenuation and cross-hearing in air-conduction audiometry. *Journal of Auditory Research, 7*, 413–424.

Cooper, J. C., Jr., Hearne, E. M., III, & Gates, G. A. (1982).

Normal tympanometric shape. *Ear & Hearing, 3,* 241–245.

Cornacchia, L., Martini, A., & Morra, B. (1983). Air and bone conducted brainstem responses in adults and infants. *Audiology, 22,* 430–437.

Dirks, D., & Malmquist, C. (1964). Changes in bone-conduction thresholds produced by masking in the non-test ear. *Journal of Speech and Hearing Research, 7,* 271–278.

Dirks, D. D. (1964). Factors related to bone-conduction reliability. *Archives of Otolaryngology, 79,* 551–558.

Feldman, A. S. (1976). Tympanometry: Application and interpretation. *Annals of Otology, Rhinology and Laryngology,* (Suppl. 25) *85,* 202–208.

Finitzo-Hieber, T., Hecox, K., & Cone, B. (1979). Brainstem auditory evoked potentials in patients with congenital atresia. *Laryngoscope, 89,* 1151–1158.

Fria, T. J., & Sabo, D. L. (1980). Auditory brainstem responses in children with otitis media with effusion. *Annals of Otology, Rhinology and Laryngology, 68,* 200–206.

Goldstein, D. P., & Hayes, C. S. (1965). The occlusion effect in bone-conduction hearing. *Journal of Speech and Hearing Research, 8,* 137–148.

Goldstein, D. P., Hayes, C. S., & Peterson, J. L. (1962). A comparison of bone-conduction thresholds by conventional and Rainville methods. *Journal of Speech and Hearing Research, 5,* 244–255.

Hall, J. W., III. (1983). Diagnostic speech audiometry. *Seminars in Hearing, 4,* 179–204.

Hall, J. W., III. (1984). Auditory brainstem response audiometry. In J. F. Jerger (Ed.), *Hearing disorders in adults.* Boston: College-Hill Press.

Hall, J. W., III. (1985). The acoustic reflex in central auditory dysfunction. In M. L. Pinheiro & F. E. Musiek (Eds.), *Assessment of central auditory dysfunction: Foundations and clinical correlates.* Baltimore: Williams & Wilkins.

Hall, J. W., III. (1987). Contemporary tympanometry. *Seminars in Hearing, 8,* 319–327.

Hall, J. W., III. (1990). *Handbook of auditory evoked responses.* Boston: College-Hill Press.

Hall, J. W., III, Huangfu, M., Gennarelli, T. A., Dolinskas, C. A., Olson, K., & Berry, G. A. (1982). Auditory evoked response, impedance measures and diagnostic speech audiometry in severe head injury. *Otolaryngology — Head and Neck Surgery, 91,* 50–60.

Hall, J. W., III, Morgan, S. H., Mackey-Hargadine, J. R., Aguilar, E. A., III, & Jahrsdoerfer, R. A. (1984). Neuro-otologic applications of simultaneous multichannel auditory evoked response recordings. *Laryngoscope, 94,* 883–889.

Harder, H., Kylen, P., Arlinger, S., & Ekvall, L. (1980). Preoperative bone conducted electrocochleography in otosclerosis. *Archives of Otolaryngology, 106,* 757–762.

Harford, E. R., Bess, F. H., Bluestone, C. D., & Klein, J. O. (1978). *Impedance screening for middle ear disease in children.* New York: Grune & Stratton.

Hicks, G. (1980). Auditory brainstem response, sensory assessment by bone conduction masking. *Archives of Otolaryngology, 106,* 392–395.

Holte, L., & Margolis, R. H. (1987). Screening tympanometry. *Seminars in Hearing, 8,* 329–337.

Hood, J. D. (1960). Principles and practices of bone conduction audiometry. *Laryngoscope, 70,* 1211–1228.

Hooks, R., & Weber, B. (1984). Auditory brainstem responses to bone conduction stimuli in premature infants: A feasibility study. *Ear & Hearing, 5,* 42–46.

Huizing, E. H. (1950). Bone conduction, the influence of the middle ear. *Acta Oto-laryngologica, Suppl., 155.*

Humes, L., & Ochs, M. (1982). Use of contralateral masking in the measurement of the auditory brainstem response. *Journal of Speech and Hearing Research, 25,* 528–535.

Jahrsdoerfer, R. A., & Hall, J. W., III. (1986). Congenital malformation of the ear. *American Journal of Otology, 7,* 267–269.

Jahrsdoerfer, R. A., Yeakley, J. W., Hall, J. W., III, Robbins, K. T., & Gray, L. C. (1985). High resolution CT scanning and ABR in congenital aural atresia — patient selection and surgical correlation. *Otolaryngology—Head and Neck Surgery, 93,* 292–298.

Jerger, J., Anthony, L., Jerger, S., & Mauldin, L. (1974). Studies in impedance audiometry. III. Middle ear disorders. *Archives of Otolaryngology, 99,* 165–171.

Jerger, J., & Hayes, D. (1976). The cross-check principle in pediatric audiometry. *Archives of Otolaryngology, 102,* 614–620.

Jerger, J., Jerger, S., & Mauldin, L. (1972). Studies in impedance audiometry. I. Normal and sensori-neural ears. *Archives of Otolaryngology, 96,* 513–523.

Jerger, J., & Tillman, T. (1960). A new method for the clinical determination of sensori-neural acuity level (SAL). *Archives of Otolaryngology, 71,* 948–955.

Jerger, J., & Wertz, M. (1959). The indiscriminate use of masking in bone-conduction audiometry. *Archives of Otolaryngology, 70,* 419–420.

Jerger, J. F. (1970). Clinical experience with impedance audiometry. *Archives of Otolaryngology, 92,* 311–324.

Jerger, J. F., & Jerger, S. (1965). Critical evaluation of SAL audiometry. *Journal of Speech and Hearing Research, 8,* 103–128.

Johansen, H. (1948). Relation of audiograms to the impedance formula. *Acta Oto-laryngologica* (Stockholm), *Suppl. 74.*

Keys, J. W., & Milburn, B. (1961). The sensorineural acuity level (SAL) technique. *Archives of Otolaryngology, 73,* 710–716.

Lempert, J., Wever, E. G., & Lawrence, M. (1947). The cochleogram and its clinical application. *Archives of Otolaryngology, 45,* 61.

Martin, F. N., & Bailey, H. A. T., Jr. (1964). Clinical comment on the sensori-neural acuity level (SAL) test. *Journal of Speech and Hearing Disorders, 29,* 326–329.

Mauldin, L., & Jerger, J. (1979). Auditory brainstem evoked responses to bone conducted signals. *Archives of Otolaryngology, 105,* 656–661.

McGee, R. J., & Clemis, J. D. (1982). Effects of conductive hearing loss on auditory brainstem response. *Annals of Otology, Rhinology and Laryngology, 91,* 304–309.

Metz, O. (1946). The acoustic impedance measured on normal and pathological ears. *Acta Oto-laryngologica* (Stockholm), *Suppl. 63.*

Michael, L. A. (1963). The SAL test in the prediction of stapedectomy results. *Laryngoscope, 73,* 1370–1376.

Naunton, R. F. (1960). A masking dilemma in bilateral conduction deafness. *Archives of Otolaryngology, 72,* 753–757.

Nober, E. H. (1964). Pseudoauditory bone-conduction thresholds. *Journal of Speech and Hearing Disorders, 29,* 469–476.

Paparella, M. M., & Shumrick, D. A. (1980). *Otolaryngology* (2nd ed.). Philadelphia: Saunders.

Rainville, M. J. (1955). Nouvelle méthode d'assourdissement pour le releve des courbes de conduction osseuse. *Journal de Francais Oto-laryngologie, 4,* 851–858.

Reid, A., & Thornton, A. R. D. (1983). The effects of contralateral masking upon brainstem electric responses. *Brit-*

ish *Journal of Audiology, 17,* 155–162.

Rosenhamer, H. J., & Holmkvist, C. (1982). Bilaterally recorded auditory brainstem responses to monaural stimulation. *Scandinavian Audiology, 11,* 197–202.

Sanders, J. W., & Rintelmann, W. F. (1964). Masking in audiometry. *Archives of Otolaryngology, 80,* 541–556.

Shanks, J. E., & Wilson, R. H. (1986). Effects of direction and rate of ear-canal pressure changes on tympanometric measures. *Journal of Speech and Hearing Research, 29,* 11–19.

Stach, B. A., & Jerger, J. F. (1987). Acoustic-reflex patterns in peripheral and central auditory system disease. *Seminars in Hearing, 8,* 369–377.

Studebaker, C. F. (1962). On masking in bone conduction testing. *Journal of Speech and Hearing Research, 5,* 215–227.

Studebaker, F. A. (1967). Intertest variability and the air-bone gap. *Journal of Speech and Hearing Disorders, 32,* 82–86.

Terkildsen, K., & Osterhammel, P. (1981). The influence of reference electrode on recordings of the auditory brainstem response. *Ear & Hearing, 2,* 9–14.

Tillman, T. W. (1963). Clinical applicability of the SAL test. *Archives of Otolaryngology, 78,* 20–32.

Tonndorf, J. (1964). Animal experiments in bone conduction: Clinical conclusions. *Annals of Otology, Rhinology and Laryngology, 73,* 659–678.

VanCamp, K. J., Margolis, R. H., Wilson, R. H., Creten, W. L., & Shanks, J. E. (1986). *Principles of tympanometry.* Rockville, MD: ASHA Press.

Ventry, I. M., Chaiklin, J. B., & Boyle, W. F. (1961). Collapse of the ear canal during audiometry. *Archives of Otolaryngology, 73,* 727–731.

Webb, K. C., & Greenberg, H. J. (1983). Bone conduction masking for threshold assessment in auditory brainstem response testing. *Ear & Hearing, 4,* 261–266.

Weber, B. A. (1983). Masking and bone conduction testing in brainstem response audiometry. *Seminars in Hearing, 4,* 343–352.

Wilson, R. H., Shanks, J. E., & Kaplan, S. K. (1984). Tympanometric changes at 226 Hz and 678 Hz across ten trials and for two directions of ear-canal pressure change. *Journal of Speech and Hearing Research, 27,* 257–266.

Zwislocki, J. (1953). Acoustic attenuation between the ears. *Journal of the Acoustic Society of America, 25,* 752–759.

GLOSSARY

Acoustic (stapedial) reflex Reflexive contraction of the stapedius muscle elicited by an acoustic signal (pure tone or noise) of usually greater than 70 to 75 dB HL (Hall, 1985).

Anotia Congenital absence of external ear (auricle).

Atelectasis In otology, the collapse (retraction) of the tympanic membrane across the middle ear space and against the promontory (lateral wall of the inner ear).

Auricle Outer, visible portion of the ear (includes the pinna).

Battle's sign Bluish discoloration ("black and blue") behind ear (postauricular) in mastoid region, indicating temporal bone trauma.

Bing test Comparison of auditory function (e.g., audiometric hearing threshold or tuning fork response) with ear unoccluded versus occluded, usually for lower-frequency signals (e.g., 500 Hz). Enhanced hearing sensitivity in the occluded state is consistent with normal middle ear function. No occlusion effect is a sign of conductive impairment.

Carhart's notch Decrease in bone conduction hearing sensitivity at 2000 Hz in otosclerosis, named after describer audiologist Raymond Carhart. Carhart (1950) actually described typical bone conduction sensitivity reductions of 5 dB at 500 Hz, 10 dB at 1000 Hz, 15 dB at 2000 Hz, and 5 dB at 4000 Hz in this patient group.

Cerebrospinal fluid Clear liquid filling the ventricles of the brain and communicating with inner ear fluids via the cochlear aqueduct.

Cerumen Ear wax.

Cholesteatoma Secondary acquired cholesteatoma, occurring in infected ear or previously infected ears, is migration of squamous epithelium into the middle ear from the external meatus through a tympanic membrane perforation.

Ecchymosis Hemorrhagic (discharge of blood into) areas of the skin, producing a "black and blue" spot.

Edema Swelling of tissue due to fluid collection, often in response to injury.

Glomus tympanicum Tumor found in middle ear space consisting of blood vessels.

Granuloma Tumor of epitheloid cells.

Hematoma Collection of blood.

Hemotympanum Collection of blood behind eardrum in middle ear space, usually after head trauma.

Iatrogenic Disease or dysfunction inadvertently caused during management of a medical problem (e.g., laceration of ear canal walls during cleaning by a physician).

Interaural attenuation "Acoustic insulation" offered by the head. Signal intensity levels of 50 to 60 dB are required before pure tone signals presented via air conduction with conventional supra-aural earphone cushions cross over from the test ear to the non-test ear. Interaural attenuation for bone conduction signals is practically 0 dB (Chaiklin, 1967).

Masking Presentation of a sound, usually white noise or narrow-band noise, to the non-test ear to eliminate its participation in perception of a signal due to acoustic cross over (Sanders and

Rintelmann, 1964; Studebaker, 1967).

Masking dilemma Intensity level necessary to mask an ear when impaired hearing exceeds air conduction interaural attenuation (usually 40–50 dB) and masks the test ear (Naunton, 1960).

Mastoidectomy Surgical removal of contents of mastoid bone (within temporal bone just behind the ear) to irradicate infection.

Meatus External auditory canal opening or channel.

Microtia Abnormally small or malformed auricle (outer ear).

Necrosis Death of tissue or bone (with destruction).

Occlusion effect Improvement in bone conduction hearing when the ear is occluded. Effect is on the order of 15 to 25 dB for lower frequencies (250 and 500 Hz), 10 dB or less at 1000 Hz, and negligible above 1000 Hz (Goldstein and Hayes, 1965).

Osteoma Benign bony tumor (arising from the ear canal walls).

Otitis externa Infection or inflammation of the external ear.

Otitis media Inflammation of the middle ear (see *Serous otitis media* and *Purulent otitis media*).

Otosclerosis Bony disorder (otospongiosis) of otic capsule (bony labyrinth) producing conductive and sometimes cochlear hearing impairment.

Purulent otitis media Bacterial infection in middle ear space characterized by pain, fever, reddish tympanic membrane, and, with exudation, tympanic membrane bulging.

Schwartze's sign Dilated blood vessels (reddish appearance) on promontory in active otosclerosis.

Sensory acuity level (SAL) Test of bone conduction hearing in which the air-bone gap is determined by subtracting air conduction hearing thresholds for pure tone or speech signals recorded with no masking from those recorded with masking noise (approximately 50–60 dB HL) presented to the forehead via bone conduction (Jerger and Jerger, 1965).

Serous otitis media Acute nonsuppurative otitis media characterized by sudden appearance of nonpurulent effusion (fluid) in the middle ear.

Sign Results of tests that are used in differential diagnosis (e.g., an air-bone gap in pure tone audiometry).

Suppurative otitis media Follows spontaneous rupture of tympanic membrane (after purulent otitis media). Small perforation of tympanic membrane is observed in pars tensa portion.

Symptom Patient complaint or description of a physical problem that is used in differential diagnosis (e.g., tinnitus).

Tinnitus Spontaneously occurring sensation of sounds (e.g., ringing, buzzing, clicking) that sometimes is localized to one or both ears.

Toynbee test (maneuver) Patient swallows with nostrils occluded (e.g., pinched). With the expected effect, negative pressure in the nasopharynx is transmitted via the eustachian tube to the middle ear space. This effect is observed otoscopically as tympanic membrane retraction or tympanometrically as negative pressure compliance peak.

Tympanic membrane Ear drum.

Tympanogram Measure of middle ear mobility (e.g., compliance or admittance) as a function of changes in air pressure in the ear canal.

Valsalva test (maneuver) Patient attempts to inflate middle ear space by blowing air against occluded nostrils and closed mouth. The expected effect on tympanic membrane (outward movement) and middle ear pressure (increase) can be observed otoscopically or recorded with tympanometry.

Ventilation tube, P.E. tube, or grommet Pressure-equalization device inserted in tympanic membrane.

Weber's test Audiometric or tuning fork procedure in which the patient lateralizes a pure tone signal (low frequency) presented via bone conduction to the forehead.

CHAPTER 9

Evaluation and Diagnosis of Cochlear Disorders

Roger A. Ruth • *Paul R. Lambert*

Hearing loss can occur as a result of many different physiologic and nonphysiologic factors. The prevalence of hearing loss, by recent estimates, is approximately 13 percent. In the United States alone there are currently over 30 million hearing-impaired individuals (Goldstein, 1984). The vast majority of these hearing losses are permanent, and of these most result from disorders of the cochlea or inner ear.

Paradoxically, most of the audiologic test procedures currently in use are designed to detect the presence of hearing loss, evaluate the conductive apparatus, or rule out the retrocochlear auditory pathways as a source of the problem. Only a few tests are devoted specifically to the examination or diagnosis of cochlear disorders. The dearth of audiologic tests designed to evaluate inner ear function results in part from the fact that the cochlea is one of the most complicated mechanical systems in the human body, with an estimated 1 million–plus moving parts. Furthermore, its location deep within the temporal bone precludes direct observation in humans. Given the complexity of the cochlea and its susceptibility to internal and external insult, it is not surprising that the majority of hearing disorders result from dysfunction of the inner ear. In spite of numerous research investigations, knowledge of the normal and abnormal function of the inner ear is relatively meager. For example, only recently have the probable function and purpose of the inner and outer hair cells begun to be understood. The auditory disorders resulting from their malfunction are less understood.

It is beyond the scope of this chapter to provide a detailed discussion of the anatomy and physiology of the cochlea. Two excellent reviews regarding the manner in which the inner ear transduces and processes sound information are highly recommended (Dallos, 1988; Lippe, 1986).

This chapter is intended to provide the reader with some insight into the various diagnostic strategies typically employed in the evaluation of sensory hearing loss (SHL). As such, issues related to the identification of a hearing disorder will not be addressed. Rather the assumption is made that hearing loss is already known to exist. Furthermore, relatively little attention is devoted to the process of ruling out a conductive and retrocochlear site of lesion in terms of their contribution to the overall hearing disorder. Thorough discussions of conductive and retrocochlear problems are dealt with elsewhere in this volume (Chapters 8 and 10).

This chapter will focus on the audiologic evaluation of cochlear disorder but will approach the discussion within the larger framework of the general evaluation of the patient with hearing loss. The contribution of audiologic assessment to the overall evaluation of SHL is, in most cases, of paramount importance; however, once conductive and retrocochlear site of lesion have been ruled out, the relative contribution of the audiologic test battery is less clear.

The chapter begins with a discussion of the clinical otologic examination and the components of the audiologic test battery designed to assist in the evaluation and differentiation of cochlear disorders. In order to introduce the reader to the process of clinical decision making, a discussion is provided of the approach to differential diagnosis of various cochlear pathologies as a function of unilateral or bilateral presenting symptoms. Finally, case studies are presented to illustrate the logical combination of various test measures.

CLINICAL EXAMINATION OF COCHLEAR HEARING LOSS

HISTORY

The evaluation of the patient with a unilateral or bilateral hearing loss begins with a history, which serves to characterize the loss in terms of its onset, duration, course, and associated symptoms. Pertinent family history and past medical history are also included in this part of the evaluation. In many instances, the information gained from the history alone will enable the examiner to narrow the diagnostic possibilities to just a few entities.

The approximate date of onset (and thus duration) of the hearing loss together with any special circumstances or activities occurring near the time of onset are initially defined. For example, was the hearing loss congenital or adult onset, and did it occur gradually or suddenly? If the onset was sudden, was it associated with straining or pressure change (e.g., barotrauma), head trauma (e.g., temporal bone fracture), illness (e.g., otitis media, meningitis), ototoxic medications (e.g., aspirin, aminoglycosides), or noise trauma? The discovery that the hearing loss was congenital or occurred within the first few years of life would raise an additional set of questions concerning prenatal or perinatal factors such as maternal illness or drug ingestion during pregnancy, birth weight, APGAR scores, or postnatal jaundice.

The course of the hearing loss after onset and its impact on the patient's life must be addressed next. Has the loss been stable or has it progressed or fluctuated over time? If the loss occurred at an early age, what effects has it had on speech, education, and social development? For the adult-onset hearing loss, what have been the consequences of the loss on speech recognition and job performance? Previous audiograms, if available, are invaluable in corroborating the patient's perception of hearing change over time.

Otologic or neurologic symptoms associated with the hearing loss, such as tinnitus, dizziness, otalgia, otorrhea, visual changes, or paresthesias, are important to elicit. Concomitant organ system disease, such as hypertension, diabetes mellitus, atherosclerotic cardiovascular disease, thyroid disease, or renal disease, may be causally related to the hearing loss and should be noted. Prior ear disease or otologic surgery is an obviously important factor that needs to be clearly defined. The history is concluded with questioning about hearing loss in the patient's immediate family and other relatives.

PHYSICAL EXAMINATION

A head and neck examination with particular attention to the ears, eyes, craniofacial development, and cranial nerves is essential in all patients with a hearing loss. When indicated, a more complete neurologic and general examination can be performed.

Although most patients with a hearing loss will have a normal examination, a number of syndromes with associated hearing loss have characteristic physical stigmata. The position and shape of the pinnae and the development of the maxilla and mandible should be noted (e.g., Crouzon's syndrome and Treacher Collins syndrome). Several features of the eye are important to note, including the intercanthal distance (increased in Waardenburg's syndrome), the sclera (blue color in osteogenesis imperfecta), the iris (heterochromia in Waardenburg's syndrome), the cornea (opacities in syphilis and Cogan's syndrome), and the retina (pigmented in Usher's syndrome). The neck should be palpated for a goiter (Pendred's syndrome). The neurologic examination should focus on cranial nerves V and VII and the cerebellum (e.g., tandem gait, Romberg test, finger-to-nose test) since tumors of the cerebellopontine angle and petrous apex frequently affect these structures.

The ear is closely inspected with a pneumatic otoscope (or operating microscope) for evidence of congenital abnormality (e.g., stenosis or atresia of the external canal), infection (e.g., herpetic vesicles of the concha or canal, otorrhea, perforated tympanic membrane, or tympanosclerosis), trauma, or active disease (e.g., cholesteatoma, middle ear effusion, or tumor). Tuning fork tests (Rinne and Weber's) can provide qualitative information regarding the hearing loss and help differentiate conductive from sensory pathology. Examination of the hard and soft palate (e.g., submucous or actual cleft) and the eustachian tube orifices in the nasopharynx completes the ear examination.

RADIOGRAPHIC EVALUATION

The advent of high-resolution computed tomography (CT) and, now, the magnetic resonance imaging (MRI) scan has refined the ability to diagnose even very small tumors of the internal auditory canal and cerebellopontine angle. The differentiation of cochlear lesions by radiographic techniques, however, is limited. The CT scan provides excellent definition of bony details, and this is helpful in diagnosing certain developmental abnormalities of the cochlea, such as Mondini's malformation; however, the CT (or MRI) scan cannot detect the more common Scheibe's malformation, which affects the membranous, not bony, portions of the labyrinth. Nevertheless, CT scanning is useful in the evaluation of many children with SHL. CT scanning can also help define infectious processes involving the middle ear and adjacent labyrinth and traumatic injuries to the ear and skull base as observed in closed head injuries.

The MRI scan uses a large superconducting magnet to create a magnetic field around the patient and affect the alignment of nuclei. In response to a radio frequency signal, these nuclei give off energy that can be processed into an image by a computer. Thus radiation is not involved. Another advantage of the MRI is that it can "see" or image structures (or tumors) within the internal auditory canal. Very small acoustic neuromas, which may have been missed by a CT scan, can be readily detected.

These new scanning techniques have largely supplanted plain x-rays (exceptions include use of plain skull films to examine for Paget's disease or eosinophilic granuloma) and, in almost all cases, tomograms of the temporal bone. In addition to CT and MRI, angiography is often necessary to define a vascular lesion involving the temporal bone or to delineate normal vascular structures contiguous with a tumor or infectious process.

LABORATORY STUDIES

Depending on how diagnostic the history and physical exam have been, laboratory studies are ordered to confirm a suspected disease process or, more commonly, to rule out a number of potential diseases when the diagnosis remains uncertain. Unfortunately, the diagnosis of only a small percentage of cochlear disorders can be investigated with peripheral blood studies. These disorders include syphilis, viral diseases (e.g., toxoplasmosis, rubella, herpes, and cytomegalic viral titers), autoimmune inner ear disease (e.g., sedimentation rate, antinuclear antibody, quantitative immunoglobulins), metabolic diseases (e.g., lipids, glucose, thyroid function tests), and Alport's syndrome (e.g., renal function tests). Blood studies are typically not helpful in the diagnosis of

Ménière's disease, noise trauma, inner ear fistula, developmental disorders, or ototoxicity (except in acute cases by measuring serum drug levels).

GENETIC WORK-UP

Genetic hearing loss is estimated to occur in as many as 0.1 percent of school-aged children and accounts for one-third to one-half of all cases of childhood deafness (Konigsmark and Gorlin, 1976). Genetic factors are also important in a significant percentage of adult-onset hearing loss. Thus, during the history the examiner should inquire about consanguinity and the presence of hearing loss in relatives. Since many children with hereditary hearing loss will have associated abnormalities (e.g., a syndrome), particular attention should be focused on physical characteristics and other organ system development. The expertise of a geneticist can be helpful in this regard and also in obtaining complete pedigrees. Audiometric testing of immediate family members and relatives may be necessary to confirm the family history data. It should be noted, however, that most childhood genetic hearing loss is autosomal recessive, and even in those cases of dominant inheritance, incomplete penetrance or expression of the trait can confound the genetic work-up.

AUDIOLOGIC EVALUATION

The audiologic portion of the clinical exam comprises a number of different tests. These individual tests are generally applied together in some grouping referred to as a *battery*. A brief description of the currently available audiologic procedures for use in assessing cochlear disorders follows:

Audiogram

The pure tone audiogram is the basic unit of virtually all hearing assessment strategies. The three primary components of the threshold audiogram available for assessment are degree of loss, slope of the configuration, and symmetry between ears. Different patterns of these audiometric characteristics will often assist in the diagnosis and prognosis of cochlear hearing loss. For instance, certain types of sensory pathology are more likely to result in unilateral deficits (e.g., Ménière's disease) whereas others generally result in bilateral symptoms (e.g., noise-induced hearing loss).

Speech Testing

A fundamental part of the core evaluation is tests involving the use of speech material as the auditory stimulus. The simplest of these measures is the speech recognition threshold, which uses two-syllable spondee words. It serves mainly as a cross check to mid-frequency pure tone threshold. Speech recognition tests that employ phonemically balanced monosyllabic words permit a rough estimate of the intelligibility of a linguistic auditory signal. Such measures are very helpful in the suprathreshold evaluation of sensory hearing disorder. Speech recognition testing can be enhanced by evaluating the intelligibility of the speech material as a function of stimulus intensity, from moderate to very high presentation levels. This latter form of speech recognition measure was first introduced by Jerger and Jerger (1971) and is commonly referred to as the *performance-intensity for phonemically balanced words function*. This test, also referred to as the *roll-over measure*, is a very effective screening tool for retrocochlear pathology. Unfortunately, its value in differentiating among various types of sensory disorder is limited.

Other forms of audiologic tests using speech material are helpful in assessing the functional integrity or capacity of the entire auditory system and the potential for benefit from some form of amplification. The synthetic speech identification test makes use of nonmeaningful sentences to determine recognition of speech material when some of the contextual cues have been minimized (Jerger, Speaks, and Trammell, 1968); however, these tests have been found to be of little value in the actual diagnosis of cochlear pathology.

Acoustic Immittance

The acoustic immittance battery contains two primary categories of tests: tympanometry and acoustic stapedial reflex. Of these, the acoustic reflex has greatest application to the assessment of sensory impairment. In addition to being a sensitive screening device for retrocochlear disorder, the acoustic reflex can provide information helpful in determining the status of the sensory portion of the hearing mechanism. For example, disorders affecting primarily the cochlea give rise to acoustic reflex threshold levels that are similar to the thresholds obtained from normal hearers. This is generally thought to be a result of the same mechanism that is responsible for the abnormally

rapid rate of loudness growth (referred to as *recruitment*) often detected in ears with cochlear impairment. Metz (1952) was the first to observe this relationship. According to his findings, the presence of an acoustic reflex at a sensation level of 60 dB or less is a positive indicator of a recruiting ear and therefore cochlear pathology.

In addition to the acoustic reflex threshold, there have also been indications that other aspects of this measure have clinical value, such as latency (Clemis and Sarno, 1980; Mangham, Lindeman, and Dawson, 1980), amplitude (Hayes and Jerger, 1982), decay (Anderson, Barr, and Wedenberg, 1970; Greisen, and Rasmussen, 1970; Olsen, Noffsinger, and Kurdziel, 1975), and ipsilateral versus contralateral response patterns (Jerger and Jerger, 1977). Although these measures may be extremely valuable in various clinical applications, such as the identification of auditory nerve and brainstem pathology, the estimation of hearing threshold levels (Jerger et al., 1974), and the evaluation of facial nerve dysfunction (Ruth, Nilo, and Mravec, 1978), by and large, they add little to our ability to differentiate from among various inner ear disorders.

Auditory Evoked Potentials

The newest major addition to the audiologic test battery involves the measurement of auditory evoked potentials. The two most frequently used auditory evoked potential tests for the evaluation of SHL are the auditory brainstem response (ABR) and electrocochleography (ECochG). The ABR is doubtless the most effective auditory screening tool in the detection of retrocochlear pathology available to the otologist and audiologist; however, the ABR provides little information that may be useful in the differential diagnosis of cochlear impairment (Hyde, 1985). On the other hand, *ECochG*, defined as a method of recording the stimulus-related electrical potentials associated with the inner ear and auditory nerve, including the cochlear microphonic, summating potential (SP), and the compound action potential (AP) of the auditory nerve (Ruth, Lambert, and Ferraro, 1988), may be of significant benefit in the differential diagnosis of certain types of sensory disorder, such as Ménière's disease or cochlear hydrops. The amplitude of the SP and AP of the auditory nerve is the measure of primary interest when evaluating an ear for possible increased endolymphatic pressure (e.g., Ménière's disease).

Vestibular Measures

Given that the vestibular system shares a common fluid chamber and cranial nerve with the hearing mechanism, it is not surprising that disorders of hearing often coexist with vestibular impairment. As with hearing loss, balance disorders may result from disturbances of the vestibular end organ proper or the more central neural pathways of the vestibular system. The basic component of the vestibular test battery is electronystagmography (ENG), which involves the measurement of spontaneous eye movement or eye movements induced by various manipulations of the peripheral vestibular system. More sophisticated methods of assessing the vestibular system include rotary and posturography testing. For a detailed account of balance disorders, see Chapter 13.

Promontory Electrical Stimulation

Promontory electrical stimulation of the cochlea is a special form of audiologic testing to determine the electrical stimulability of the peripheral auditory system in patients with profound hearing impairment. As such, an electrical instead of acoustic stimulus is delivered to the ear. This electrical signal is meant to simulate, to a first approximation, the manner of stimulation that results from an actual cochlear implant. The test is typically performed by observing a subject's behavioral responses to various levels and frequencies of electrical pulse stimulation. Evoked potentials can also be obtained in response to this electrical stimulation (Kileny and Kemink, 1987).

Promontory testing is generally accomplished by placing a needle electrode through the tympanic membrane to the promontory wall of the middle ear. In some cases it is necessary to use a small ball electrode placed directly on the round window. The round window electrode is more invasive (i.e., must lift tympanic membrane for sufficient exposure), but it generally results in somewhat more effective stimulation to the neural elements deep within the inner ear. Promontory electrical testing is intended to provide information regarding the viability of these remaining neural elements in order to more accurately predict which profoundly hearing-impaired ears may likely benefit from a cochlear implant (Lambert, Ruth, and Hodges, 1987).

CLINICAL PRESENTATION

On the basis of the pure tone audiogram, patients with SHL can be classified into the following categories: unilateral SHL, bilateral symmetric SHL, bilateral asymmetric SHL, and mixed conductive and SHL. In addition to being descriptive, these categories are important in helping to formulate a differential diagnosis, which, in turn, is important in directing further test strategy.

Although the etiology of the hearing loss cannot be ascertained with certainty from the audiogram, its configuration can suggest certain disease processes. For example, Ménière's disease most commonly produces a flat or rising sloping loss (this diagnosis is further strengthened by the observation of a fluctuating bone line measured on sequential audiograms); chronic noise exposure characteristically affects those frequencies above 1000 Hz and often produces the greatest loss (a "notch") at around 4000 to 6000 Hz; presbycusis typically causes a down-sloping loss; a recessive genetic hearing loss is usually associated with a down-sloping loss, whereas most adult-onset hereditary hearing loss, which is dominantly inherited, typically produces a flat or basin-shaped audiogram (Konigsmark and Gorlin, 1976; Paparella et al., 1975).

Occasionally, the pure tone audiogram will provide prognostic information. For example, the patient with a sudden idiopathic rising sloping pattern is more predictive of recovery than a down-sloping configuration (Mattox and Simmons, 1977). Obviously, the degree of additional loss at interval audiometric testing can be extrapolated and used to broadly predict prognosis. For example, documentation of several episodes of repeated fluctuating hearing thresholds in patients with Ménière's disease would likely give rise to a somewhat poorer prognosis (Eggermont and Schmidt, 1985).

SPECIFIC AUDIOMETRIC PATTERNS

Unilateral or Bilateral Asymmetric SHL

For the patient with unilateral SHL or a bilateral asymmetric SHL, the principal role of the audiologic evaluation is to rule out a retrocochlear lesion. In this regard, various audiologic tests serve a valuable purpose; however, it is generally believed that no one audiologic test is sufficiently effective to stand alone as a screening tool for a retrocochlear disorder. As such, several different tests are generally used in a battery in order to strengthen their overall predictive accuracy (Jerger, and Jerger, 1983). Turner and colleagues (Turner and Nielson, 1984; Turner, Frazier, and Shepard, 1984; Turner, Shepard, and Frazier, 1984) have recently summarized methods by which audiologic tests may be evaluated in terms of their sensitivity and specificity for a particular disorder in relation to the prevalence of the disease in question. In their presentations, these authors criticize the widely held belief that a test battery is better merely because it contains a larger number of different tests. Schwartz (1987) also questions the relative power and actual benefit of what often amounts to cumbersome test batteries proposed by various investigators in the field. Clearly, the sensitivity of an individual test measure to a particular disorder must be considered along with the time efficiency of the test in order to justify its inclusion in the clinical examination. A summary of predictive test strategy is found in Chapter 14.

Over the past 30 years, a great deal of attention has been paid to the development of tests designed to differentiate cochlear from retrocochlear site of lesion (Miller, 1985). Most of these audiologic tests were based either on the detection of recruitment (abnormally rapid rate of loudness growth) or excessive adaptation in the perception of an auditory signal. Table 9-1 lists the various psychophysical tests typically employed in the conventional cochlear versus retrocochlear battery. By and large, these procedures have given way to more efficient tests, both in terms of overall accuracy and time.

The authors' approach to the current neurodiagnostic audiologic test battery is summarized in

TABLE 9-1. CONVENTIONAL NEUROAUDIOLOGIC TEST BATTERIES BASED ON RECRUITMENT OR ADAPTATION

Recruitment

    Alternate Binaural Loudness Balance (ABLB)
      (Fowler, 1937)

    Short-Increment Sensitivity Index (SISI)
      (Jerger, Shedd, and Harford, 1959)

    Difference Limen Intensity (DLI)
      (Luscher and Zwislocki, 1949)

Adaptation

    Tone Decay Test (TDT)
      (Carhart, 1957; Hood, 1956)

    Suprathreshold Adaptation Test (STAT)
      (Jerger and Jerger, 1975)

    Bekesy (Jerger, 1960)

    Bekesy Comfortable Loudness (BCL)
      (Jerger and Jerger, 1974)

Table 9-2. Note that a two-tiered screening protocol is advocated. The first level comprises speech recognition and acoustic reflex measures that are essentially part of our comprehensive audiologic evaluation. The second level of screening is proceeded to if the preponderance of evidence from the first level screening and case history suggests a retrocochlear disorder. The virtues of ABR are discussed elsewhere (Chapter 7), but suffice it to say that ABR is clearly the most powerful tool currently available to the audiologist for differentiating cochlear from retrocochlear pathology in unilateral or bilateral asymmetric SHL. A positive ABR should be followed by a CT or MRI scan. If the ABR is unobtainable because of the severity of the hearing loss, or if it is negative yet clinical suspicion for retrocochlear lesion is high, a CT or MRI scan is necessary. As indicated in the section on radiographic evaluation, the MRI, because of its ability to image very small acoustic tumors within the internal auditory canal, is the more powerful diagnostic tool, and is the radiographic procedure of choice.

A flow diagram of a typical diagnostic strategy applied to unilateral or bilateral asymmetric SHL is illustrated in Figure 9-1. If the work-up suggests a cochlear rather than retrocochlear site of lesion, attention must be paid to differentiating among various sensory disorders. As previously indicated, few audiologic procedures contribute to the differential diagnosis of cochlear disorders. Ménière's disease is an excellent example. A hallmark of Ménière's disease is its variable expression from one patient to the next or even in the same patient over time. The array of terms applied to this disorder such as *Ménière's-like syndrome, vestibular hydrops,* and *cochlear hydrops* reflect this diagnostic uncertainty. Unfortunately, an objective test with excellent sensitivity and specificity for Ménière's disease is not currently available. The audiometric pattern of the SHL, for example, is highly variable, al-

TABLE 9-2. CURRENT NEUROAUDIOLOGIC TEST BATTERY

First-Level Screening

    Speech recognition (Owens, 1971)

    Phonemically balanced rollover (Jerger and Jerger, 1971)

    Acoustic reflex threshold (Jerger and Jerger, 1977)
      Ipsilateral stimulation
      Contralateral stimulation

    Acoustic reflex decay (Anderson, Barr, and
      Wedenberg, 1970)

Second-Level Screening

    ABR (Selters and Brackmann, 1977)

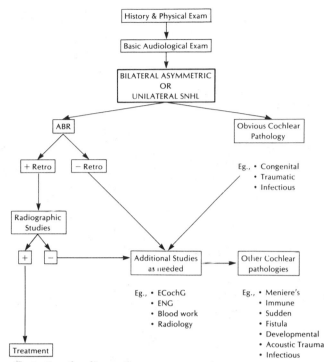

Figure 9-1. Flow diagram illustrating the diagnostic decision strategy most frequently employed in cases of unilateral or bilateral asymmetric SHL. Once retrocochlear pathology has been ruled out, additional studies are often needed in order to isolate the probable cause of the SHL. Several of these additional studies are listed in this flow chart as are the more likely cochlear pathologies from which a differential diagnosis is made.

though documentation of hearing fluctuation points to this disorder (Pfaltz and Matefi, 1981). ENG and sinusoidal harmonic acceleration testing have not revealed a characteristic vestibular deficit (Stahle, 1976; Wolfe, Engelken, and Olson, 1981). Although conceptually appealing, dehydration testing has a high false-negative rate, particularly in patients older than 50 years, and side effects from administration of these agents are often unpleasant (Imoto and Stahle, 1983; Klockhoff, 1981; Klockhoff and Lindblom, 1966).

In recent years, attention has focused on ECochG as a relatively noninvasive test for Ménière's disease. Studies have found that patients with Ménière's disease have distinctive changes in the ECochG response, specifically an enlarged SP relative to the amplitude of the AP (Coats, 1981; Dauman et al., 1988; Eggermont, 1979; Ferraro, Arenberg, and Hassanien, 1985; Gibson, Moffat, and Ramsden, 1977; Schmidt, Eggermont, and Odenthal, 1974). It has been postulated that an in-

crease in endolymph volume alters the mechanical characteristics of basilar membrane vibration. Since the SP is thought to result from distortion products associated with the cochlear transduction process, the enhanced asymmetry of basilar membrane movement resulting from increased endolymphatic pressure apparently causes an even larger SP. Thus, the enlargement of SP is viewed as a physiologic manifestation of endolymphatic hydrops. Most investigators have found an abnormally enlarged SP-to-AP ratio in approximately two-thirds of patients with Ménière's disease (Ruth et al., 1988). Ferraro et al. (1985) noted a high correlation between enlarged SP relative to AP amplitude and the presence of symptoms at the time of recording, especially fullness or aural pressure and some degree of hearing loss.

Bilateral Symmetric SHL

Retrocochlear pathology rarely, if ever, causes bilateral symmetric SHL. Even von Recklinghausen's disease with bilateral acoustic neuromas typically affects one ear more than the other. Thus, symmetric SHL strongly suggests cochlear pathology. Furthermore, this type of loss points toward a disease process with the potential of affecting both ears equally and not toward a more intrinsic problem such as an inner ear fistula, labyrinthitis from otitis media or cholesteatoma, idiopathic sudden SHL, or temporal bone trauma. Although Ménière's disease, cochlear otosclerosis, and autoimmune inner ear disease can cause bilateral disease, the hearing loss is usually not symmetric. Those diseases or conditions usually causing symmetric SHL include ototoxicity, chronic noise exposure, presbycusis, and genetic hearing loss.

If the audiogram shows a bilateral symmetric SHL, further audiometric testing rarely provides additional diagnostic information. ENG and other vestibular function tests (e.g., rotary chair), however, can be helpful in documenting coexisting vestibular pathology. Many types of drugs, for example, will damage the vestibular end organs, and the finding of reduced peripheral vestibular function would be consistent with ototoxic-induced SHL. Possible sources of bilateral symmetric SHL are shown in Figure 9-2 along with a listing of studies that may be helpful in arriving at a final diagnosis.

Mixed-Conductive and SHL

Few disease processes affect both the middle ear system and the cochlea. Those that could, include otosclerosis (stapedial and cochlear), inflammatory conditions (e.g., otitis media or cholesteatoma with labyrinthitis), or tumors of the middle ear (e.g., squamous cell carcinoma or, rarely, a glomus tumor). Otosclerosis and inflammatory disease would be the most commonly encountered conditions, and aural acoustic immittance measures can be useful in their differentiation. A flow diagram of the diagnostic approach to the evaluation of mixed-type hearing loss is illustrated in Figure 9-3.

SUMMARY

In the clinical assessment of SHL an attempt is made to differentiate cochlear from retrocochlear disorders; however, in reality the difference is not always clear-cut. For example, it has been suggested that tumors of the auditory nerve can dis-

Figure 9-2. Flow diagram illustrating the diagnostic decision strategy most frequently employed in cases of bilateral symmetric SHL. Several additional studies are listed as are some of the more likely sources of the hearing disorder.

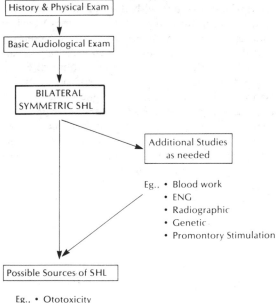

Figure 9-3. Flow diagram illustrating the diagnostic decision strategy most frequently employed in cases of mixed-type hearing loss. Additional studies are listed as well as possible sources of the hearing disorder.

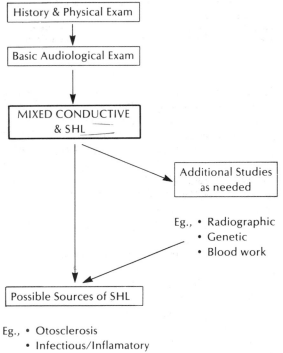

rupt the vascular supply to the cochlea, thus causing a sensory hearing impairment as well as a retrocochlear disorder. This situation most likely accounts for the reason that some of the early psychophysical tests sensitive to sensory impairment, such as the alternate binaural loudness balance and the short-increment sensitivity index tests, often missed the presence of an acoustic tumor. Likewise, it is well known that disorders resulting in damage to the hair cells of the cochlea will ultimately cause some degree of retrograde degeneration of auditory nerve fibers (Spoendlin, 1975). In this sense, it would be difficult if not impossible to isolate a single area of the peripheral auditory system that is solely responsible for a hearing impairment. Given that the sites of lesion may well be mixed between cochlea and auditory nerve in many cases, it seems reasonable that some confusion would result from audiologic tests designed for one or the other type of pathology.

This chapter illustrates the diagnostic strategies frequently used in the evaluation of cochlear disorders and the contribution of various audiologic tests to the overall evaluative process. Case studies follow to illustrate the manner in which various audiologic tests are used with other types of information in the diagnosis and evaluation of inner ear disease.

ILLUSTRATIVE CASES

The following cases are intended to demonstrate the manner in which various diagnostic procedures are combined in the assessment of SHL.

CASE 1: MÉNIÈRE'S DISEASE

A 51-year-old woman was referred with a 12-year history of right-sided hearing loss, tinnitus, aural fullness, and dizziness varied in nature at different times ranging from an unsteadiness to actual vertigo. She also reported a "numbness" of her head during many of the attacks. During the past 6 months, the dizziness was more an unsteadiness that occurred daily. Physical examination was normal. The audiogram (Figure 9-4) revealed a moderate to severe relatively flat SHL in the right ear. Speech recognition was within normal limits bilaterally with no evidence of roll over in either ear. Acoustic reflexes were within normal limits bilaterally with no evidence of reflex decay. Because of the facial paresthesia and atypical dizziness, a CT scan with contrast was ordered and was found normal. Results of ECochG testing are shown in Figure 9-5. The abnormal SP-to-AP relationship suggested Ménière's disease and the patient was started on a medical regimen. This therapy was unsuccessful, however, and the patient eventually elected to undergo endolymphatic sac decompression. Postoperatively, her symptoms of dizziness improved significantly but did not completely resolve.

Comment: This patient had unilateral fluctuating SHL in the right ear accompanied by a vague, atypical pattern of dizziness. ECochG was helpful in establishing the diagnosis of Ménière's disease by demonstrating the presence of a grossly abnormal SP-to-AP amplitude relationship. An enlarged SP relative to AP amplitude has been shown to be associated with increased endolymphatic pressure.

CASE 2: SUDDEN SHL

A 39-year-old man with no prior history of ear disease noted the sudden (1–2 day) onset of left ear tinnitus and

Figure 9-4. Results of audiologic evaluation from case 1.

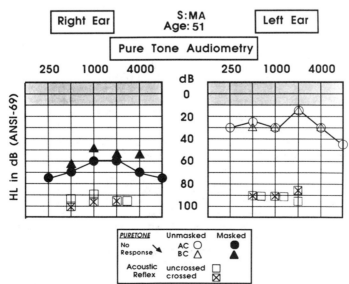

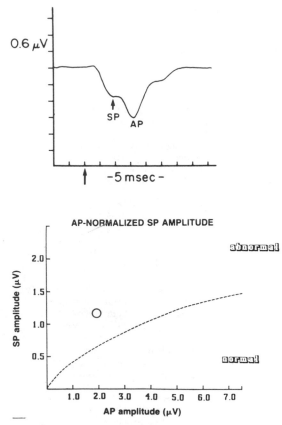

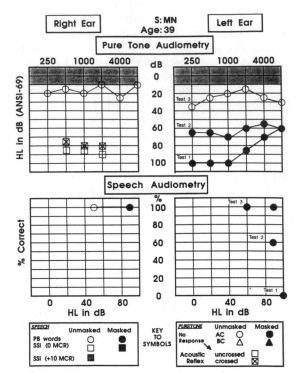

Figure 9-6. Results of audiologic evaluation from case 2. Results are shown for three different test sessions: Test 1 — initial results obtained within 3 days of onset of sudden hearing loss. Test 2 — follow-up testing 5 days later. Test 3 — audiogram obtained 2 weeks after the second visit. Note the degree of improvement in both hearing sensitivity and speech recognition in the left ear over the course of 3 weeks.

Figure 9-5. Electrocochleographic recording from the right ear of case 1 obtained with a tympanic membrane electrode. The arrow along the horizontal axis indicates the point in time at which a 90 dB HL alternating polarity click stimulus was delivered to the right ear via an insert transducer. Note the enlarged SP amplitude relative to AP amplitude in the ECochG tracing in the upper portion. The graph in the lower portion shows the SP amplitude plotted against AP amplitude. Values falling above the dashed line indicate an abnormally large SP amplitude consistent with increased endolymphatic pressure.

hearing loss. There was no associated ear pain, drainage, or dizziness. Past history was negative for barotrauma, head trauma, toxin exposure, or family history of hearing loss. Physical examination was normal with the exception of tuning fork lateralization to the right (Weber's test). The basic audiologic evaluation obtained 3 days postonset showed a left SHL with absent acoustic reflexes, but normal tympanometry (Figure 9-6). Blood studies were normal and the patient was started on a tapering dose of prednisone. A repeat audiogram 5 days later showed an improvement in the pure tone average and the presence of an acoustic reflex at 500 and 1000 Hz. An ABR was obtained and found normal (Figure 9-7). Two weeks later the hearing returned to normal with 100 percent speech recognition, no roll over, and crossed and uncrossed acoustic reflexes within normal limits. One and one-half years later, the patient reports the ear to be asymptomatic.

Comment: The cause of SHL is uncertain, although temporal bone histopathologic studies suggest a viral etiology (e.g., viral labyrinthitis) (Schuknecht, Kimura, and Naufal, 1973). Typically this problem develops in previously healthy individuals of any age group and involves one ear only. Hearing recovery (partial or complete) occurs in up to 65 percent of patients. Prognosis can be predicted by the shape of the initial audiogram, as the chance for hearing recovery is better in up-sloping rather than down-sloping losses (Mattox and Simmons, 1977).

CASE 3: AUTOIMMUNE INNER EAR DISEASE

A 73-year-old man presented with an 8-month history of dizziness and progressive hearing loss. He had a longstanding moderate-degree SHL but recently noted a marked decrease in hearing bilaterally with fluctuation in sensitivity. The dizziness was described as more an unsteadiness, especially with position change, than actual vertigo. It occurred intermittently, lasting minutes to days. Intermittent tinnitus was also noted. The tinnitus and hearing fluctuation did not correlate temporally with the dizziness. The patient was on no medications and had no prior history of ear disease other than the high-frequency SHL. Examination of the ears and a general physical examination were normal. Ophthalmologic examination was also nor-

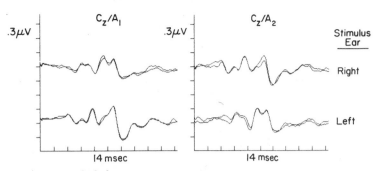

Figure 9-7. ABR obtained from case 2, 8 days postonset of a sudden SHL in the left ear.

mal. The initial work-up included an audiogram, ENG, MRI, and blood studies. The audiogram showed a moderate low- to mid-frequency SHL with a more severe loss in the high frequencies (Figure 9-8). The ENG revealed a right spontaneous and positional nystagmus. The MRI was negative. Laboratory studies were positive for an elevated sedimentation rate and antinuclear antibody titer.

The patient's symptoms of fluctuating hearing loss and dysequilibrium and the objective findings of SHL, vestibular dysfunction, and positive immunologic screening blood tests all suggested the diagnosis of autoimmune inner ear dis-

Figure 9-8. Results of initial (test 1) and follow-up (test 2) audiologic evaluation from case 3. Acoustic reflexes were absent under all conditions in the initial evaluation but returned in the follow-up evaluation and are reflected on the audiogram. Acoustic reflex decay was negative bilateral at 1000 Hz (crossed condition).

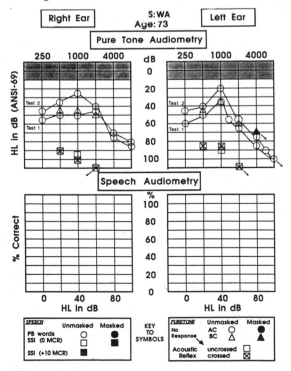

ease. The patient was begun on prednisone and within 1 week noted an improvement in his dysequilibrium. An audiogram 2 weeks later showed a significant improvement in the mid-frequency range. A repeat ENG showed resolution of the spontaneous nystagmus but continued presence of the positional nystagmus. The patient has been maintained on long-term (2 years), low-dose prednisone with stabilization of his hearing, an "80 percent improvement" in his dysequilibrium, and normalization of the sedimentation rate.

Comment: Autoimmune inner ear disease was first described by McCabe in 1979 and recently has been the subject of intense investigation (Harris, 1987; Hughes, Barna, and Kinney, 1986; Hughes et al., 1984). Although the exact mechanism of injury to the auditory and vestibular systems is unclear, various forms of treatment have been utilized with some degree of success. In this disease process, for example, patients often do respond to steroids. Serial audiograms and ENGs provide objective data that are helpful in assessing response to medical treatment and in regulating steroid dose.

CASE 4: MENINGITIS

A 49-year-old woman was referred for evaluation of profound bilateral hearing loss. Three years previously she suffered streptococcal meningitis, apparently secondary to a spontaneous cerebrospinal fluid leak in the cribriform plate (anterior skull base). This cerebrospinal fluid leak was subsequently repaired. Prior to the meningitis, the patient reported normal hearing. The ear examination and physical examination were normal with the exception of apparent profound deafness bilaterally (Figure 9-9). Speech was normal and the patient demonstrated fair lip-reading skills. The CT scan showed the cochleas to be patent bilaterally.

A cochlear implant evaluation was carried out and revealed essentially no benefit from optimally fit amplification devices in terms of open or closed set speech recognition tests or speech-reading ability. Promontory electrical stimulation of both ears indicated that an auditory sensation could be elicited using electrical stimulation (Table 9-3). Based on audiologic results, this patient was deemed to be a good candidate for cochlear implantation.

The patient wished to proceed with a cochlear implant, and a multichannel device was implanted. The patient is now 6 months postsurgery and has demonstrated a marked improvement in speech-reading skills and some open set word recognition.

Comment: SHL is a relatively common complication of bacterial meningitis, occurring in 5 to 30 percent of cases (Dodge et al., 1984; Keane et al., 1979; Nadol, 1978). Most commonly this occurs by spread of the infection from the subarachnoid space into the cochlea through the cochlear aqueduct or along the vascular and nerve channels of the interior auditory canal. This results in a purulent labyrinthitis

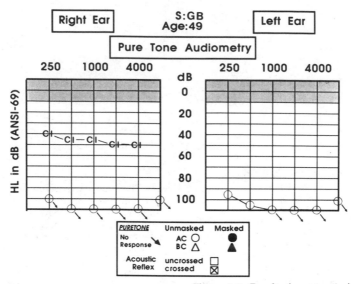

Figure 9-9. Results (preoperative) of audiologic evaluation from case 4. Note this patient has virtually no residual hearing in either ear. Postimplant sound field thresholds are indicated by *CI*.

TABLE 9-3. PROMONTORY ELECTRICAL STIMULATION TEST RESULTS FOR CASE 4

	Frequency (Hz)			
	50	100	200	400
Threshold (Amp)	12.8	9.0	15.0	52.0
Uncomfortable loudness (Amp)	29.1	22.5	25.0	83.0
Dynamic range (Amp)	16.3	13.5	10.0	31.0
Gap detection threshold (at 100 Hz) — 20 msec				

with degeneration of the organ of Corti. Occasionally the labyrinthitis will induce bone growth within the fluid spaces of the cochlea, which, if extensive, can cause ossification of the inner ear (labyrinthitis ossificans). The CT, therefore, is an important part of the cochlear implant evaluation in meningitis patients to determine if the cochlea is patent.

In addition, promontory electrical stimulation testing is viewed as a necessary measure of the extent and viability of excitable auditory nerve elements. The absence of an auditory percept in response to promontory electrical stimulation strongly suggests that a patient may not be a suitable candidate for cochlear implantation (Lambert et al., 1987).

CASE 5: COCHLEAR OTOSCLEROSIS

A 53-year-old woman was evaluated for a 20-year history of progressive hearing loss in each ear. There was no history of ear infections, head trauma, ototoxic medications, vertigo, or tinnitus. The family history revealed that her father began wearing hearing aids as a young man and that several siblings had a hearing loss, though not as severe as hers. Examination of the ears and a general physical examination were normal except for the tuning fork tests. Bone conduction was greater than air conduction with the 512 Hz and 1024 Hz tuning forks, and both forks were referred to the left ear on the Weber test.

The audiogram showed a severe flat hearing loss by air conduction and a moderate sloping SHL by unmasked bone conduction (Figure 9-10). Because of the masking dilemma, lateralization of the sensory loss was not possible. An ABR

was obtained using ear canal electrodes to better characterize cochlear function in each ear and to rule out retrocochlear pathology (Figure 9-11). Wave I was readily identified bilaterally and the I to V interwave interval was normal bilaterally. Given these results, the tentative diagnosis was bilateral otosclerosis with involvement of both the stapes (conductive loss) and cochlea (sensory loss). A left middle ear exploration was performed with findings of otosclerosis. A stapedectomy significantly improved the patient's hearing.

Comment: Although otosclerosis is usually confined to the stapes footplate, it can involve the cochlea in combination with stapes fixation or, less commonly, as an isolated process (Balle and Linthicum, 1984). Because of the masking dilemma, it was not possible by routine air and bone conduction studies to assess the degree of sensory loss in each ear. This information is important in attempting to reach a diagnosis and in deciding which, if either, ear should be operated on. In this case the ABR was able to determine the cochlear function was nearly symmetric, thus lending support to the provisional diagnosis of otosclerosis that was suggested by the patient's history, exam, and family history. If wave I of the ABR had not been present for both right and left ear stimulation, ECochG would have been the next diagnostic test employed.

CASE 6: INNER EAR FISTULA

A 6-year-old girl was evaluated for progressive bilateral SHL. Her parents were first aware of the loss at age 3 because of poor language development. Yearly audiometric studies have shown a significant incremental loss of hearing (Figure 9-12). The patient denied tinnitus but did complain of intermittent, mild dizziness. The patient's prenatal and perinatal histories were unremarkable. As a young child she had no history of meningitis, ear infections, head trauma, or ototoxic medications. Her family history was notable only for a parental grandmother who began wearing hearing aids as an adult. The patient's ear examination and general physical examination were normal.

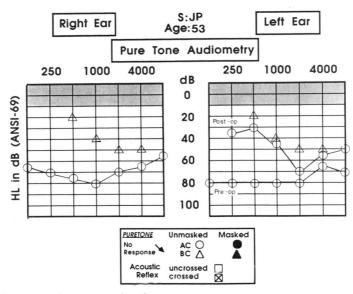

Figure 9-10. Pre- and poststapedectomy results of audiologic evaluation from case 5. Bone conduction results remain constant for both evaluations.

An ear canal pressure–induced perilymph fistula test was performed with negative findings bilaterally. A CT scan demonstrated normal development of the cochlea and semicircular canals and no evidence of retrocochlear pathology. Blood studies were all normal. The tentative diagnosis was SHL (cochlear) secondary either to genetic factors or to perilymph fistulas. The patient underwent a left middle ear exploration with findings highly suggestive of a round window fistula. Findings during a right middle ear exploration 2 months later were equivocal for a perilymph fistula. During a 2-year follow-up, hearing sensitivity was relatively unchanged in each ear.

Figure 9-11. ABR recording from case 5 using ear canal electrodes. Both right and left ear responses have a clear wave I, most likely indicating some degree of peripheral or cochlear function bilaterally.

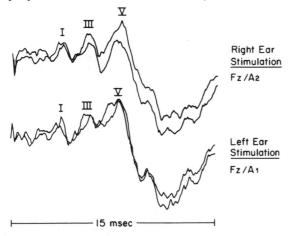

Comment: This young patient had progressive, bilaterally symmetric SHL. Given her history and examination, the most likely diagnosis is genetic hearing loss. The negative family history is not surprising since the majority of these losses are recessive (Konigsmark and Gorlin, 1976). The other principal consideration in the differential diagnosis is perilymph fistulas. Although uncommon, they can be a cause of progressive SHL in children (Seltzer and McCabe, 1986; Supance and Bluestone, 1983). The CT scan was obtained to examine for cochlear malformation, especially the Mondini deformity. This deformity is the most common structural abnormality of the cochlea identified radiographically, and it is often associated with a perilymph fistula (Jackler, Luxford, and House, 1987). Despite the negative CT scan, the ears were explored and a positive round window fistula was found on one side. The oval window and round window of each ear were patched with adipose tissue, and, although long-term follow-up is not available, the patient has demonstrated stable hearing for 2 years.

CASE 7: AMINOGLYCOSIDE TOXICITY

A 42-year-old man was admitted to the hospital for third-degree burns. He developed *Pseudomonas* infection and was placed on several antibiotics, including gentamicin. A baseline audiogram (Figure 9-13) was obtained prior to treatment and then at biweekly intervals for 3 weeks. After 2 weeks of antibiotic treatment, a bilateral high-frequency SHL was noted (test 2). Subjectively, the patient noted tinnitus in each ear. The patient was not ambulatory and did not describe dizziness. There was no spontaneous or gaze-induced nystagmus present. At 3 weeks (test 3) the high-frequency hearing loss had worsened and the gentamicin was stopped. The infection had largely cleared, although the patient was continued on the other antibiotics for an additional week. Six months after discharge from the hospital, the bilateral SHL persisted and was consistent with the previous audiometric results (test 3).

Comment: Aminoglycosides can cause hearing loss by destroying the cochlear hair cells (Fee, 1980; Keane and Hawke, 1981; Ylikoski, 1974). They are also toxic to the vestibular sensory epithelium. Hair cell loss begins in the base

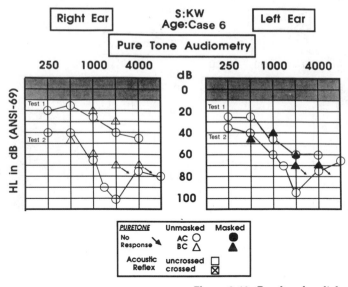

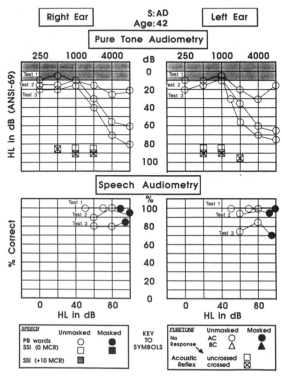

Figure 9-12. Results of audiologic evaluation from case 6 at age 3 years 11 months (test 1) and age 5 years 1 month (test 2). Thresholds were obtained using conditioned play audiometry procedures and were judged to be very reliable. Acoustic reflexes were absent bilaterally (test 2), and speech recognition was consistent with hearing loss.

Figure 9-13. Baseline audiologic results (test 1) from case 7. Test 2 and test 3 represent subsequent audiometric results after antibiotic treatment (see text for description). Acoustic reflexes are plotted from initial test evaluation. Speech recognition scores show decrease consistent with reduction in high-frequency thresholds.

of the cochlea and extends apically over time and with continued drug administration. The outer hair cells are the structures principally affected, and the hearing loss is usually incomplete, although total deafness can occur. Occasionally hearing recovery from the cochlear injury has been observed in patients over the course of weeks to months (Fee, 1980; Moffat and Ramsden, 1977). Experimental studies in birds have shown evidence for cochlear hair cell regeneration, but whether this occurs in humans is unknown (Cruz, Lambert, and Rubel, 1987).

Because the hearing loss after aminoglycoside toxicity initially occurs in the high frequencies, periodic audiometric testing can be useful in detecting cochlear injury before it becomes widespread. In some cases the infection is life-threatening, and continued aminoglycoside administration is essential; in other cases, however, a different antibiotic can be substituted and the hearing preserved.

CASE 8: CYTOMEGALOVIRUS

This child's past history was significant for cytomegalovirus (CMV) infection. At birth he was noted to have petechiae, mild hepatosplenomegaly, and to be small in size and weight for gestional age. CMV was cultured from his urine. He passed an ABR screen at 30 dB HL in both ears prior to discharge from the hospital. At 12 months of age a follow-up ABR test was performed with responses present down to a level of 30 dB HL bilaterally, indicating hearing most probably within or near normal limits (Figure 9-14). Visual reinforcement operant conditioning audiometry procedures confirmed the ABR results (Figure 9-15). At 2 years 7 months of age, the child returned to the authors' clinic for evaluation of speech and language delay. The audiogram obtained during this visit showed a mild SHL on the right and a moderate SHL on the left (test 2). Except for the de-

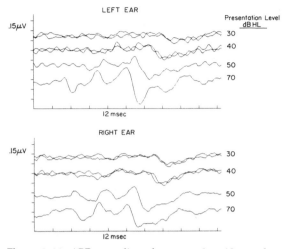

Figure 9-14. ABR recordings from case 8 at 12 months of age. Note responses were present down to a level of 30 dB HL bilaterally.

layed speech and language, development had otherwise been normal. The otologic and general physical examination were also normal. Amplification was recommended for the left ear. Hearing loss has remained stable in both ears for nearly 2 years.

Comment: CMV is the most common congenital viral infection in humans, infecting 1 to 2 percent of all newborn infants. Although most of these infants are asymptomatic,

Figure 9-15. Audiologic results from case 8 at 12 months of age (test 1) and 2 years 7 months (test 2). Thresholds were obtained by means of visual reinforcement operant-conditioning audiometry procedures (test 1). Acoustic reflex thresholds represent second visit. Note the progressive loss of hearing in the left ear.

a small percentage will manifest severe neurologic sequelae. In the group of initially asymptomatic children, progressive SHL can occur in 20 to 50 percent (Davis, 1981; Strauss, 1985), thus CMV is the most common cause of congenital and viral-induced deafness and probably accounts for a large proportion of children previously classified with congenital hearing loss of unknown etiology. To date, no antiviral therapy or treatment of CMV-induced hearing loss exists.

REFERENCES

Anderson, H., Barr, B., & Wedenberg, E. (1970). Early detection of the eighth nerve tumors by acoustic reflex tests. *Acta Oto-laryngologica.* Supplement (Stockholm), *263,* 232–237.

Balle, V., & Linthicum, F. H. (1984). Histologically proven cochlear otosclerosis with pure sensorineural hearing loss. *Annals of Otology, Rhinology, and Laryngology, 93,* 105–111.

Carhart, R. (1957). Clinical determination of abnormal auditory adaptation. *Archives of Otolaryngology, 65,* 32–39.

Clemis, J. D., & Sarno, C. N. (1980). The acoustic reflex latency test: Clinical applications. *Laryngoscope, 90,* 601–611.

Coats, A. (1981). The summating potential and Ménière's disease: I. Summating potential amplitude in Ménière's and non-Ménière's ears. *Archives of Otolaryngology, 107,* 199–208.

Cruz, R., Lambert, P., & Rubel, E. (1987). Light microscopic evidence of hair cell regeneration after gentamicin toxicity in chick cochlea. *Archives of Otolaryngology — Head and Neck Surgery, 113,* 1058–1062.

Dallos, P. (1988). Cochlear neurobiology: Revolutionary developments. *Journal of the American Speech and Hearing Association, June/July,* 50–56.

Dauman, R., Aran, J., Savage, R., & Portmann, M. (1988). Clinical significance of the summating potential in Ménière's disease. *American Journal of Otology, 9,* 31–38.

Davis, G. (1981). In vitro models of viral-induced congenital deafness. *American Journal of Otology, 3,* 56–160.

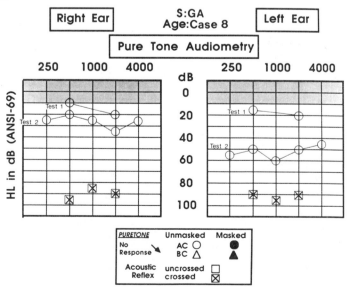

Dodge, P. R., Davis, H., Feigin, R. D., Holmes, S. J., Kaplan, S. L., Jubelirer, D. P., Stechenberg, B. W., & Hirsh, S. K. (1984). Prospective evaluation of hearing impairment as a sequela of acute bacterial meningitis. *New England Journal of Medicine, 311,* 869–874.

Eggermont, J. (1979). Summating potentials in Ménière's disease. *Archives of Otolaryngology, 222,* 65–75.

Eggermont, J. J., & Schmidt, P. H. (1985). Ménière's disease: A long-term follow-up study of hearing loss. *Annals of Otology, Rhinology, and Laryngology, 94,* 1–9.

Fee, W. E. (1980). Aminoglycoside ototoxicity in the human. *Laryngoscope, 90*(Suppl. 24), 1–19.

Ferraro, J., Arenberg, I., & Hassanien, R. (1985). Electrocochleography and symptoms of inner ear dysfunction. *Archives of Otolaryngology, 111,* 71–74.

Fowler, P. E. (1937). The diagnosis of disease of the neural mechanism of hearing by the aid of sounds well above threshold. *Transactions of the American Otolaryngology Society, 27,* 207–219.

Gibson, W., Moffat, D., & Ramsden, R. (1977). Clinical electrocochleography in the diagnosis and management of Ménière's disease. *Audiology, 16,* 389–401.

Goldstein, D. P. (1984). Hearing impairment, hearing aids and audiology. *Journal of the American Speech and Hearing Association, September,* 24–38.

Greisen, O., & Rasmussen, P. E. (1970). Stapedius reflexes and oto-neurological examinations in brain-stem tumors. *Acta Oto-laryngologica,* (Stockholm), 70, 366–370.

Harris, J. P. (1987). Experimental autoimmune sensorineural hearing loss. *Laryngoscope, 97,* 63–76.

Hayes, D., & Jerger, J. F. (1982). Signal-averaging of the acoustic reflex: Diagnostic applications of amplitude characteristics. *Scandinavian Audiology.* Supplementum, 17, 31–36.

Hood, J. D. (1956). Fatigue and adaptation of hearing. *British Medical Bulletin, 12,* 125–130.

Hughes, G. B., Barna, B. P., & Kinney, S. E. (1986). Predictive value of laboratory tests in autoimmune inner ear disease: Preliminary report. *Laryngoscope, 96,* 502–505.

Hughes, G. B., Kinney, S. E., Barna, B. P., & Calabresse, L. H. (1984). Practical versus theoretical management of autoimmune inner ear disease. *Laryngoscope, 94,* 758–767.

Hyde, M. L. (1985). The effect of cochlear lesions on the ABR. In J. Jacobson (Ed.), *The auditory brainstem response.* Boston: College-Hill Press.

Imoto, T., & Stahle, J. (1983). Glycerin and urea tests in Ménière's disease. *Otolaryngology Clinics of North America, 16,* 37–48.

Jackler, R. K., Luxford, W. M., & House, W. F. (1987). Congenital malformations of the inner ear: A classification based on embryogenesis. *Laryngoscope, 97*(Suppl. 40), 2–14.

Jerger, J. F. (1960). Bekesy audiometry in analysis of auditory disorders. *Journal of Speech and Hearing Research, 3,* 275–287.

Jerger, J. F., & Jerger, S. W. (1971). Diagnostic significance of PB word functions. *Archives of Otolaryngology, 93,* 573–580.

Jerger, J. F., & Jerger, S. W. (1974). Diagnostic value of Bekesy comfortable loudness tracings. *Archives of Otolaryngology, 99,* 351–360.

Jerger, J. F., & Jerger, S. W. (1975). A simplified tone decay test. *Archives of Otolaryngology, 101,* 403–407.

Jerger, J. F., & Jerger, S. W. (1977). Diagnostic value of crossed vs. uncrossed acoustic reflexes. *Archives of Otolaryngology, 103,* 445–453.

Jerger, J. F., Burney, P., Mauldin, L., & Crump, B. (1974). Predicting hearing loss from the acoustic reflex. *Journal of Speech and Hearing Disorders, 39,* 11–17.

Jerger, J. F., Shedd, J., & Harford, E. (1959). On the detection of extremely small changes in sound intensity. *Archives of Otolaryngology, 69,* 200–211.

Jerger, J. F., Speaks, C., & Trammell, J. A. (1968). A new approach to speech audiometry. *Journal of Speech and Hearing Disorders, 33,* 318–328.

Jerger, S. W., & Jerger, J. F. (1983). Evaluation of diagnostic audiometric tests. *Audiology, 22,* 144–161.

Keane, M., & Hawke, M. (1981). Pathogenesis and detection of aminoglycoside ototoxicity. *Journal of Otolaryngology, 10,* 228–236.

Keane, W. M., Potsic, W. P., Rowe, L. D., & Konkle, D. F. (1979). Meningitis and hearing loss in children. *Archives of Otolaryngology — Head and Neck Surgery, 105,* 39–44.

Kileny, P. R., & Kemink, J. L. (1987). Electrically evoked middle-latency auditory potentials in cochlear implant candidates. *Archives of Otolaryngology, 113,* 1072–1077.

Klockhoff, I. (1981). Some remarks after 15 years experience. In K. Vosteen, H. Schuknecht, C. Pfaltz, J. Wersäll, R. Kimura, C. Morganstern, & S. John (Eds.), *Ménière's disease: Pathogenesis, diagnosis and treatment* (pp. 148–151). New York: Thieme-Stratton.

Klockhoff, I., & Lindblom, U. (1966). Endolymphatic hydrops revealed by glycerol test. *Acta Oto-laryngologica* (Stockholm), 61, 399–402.

Konigsmark, B., & Gorlin, R. (1976). *Genetic and metabolic deafness* (pp. 1–6). Philadelphia: Saunders.

Lambert, P., Ruth, R., & Hodges, A. (1987). Meningitis and facial paresis: Implications for cochlear implantation. *Archives of Otolaryngology, 113,* 1101–1103.

Lippe, W. R. (1986). Recent developments in cochlear physiology. *Ear & Hearing, 7,* 233–239.

Luscher, E., & Zwislocki, J. (1949). A simple method of indirect monaural determination of the recruitment phenomenon (difference limen in intensity in different types of deafness). *Acta Oto-laryngologica* (Stockholm), 78, 156–168.

Mangham, C. A., Lindeman, R. C., & Dawson, W. R. (1980). Stapedius reflex quantification in acoustic tumor patients. *Laryngoscope, 90,* 242–250.

Mattox, D., & Simmons, F. (1977). Natural history of sudden sensorineural hearing loss. *Annals of Otology, Rhinology, and Laryngology, 86,* 463–480.

McCabe, B. F. (1979). Autoimmune sensorineural hearing loss. *Annals of Otology, 88,* 585–589.

Metz, O. (1952). Threshold of reflex contractions muscles of the middle ear and recruitment of loudness. *Archives of Otolaryngology, 55,* 536–543.

Miller, M. (1985). The integration of audiologic findings. In J. Katz (Ed.), *Handbook of clinical audiology* (pp. 259–272). Baltimore: Williams & Wilkins.

Moffat, D., & Ramsden, R. (1977). Profound bilateral sensorineural hearing loss during gentamicin therapy. *Journal of Laryngology and Otology, 91,* 511–516.

Nadol, J. B. (1978). Hearing loss as a sequela of meningitis. *Laryngoscope, 88,* 739–755.

Olsen, W. O., Noffsinger, D., & Kurdziel, S. (1975). Acoustic reflex and reflex decay. *Archives of Otolaryngology, 101,* 622–625.

Owens, E. (1971). Audiologic evaluation of cochlear versus retrocochlear lesions. *Acta Oto-laryngologica.* Supplement (Stockholm), 283, 1–45.

Paparella, M., Hanson, D., Rao, K., & Ives, R. (1975). Genetic sensorineural deafness in adults. *Annals of Otology, Rhinology, and Laryngology, 84,* 459–472.

Pfaltz, C., & Matefi, L. (1981). Ménière's disease — or syndrome? A critical review of diagnostic criteria. In K. Vosteen, H. Schucknecht, C. Pfaltz, J. Wersäll, R. Kimura, C. Morganstern, & S. John (Eds.), *Ménière's disease: Pathogenesis, diagnosis and treatment* (pp. 1–10). New York: Thieme-Stratton.

Ruth, R. A., Lambert, P. R., & Ferraro, J. A. (1988). Electrocochleography: Methods and clinical applications. *American Journal of Otology, 9,* 1–11.

Ruth, R. A., Nilo, E. R., & Mravec, J. J. (1978). Consideration of acoustic reflex magnitude (ARM) in cases of idiopathic facial paralysis. *Journal of Otolaryngology, 86,* 215–220.

Schmidt, P., Eggermont, J., & Odenthal, D. (1974). Study of Ménière's disease by electrocochleography. In J. Eggermont, D. Odenthal, P. Schmidt, & A. Spoor (Eds.), *Electrocochleography: Basic principles and clinical applications. Acta Oto-laryngologica* (Stockholm), Suppl. *316,* 75–84.

Schuknecht, H., Kimura, R., & Naufal, P. (1973). The pathology of sudden deafness. *Acta Oto-laryngologica* (Stockholm), *76,* 75–82.

Schwartz, D. M. (1987). Neurodiagnostic audiology: Contemporary perspectives. *Ear & Hearing, 8* (Suppl.), 43–48.

Selters, W. A., & Brackmann, D. E. (1977). Acoustic tumor detection with brainstem electric response audiometry. *Archives of Otolaryngology, 103,* 15–24.

Seltzer, S., & McCabe, B. F. (1986). Perilymphatic fistula. The Iowa experience. *Laryngoscope, 96,* 37–49.

Spoendlin, H. (1975). Retrograde degeneration of the cochlear nerve. *Acta Oto-laryngologica* (Stockholm), *79,* 266–275.

Stahle, J. (1976). Advanced Ménière's disease. *Acta Oto-laryngologica* (Stockholm), *81,* 113–119.

Strauss, M. (1985). A clinical pathologic study of hearing loss in congenital cytomegalovirus infection. *Laryngoscope, 95,* 951–962.

Supance, J. S., & Bluestone, C. D. (1983). PLF in infants and children. *Otolaryngology — Head and Neck Surgery, 92,* 663–671.

Turner, R. G., & Nielson, D. W. (1984). Application of clinical decision analysis to audiological tests. *Ear & Hearing, 5,* 125–133.

Turner, R. G., Frazier, G. J., & Shepard, N. T. (1984). Formulating and evaluating audiological test protocols. *Ear & Hearing, 5,* 321–330.

Turner, R. G., Shepard, N. T., & Frazier, G. J. (1984). Formulating and evaluating audiological test protocols. *Ear & Hearing, 5,* 187–194.

Wolfe, J., Engelken, E., & Olson, W. E. (1981). Vestibular responses to bithermal caloric and harmonic acceleration in patients with Ménière's disease. In K. Vosteen, H. Schucknecht, C. Pfaltz, J. Wersäll, R. Kimura, C. Morganstern, & S. John (Eds.), *Ménière's disease: Pathogenesis, diagnosis and treatment* (pp. 170–177). New York: Thieme-Stratton.

Ylikoski, J. (1974). Guinea pig hair cell pathology from ototoxic antibiotics. *Acta Oto-laryngologica* (Stockholm), (Suppl. 236), 5–59.

CHAPTER 10

Acoustic Neuroma: Diagnosis and Management

Paul R. Kileny • Steven A. Telian • John L. Kemink

Recent advances in clinical neurophysiology, central nervous system imaging, and microsurgical techniques have collectively contributed to the earlier diagnosis and management of tumors of the cerebellopontine angle (CPA). This is the result of a cooperative interdisciplinary effort involving the disciplines of audiology, radiology, neurotology, and neurosurgery. From the patient's point of view, the net result is safer and more effective surgical management with reduced morbidity and low rates of mortality.

This chapter provides an overview of contemporary diagnosis and management of acoustic neuromas. In order to place the current state of the art into perspective, the historical evolution leading to contemporary diagnostic methods is also summarized. The diagnostic modalities addressed include audiologic (with a strong emphasis on electrophysiology) and radiographic imaging techniques, since in practice they are complementary.

Approximately 11 percent of diagnosed intracranial tumors occur in the CPA; most of those (75%) arise from the eighth cranial nerve (Nager, 1969; Pool, Pava, and Greenfield, 1970). Although the reported prevalence of tumors of the eighth cranial nerve found at autopsy is about 1 percent, the diagnosed clinical incidence was reported to be approximately 1 in 100,000 (Moberg, Anderson, and Wedenberg, 1969; Morrison, 1975). Clearly, many cases are asymptomatic or undiagnosed due to the predominance of cochlear site of lesion signs and symptoms. Contemporary diagnostic techniques may result in an apparent increase in the prevalence of CPA tumors due to their higher sensitivity, which contributes to the detection of increasingly smaller tumors.

Acoustic neuromas are benign, encapsulated neoplasms originating from the Schwann cells of the distal intracanalicular portion of the vestibular division of the eighth cranial nerve, thus the alternate term *vestibular schwannoma* proposed by Schuknecht (1974). Frequently, acoustic neuromas originate from the superior vestibular division and occasionally from the inferior vestibular or the cochlear divisions of the eighth cranial nerve. Regardless of the nerve of origin, acoustic neuromas are contained within the internal acoustic meatus (IAM) in the early stages, and as they grow, they extend medially until they emerge from the IAM into the posterior cranial fossa. If undetected, they may compress the brainstem and the cerebellum. Therefore, the most common early symptoms associated with an acoustic neuroma are related to the auditory or vestibular systems, or both. The extension of the tumor into the CPA is associated with brainstem and cerebellar neurologic signs and symptoms. Other tumors that originate in rather than extend into the CPA are meningiomas, epidermoids (primary cholesteatomas), and glomus jugular tumors. Since their origin is not from the eighth cranial nerve, the initial symptoms are rarely auditory or vestibular.

House (1979) reviewed the history of the diagnosis and management of acoustic tumors from the early nineteenth century to the first half of the twentieth century. Important advances in the understanding of cranial nerve function took place during the nineteenth century. The foundation of this work was laid earlier by the noted English surgeon and comparative anatomist John Hunter who died in 1793. His methods, based on accurate clinical observations and an appreciation of the importance of anatomic studies, were carried on by Sir Charles Bell who in 1830 published a clinical and autopsy report on a patient with an acoustic neuroma. Bell emphasized the involvement of cranial nerves V and VII leading to a relationship between deafness and acoustic tumors.

Helmholz's invention of the opthalmoscope was an important milestone in the diagnosis of intracranial tumors. The opthalmoscope enabled physicians to diagnose intracranial tumors based on patient symptoms (e.g., headaches) and objective signs (e.g., papilledema) and their site relative to the tentorium based on the presence or absence of cerebellar signs.

The noted neurosurgeon Harvey Cushing's interest in tumors of the CPA during the early part of the twentieth century laid the foundation for contemporary diagnostic and treatment strategies. During that era, most diagnoses were made at advanced stages after the appearance of significant neurologic deficits. Through careful observation and attention to case histories, Cushing was able to reconstruct the sequence of symptoms associated with acoustic tumors. In his monograph published in 1917, he correctly identified auditory and vestibular symptoms followed by a hierarchy of other neurologic events. He also recognized the significance of a unilateral hearing loss in the diagnosis of acoustic neuroma.

Although today some acoustic neuromas remain undiagnosed until the appearance of neurologic sequelae beyond auditory symptoms, there is an increased appreciation of the relationship between an unexplained asymmetric sensory hearing loss (SHL) and the suspicion of an acoustic neuroma. Therefore, often a hearing assessment is the first diagnostic test administered to patients suspected to have an acoustic neuroma. Beyond the tests dealing primarily with hearing sensitivity, various site of lesion diagnostic test batteries have been used and advocated. Most of the recent diagnostic emphasis has been directed toward the development of test modalities or test batteries with high sensitivity and specificity. Nevertheless, attention to the history and high clinical suspicion are as important today as during the Cushing era.

CLINICAL PRESENTATION

Many attempts have been made to synthesize a typical clinical profile of the acoustic neuroma patient (Graham, 1979; Johnson, 1979). Graham (1979) reviewed 35 surgically confirmed acoustic neuroma cases. Twenty-eight of the patients (80%) presented with progressive SHL ranging in duration from 3 months to 24 years on the affected side. Only seven patients (20%) presented with a sudden hearing loss on the affected side or did not relate a history of progressive hearing im-

pairment. In 25 of these cases (71%), there was also a complaint of tinnitus on the affected side. Eighteen patients (51%) also presented with a history of vestibular symptoms (unsteadiness, dizziness). Pain on the affected side, facial numbness, and visual disturbance occurred in a minority of these patients. Tumor size in this series ranged from a small intracanalicular tumor (70 dB pure tone average on the affected side) to a 5 cm tumor (with a flat 35 dB SHL on the affected side). The next largest was a 4.5 cm tumor associated with a 15 dB pure tone average. In six of these cases, with tumor size ranging from 1.5 to 3.5 cm, hearing sensitivity was beyond the limits of the audiometer (110 dB). Using the complete data set (n = 35), the authors calculated the correlation coefficient (r) between tumor size and pure tone average. This resulted in a low r value of 0.01, indicating that, at least in this series, hearing sensitivity was not a reliable predictor of tumor size. It should be noted, however, that all patients shared the common feature of some degree of SHL on the affected side, which in the majority of cases (80%) was progressive in nature.

AUDIOLOGIC DIAGNOSIS

The recognition that the earliest symptoms indicating the presence of an acoustic neuroma involved the auditory system has brought about attempts to devise auditory tests and test batteries to facilitate early diagnosis of acoustic neuromas. Attempts at acoustic neuroma diagnosis from the pure tone audiometric pattern have by and large failed, since no specific pattern has been established (Johnson, 1979). Threshold shift (abnormal adaptation or tone decay) with prolonged stimulation was observed as early as 1893 (Johnson, 1979). It was noted that patients with acoustic neuromas were able to hear a vibrating tuning fork for only a few seconds. Later, Carhart (1957) developed the notion of *tone decay*, or excessive adaptation to prolonged pure tone stimuli.

Johnson (1979) reviewed 500 patients with surgically confirmed unilateral acoustic neuromas. In 78 of these patients (16%), hearing sensitivity exceeded audiometric limits on the affected side. In the remaining cases, a statistically significant relationship was demonstrated between pure tone thresholds and tumor size, that is, the larger the tumor, the more elevated the pure tone threshold average. Based on diagnostic audiologic tests, tone decay exhibited the next highest sensitivity;

test results were positive in 77 percent of acoustic neuroma patients tested. Acoustic reflexes were tested in a subset of 117 patients of this series; positive results (absence of reflexes or abnormal reflex decay) were obtained in 81 percent, slightly exceeding the sensitivity of the tone decay test.

Selters and Brackmann (1977, 1979) reported the earliest auditory brainstem response (ABR) results on large series of surgically confirmed acoustic neuroma cases (n = 35 and 94, respectively). Using the interaural latency difference of wave V (IT_5 or ILD-V) as an indicator, after correcting for hearing loss at 4000 Hz, they reported a hit rate of 96 percent and a false-positive rate of 8 percent. They considered this new electrophysiologic test modality a "significant addition to the acoustic tumor detection test battery" and advocated its use as a primary screening test for acoustic neuroma detection. The advantages of the ABR as a diagnostic test for the detection of eighth nerve disorders were also demonstrated by Jerger (1983) who applied decision matrix and information theory analyses to evaluate the efficacy of neuroaudiologic diagnostic tests. The performance of the ABR exceeded the performance of acoustic reflex studies, Bekesy audiometry, and performance-intensity functions for phonetically balanced (PI-PB) monosyllabic words with a sensitivity of 97 percent, specificity of 88 percent, and an efficiency of 91 percent. Acoustic reflex studies followed with a sensitivity of 85 percent, specificity of 70 percent, and an efficiency rating of 78 percent (efficiency was calculated as the ratio between the sum of all true-negative and true-positive cases, including cochlear and retrocochlear diagnoses). In the authors' experience, normal acoustic reflex study results and tone decay results compatible with a cochlear site of lesion and normal PI-PB scores are far more frequent in patients with confirmed acoustic neuromas than normal ABR results. Therefore, we generally rely on the ABR as the definitive audiologic test for the detection and diagnosis of an acoustic neuroma.

The characteristics of an ideal diagnostic test are a high rate of correct diagnoses (hit rate, a low rate of missed diagnoses [false-negatives]) and a low rate of incorrect diagnoses of individuals not presenting with the particular pathology (false-positives). A large percentage of false-negatives would result in many undiagnosed and untreated patients whereas a high percentage of false-positives may result in a large number of patients treated or followed for a disease they do not have. In the diagnosis of tumors of the CPA, there has

been a steady improvement of diagnostic modalities, which culminated with the use of the ABR. Due to the superiority of the ABR as a diagnostic test for acoustic neuroma diagnosis, the remainder of the discussion on audiologic diagnosis of acoustic neuromas will focus on the ABR.

ACOUSTIC NEUROMA DIAGNOSIS WITH THE ABR: PRINCIPLES AND PRACTICES

The ABR is the averaged surface-recorded manifestation of the neuroelectrical activation of auditory neural generators extending from the cochlea to the upper brainstem or lower midbrain level (Moller and Jannetta, 1985; Moller, Jannetta, and Sekhar, 1988). The principle underlying the diagnostic use of the ABR in acoustic neuroma detection is seemingly a simple one: Depending on its size, relative location, and anatomic orientation, a space-occupying lesion in the vicinity of auditory pathways contributing to the genesis of the ABR will either result in the complete absence of an ABR component, or will attenuate its amplitude or delay its latency, or both. This rather simplistic view (which is applicable in some cases) is based in part on the nerve conduction model and on a simplified view of the anatomy of the auditory pathway. Often these principles do not apply because the auditory system is a complex receptor that in itself affects the configuration of the ABR (Keith and Greville, 1987). The complexity of the central auditory pathways further contributes to difficulty in ABR interpretation (Moller et al., 1981). Therefore, when analyzing the ABR for diagnostic purposes, the interaction between the patient's hearing status and the ABR needs to be taken into consideration. A simple example is the total absence of the ABR to an 85 dB nHL click in a patient whose pure tone thresholds exceed 85 dB HL. A lack of attention to the patient's hearing status may result in reporting "an absence of any typical replicable ABR waveforms indicating a high probability of an eighth nerve or brainstem lesion." In order to avoid such haphazard statements, every effort needs to be made to separate end organ from central effects or to compensate for end-organ involvement in order to investigate retrocochlear status.

Differential diagnosis with the ABR involves a hierarchic interpretation strategy. This hierarchy depends on the overall configuration of the response and on hearing status. The first and most basic level of this hierarchy is to determine the presence or absence of an ABR evoked by an appropriate effective stimulus. For instance, if the patient has little or no measurable hearing at frequencies exceeding 500 Hz, one can hardly expect a morphologically "well-defined" response to a 75 dB nHL click. In 93 cases of acoustic neuroma with adequate ABR studies managed at the University of Michigan Medical Center, 25 (27%) cases presented with profound SHL on the affected side, resulting in an inablity to evoke an ABR by stimuli presented at 95 to 100 dB nHL (Telian et al., 1989). The following case is representative of this group:

A 65-year-old woman presented with a 4-year history of progressive bilateral mild to moderate

SHL, low frequency in the right ear, severe to profound on the left. Her audiogram and ABRs are illustrated in Figure 10-1A and Figure 10-1B, respectively. A speech recognition score of 64 percent was obtained in the right ear, whereas no speech information could be obtained from the left. The ABR evoked by right ear stimulation is characterized by normal peak and interpeak latencies and a reduced wave V amplitude. With left ear stimulation at the limits of the equipment (95 dB nHL), there was no response with the exception of a very low amplitude vertex-positive peak with a latency of 10.5 msec. Although the absence of a response with left ear stimulation might have

Figure 10-1. Audiogram (A) and ABR (B) from 65-year-old female patient with a 4-year history of progressive hearing loss and a 3.5-cm left-sided acoustic neuroma.

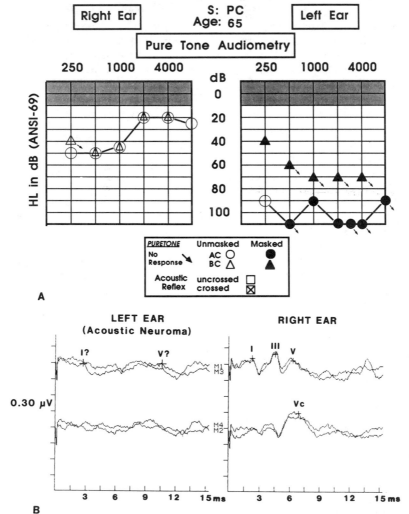

been attributed to the high-frequency hearing loss, the investigation was continued and a 3.5-cm acoustic neuroma was diagnosed by computed tomography (CT).

The second level of the ABR evaluative hierarchy involves an assessment of the morphology of the ABR (determining the presence of all major component peaks and their replicability). Assuming that the recorded waveforms are of an adequate technical quality, the following rules apply. Wave V is the most robust ABR component peak that, in normal-hearing subjects and patients with cochlear pathology, is preserved at near threshold stimulus levels. Wave I is less robust and as a rule is no longer resolved at levels of 40 to 50 dB sensation level. An absent or poorly resolved wave I (with waves III and V present) in moderate to severe SHL is an acceptable deficiency and has no site of lesion diagnostic implications; however, an absence of waves III or V, or both, with a robust and well-defined wave I, is pathognomonic of a lesion affecting auditory brainstem structures medial to the porus acousticus. Absence of components beyond wave I can occur in cases of acoustic neuroma with or without significant hearing loss as illustrated by the two following examples:

The first patient was a 29-year-old woman with a complaint of paresthesia involving the left side of her face. A neurologic evaluation including cerebrospinal fluid studies was unremarkable. The audiometric evaluation was unremarkable as illustrated in Figure 10-2A with the exception of a mild low-frequency SHL in the left ear. Speech audiometry and acoustic reflex studies were normal bilaterally. The ABR illustrated in Figure 10-2B was normal on the right and consisted of wave I only on the left. A magnetic resonance imaging (MRI) scan demonstrated a 5-cm acoustic neuroma, which was resected in two stages through a suboccipital approach (see Figure 10-9).

The next example is a 13-year-old girl who demonstrated progressive clumsiness, ataxia, and a left-sided SHL. She initially presented with a profound SHL in her left ear, illustrated in Figure 10-3A. Hearing in the right ear was normal. The ABR evoked with right ear stimulation exhibited a good morphology with an increased III–V interpeak interval. An attempt to evoke an ABR from the left ear by 95 dB nHL clicks resulted in a well-defined and replicated wave I that was still present at 75 dB nHL (Figure 10-3B). The paradoxical presence of wave I on the left at levels below audiometric thresholds with the absence of the later components coupled with an increased contralat-

eral III–V interpeak latency indicated a high likelihood of a space-occupying lesion involving the left auditory pathway. CT with intravenous contrast confirmed a 5-cm left-sided acoustic neuroma that was subsequently resected in two stages via a suboccipital approach. This case illustrates the value of attempting electrophysiologic testing even if audiometric results suggest that it may be unproductive to do so. The discrepancy between pure tone thresholds and the threshold of wave I (peripheral threshold) demonstrates a true retrocochlear hearing loss.

The third level in the interpretative hierarchy is more objective and quantitative involving the measurement and categorization of absolute and interpeak latencies. If the morphology of the response allows the measurement of I to III and III to V interpeak latencies, these values are compared to the available normative data and are classified as within or outside "normal limits." If wave I is not available, the quantitative evaluation of the ABR usually consists of the measurement of the absolute latency of wave V and a calculation of the ILD-V. Since any type of hearing loss (conductive, cochlear, or retrocochlear) affects the absolute latency of wave V, hearing status needs to be taken into consideration when the interpretation of the ABR is based on ILD-V, which is assessed as a rule with consideration to the magnitude of the hearing loss at 4000 Hz. Selters and Brackmann (1979) recommended to consider an ILD-V of equal to or less than 0.2 msec normal, after a latency adjustment accounting for the effect of high-frequency hearing loss. This was accomplished by subtracting 0.1 msec from the measured latency of wave V for every 10 dB of hearing threshold exceeding 50 dB at 4000 Hz. This latency adjustment decreased the false-positive rate from 24 percent in the uncorrected condition to 8 percent in a group of 266 patients with unilateral SHL. In a group of 94 confirmed acoustic neuroma cases, the same criterion with correction for hearing loss at 4000 Hz resulted in a false-negative rate of 2.3 percent (three patients) (Selters and Brackmann, 1979). Rosenhamer, Lindstrom, and Lundborg (1981) suggested a correction of 0.1 msec for each 10 dB exceeding 30 dB at 4000 Hz. In cases with an intact ABR, the typical and often earliest ABR manifestaton of a CPA tumor is an increase in the I to III interpeak latency on the affected side (Beck et al., 1986; Musiek et al., 1986). The following examples illustrate changes in the I to III interpeak latency in four patients with surgically confirmed acoustic neuromas. Hearing sensitivity in the affected ear

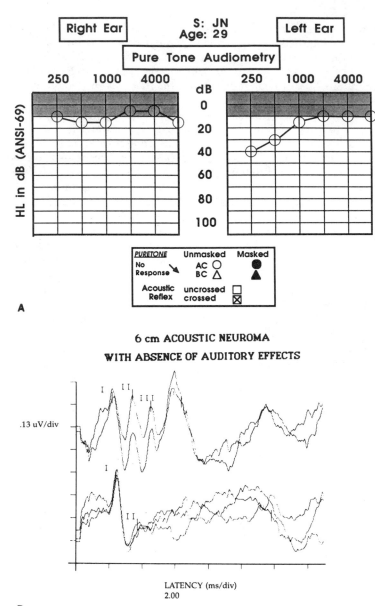

A

6 cm ACOUSTIC NEUROMA

WITH ABSENCE OF AUDITORY EFFECTS

B

Figure 10-2. Audiogram (A) and ABR (B, top trace right ear, bottom trace left ear) from 29-year-old female patient with no auditory complaints and a 6.0-cm left-sided acoustic neuroma.

ranged from normal to moderate to severe high-frequency SHL. The I to III interpeak intervals ranged from 2.70 msec in a case with moderate mid-frequency SHL and a 1.5-cm tumor to 3.60 msec in a case with moderate high-frequency SHL and a 2.5 cm tumor.

Figure 10-4 displays the ABRs from the affected side recorded from the four patients to be discussed in this context. The top left-hand set of ABR traces (Figure 10-4A) are from a 33-year-old female patient with a 2-cm right-sided acoustic neuroma. She presented with a moderate mid-

frequency SHL on the affected side with normal hearing at 250, 500, 4000, and 8000 Hz. Speech recognition was 80 percent with an absence of PB roll over. The patient reported buzzing tinnitus and decreased hearing sensitivity on the affected side. At first glance, her ABR exhibits excellent morphology; however a measurement of the interpeak intervals revealed a prolonged I to III

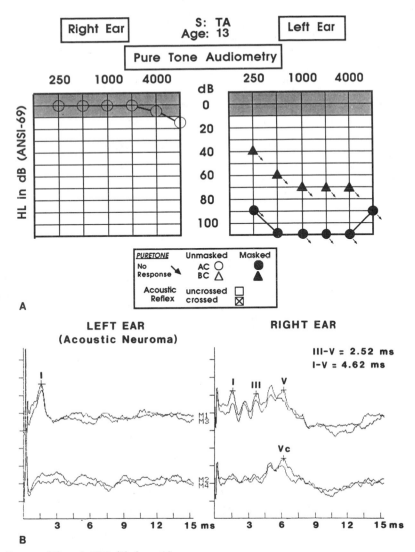

Figure 10-3. Audiogram (A) and ABR (B) from 13-year-old girl with progressive ataxia, left-sided SHL, and a 5.0-cm left-sided acoustic neuroma.

interval (2.70 versus 2.28 msec on the uninvolved side) and hence a prolonged I to V interval (4.56 versus 4.20 msec on the unaffected side) and a normal III to V interval (1.86 msec).

The top right-hand set of replicated ABRs (Figure 10-4B) is from a 24-year-old female patient with a 2.5-cm right-sided acoustic neuroma. The audiogram on the affected side indicated a mild to moderate high-frequency SHL with good speech recognition (72%). As in the previous case, the ABR exhibits excellent morphology (all major component peaks present and well replicated) but an excessively prolonged I to III interpeak interval (3.60 versus 2.04 msec on the uninvolved side).

The bottom left-hand set of replicated ABRs (Figure 10-4C) are from a 35-year-old female patient with a 10-year history of occasional unsteadiness. The frequency and severity of these episodes had increased in the months preceding her first examination. The patient's only hearing-related complaint was a muffled quality of sounds in her left ear with no changes in acuity. Pure tone thresholds were normal with excellent speech recognition scores and normal acoustic reflex studies bilaterally. A CT scan with air contrast demonstrated an intracanalicular acoustic neuroma, about 1 cm in diameter with evidence of bone erosion on the left side. The ABR was characterized by poor overall morphology. The amplitude of wave I was reduced and only partially replicated, whereas the identity of wave III was uncertain. If

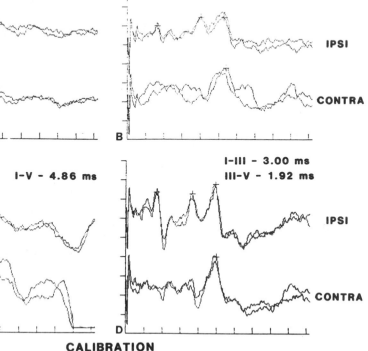

CALIBRATION
1.5 ms and 0.30 uV/div.

Figure 10-4. ABRs from the affected side of four patients with acoustic neuroma. A and B were obtained with supra-aural earphones; C and D were obtained with insert transducers. (A) 2.0-cm right-sided acoustic neuroma; (B) 24-year-old patient with 2.5-cm right-sided acoustic neuroma; (C) 35-year-old patient with 1.0-cm intracanalicular acoustic neuroma; (D) 29-year-old patient with 3.5-cm acoustic neuroma.

wave I is correctly identified, the I to V interpeak latency is 4.86 msec, exceeding the one standard deviation limit used in the authors' laboratory (4.40 msec).

The bottom right-hand set of replicated ABRs (Figure 10-4D) are from a 29-year-old female with a 3.5-year history of progressive hearing loss and tinnitus in her left ear and complaints of nausea, fatigue, and headaches. Her audiogram indicated normal pure tone thresholds in her left ear and a moderate to severe mid-frequency hearing loss on the right. The morphology of the ABR was excellent on the affected side; however, the I to III interpeak interval was prolonged (3.00 versus 1.98 msec on the unaffected side). A 3.5-cm acoustic neuroma was diagnosed by CT and resected by the translabyrinthine approach.

Although in these cases the I to III interpeak latency did not appear to be influenced by the specific audiometric configuration or tumor size, recent evidence shows that the I to V interpeak latency is affected by audiometric configuration. Keith and Greville (1987) found increased I to V

interpeak latencies in patients with notched high-frequency hearing loss with no CPA mass. This is probably due to the higher-frequency neural generators responsible for wave I than for wave V. In the authors' experience the I to III interpeak latency is affected to a lesser extent by the specific audiometric profile and is therefore recommended for neurotologic diagnostic applications whenever those two component peaks are available.

Attention to audiometric configuration and the appropriate use of spectrally constrained tonal stimuli become of the greatest importance especially when the morphology of the ABR does not allow for the measurement of wave I–referenced interpeak latencies. To take advantage of better thresholds at 1000 Hz and attempt to evoke the

ABR with 1000 Hz tone pips to supplement the click evoked ABR, the use of 1000 Hz tone pips gated with a nonlinear function (Blackman) using a 1 msec rise-fall time and a very brief plateau (100 msec) is advocated. At 75 dB nHL, mean wave V latency in a normal-hearing control group was nearly identical to mean wave V latency in a group of patients with high-frequency SHL of cochlear origin with unaffected hearing at 1000 Hz (6.35 msec $\pm$ 0.29 and 6.42 msec $\pm$ 0.16, respectively). In selected cases, the authors have found the use of 1000 Hz tone pips helpful in circumventing the effects of elevated thresholds in the 2000 to 4000 Hz range on the click evoked ABR. Of 17 patients with surgically confirmed acoustic neuromas, 15 of which presented with sloping high-frequency SHL, reliable evidence of retrocochlear involvement could be made from the click evoked ABR in only five cases based on abnormal interpeak latencies and ILD-V. In two patients, wave V was the only replicable and identifiable component for both clicks and the 1000 Hz tone pips, and the diagnosis of retrocochlear involvement was based on prolonged ILD-V for both stimuli. In the remaining 10 patients, the 1000 Hz tonal ABRs were very helpful in the diagnosis of retrocochlear involvement. Some of these were cases where click responses were absent and the diagnosis was based on the significant prolongation of wave V latency for tone pips. In other cases, despite the fact that the ILD-V for clicks normalized after correcting for hearing loss at 4000 Hz as recommended by Selters and Brackmann (1979), the ILD-V for tone pips was significantly prolonged in spite of symmetric hearing sensitivity at 1000 Hz as illustrated by the following case (Telian and Kileny, 1989).

A 38-year-old man came to the authors' clinic with complaints of hearing loss and tinnitus in his left ear. Pure tone audiometry (Figure 10-5A) indicated normal hearing in his right ear and a sloping high-frequency SHL in the left ear. The click evoked ABR had a normal morphology as well as peak and interpeak latencies with right ear stimulation and exhibited a delayed wave V and an absence of a replicable wave I in the patient's left ear (Figure 10-5B). The ILD-V was 0.54 msec for clicks and was reduced to 0.09 msec after correcting for hearing loss at 4000 Hz. Despite better hearing at 1000 Hz, the ILD-V was 1.62 msec for the 1000 Hz tone pips. In addition, the absolute latency of wave V in the left ear exceeded the normative mean value by more than two standard deviations. This was considered to be highly suspicious for a retro-

cochlear lesion, and an acoustic neuroma was confirmed by CT. The patient underwent an uncomplicated translabyrinthine resection.

MEASUREMENT CRITERIA

The diagnostic sensitivity and specificity of latency and interpeak latency measures will depend on the criteria chosen for the definition of normal limits. A conservative criterion such as $\pm$ one standard deviation range for instance will result in few missed cases and a larger number of "false-positive" findings.

An excellent example of the effects of the criteria choice on diagnostic outcome was presented by Thomsen, Terkildsen, and Osterhammel (1978). These authors reviewed ILD-V values in 27 patients with surgically confirmed acoustic neuromas and 70 patients with Ménière's disease. A criterion of ILD-V more than 1.0 msec resulted in 0 percent false-positives and 15 percent false-negatives (i.e., tumor cases classified as nontumor). When an ILD-V criteria of greater than or equal to 0.5 msec was chosen, there was an increase in the false-positive rate to 11 percent and a reduction of the false-negative rate to 4 percent (one tumor case classified as nontumor). An ILD-V criterion of 0.3 msec left the false-negative rate at 4 percent but raised the false-positive rate further to 23 percent, clearly an undesirable effect.

Mangham (1987) investigated the performance of ABR and sinusoidal harmonic acceleration tests and their cost-effectiveness in the diagnosis of acoustic neuroma. The study included 74 patients with acoustic tumors and 78 controls. Overall, the ABR outperformed single harmonic acceleration alone or in combination with the ABR and proved to be more cost-effective than a protocol including both ABR and sinusoidal harmonic acceleration. Using the Selters and Brackmann criterion for ABR positivity (ILD = V > 0.2 msec), Mangham found that the sensitivity of the ABR alone was 94 percent and its specificity was 79 percent. In a hypothetical case with a posterior probability for an acoustic tumor of 0.01, an ILD-V of 0.2 msec increases the probability of an acoustic neuroma to 0.047. The probability of a tumor increases monotonically until the ILD-V reaches a value of 0.7 msec, at which point there is little increase in the posterior probability for a tumor. Cashman and Rossman (1983) compared ABR results between patients with cochlear hearing loss and patients with confirmed acoustic neuromas. If the upper limit for a "normal" ILD-V was considered to be 0.2

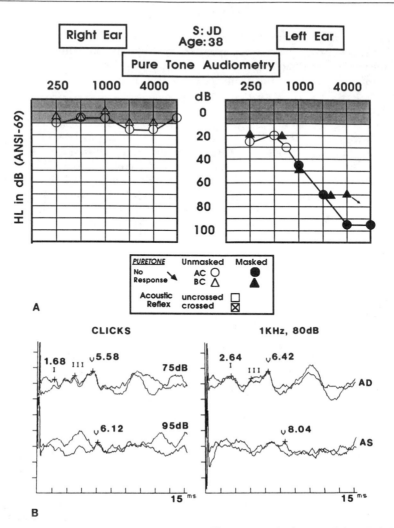

Figure 10-5. Audiogram (A) and click and 1-kHz tonal ABR (B) from a 38-year-old male patient with left-sided acoustic neuroma.

msec, all patients with confirmed tumors of the CPA and 7 percent of the patients with no tumors were classified as "retrocochlear." If the upper limit was raised to 0.4 msec, only 3 percent of patients without tumors were misclassified as "retrocochlear" along with all confirmed tumors still detected. Based on normative data collected in the authors' laboratory and our experience with confirmed acoustic neuromas, our criteria for a positive test result are as follows:

I–III ≥ 2.3 msec; III–V ≥ 2.1 msec;
I–V ≥ 4.4 msec; ILD-V ≥ 0.4 msec;
ILD-V (1000 Hz tone pips) ≥ 0.60 msec.

The incidence of false-negative ABR in acoustic neuroma patients in the authors' series was 2 percent (Telian et al., 1989). This compares favorably

with other large series. Selters and Brackmann (1979) found a 4 percent false-negative rate in a series of 94 patients with surgically confirmed acoustic tumors. Glasscock et al. (1985) presented a series of 49 acoustic neuromas in which there was one false-negative ABR (2%). This patient had normal hearing and was being evaluated for unilateral tinnitus. A 1.5-cm tumor was discovered using a posterior fossa myelogram. Barrs et al. (1985) reported on the diagnostic evaluation of a series of 305 acoustic neuromas. Five false-negative ABRs occurred out of 229 patients tested for a rate of 2 percent. Four of these patients had abnormalities on a CT scan of the temporal bone with intravenous contrast enhancement. In the fifth case, further diagnostic evaluation was pursued because of a family history of bilateral acoustic neuromas, and a tiny intracanalicular acoustic neuroma was found. It is conceivable that with less invasive imaging modalities available, more acoustic tumors will be identified before they produce suspicious ABR findings, leading to an increase in the incidence of "false-negative" ABRs.

RADIOGRAPHIC IMAGING IN THE EVALUATION OF RETROCOCHLEAR PATHOLOGY

Since the mid-1970s, remarkable advances have been made in radiographic imaging of the auditory system. The development of CT, coupled with refinements of software to process the images, has resulted in the ability to display the temporal bone in fine detail. The CT has become the imaging modality used almost exclusively for the radiographic evaluation of the temporal bone and is also useful in imaging the rest of the auditory pathway but recently has been supplanted in quality by MRI. This discussion will center on the diagnosis of acoustic neuroma, which composes greater than 80 percent of posterior fossa lesions and presents the most complex radiographic challenges.

HISTORICAL DEVELOPMENT OF ACOUSTIC TUMOR IMAGING

Shortly after the development of the diagnostic use of x-rays, these techniques were applied to the study of the temporal bone, and radiographic evidence of internal auditory canal (IAC) erosion could be detected (Lysholm, 1928). The next major development was the design of special x-ray units for examination of the head. As early as 1936, 80 percent of acoustic tumors removed surgically had detectable abnormalities on x-rays of the petrous pyramid (Ebenius, 1934).

In the late 1930s tomography of the temporal bone was introduced, providing a more precise visualization of deeper structures. In 1950, the Polytome machine was introduced, which improved the image quality of tomography by using a hypocycloidal trajectory. These two techniques were far superior to plain x-rays for the diagnosis of chronic otitis media, but considerable debate centered on whether any additional benefit in acoustic tumor diagnosis was obtained. The early

experience from the Otologic Medical Group in the mid-1960s indicated that plain x-rays were adequate, demonstrating abnormalities in 85 percent of tumors (Crabtree and Gardner, 1979). Valvassori (1974) advocated the use of tomography to overcome problems of superimposition of superficial structures on the IAC but only demonstrated abnormal findings in 78 percent of the tomographic films obtained from acoustic neuroma patients. His criteria for a positive study were based on evidence of bone erosion or a 2-mm difference in the width of the suspect IAC. Meanwhile, Crabtree and Gardner (1979) demonstrated that high-quality plain films were normal in only 8.9 percent of 688 acoustic neuroma patients. They considered that high-quality plain films, including a Stenver's, transorbital, and fronto-occipital views were equivalent in sensitivity to tomography. The shortcoming of both plain x-rays and tomography is failure to detect tumors in the CPA that had not yet produced erosion of the IAC.

The next major development was the introduction of positive contrast material, which was instilled into the cerebrospinal fluid through a lumbar puncture. Iophendylate (Pantopaque) was introduced for use in the posterior fossa in 1955. Initially, approximately 10 cc was injected and the posterior fossa examined using fluoroscopy. This technique was later refined so that only 1 cc of contrast was injected and directed toward the IAC by positioning of the patient, followed by polytomography of the IAC (Hitselberger and House, 1968). This study was used to confirm the presence of a mass lesion when audiologic findings or routine x-rays suggested an acoustic neuroma. Although this test was not ideal because it involved an invasive procedure, as well as the risk of severe headache and back pain in approximately 5 percent of patients, it was very specific with only one false-positive in 2500 cases (Britton, 1979). It also carried a very small risk of serious neurologic complications.

COMPUTED TOMOGRAPHY

CT was introduced in the mid-1970s. The radiographic images produced by the first-generation scanners were extremely crude, and only the largest acoustic neuromas could be reliably identified. Although 95 percent of tumors larger than 2.5 cm could be detected, smaller tumors were usually overlooked (Wong and Brackmann, 1981). Modern CT scans can take thin sections

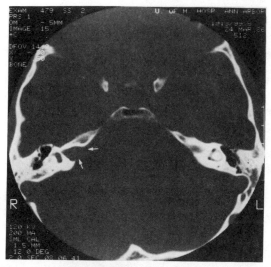

Figure 10-6. High resolution CT scan of temporal bone using algorithm designed to demonstrate bony detail. Findings include widening of internal auditory meatus on the right (small arrows) and faint tumor blush in canal.

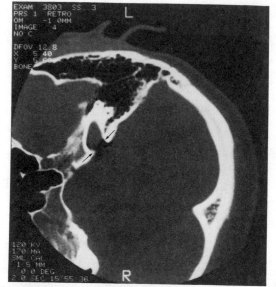

Figure 10-7. Air contrast CT meatography demonstrating tumor in internal auditory canal and air outlining the neurovascular bundle in the cerebellopontine angle (arrows). This tumor was not detected on a routine CT with intravenous contrast.

through the posterior fossa and reliably identify greater than 90 percent of tumors larger than 1.5 cm, as illustrated in Figure 10-6 (axial section, approximately parallel to an imaginary line drawn between lateral canthus and external ear canal; patient's feet are pointing to the viewer, therefore the patient's right side is on the left side of the figure). The combined use of ABR testing and a high-quality CT scan with intravenous contrast will detect greater than 99 percent of acoustic neuromas (Barrs et al., 1985).

COMPUTED TOMOGRAPHY WITH AIR CONTRAST

After the refinement of CT, iophendylate myelography was rapidly replaced by the use of air contrast studies. A small amount (2–4 cc) of oxygen or carbon dioxide is injected via a lumbar puncture and directed toward the CPA. If no tumor is present, the gas fills the IAC and outlines the eighth nerve trunk entering the temporal bone. Figure 10-7 illustrates the air contrast CT myelography imaging of a small intracanalicular tumor. The outline of the neurovascular bundle in the CPA demonstrates that the tumor is confined to the IAC (axial section of left temporal bone and CPA; the patient's left ear is at the top and the occipital bone on the right side). A normal study is considered to be highly reliable in excluding mass lesions. Although this technique significant-

ly decreased the incidence of headache and other complications of iophendylate injection, it had a higher incidence of false-positive findings (Barrs et al., 1984). As in iophendylate studies, it still requires that the patient submit to a lumbar puncture.

MAGNETIC RESONANCE IMAGING

In the mid-1980s, MRI was introduced. This noninvasive imaging modality is capable of identifying even the tiniest tumors. Figure 10-8 shows the MRI of the case illustrated in Figure 10-7 (axial section). A portion of the neuroepithelium of the semicircular canals and ampullae is visible on the right side; on the left side, the lateral semicircular canal, utricle, and tumor are clearly visible. Patients who have implanted metallic devices or who are extremely claustrophobic cannot undergo MRI testing. In all other patients, MRI is the diagnostic modality of choice in the diagnosis of acoustic neuroma when CT scan is equivocal or the patient is allergic to intravenous contrast material. Because of the increased availability of MRI imaging facilities, this modality is quickly replacing CT as the initial study performed when acoustic neuroma is suspected. In 1989, the use of gadolinium-DPTA, a paramagnetic contrast agent, was approved for clinical purposes. The use of gadolinium has allowed detection of acoustic

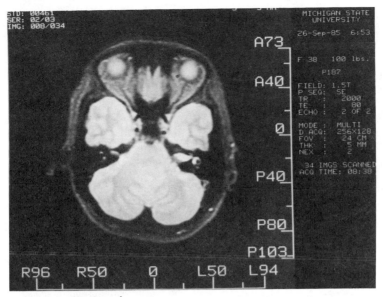

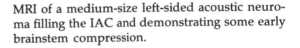

Figure 10-8. Magnetic resonance imaging of same patient as in Figure 10-7 shows high-signal intensity on T_2-weighted images typical of acoustic neuroma.

MRI of a medium-size left-sided acoustic neuroma filling the IAC and demonstrating some early brainstem compression.

RADIOGRAPHIC TEST SELECTION

Although most patients with acoustic neuroma will present with an SHL in the affected ear and an abnormal ABR, approximately 5 percent of patients will have a normal pure tone audiogram, and at least 2 percent of patients will have a normal ABR. It is desirable to establish the diagnosis of acoustic neuroma early on in every case where such a tumor is causing auditory or vestibular symptoms. Although the ABR is a very sensitive tool in the neurotologic evaluation in qualified hands, it does not replace appropriate radiographic investigation. Because of the small rate of false-negative ABRs in acoustic tumors, and the much larger rate (25%) in other posterior fossa lesions, it is the authors' opinion that radiographic evaluation should not be deferred in the face of a normal ABR when other signs and symptoms suggest the possibility of a mass lesion. The choice of CT or MRI should be individualized depending on the nature of the clinical problem and the results of audiologic testing. Local considerations, such as availability, cost, and technical quality, are factors that must be considered. If there is a family history of bilateral acoustic tumors, evaluation with MRI is preferred. It will be interesting to see how much the false-negative ABR rate increases in series of tumors identified using advanced imaging techniques, such as MRI.

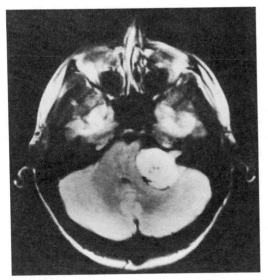

Figure 10-9. Axial section of a large acoustic neuroma demonstrated on MRI (same patient illustrated in Figure 10-2).

neuromas as small as 2 mm in size. Figure 10-9 illustrates the MRI of a large acoustic neuroma from the patient whose ABR and audiogram are shown in Figure 10-2. This is a large left-sided cerebellopontine mass compressing the brainstem and cerebellum (axial section, the patient is supine). Figure 10-10 illustrates a coronal section

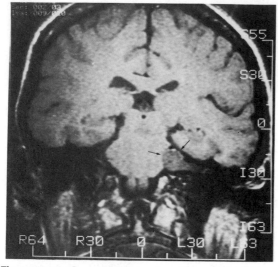

Figure 10-10. Coronal section of medium-size acoustic neuroma demonstrated on MRI and showing the involvement of the internal auditory canal and early brainstem compression (arrows).

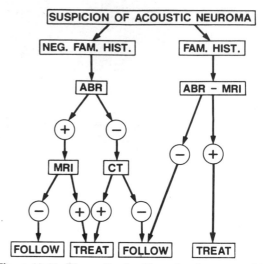

Figure 10-11. Diagnostic algorithm, showing approach to patient with suspected acoustic neuroma.

It is clear at the present time that a normal ABR does not completely exclude the diagnosis of acoustic neuroma. In addition, it is much more common for lesions of the CPA other than acoustic neuroma to present with normal ABRs.

The authors' 1988 diagnostic algorithm is pictured in Figure 10-11. It is our opinion that patients with a family history of bilateral acoustic neuromas should undergo MRI testing regardless of their audiologic findings because of the high priority of identifying and removing tiny tumors in this population. In patients without such a history, a normal ABR and a negative high-quality CT scan with intravenous contrast enhancement constitute an adequate evaluation for acoustic neuroma. When the ABR suggests retrocochlear pathology, a CT scan with intravenous contrast will identify most of the patients with acoustic neuroma. A small fraction of patients will have tiny tumors that will result in a negative or equivocal CT scan. These patients should then undergo an MRI study. Increasingly, MRI is being used as the initial study in the investigation of a suspected acoustic neuroma because of its high sensitivity rate and lack of radiation exposure. The major drawback to adopting this protocol on a routine basis is the higher cost of the study and limited availability in certain geographic regions. An air CT or Pantopaque myelogram is required only in the rare event that the MRI is equivocal. Since the introduction of gadolinium enhance-

ment, this problem has been virtually eliminated. Patients with intravenous contrast allergy should undergo MRI as the initial radiographic modality.

The extent of the radiographic work-up depends somewhat on the philosophy of the surgeon regarding the management of tiny tumors. Those who feel that early resection is desirable, resulting in higher rates of facial nerve preservation and a chance for preservation of hearing, will pursue the diagnosis of small tumors. Obviously, if the surgeon does not endorse resection of tiny tumors, or if the patient is elderly, it is not necessary to pursue further evaluation if the CT scan is negative.

SURGICAL MANAGEMENT

Recent advances in the management of CPA tumors have allowed contemporary surgeons the ability to significantly reduce postoperative morbidity and mortality. Increased physician awareness, advances in audiologic and radiologic techniques for early diagnosis of tumors, improved surgical approaches and instrumentation, and safer anesthetic techniques have combined to allow more effective extirpation of tumors in the CPA.

Philosophically, the neurosurgeon and neurotologist are increasingly aware of the benign biologic behavior of most CPA, and thus desire to minimize postoperative neurologic residue. During the past 20 years, techniques to improve postoperative facial nerve function have rapidly improved, and in recent years hearing has also been preserved in a limited number of patients with acoustic neuroma. Increased knowledge of the natural history of these lesions permits careful observation of small tumors or subtotal removal of large tumors in the elderly.

Multiple surgical approaches are available to the surgeon for removal of CPA tumors. In general, although surgeons increasingly agree that the surgical approach for removal of these lesions should be determined by the tumor size and preoperative hearing levels, legitimate differences of opinion still remain. The most common contemporary surgical approaches used are the middle cranial fossa, the translabyrinthine, and the suboccipital/retrosigmoid.

MIDDLE FOSSA APPROACH

The middle fossa route is recommended for those patients with useful hearing and small tumors confined to the IAC. If the acoustic neuroma extends into the posterior fossa, the middle fossa approach is inadequate, due to its limited access to the CPA. The IAC must be widely opened, especially in the lateral extent, to allow identification and dissection of the facial nerve. One disadvantage of this approach is that the facial nerve is frequently superior to the tumor surface and the surgeon must work past the facial nerve to remove the tumor from its deep surface. Hearing preservation requires maintenance of the cochlear nerve and intact cochlear blood supply via the internal auditory artery. Extirpation of the tumor usually proceeds medially after identification of the facial nerve in the lateral fundus of the canal. The anterior inferior cerebellar artery may present in the canal and must be preserved.

Large series suggest that few tumors are amenable to removal by this route. Glasscock et al. (1982) attempted middle fossa excision of acoustic neuroma in only 10 of this series of 139 cases and preserved hearing in 6. House (1961) found only 5 cases of tumor confined to the IAC in a series of 200 cases, and in 4, preserved hearing. House attempted middle fossa removal of acoustic tumors in 14 additional patients with some degree of tumor extension into the CPA. Hearing was preserved in only 3 patients, leading him to recommend translabyrinthine excision of such tumors in the future.

Preservation of cochlear function assumes greatest priority in an only hearing ear or in the patient with bilateral acoustic neuromas. The latter group tends to be young (in the second or third decades) with a familial history of bilateral acoustic neuromas, but often without the cutaneous stigmata of neurofibromatosis. Histologically, bilateral tumors tend to be neurofibromas rather than neuromas and are more infiltrative into the substance of the auditory nerve. Thus, hearing preservation is considered to be more difficult, and there is an increased risk of leaving residual microscopic tumor.

TRANSLABYRINTHINE APPROACH

For most otolaryngologists, the translabyrinthine approach to the CPA has provided a new standard for the reduction of postoperative morbidity and mortality in acoustic tumor surgery. This approach appears to have achieved a real reduction in patient morbidity, particularly postoperative facial nerve dysfunction, while retaining a high percentage of complete tumor removal. Although this approach has a higher incidence of postoperative cerebrospinal fluid leaks and meningitis, most commonly these are easily controlled. Since House (1979) popularized this approach, many surgeons have considered this the preferred surgical approach for the removal of small to large tumors with diminished hearing. With the translabyrinthine approach, the vestibular labyrinth is removed, resulting in an obligatory loss of residual hearing. Although presently there is interest in the preservation of hearing, many surgeons will not attempt hearing preservation unless the speech recognition threshold is at least 30 dB, with a speech recognition score of 70 percent or better, and unless the tumor is less than 2 cm. Historically, one advantage of the translabyrinthine approach is the improved ability to preserve facial nerve integrity. Intraoperative electrophysiologic monitoring of facial function has improved the preservation of the integrity of the facial nerve (Niparko et al., 1989).

SUBOCCIPITAL/RETROSIGMOID APPROACH

The suboccipital retrosigmoid approach to the CPA is a classic neurosurgical approach to this area described by Cushing and later refined by Dandy. Their innovations in management of these tumors during the early 1900s resulted in decreased mortality rates from 80 to 10 percent. Subsequently, the introduction of microneurosurgical techniques has continued the improvement in postoperative mortality and morbidity rates. Although many neurosurgical and combined neurosurgical-neurotologic teams continue to use the suboccipital route as their standard approach to acoustic tumors, others have returned to this approach as a method of hearing preservation for removal of selected extracanalicular acoustic neuromas.

The decision to attempt hearing preservation in the patient with a unilateral acoustic neuroma depends largely on the size of the tumor, residual hearing in the affected ear, and the status of the contralateral ear. Clemis (1984) discussed these issues and noted that some advocates of hearing preservation surgery fail to recognize that most patients benefit only minimally from preservation of their residual hearing because of the degree of their loss. In addition, efforts to preserve hearing in tumors extending into the CPA are presently at best 50 percent successful or less, depending on the size of the tumor. This may relate to the amount of trauma to the cochlear nerve or to disruption of the cochlear blood supply during tumor dissection. Because of the difficulties in reliably preserving hearing by the suboccipital route, and the low incidence of suitable candidates for hearing preservation, many authors feel that all unilateral tumors outside the IAC should be approached via the translabyrinthine route instead of the suboccipital approach, regardless of hearing status. Tos and Thomsen (1982) cited the difference in mortality rates, incidence of morbid complications, and rates of functional preservation of the facial nerve as adequate reasons to abandon efforts at hearing preservation; however, recent series of suboccipital removals have mortality rates that compare favorably with large neurotologic series. It is likely that mortality figures in many older series are influenced by a disproportionate number of larger tumors. It is reasonable to expect that suboccipital removal can theoretically be accomplished with morbidity rates comparable to the translabyrinthine approach.

REFERENCES

Barrs, D. M., Brackmann, D. E., Olson, J. E., & House, W. F. (1985). Changing concepts of acoustic neuroma diagnosis. *Archives of Otolaryngology, 111*, 17–21.

Barrs, D. M., Luxford, W. M., Becker, T. S., & Brackmann, D. E. (1984). Computed tomography with gas cisternography for detection of small acoustic tumors. *Archives of Otolaryngology, 110*, 535–537.

Beck, H. J., Beatty, C. W., Harner, S. G., & Ilstrup, D. M. (1986). Acoustic neuromas with normal pure tone hear-

ing levels. *Otolaryngology — Head and Neck Surgery, 94*, 96–103.

Britton, B. H. (1979). Lophendylate examination of the posterior fossa in diagnosis of cerebellopontine angle tumors. In W. F. House & C. M. Luetje (Eds.), *Acoustic tumors: Vol. I. Diagnosis* (pp. 279–290). Baltimore: University Park Press.

Carhart, R. (1957). Clinical determination of abnormal auditory adaptation. *Archives of Otolaryngology, 65*, 32–39.

Cashman, M. Z., & Rossman, R. N. (1983). Diagnostic features of the auditory brainstem response in identifying cerebellopontine angle tumors. *Scandinavian Audiology, 12*, 35–41.

Clemis, J. D. (1984). Hearing conservation in acoustic tumor surgery: Pros and cons. *Otolaryngology — Head and Neck Surgery, 92*, 15–161.

Crabtree, J. A., & Gardner, G. (1979). Radiographic findings in cerebellopontine angle tumors. In W. F. House & C. M. Luetje (Eds.), *Acoustic tumors: Vol. I. Diagnosis* (pp. 241–252). Baltimore: University Park Press.

Cushing, H. (1917). *Tumors of the nervous acusticus and the syndrome of the cerebellopontine angle.* Philadelphia: Saunders.

Ebenius, B. (1934). The results of examination of the petrous bone in auditory nerve tumors. *Acta Radiologica, 15*, 284–290.

Glasscock, M. E., Hays, J. W., Josey, A. F., Jackson, C. G., & Whitaker, S. R. (1982). Middle fossa approach for acoustic tumor removal and preservation of hearing. In D. E. Brackmann (Ed.), *Neurological surgery of the ear and skull base* (pp. 223–226). New York: Raven Press.

Glasscock, M. E., Jackson, C. G., Josey, A. F., Dickens, J. R. E., & Wiet, R. J. (1985). Brainstem evoked response audiometry in a clinical practice. *Laryngoscope, 89*, 1021–1035.

Graham, M. D. (1979). Acoustic tumors: Selected histories and patient reviews. In W. F. House & C. M. Luetje (Eds.), *Acoustic tumors: Vol. I. Diagnosis* (pp. 151–198). Baltimore: University Park Press.

Hitselberger, W. E., & House, W. F. (1968). Polytome-Pantopaque: A technique for the diagnosis of small acoustic tumors. *Acta Otolaryngologica* (Stockholm), *65*, 555–564.

House, W. F. (1961). Surgical exposure of the internal auditory canal and its contents through the middle cranial fossa. *Laryngoscope, 71*, 1363–1385.

House, W. F. (1968). Case summaries. *Archives of Otolaryngology, 88*, 689.

House, W. F. (1979). A history of acoustic tumor surgery. In W. F. House & C. M. Luetje (Eds.), *Acoustic tumors: Vol. I. Diagnosis* (pp. 3–32). Baltimore: University Park Press.

Jerger, S. (1983). Decision matrix and information theory analyses in the evaluation of neuroaudiologic tests. *Seminars in Hearing, 4*, 121–131.

Johnson, E. W. (1979). Results of auditory tests in acoustic tumor patients. In W. F. House & C. M. Luetje (Eds.), *Acoustic tumors: Vol. I. Diagnosis* (pp. 209–224). Baltimore: University Park Press.

Keith, W. J., & Greville, K. (1987). Effects of audiometric configuration on the auditory brainstem response. *Ear & Hearing, 8*, 49–55.

Lysholm, E. (1928). Contribution to the technique of projection in roentgenological examination of pars petrosa. *Acta Radiologica, 9*, 54–66.

Mangham, C. A. (1987). Decision analysis of auditory brainstem responses and rotational vestibular tests in acoustic tumor diagnosis. *Otolaryngology — Head and Neck Surgery, 96*, 22–29.

Moberg, A., Anderson, H., & Wedenberg, E. (1969). In C. A. Hamberger & J. Wersall (Eds.), *Nobel Symposium 10: Disorders of the skull base region*. Stockholm: Almqvist & Wiksell.

Moller, A. R., & Jannetta, P. J. (1985). Neural generators of the auditory brainstem response. In J. T. Jacobson (Ed.), *The auditory brainstem response* (pp. 13–31). Boston: College-Hill Press.

Moller, A. R., Jannetta, P. J., & Sekhar (1988). Contributions from the auditory nerve to the brain-stem auditory evoked potentials (BAEPs): Results of intracranial recordings in man. *Electroencephalography and Clinical Neurophysiology, 71*, 198–211.

Moller, A. R., Jannetta, P. J., Bennett, M., & Moller, M. B. (1981). Intracranially recorded responses from the human auditory nerve: New insights into the origin of brainstem evoked potentials. *Electroencephalography and Clinical Neurophysiology, 52*, 18–27.

Morrison, A. W. (1975). *Management of sensorineural deafness*. London: Butterworths.

Musiek, F. E., Kibbe-Michal, K., Geurkink, N. A., Josey, A. F., & Glasscock, M. E., III. (1986). ABR results in patients with posterior fossa tumors and normal pure tone hearing. *Otolaryngology — Head and Neck Surgery, 94*, 568–573.

Nager, G. T. (1969). Acoustic neuromas. Pathology and differential diagnosis. *Archives of Otolaryngology, 89*, 252.

Niparko, J. K., Kileny, P. R., Kemink, J. L., Lee, H. M., & Graham, M. D. (1989). Neurophysiological intraoperative monitoring II. Facial nerve function. *American Journal of Otology, 10*, 55–61.

Pool, J. L., Pava, A. A., & Greenfield, E. C. (1970). *Acoustic nerve tumors. Early diagnosis and treatment*. Springfield, IL: Charles Thomas.

Rosenhamer, J. H., Lindstrom, B., & Lundborg, T. (1981). On the use of click evoked electric brainstem responses in audiological diagnosis. III. Latencies in cochlear hearing loss. *Scandinavian Audiology, 10*, 3–11.

Schuknecht, H. (1974). *Pathology of the ear*. Cambridge: Harvard University Press.

Selters, W. A., & Brackmann, D. E. (1977). Acoustic tumor detection with brainstem electric response audiometry. *Archives of Otolaryngology, 103*, 181–187.

Selters, W. A., & Brackmann, D. E. (1979). Brainstem electric response audiometry in acoustic tumor detection. In W. F. House & C. M. Luetje (Eds.), *Acoustic tumor: Vol. I. Diagnosis* (pp. 225–236). Baltimore: University Park Press.

Telian, S. A., & Kileny, P. R. (1989). Usefulness of 1000 Hz tone-burst evoked responses in the diagnosis of acoustic neuroma. *Otolaryngology — Head and Neck Surgery, 101*, 466–471.

Telian, S. A., Kileny, P. R., Niparko, J. K., Kemink, J. L., & Graham, M. D. (1989). Normal auditory brainstem response in patients with acoustic neuroma. *Laryngoscope, 99*, 10–14.

Thomsen, J., Terkildsen, K., & Osterhammel, P. (1978). Auditory brainstem responses in patients with acoustic neuroma. *Scandinavian Audiology, 7*, 179.

Tos, M., & Thomsen, J. (1982). The price of preservation of hearing in acoustic neuroma surgery. *Annals of Otology, Rhinology, and Laryngology, 91*, 240–245.

Valvassori, G. E. (1974). Benign tumors of the temporal bone. *Radiology Clinics of North America, 12*, 533–542.

Wong, M. L., & Brackmann, D. E. (1981). Computed cranial tomography in acoustic tumor diagnosis. *Journal of the American Medical Association, 245*, 2497–2500.

CHAPTER 11

Central Auditory Disorders

Robert W. Keith • Susan Jerger

The clinical focus of central auditory testing in adults and children has taken very different approaches. While early research on adults was conducted with known central lesions, investigations on children were generally directed toward populations with language and learning difficulties and, presumably, disorders of auditory perception. In few studies was a known lesion identified, although the presence of abnormalities of the auditory pathway was often inferred. Thus, while studies of adults proceeded from the identification of central auditory lesions to functional auditory processing, studies of children developed from the identification of auditory perceptual disorders, with little documentation of the presence or locus of known central lesions. The difficulty of relating central auditory findings in these two populations lies fundamentally with the plasticity of the developing brain in younger subjects. With lesions in the maturing auditory system, other areas of the brain may take over functions usually supported by the impaired region. In addition, different rates of maturation, genetics, and other factors have far different implications for interpretation of results from children than from adult populations.

This chapter will summarize the research on testing for lesions of the central auditory pathways of adult patients, review the literature on the assessment of auditory processing disorders in adults, and discuss future applications for central auditory testing. In addition, the value of identifying patterns of test results in children with known lesions of the central auditory pathway will be discussed. Understanding those relationships leads to a better understanding of children with language and learning disorders who have no known organic basis for their learning problem.

TESTING FOR CENTRAL AUDITORY LESIONS IN ADULTS

HISTORICAL ORIENTATION

Speech audiometry has been used in the assessment of central auditory disorders for many years. As early as 1954, Bocca, Calearo, and Cassinari stated that "modifications of the audiometric threshold for pure tones are only rarely demonstrable in cases of temporal lobe tumors." In subsequent research spanning several years, Bocca et al. reported their systematic investigations of the ability to detect cortical and brainstem lesions using sensitized speech audiometry. These studies began an era of investigation of central auditory testing that sparked widespread and continued interest among audiologists and other professionals. What followed was a series of publications documenting the stimulus and response parameters that resulted in identification of lesions of the central auditory pathways. These studies also demonstrated the sensitivity and specificity of test results for identifying the presence of auditory pathway pathology, the site of lesion, and the affected hemisphere.

Recently studies of auditory processing abilities in patients with diffuse brain pathology have been conducted. These studies represent a different approach to the assessment of communication disorders in the adult population. They are among the categories mentioned by Jerger (1970) when central auditory testing was emerging from its infancy stage. Jerger stated that the purposes of speech audiometry included both medical diagnosis and assessment of handicap.

In a review of their own germinal studies, Calearo and Antonelli (1973) stated that "the approach to the problem of hearing function in central nervous system (CNS) disease may be aimed toward two different targets: either clinic/diagnostic, or experimental research on hearing integration." They defined *hearing integration* as the evaluation of auditory performance when a lesion disrupts the normal flow of the hearing process.

PRINCIPLES

The principle that pure tone and undistorted speech audiometry is ineffective in identifying central auditory pathway lesions was well known in the early days of central auditory testing. The need for presenting speech material with reduced normal speech redundancy was established by the early 1960s. The concept of *sensitized speech tests* was summarized by Teatini (1970) as follows: Normal speech is highly redundant in terms of frequency content, intensity, and linguistic content. Similarly, the neural pathway of the normal human auditory system is also physiologically redundant with the number of neurons, and opportunity for interneural connections. Therefore, the practical implication for identification of central pathway lesions or auditory processing disorders is that a speech signal of reduced acoustic (extrinsic) redundancy must be put in series with an auditory pathway of reduced (intrinsic) redundancy in order for speech intelligibility to suffer. This principle is shown in Table 11-1.

The redundancy of the speech signal can be reduced in several ways. Monaural speech tests are sensitized by electronic filtering, interruption of the speech signal, time compression, and presentation of the speech in noise. Other methods of challenging the central auditory system, presumably at the level of the brainstem, include binaural fusion of low- and high-pass filtered speech presented to separate ears (Matzker, 1959), Speech with Alternating Masking (Jerger, 1964), and Synthetic Sentence Identification with Ipsilateral Competing Message (SSI-ICM) (Jerger, 1973). Tests of cortical integrity include binaural switching of the speech signal and a number of competing (dichotic) speech tests with signals ranging from consonant-vowel (CV) syllables (Kimura, 1961), digits (Stephens and Thornton, 1976), monosyllabic words (Keith, 1986), spondees (Katz, 1962), sentences (Willeford, 1977), and Synthetic Sentence Identification with Contralateral Competing Message (SSI-CCM) (Jerger, 1970).

ANATOMY AND PHYSIOLOGY OF THE AUDITORY SYSTEM

Before performing tests of central auditory function, whether for purposes of site of lesion diagnosis in the central auditory nervous system (CANS) or determining auditory perceptional abilities, it is important to be familiar with the neuroanatomy of the auditory system. At the precortical level, the auditory signals travel from the cochlear hair cells through the various pathways of the brainstem to the medial geniculate body then rise homolaterally to the auditory cortex. At the cortical level, the signal is processed through the primary auditory reception area in the temporal lobe transverse gyrus of Heschl to the association areas of the brain. Also interhemispheric transfer of information occurs through the corpus callosum, the large body of myelinated fibers that connects the two cerebral hemispheres. Figure 11-1 shows the major neural auditory pathways of the brainstem and auditory cortex.

Some of the physiologic functions important for processing neural signals include tonotopic organization; tuning; frequency selectivity of single neural units; inhibition of one stimulus as a result of ·a second stimulus; adaptation; intensity coding represented by the number of participating fibers; temporal coding by phase-locked neural discharge or volley; and binaural interaction through neural integration for spatial representa-

TABLE 11-1. PRINCIPLE OF REDUCED REDUNDANCY UNDERLYING SENSITIZED SPEECH TESTS

Redundancy of message	Redundancy of subject	Intelligibility
(Extrinsic)	(Intrinsic)	
Normal	Normal	Good
Reduced	Normal	Rather good
Normal	Reduced	Rather good
Normal	Reduced	Poor

Source: Adapted from Teatini, G. P. (1970). Sensitized speech tests: Results in normal subjects. In C. Rojskjaer (Ed.), *Speech audiometry*. Odense, Denmark: Danavox.

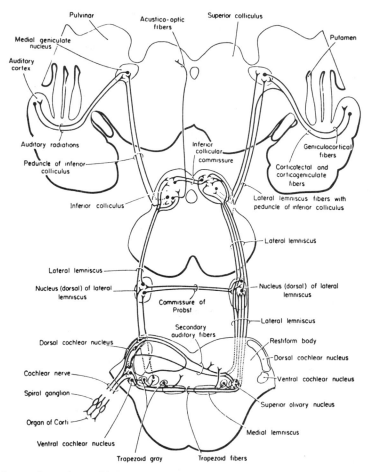

Figure 11-1. Auditory pathways from the cochlea to the cerebral cortex. (From Keith, R. W. [1988]. Central auditory tests. In N. J. Lass et al. [Eds.], *Handbook of speech-language pathology and audiology* [p. 1216]. Toronto: B. C. Decker. With permission.)

tion. In addition to the afferent pathways, an efferent system feeds back from higher auditory levels to the cochlea.

In summary, the auditory nervous system presents a complex interaction of neural signals that integrate acoustic signals from the auditory periphery at nearly all levels of the CANS. It is important to remember that this pathway is not a simple passive conductor of electrical signals, rather a complex functioning of processing occurring at all levels of the auditory system. At the cortical level, this analysis results in meaning something that was not present in the acoustic signal. It is equally important to remember that these neural structures are located within compact spaces and are susceptible to pressure and displacement from space-occupying lesions. These anatomic

and physiologic facts have significant implications for the difficulty of determining the precise site of lesion using behavioral audiometric tests. They also indicate the many possibilities for perceptual dysfunction resulting from neurologic abnormalities at any level of the auditory system.

PRECAUTIONS

Specific techniques for administering a central auditory test battery are beyond the scope of this chapter. Instructions on test procedures can be found in original references in the scientific literature, in test manuals, and in chapters of several textbooks on this subject (Arnst and Katz, 1982; Keith, 1977; Lasky and Katz, 1983; Pinheiro and Musiek, 1985; Willeford and Burleigh, 1985). The general principles of test administration are familiar to audiologists. Both monaural and binaural tests of sensitized speech materials are subject to influences of equipment, examiner, and patient that have nothing to do with central lesions. For example, results are affected by the quality of recorded materials, the playback equipment, and stimulus intensity. They are also affected by such subject variables as peripheral hearing impairment (both conductive and sensory), linguistic background, motivation, and intellectual ability.

When a peripheral hearing loss is present, it is difficult to determine whether poor performance is the result of peripheral (cochlear) distortion or central factors. For example, although some authors are willing to correct the Staggered Spondee Word (SSW) results for patients with cochlear losses and errors of speech recognition (Arnst and Katz, 1982), many clinicians prefer to administer central auditory tests only when peripheral hearing is "normal," in the belief that it is difficult to separate cochlear from retrocochlear influences on the results of the central auditory test. Only one test has been specifically designed to be administered to patients with a peripheral hearing loss — the Dichotic Sentence test (Fifer et al., 1983). The problem of possible contamination of central auditory test results is not trivial, especially when one considers an older population of subjects in whom hearing loss is especially prevalent.

Finally, nonnative English-speaking subjects are likely to yield poor scores on an English language central test battery, based on their linguistic background, even though they have used English as a primary language for communication (Gat and Keith, 1978; Keith et al., 1987; Keith, Tawfik, and Katbamna, 1985).

INTERPRETATION OF RESULTS

Results of sensitized speech tests in normal adults do not show a dominance effect. The possible exception to this is the dichotic CV test that yields a small right ear advantage in normal adults. For adult patients with central lesions, a review of the available literature finds some general consensus, regardless of the test approach used. For example, according to Lynn and Gilroy (1977), there is a distinctive laterality pattern of abnormal auditory findings in patients with temporal lobe lesions known as the *contralateral ear effect*. The pattern performance is relatively normal in the ear ipsilateral to the lesion, with decreased auditory performance in the ear opposite the involved hemisphere.

When lesions of the temporal lobe extend deep toward the midline, there is a *paradoxical ipsilateral ear effect* (Jerger and Jerger, 1981; Lynn and Gil-

roy, 1977; Musiek and Baran, 1987; Olsen, 1983). According to Jerger (1987), this finding results from interruption of the interhemispheric auditory pathways.

When a lesion involves the auditory tracts that decussate via the posterior portion of the corpus callosum, no ipsilateral or contralateral ear effect occurs. There is, however, decreased performance in the ear opposite the nondominant hemisphere (Musiek, 1986; Musiek, Reeves, and Baran, 1985).

Finally, although sites of involvement can be postulated, it is uncertain whether audiologic tests can determine the laterality of a lesion. Olsen (1983) reported that the central auditory system is too complex to allow single patterns of results to be associated with involvement of one hemisphere or the other using dichotic CV tests. A specific example of this is the ipsilateral ear effect seen with patients who have deep lesions involving the cerebral cortex. All of these factors make the identification of the specific site of central lesion difficult, based on the currently available CANS assessment materials.

SENSITIVITY AND SPECIFICITY OF RESULTS

The *sensitivity* of a test battery is defined as "the percent of individuals with a certain problem who are so specified by the test (true positive)." *Specificity* is defined as "the percent of individuals who do not have a certain problem who are so specified by the test (true negative)" (Jerger, 1983; Keith, 1988). Mueller, Sedge, and Salazar (1986) pointed out that most of the auditory studies available on this subject address cochlear versus eighth nerve pathology and few investigations are available that evaluate the question of the central auditory test battery sensitivity and specificity. Lynn and Gilroy (1977) described the relative efficiency of various central auditory tests. They found that in a group of 35 patients with temporal lobe lesions, 85 percent were correctly identified using the SSW test, 74 percent were correctly identified with a low-pass filtered word test, whereas abnormality was identified only in 57 percent with competing sentence material. Results were similar in patients with parietal lesions, but findings were less consistent in patients with brainstem lesions. Lynn and Gilroy did not report attempts to calculate test specificity.

In the single publication available on this subject, Mueller et al. (1986) reported operating characteristics of right ear scores obtained using the SSW, dichotic digit, and CV tests. Their patients had suffered penetrating head injuries and had longstanding documented brain injury. Results indicated that different cutoff scores were required for each of the three tests to obtain maximum sensitivity because of the relative difficulty of the measures. For each test, high sensitivity was obtained at the cost of poor specificity. The best combined effectiveness of the SSW occurred when the cutoff score for the right ear was below 96 percent, for the dichotic digit below 90 percent, and for the CV 63 percent. Mueller et al. cautioned that care should be taken when predicting the presence or absence of injury in individual subjects. Much more research is needed to document sensitivity and specificity of central auditory tests before valid and reliable conclusions may be drawn. Thus, the routine use of such tests in central auditory disorders should be interpreted with caution.

TESTING FOR AUDITORY PROCESSING DISORDERS IN ADULTS

The need for central auditory testing in the future will be to describe functional auditory abilities and breakdown of auditory processing in patients with various brain lesions. These tests complement sophisticated imaging techniques that identify anatomic structure without describing functional disorders related to specific lesions.

There are a number of etiologies of auditory processing disorders in adults including those associated with aging, parkinsonism, chronic alcoholism, Alzheimer's disease, multiple sclerosis, head trauma, stroke, and possibly acquired immunodeficiency syndrome. Further, the identification of auditory perceptual disorders in previously undiagnosed learning-disabled adults can add to the understanding of their social and vocational problems and enhance their ability to compensate for auditory processing deficits. Mueller et al. (1986) stated that results of central auditory tests are useful in detecting injury to the auditory areas of the brainstem or cortex and "can be used to monitor recovery of auditory processing skills and provide a framework for counseling the patient (and the patient's family) concerning their communication capabilities." That application has been addressed in the literature by Grimes et al. (1985) who studied patients with Alzheimer's disease and Bergman et al. (1987) who studied patients with head injury and stroke in order to determine "functional disorders of communication."

When attempting to evaluate the auditory processing abilities of the aging patient, one of the greatest difficulties encountered is separating peripheral from central factors. Nevertheless, a review of the literature indicates that some elderly patients have greater difficulty with sensitized speech tasks, including time-compressed speech and speech in noise, than others with similar audiometric configurations. Marshall (1981) described these dilemmas in detail and discussed the need for further investigation of this population in order to be able to describe the auditory problems of each elderly individual to better serve their rehabilitation needs. Stach, Jerger, and Fleming (1985) reported a longitudinal case study of a patient with central presbycusis. Although their patient showed little change in peripheral hearing sensitivity over a 9-year interval, central auditory function declined substantially. The patient's diminished success as a hearing aid user seemed to parallel the change in central function. This case report points out an important contribution of the central auditory test battery in tracking auditory processing skills in patients and in providing insight to their rehabilitation needs and problems.

In a study with Alzheimer's disease, Grimes et al. (1985) found that central auditory function was measurably poorer than in normal subjects. Significant relationships were observed between dichotic scores and intelligence quotient, cortical atrophy, and glucose metabolism in the left temporal lobe. Their findings of contralateral ear effects of dichotic performance were consistent with models of dichotic listening in other forms of temporal pathology. Grimes et al. suggested that dichotic speech measures may be useful in assessing progression of temporal lobe involvement. These tests can also provide insight into functional impairment in this disease population.

In an early study of 16 patients with Parkinson's disease, Jerger et al. (1960) found that patients performed less well than a comparison group of noninvolved subjects. The differences were not due to peripheral hearing levels. Similarly, Spitzer and Ventry (1980) studied 15 patients identified as chronic gamma-stage alcoholics who were undergoing rehabilitation. They were age matched with 15 control subjects. Significant differences not attributable to peripheral hearing between groups were found on several measures, indicating both cortical and brainstem pathology in this population.

Finally, Hasbrouk (1983) examined 24 adults who complained of general difficulties in hearing, understanding, and remembering. Five areas of auditory perception were assessed with the studies indicating problems in auditory memory, auditory figure-ground, and auditory discrimination among others. The results indicated the positive benefits of studying auditory perception in adults with previously undiagnosed learning disabilities to provide information, reduce anxiety, suggest environmental modifications, and otherwise implement remediation procedures.

Although more studies are necessary, all of the examples given indicate that further investigation of auditory processing abilities in adult patients is needed.

CENTRAL AUDITORY DISORDERS IN CHILDREN

HISTORICAL ORIENTATION

Central auditory dysfunction in children became a prominent audiologic concern approximately 10 years ago when an influential conference on the subject (Keith, 1977) stimulated interest in pediatric central auditory processing disorders (CAPDs). Since then, "sensitized" pediatric tests have been widely used throughout the United States, e.g., Test of Auditory Discrimination (Goldman, Fristoe, and Woodcock, 1974), Competing Spondaic Words (Katz and Illmer, 1972), Competing Sentences (Willeford, 1977), Time-Compressed Speech (Beasley, Maki, and Orchick, 1976; Manning, Johnson, and Beasley, 1977; Oelschlaeger and Orchik, 1977), Filtered Speech (Martin and Clark, 1977), Pitch Pattern Sequencing (Pinheiro, 1977), and Masking Level Difference (Sweetow and Reddell, 1978).

These initial efforts were distinguished by two different orientations to the problem of "sensitizing" pediatric evaluative procedures. In one approach, existing adult central auditory tests were adjusted for use with children, usually by modifying the expected range of normal performance. In the second approach, new central auditory test materials and testing paradigms that conformed to children's interests and abilities were developed and standardized. During the next decade (1977–1987), research in the auditory domain continued from both of these orientations (Berrick et al., 1984; Farrer and Keith, 1981; Ferre and Wilber, 1986; Jerger, Jerger, and Abrams, 1983; Jerger,

Martin, and Jerger, 1987; Musiek, Geurkink, and Kietel, 1982; Plakke, Orchik, and Beasley, 1981). Interested readers will find up-to-date analyses of contemporary pediatric central auditory assessment batteries in several sources (Jerger, 1984; Pinheiro and Musiek, 1985).

One example of a screening battery that emerged from the research mentioned above is SCAN: A Screening Test for Auditory Processing Disorders (Keith, 1986). According to the author, the purposes of this test are (1) to determine possible disorders of central nervous functions by assessing auditory maturation, (2) to identify children who may be at risk for auditory processing or receptive language problems who may require additional audiologic and language testing, and (3) to identify children who may benefit from specific management strategies. The battery includes three subtests: low-pass filtered words, auditory figure-ground, and competing monosyllable word pairs presented dichotically with simultaneous onset times. As a norm-referenced test, SCAN was standardized on 1034 children between the ages of 3 and 11 years. It can be administered in quiet environments using a high-fidelity portable stereo cassette player and two quality headphones.

Validation studies indicate that children with language and learning problems (Keith et al., 1988) and learning-disabled children with hyperactivity (Johnson, 1988) have poorer performance on subtests of SCAN than normal subjects. In addition, results of research on children with elevated blood lead levels indicate that their performance is poorer than children with low blood lead levels of equivalent age, intelligence, and socioeconomic status (Deitrich, 1988, personal communication). Although additional validation is required, it appears possible to identify children with auditory processing disorders with a battery of speech tests. The implication is that test batteries that measure other auditory processing abilities can be developed, although they need to be carefully designed and standardized.

FUTURE PERSPECTIVES

In the coming decade, the trend in pediatric central auditory assessment is predicted to center around dissecting the concept of CAPD into different types of abnormalities. Presently, *CAPD* may be only broadly defined as an impaired ability to discriminate, identify, or otherwise process auditory information that cannot be attributed to impaired hearing sensitivity or impaired intellectual function. The challenge to differentiate the concept of CAPD is reminiscent of the two-stage history characterizing the concept of *retrocochlear* disorder. Whereas the initial stage was marked by interest in detecting retrocochlear dysfunction, the following stage was distinguished by the realization that the term *retrocochlear* did not represent a unitary concept. Today, the word *retrocochlear* has been replaced by more specific terminology. By the year 2000, the term *CAPD* may also be considered antiquated if the trend toward developing a taxonomy of the disorder succeeds.

Audiologists' ability to elucidate the important characteristics of pediatric central auditory dysfunction during the coming years hinges, at least in part, on applying existing knowledge to formulate more meaningful questions and more sensitive experimental approaches to the problem. Thus, close examination and understanding of prior pediatric auditory research — its strategies and assumptions — are important.

STRATEGY AND ASSUMPTIONS OF RESEARCH

The predominant strategy of research within the auditory domain has been to relate performance in children with suspected central dysfunction to results in adults with known CNS lesions (Musiek, Gollegly, and Baran, 1984). This approach is based on the assumption that the child with central dysfunction has developmental immaturity or abnormality of the central auditory system and thus functions as if she or he has a CNS lesion. Support for this inference exists within both human and animal fields of study (see Caramazza and Zurif, 1978 and Rose, 1980 for discussion). An additional assumption of this approach has been that behavioral test results in adults with CNS lesions may be generalized to behavioral results in children with suspected disorders. Thus, validation of central auditory tests in children with CNS lesions is unnecessary. This latter assumption rests on a sparse body of equivocal data in the literature.

Prior Evidence in Adult versus Childhood Central Nervous System Lesions

At least two lines of evidence suggest that results in brain-lesioned children may differ from findings in brain-lesioned adults, either in terms of the specificity or the severity of deficits. Hynd and Cohen (1983) report that the cognitive deficits accompanying CNS lesions are less specific in children than in adults. Transferred to the auditory domain, this line of reasoning suggests that the auditory deficits in a young child with a CNS lesion may be more generalized than the ear-specific patterns of deficits seen in adults. With regard to the severity of deficits, many studies suggest that the behavioral deficits associated with some childhood CNS disorders are less severe than the deficits characterizing comparable adult CNS lesions. Examples of this evidence are findings on dichotic auditory tasks showing that some subjects with callosal agenesis or with early unilateral cerebral lesions or hemispherectomies do not show the pronounced ear deficits typically observed in adults with commissurotomies or unilateral hemispheric lesions (Bogen, 1985; Bruyer et al., 1985; Bryden and Zurif, 1970; Netley, 1972; Pirozzolo, Pirozzolo, and Ziman, 1979; Woods, 1984). These observations suggest that the immature brain is capable of functional reorganization that tends to normalize perceptual function. Both these lines of evidence caution against casual inferences from results in adults to results in children.

An equally strong, contrary line of evidence suggests that the behavioral auditory manifestations of childhood and adult brain lesions do not differ appreciably. Examples of this viewpoint are studies indicating that children and adults with unilateral brain lesions exhibit similar patterns of ear deficits on dichotic and other auditory tasks (Bergman et al., 1984; Goodglass, 1967; Jerger, 1987; Jerger and Zeller, 1989; Murray, 1987; Nass, 1984; Pohl, 1979). This latter group of studies supports the inference that audiologic findings in children may be interpreted according to the principles that guide the interpretation of corresponding results in adults. Further investigation of behavioral auditory test results in children with known CNS lesions is needed, however, before this conclusion can be accepted with confidence.

Application of Auditory Results in Children with Confirmed Central Nervous System Lesions

A stong database of auditory results in children with documented CNS lesions is critical for determing whether behavioral test results in developing children are as contingent on site of disorder as they are in adults. Encouragingly, some

242

II. AUDITORY ASSESSMENT

audiologic evidence to date suggests that the patterns of auditory abnormalities in children are consistent with the principles describing the abnormalities of auditory function in adults with comparable lesions (Jerger, 1987). If this is indeed the case, then strong interpretations of auditory results in children with suspected central auditory disorders are possible.

Thus, three steps will be important in determining whether CAPD represents a homogeneous disorder or many different types of abnormalities: (1) establishing a database of auditory results in children with confirmed lesions, (2) establishing the relation between this database and results in children with suspected central disorders, and (3) establishing the relation between a pattern of auditory results and associated functional deficits. Preliminary work toward these goals has already begun (Harris, Keith, and Novak, 1983; Jerger, Johnson, and Loiselle, 1988; Keith and Novak, 1984; Sanger, Keith, and Maher, 1987), and the future offers exciting opportunities as imaging techniques allow more precise documentation and specification of CNS lesions and developmental abnormalities.

The following section briefly summarizes the background knowledge that will guide future audiologic studies in children with documented or suspected central auditory dysfunction. Previous investigations separate into those studies based on (1) adult procedures that were generalized to children and (2) pediatric procedures and materials.

Application of Adult Methodologies to Central Auditory Evaluations in Children

A primary thrust of research with adult tests (described earlier) has been to address the question of whether a specific test yields normal results in "nonsuspect" children (with no evidence of abnormality) and abnormal results in "suspect" children. The success of this research strategy, of course, depends on correctly categorizing nonsuspect and suspect children. And, if a perfect *a priori* criterion for classifying normal and suspect children existed, tests for identifying normal and abnormal auditory function would not be necessary. In spite of this limitation, previous research has yielded interesting findings.

Results of the studies with adult test materials and procedures may be best understood by considering group data and individual data separately. In terms of average results between groups, it

has been well established that children with suspected central auditory disorder perform more poorly than normal children (Bamford and Saunders, 1985; Johnson, Enfield, and Sherman, 1981; Stubblefield and Young, 1975; Tobey et al., 1979; Willeford, 1985; but see Roeser, Millay, and Morrow, 1983 for a precaution). In terms of individual results, however, considerable overlap occurs in the performance of the normal and suspect subjects (Berrick et al., 1984; Musiek et al., 1982; Willeford and Billger, 1978). A wide range of absolute performance scores, i.e., overlap between the groups, lessens the specificity of a single test procedure. Both false-positive results in normal children and false-negative results in suspect children are observed. Thus, no single test procedure has proved a conclusive indicator of central auditory disorder in individual children.

A common strategy for handling the problem of variable performance in individual children has been to recommend a test battery approach for clinical evaluations. The normalcy or abnormalcy of central auditory function in a child is defined with an array of tests, rather than a single procedure. As noted earlier, interpretation of the normalcy or abnormalcy of results on a test is based on previous findings in adults with documented lesions, with the constraint that the range of normal findings may be adjusted for children. A broad variety of test batteries representing site of lesion approaches, type of dysfunction approaches, and "shotgun" approaches (individual tests formed into a battery without an underlying conceptual framework) are commonly used. To some clinicians, the current state of affairs presents a "confusing array of choices" (Sloan, 1986, p. 36).

To recapitulate, adult test materials and procedures seem sensitive to the presence of central auditory disorder in children. Individual data, however, have indicated a large degree of variability or overlap between normal and suspect children's performance, perhaps due to some of the nonauditory cognitive skills required by the tasks. In an attempt to counteract the problem of performance variability, a test battery approach has been advocated for individual evaluations.

Application of Pediatric Methodologies to Central Auditory Evaluations in Children

Research with pediatric tests of central auditory function accelerated in the 1980s as audiologists became increasingly aware of the importance of controlling the influence of nonauditory, cognitive factors on task performance (Bamford and Saunders, 1985; Keith, 1982; Keith et al., 1985). To reiterate the problem in evaluating central auditory status in the presence of immature cognitive abilities, a test instrument must be (1) sufficiently easy in terms of linguistic-cognitive demands and mode of responding to be insensitive to developmental differences in cognitive skills but (2) sufficiently difficult in terms of auditory perceptual demands to be sensitive to the presence of central auditory deficits. Several pediatric procedures have been constructed that attempt to accomplish the first goal (Elliott and Katz, 1980; Finitzo–Hieber et al., 1980; Ross and Lerman, 1970); fewer investigators, however, have been interested in both of the above aims (Farrer and Keith, 1981; Ferre and Wilbur, 1986; Jerger and Jerger, 1984).

One of the above approaches that has attempted to meet both aims is the Pediatric Speech Intelligibility (PSI) test (Jerger and Jerger, 1984), which consists of monosyllabic word and sentence materials composed by normal children between 3 and 6 years old. Testing is carried out by presenting a sentence or word target and requiring the child to point to the picture corresponding to the sentence or word that was heard. The basic procedures of the PSI test are performance-intensity functions and message-to-competition ratio (MCR) functions.

Recently, Jerger and colleagues investigated the validity of the MCR component of the PSI test in detecting and differentiating central auditory dysfunction in children with confirmed CNS lesions or suspected developmental abnormalities (Jerger, 1987; Jerger and Zeller, 1989; Jerger et al., 1988). Subjects were 10 children with lesions in areas of the brain anatomically remote from auditory nuclei and pathways (nonauditory CNS disorders), 9 children with circumscribed lesions in areas of the brain important for auditory function (CNS auditory disorders), and 11 children with suspected CAPDs (with no known brain lesion). Ages ranged from 3 to 8 years. The normalcy or abnormalcy results was determined on the basis of 95 percent normal confidence intervals that were established in normal children of comparable ages.

Results of the Jerger studies indicated that the MCR component of the PSI test accurately distinguished between children with central auditory versus nonauditory CNS lesions. All children with CNS lesions in the areas of the brain important for auditory perceptual function (cochlear nucleus, superior olivary complex, lateral lemniscus, inferior colliculus, medial geniculate body, temporal lobe, or corpus callosum) had abnormal PSI results. Children with nonauditory CNS lesions consistently had normal PSI performance. No children had false-negative or false-positive findings. These results were interpreted as indicating that the PSI test was a valid index of central auditory function and that abnormal PSI results were specific to involvement of the central auditory pathways.

The finding that the PSI test was an accurate detector of central auditory lesions encouraged further analysis to determine whether PSI results could also differentiate between brainstem versus temporal lobe sites of disorder and between right- versus left-sided lesions. Data for this analysis were the relation between MCR functions in the presence of an ICM versus a CCM. Historically, the relation between ICM and CCM conditions (a degraded monotic versus a dichotic task) has been effective in differentiating brainstem and temporal lobe lesions in adults (Jerger and Jerger, 1975; Keith, 1977; Speaks, 1980). Jerger and associates reasoned therefore that the ICM-CCM relation on the PSI test might also be effective in differentiating the site of disorder in children if PSI results are consistent with the principles that guide the interpretation of corresponding results in adults.

Figure 11-2 summarizes the normalcy and abnormalcy of ICM and CCM results in the nine children from the Jerger study with circumscribed CNS lesions affecting the central auditory pathways. The configuration of results for ICM versus CCM conditions differed between children with brainstem and temporal lobe lesions. For children with brainstem lesions, performance was typically abnormal for ICM and normal for CCM. In contrast, children with temporal lobe lesions showed either normal ICM or abnormal CCM or abnormality on both measures. In the temporal lobe subjects with performance deficits on both measures, the degree of abnormality was consistently greater for the CCM task than for the ICM task. The similarity between findings in the children and findings in adults with comparable lesions (Berlin et al., 1972; Jerger and Jerger, 1974; Speaks et al., 1975) was notable.

With one exception, performance deficits for the ICM and CCM conditions were observed either on both ears or on the ear contralateral to the lesion (i.e., the right ear for the left-sided lesion and vice versa). Again, this pattern of results

SUBJECTS				RIGHT EAR		LEFT EAR	
LESION SITE	SIDE	AGE	SEX	PSI-ICM	PSI-CCM	PSI-ICM	PSI-CCM
EXTRA-AXIAL BRAINSTEM	R	6-4	F	●	○	●	○
INTRA-AXIAL BRAINSTEM	R	8-4	M	○	○	●	●
	R	6-8	F	○	○	●	○
	R	5-11	M	●	○	●	○
TEMPORAL LOBE	R	8-1	M	○	○	○	●
	L	3-2	M	○	●	○	●
	R	7-9	M	○	●	●	●
	L	4-0	M	●	●	●	●
THALAMUS	L	4-11	F	○	○	○	●
KEY TO SYMBOLS				○ NORMAL		● ABNORMAL	

agrees with previous observations in adults (Jerger and Jerger, 1975; Lynn and Gilroy, 1977; Mueller et al., 1986; Olsen, 1983; Speaks, 1980). The exception to this general pattern was the isolated CCM abnormality on the ipsilateral (left) ear only in the child with a deep-seated thalamic glioma (4–11 year girl). A "paradoxical" ipsilateral ear effect on dichotic testing has been noted repeatedly in adults with deep-seated left hemispheric lesions (Damasio and Damasio, 1979; Denes and Caviezel, 1981; Jerger and Jerger, 1981; Musiek, 1983; Sparks, Goodglass, and Nickel, 1970; Speaks, 1980). The results in this unusual child have been highlighted in a case study (Jerger and Zeller, 1989).

Although strong interpretations of the data were limited by the small number of children, these results were interpreted as generally consistent with the adult principle that subjects with brainstem lesions have poorer performance on the ICM task and subjects with temporal lobe lesions have poorer performance on the CCM task or on both ICM and CCM tasks; however, as in adults, the laterality of the abnormality could not be predicted with certainty from the ICM and CCM measures. An isolated CCM deficit on the left ear only was observed, for example, in the presence of either a right or a deep-seated left hemispheric lesion (subjects 8–6 year boy and 4–11 year girl, respectively). Likewise, the presence of bilateral CCM deficits was observed in the presence of either a right or left temporal lobe lesion (subjects 7–9 year boy and 3–2 year boy, respectively).

In order to investigate the relation between results in children with confirmed versus suspected lesions, the above PSI protocol was administered to 11 children with suspected CAPDs. Figure 11-3

Figure 11-2. Distribution of normal and abnormal results for PSI sentences in the presence of an ipsilateral competing message (ICM — degraded monotic condition) and a contralateral competing message (CCM — dichotic condition) for nine children with confirmed, localized CNS lesions. (From Jerger, S., Johnson, K., and Loiselle, L. [1988]. Pediatric central auditory dysfunction: Comparison of children with confirmed lesions versus suspected processing disorders. *American Journal of Otology, 9*[Suppl.], 63–71. With permission.)

summarizes the results. Performance was typically normal for the ICM condition and abnormal for the CCM condition. The performance deficit was observed only on the left ear in 7 (64%) children and on both ears in 3 (27%) children. One child performed normally on both measures. Jerger and colleagues concluded that results in the CAPD group were more similar to findings in the temporal lobe group than to findings in either the nonauditory CNS or brainstem groups. This observation suggested that the children with CAPDs have developmental or pathologic dysfunction at the level of the auditory cortex. Supporting this supposition was the presence of normal auditory brainstem responses in all the subjects with CAPDs. Data in the Jerger series encourage further studies to support or deny the preliminary finding of relatively homogeneous and predictable results for dichotic versus degraded monotic sentence tasks in children with documented brain lesions or suspected CAPDs.

SUMMARY

The application of central auditory tests on adult patients can achieve a number of goals. The first is

SUBJECTS		RIGHT EAR		LEFT EAR	
AGE	SEX	PSI-ICM	PSI-CCM	PSI-ICM	PSI-CCM
5-2	M	○	○	○	○
7-6	F	○	○	○	●
4-9	M	○	○	○	●
4-6	M	○	○	○	●
4-7	F	○	○	○	●
5-7	M	○	○	○	●
7-1	M	○	○	○	●
5-6	M	○	●	○	●
4-0	M	○	●	○	●
6-6	M	○	●	○	●
5-11	F	○	○	●	●
KEY		○ NORMAL		● ABNORMAL	

Figure 11-3. Distribution of normal and abnormal results for PSI sentences in the presence of an ipsilateral competing message (ICM — degraded monotic condition) and a contralateral competing message (CCM — dichotic condition) for 11 children with suspected central auditory processing disorders. (From Jerger, S., Johnson, K., and Loiselle, L. [1988]. Pediatric central auditory dysfunction: Comparison of children with confirmed lesions versus suspected processing disorders. *American Journal of Otology,* 9[Suppl.], 63–71. With permission.)

to identify the presence of auditory processing disorders that may be related to problems of receptive communication. Auditory test batteries are appropriately administered to a number of patient populations including those with head trauma, neurologic disease, stroke, alcoholism, and old age. In certain patients, test results can be used to document progression or improvement of auditory processing ability.

When auditory processing disorders are identified, test results can be used to counsel professionals, families, and friends to help them understand the communication disorder and to develop remediation strategies that can be implemented to assist that individual. For example, Cohen (1987) presented several specific suggestions for improving speech material for the elderly listener by structuring the information, repeating main ideas, and stating facts explicitly rather than being left for the listener to infer. Similarly,

Cohen suggested use of stress and intonation to direct listener's attention to the most important words and facilitate decoding.

Another way in which central auditory test findings are helpful in adult populations is to identify previously undiagnosed learning disabilities. In those individuals, as with other patient populations, results can be used to establish recommendations for educational needs and vocational counseling. At times, the results of testing may be helpful in advising employers regarding the ability of employees to communicate under difficult listening conditions. Finally, in some individuals, results of central auditory tests have useful implications regarding recommendations for wearable hearing aids and assistive listening devices.

Similarly, when testing children, the central auditory test battery can help identify whether the auditory system is functioning normally. Results can provide information whether there appears to be a neurologic basis for a language-learning disorder as shown by reversed cerebral dominance, depressed overall performance, immature auditory receptive abilities, or failure of interhemispheric transfer of information. In some situations results can provide information that a lesion of the auditory system exists.

More commonly, central auditory testing in children is used to determine functional auditory ability. It is used to describe a child's ability to process speech under various difficult listening conditions including noise or other distortions of frequency or time. Results can describe the child's ability to recognize speech, to attend to auditory information, to inhibit irrelevant auditory input, and to recall auditory information. When these abilities are known, it is possible to determine what steps can be taken to ameliorate the negative effects of a central auditory disorder on the child's life, learning, vocational goals, and social development. The central auditory test battery administered to children should determine whether a neurologic abnormality exists, provide a description of the child's functional auditory and auditory-language ability, and establish avenues of possible remediation.

In children, a better understanding of different subgroups of central auditory disorders is needed. It is important to understand the implications of early brain lesions on cognition and how the plasticity of the developing brain results in different outcomes of auditory processing than adults with similar brain lesions. Finally, research should provide new insights on the relationships that exist between a pattern of auditory test results and functional auditory deficits.

For the testing of both adults and children, there is a need to continue to develop better tests of central auditory function with appropriate norms, and validation. Future research should provide clinicians insight into the questions addressed in this chapter and more specific information about auditory processing disorders and their remediation.

REFERENCES

Arnst, D., & Katz, J. (1982). *Central auditory assessment. The SSW test: Development and clinical use.* Boston: College-Hill Press.

Bamford, J., & Saunders, E. (1985). *Hearing impairment, auditory perception and language disability.* London: Edward Arnold.

Beasley, D., Maki, J., & Orchik, D. (1976). Children's perception of time-compressed speech using two measures of speech discrimination. *Journal of Speech and Hearing Disorders, 41,* 216–225.

Bergman, M., Costeff, H., Koren, V., Koifman, N., & Reshef, A. (1984). Auditory perception in early lateralized brain damage. *Cortex, 20,* 233–242.

Bergman, M., Hirsch, S., Solzi, P., & Mankowitz, Z. (1987). The threshold-of-interference test: A new test of interhemispheric suppression in brain injury. *Ear & Hearing, 8,* 147–150.

Berlin, C., Lowe–Bell, S., Jannetta, P., & Kline, D. (1972). Central auditory deficits after temporal lobectomy. *Ar-*

chives of Otolaryngology, 96, 4–10.

Berrick, J., Shubow, G., Schultz, M., Freed, H., Fournier, S., & Hughes, J. (1984). Auditory processing tests for children: Normative and clinical results on the SSW test. *Journal of Speech and Hearing Disorders, 49,* 318–325.

Bocca, E., Calearo, C., & Cassinari, V. (1954). A new method for testing hearing in temporal lobe tumours. *Acta Oto-laryngologica* (Stockholm), *44,* 219–221.

Bogen, J. (1985). The stabilized syndrome of hemisphere disconnection. In D. Benson & E. Zaidel (Eds.), *The dual brain: Hemispheric specialization in humans* (pp. 247–261). New York: Guilford Press.

Bruyer, R., Dupuis, M., Ophoven, E., Rectem, D., & Reynaert, C. (1985). Anatomical and behavioral study of a case of asymptomatic callosal agenesis. *Cortex, 21,* 417–430.

Bryden, M., & Zurif, E. (1970). Dichotic listening performance in a case of agenesis of the corpus callosum. *Neuropsychologia, 8,* 371–377.

Calearo, C., & Antonelli, A. (1973). Disorders of the central auditory nervous system. In M. Paparello & D. Shumrick (Eds.), *Otolaryngology* (Vol. 2). Philadelphia: Saunders.

Caramazza, A., & Zurif, E. (Eds.). (1978). *Language acquisition and language breakdown: Parallels and divergencies.* Baltimore: Johns Hopkins University Press.

Cohen, G. (1987). Speech comprehension in the elderly: The effects of cognitive changes. *British Journal of Audiology, 21,* 221–226.

Damasio, H. & Damasio, A. (1979). "Paradoxic" ear extinction in dichotic listening: Possible anatomic significance. *Neurology, 29,* 644–653.

Denes, G., & Caviezel, F. (1981). Dichotic listening in crossed aphasia: "Paradoxical" ipsilateral suppression. *Archives of Neurology, 38,* 182–185.

Elliott, L., & Katz, D. (1980). *Development of a new children's test of speech discrimination.* St. Louis: Auditec.

Farrer, S., & Keith, R. (1981). Filtered word testing in the assessment of children's central auditory abilities. *Ear & Hearing, 2,* 267–269.

Ferre, J., & Wilber, L. (1986). Normal and learning disabled children's central auditory processing skills: An experimental test battery. *Ear & Hearing, 7,* 336–343.

Fifer, R., Jerger, J., Berlin, C., Tobey, E., & Campbell, J. (1983). Development of a dichotic sentence identification test for hearing impaired adults. *Ear & Hearing, 4,* 300–305.

Finitzo–Hieber, T., Gerling, I., Matkin, N., & Cherow–Skalka, E. (1980). A sound effects recognition test for the pediatric audiological evaluation. *Ear & Hearing, 1,* 271–276.

Gat, I., & Keith, R. W. (1978). An effect of linguistic experience: Auditory word discrimination by native and non-native speakers of English. *Audiology, 17,* 339–346.

Goldman, R., Fristoe, M., & Woodcock, R. (1974). *Goldman–Fristoe–Woodcock Auditory Skills Battery.* Circle Pines, MN: American Guidance Services.

Goodglass, H. (1967). Binaural digit presentation and early lateral brain damage. *Cortex, 3,* 295–306.

Grimes, A., Grady, C., Foster, N., Sunderland, T., & Patronas, N. (1985). Central auditory function in Alzheimer's disease. *Neurology, 35,* 352–358.

Harris, V., Keith, R., & Novak, K. (1983). Relationship between two dichotic listening tests and the token test for children. *Ear & Hearing, 4,* 278–282.

Hasbrouk, J. (1983). Diagnosis of auditory perceptual disorders in previously undiagnosed adults. *Journal of Learning Disabilities, 16,* 206–208.

Hynd, G., & Cohen, M. (1983). *Dyslexia: Neuropsychological theory, research, and clinical differentiation.* New York: Grune & Stratton.

Jerger, J. (1964). Auditory tests for disorders of the central auditory mechanism. In W. Fields & B. Alford (Eds.), *Neurological aspects of auditory and vestibular disorders.* Springfield, IL: Charles C. Thomas.

Jerger, J. (1970). Development of the synthetic sentence identification (SSI) as a tool for speech audiometry. In C. Rojskjaer (Ed.), *Speech audiometry.* Odense, Denmark: Danavox.

Jerger, J. (1973). Audiological findings in aging. *Advances in Otorhinolaryngology, 20,* 115–124.

Jerger, J. (Ed.). (1984). *Pediatric audiology: Current trends.* Boston: College-Hill Press.

Jerger, J. & Jerger, S. (1974). Auditory findings in brain stem disorders. *Archives of Otolaryngology, 99,* 342–350.

Jerger, J. & Jerger, S. (1975). Clinical validity of central auditory tests. *Scandinavian Audiology, 4,* 147–163.

Jerger, J., Mier, M., Boshes, B., & Canter, G. (1960). Auditory behavior in Parkinsonism. *Acta Oto-laryngologica* (Stockholm), *52,* 541–550.

Jerger, S. (1983). Decision matrix and information theory analyses in the evaluation of neuroaudiological tests. *Seminars in Hearing, 4,* 121–132.

Jerger, S. (1984). Speech audiometry. In J. Jerger (Ed.), *Pediatric audiology: Current trends* (pp. 71–93). Boston: College-Hill Press.

Jerger, S. (1987). Validation of the pediatric speech intelligibility test in children with central nervous system lesions. *Audiology, 26,* 298–311.

Jerger, S., & Jerger, J. (1981). *Auditory disorders: A manual for clinical evaluation.* Boston: Little, Brown.

Jerger, S., & Jerger, J. (1984). *Pediatric speech intelligibility test: Manual for administration.* St. Louis: Auditec.

Jerger, S., & Zeller, R. (1989). Dichotic listening in a child with a cerebral lesion: The "paradoxical" ipsilateral ear deficit. *Ear & Hearing, 10,* 167–172.

Jerger, S., Jerger, J., & Abrams, S. (1983). Speech audiometry in the young child. *Ear & Hearing, 4,* 56–66.

Jerger, S., Johnson, K., & Loiselle, L. (1988). Pediatric central auditory dysfunction: Comparison of children with confirmed lesions versus suspected processing disorders. *American Journal of Otology, 9,* 63–71.

Jerger, S., Martin, R., & Jerger, J. (1987). Specific auditory perceptual dysfunction in a learning disabled child. *Ear & Hearing, 8,* 78–86.

Johnson, D., Enfield, M., & Sherman, R. (1981). The use of the Staggered Spondaic Word test and the Competing Environmental Sounds test in the evaluation of central auditory function in hearing disabled children. *Ear & Hearing, 2,* 70–77.

Johnson, Y. (1988). *Auditory vigilance and auditory processing abilities in adolescents with learning disabilities.* Unpublished master's thesis, University of Cincinnati.

Katz, J. (1962). The use of the staggered spondaic words for assessing the integrity of the central auditory nervous system. *Journal of Auditory Research, 2,* 327.

Katz, J., & Illmer, R. (1972). Auditory perception in children with learning disabilities. In J. Katz (Ed.), *Handbook of clinical audiology* (pp. 540–563). Baltimore: Williams & Wilkins.

Keith, R. (Ed.). (1977). *Central auditory dysfunction.* New York: Grune & Stratton.

Keith, R. (1982). Central auditory tests. In N. Lass, L. McReynolds, J. Northern, & D. Yoder (Eds.), *Speech, language, hearing: Vol. 3. Hearing disorders* (pp. 1015–1038). Philadelphia: Saunders.

Keith, R. (1986). *SCAN, A Screening Test for Auditory Processing Disorders.* San Antonio: Psychology Corp.

Keith, R. (1988). Central auditory tests. In N. Lass, L. McReynolds, J. Northern, & D. Yoder (Eds.), *Handbook of speech-language pathology and audiology.* Toronto: B.C. Decker.

Keith, R. & Novak, K. (1984). Relationships between tests of central auditory function and receptive language. *Seminars in Hearing, 5,* 243–250.

Keith, R., Katbamna, B., Tawfik, S., & Smolak, L. (1987). The effect of linguistic background on staggered spondaic word and dichotic consonant vowel scores. *British Journal of Audiology, 21,* 21–26.

Keith, R., Rudy, J., Donahue, P., & Schwallie, L. (1988). *Validation of SCAN with other auditory and language measures.* Paper presented at the annual convention of the American-Speech-Language-Hearing Association, Boston.

Keith, R., Tawfik, S., & Katbamna, B. (1985). Performance of adults on directed listening tasks using a dichotic CV test. *Ear & Hearing, 6,* 270–273.

Kimura, D. (1961). Some effects of temporal lobe damage on auditory perception. *Canadian Journal of Psychology, 15,* 166–171.

Lasky, E., & Katz, J. (1983). *Central auditory processing disorders.* Baltimore: University Park Press.

Lynn, G., & Gilroy, J. (1977). Evaluation of central auditory dysfunction in patients with neurological disorders. In R. Keith (Ed.), *Central auditory dysfunction.* New York: Grune & Stratton.

Manning, W., Johnson, K., & Beasley, D. (1977). The performance of children with auditory perceptual disorders on a time-compressed speech discrimination measure. *Journal of Speech and Hearing Disorders, 42,* 77–84.

Marshall, L. (1981). Auditory processing in aging listeners. *Journal of Speech & Hearing Disorders, 46,* 226–240.

Martin, F., & Clark, J. (1977). Audiologic detection of auditory processing disorders in children. *Journal of the American Audiological Society, 3,* 140–146.

Matzker, J. (1959). Two new methods for the assessment of central auditory functions in cases of brain disease. *Annals of Otolaryngology, 68,* 1185.

Mueller, H., Sedge, R., & Salazar, A. (1986). Auditory assessment of neural trauma. In M. Miner & K. Wagner (Eds.), *Neurotrauma: Treatment, rehabilitation and related issues* (pp. 155–158). Boston: Butterworths.

Murray, G. (1987). *Auditory processing in children with acquired unilateral lesions.* Unpublished doctoral dissertation, Case Western Reserve University, Cleveland.

Musiek, F. (1983). Results of three dichotic speech tests on subjects with intracranial lesions. *Ear & Hearing, 4,* 318–323.

Musiek, F. (1986). Neuroanatomy, neurophysiology, and central auditory assessment. Part III: Corpus callosum and efferent pathways. *Ear & Hearing, 7,* 349–358.

Musiek, F., & Baran, J. (1987). Central auditory assessment: Thirty years of challenge and change. *Ear & Hearing, 8,* 22S–35S.

Musiek, F., Geurkink, N., & Kietel, S. (1982). Test battery assessment of auditory perceptual dysfunction in children. *Laryngoscope, 92,* 251–257.

Musiek, F., Gollegly, K., & Baran, J. (1984). Myelination of the corpus callosum and auditory processing problems in children: Theoretical and clinical correlates. *Seminars in Hearing, 5,* 231–241.

Musiek, F., Reeves, A., & Baran, J. (1985). Release from central auditory competition in the split-brain patient. *Neurology, 35*(7), 983–987.

Nass, R. (1984). Case report: Recovery and reorganization after congenital unilateral brain damage. *Perceptual and Motor Skills, 59,* 867–874.

Netley, C. (1972). Dichotic listening performance of hemispherectomized patients. *Neuropsychologia, 10,* 233–240.

Oelschlaeger, M., & Orchik, D. (1977). Time-compressed speech discrimination in central auditory disorder: A pediatric case study. *Journal of Speech and Hearing Disorders, 42,* 483–486.

Olsen, W. (1983). Dichotic test results for normal subjects and for temporal lobectomy patients. *Ear & Hearing, 4,* 324–330.

Pinheiro, M. (1977). Tests of central auditory function in children with learning disabilities. In R. Keith (Ed.), *Central auditory dysfunction* (pp. 223–256). New York: Grune & Stratton.

Pinheiro, M., & Musiek, F. (1985). *Assessment of central auditory dysfunction.* Baltimore: Williams & Wilkins.

Pirozzolo, F., Pirozzolo, P., & Ziman, R. (1979). Neuropsychological assessment of callosal agenesis: Report of a case with normal intelligence and absence of the disconnexion syndrome. *Clinical Neuropsychology, I,* 13–16.

Plakke, B., Orchik, D., & Beasley, D. (1981). Children's performance on a binaural fusion task. *Journal of Speech and Hearing Research, 24,* 520–525.

Pohl, P. (1979). Dichotic listening in a child recovering from acquired aphasia. *Brain and Language, 8,* 372–379.

Roeser, R., Millay, K., & Morrow, J. (1983). Dichotic consonant-vowel (CV) perception in normal and learning-impaired children. *Ear & Hearing, 4,* 293–299.

Rose, D. (1980). Some functional correlates of the maturation of neural systems. In D. Caplan (Ed.), *Biological studies of mental processes* (pp. 27–43). Cambridge: MIT Press.

Ross, M., & Lerman, J. (1970). A picture identification test for hearing-impaired children. *Journal of Speech and Hearing Research, 13,* 44–53.

Sanger, D., Keith, R., & Maher, B. (1987). An assessment technique for children with auditory-language processing problems. *Journal of Communication Disorders, 20,* 265–279.

Sloan, C. (1986). *Treating auditory processing difficulties in children.* Boston: College-Hill Press.

Sparks, R., Goodglass, H., & Nickel, B. (1970). Ipsilateral versus contralateral extinction in dichotic listening resulting from hemispheric lesions. *Cortex, 6,* 249–260.

Speaks, C. (1980). Evaluation of disorders of the central auditory system. In M. Paparella & D. Shumrick (Eds.), *Otolaryngology: Vol. 2. The ear* (2nd ed., pp. 1846–1860). Philadelphia: Saunders.

Speaks, C., Gray, G., Miller, J., & Rubens, A. (1975). Central auditory deficits and temporal-lobe lesions. *Journal of Speech and Hearing Disorders, 40,* 192–205.

Spitzer, J., & Ventry, I. (1980). Central auditory dysfunction among chronic alcoholics. *Archives of Otolaryngology, 106,* 224–229.

Stach, B., Jerger, J., & Fleming, K. (1985). Central presbyacusis: A longitudinal case study. *Ear & Hearing, 6,* 304–306.

Stephens, S., & Thornton, A. (1976). Subjective and electrophysiologic tests in brain stem lesions. *Archives of Otolaryngology, 102,* 608–613.

Stubblefield, J., & Young, C. (1975). Central auditory dysfunction in learning disabled children. *Journal of Learning Disabilities, 8,* 89–94.

Sweetow, R., & Reddell, R. (1978). The use of masking level differences in the identification of children with perceptual problems. *Journal of the American Audiological Society, 4,* 52–56.

Teatini, G. P. (1970). Sensitized speech tests: Results in normal subjects. In C. Rojskjaer (Ed.), *Speech audiometry.* Odense, Denmark: Danavox.

Tobey, E., Cullen, J., Rampp, D., & Fleischer–Gallagher, A. (1979). Effects of stimulus-onset asynchrony on the dichotic performance of children with auditory processing disorders. *Journal of Speech and Hearing Research, 22,* 197–211.

Willeford, J. (1977). Assessing central auditory behavior in children: A test battery approach. In R. Keith (Ed.), *Central auditory dysfunction* (pp. 43–72). New York: Grune & Stratton.

Willeford, J. (1985). Assessment of central auditory disorders in children. In M. Pinheiro & F. Musiek (Eds.), *Assessment of central auditory dysfunction: Foundations and clinical correlates* (pp. 239–255). Baltimore: Williams & Wilkins.

Willeford, J., & Billger, J. (1978). Auditory perception in children with learning disabilities. In J. Katz (Ed.), *Handbook of clinical audiology* (pp. 410–425). Baltimore: Williams & Wilkins.

Willeford, J., & Burleigh, J. (1985). *Handbook of central auditory processing disorders in children.* Orlando: Grune & Stratton.

Woods, B (1984). Dichotic listening ear preference after childhood cerebral lesions. *Neuropsychologia, 22,* 303–310.

PART III

Special Considerations

CHAPTER 12

Assessment of Infants for Hearing Impairment

Deborah Hayes • Nigel R. T. Pashley

One of the most challenging and rewarding aspects of clinical audiology is evaluation of infants and young children. Pediatric audiology is a rapidly evolving field. Less than 40 years ago, a noted investigator wrote, "Only rarely is it possible to use a hearing aid of any kind before the child is two years of age...." (Myklebust, 1950). Today, the recognized goal of infant assessment is identification and habilitation, including amplification, by age 6 months (American Speech-Language-Hearing Association, 1982). Recent advances in techniques for evaluation and technology for habilitation mean that every infant with hearing impairment should be identified and should receive appropriate habilitation at an early age. At the present time, unfortunately, this simply does not occur (Coplan, 1987; Elssmann, Matkin, and Sabo, 1987; Stein, Clark, and Kraus, 1983).

The well-documented and devastating effects of childhood hearing impairment provide a compelling argument for early identification and habilitation. Many hearing-impaired children not only suffer from severe delays in all aspects of receptive and expressive language, but they also show only negligible growth in language skills and academic achievement after 12 to 13 years of age (Allen, 1986; Osberger, 1986). As a consequence, many hearing-impaired children do not reach economic equality in their productive adult years (Northern and Downs, 1984).

In 1986, the federal government recognized the importance of early identification and habilitation of all childhood handicapping conditions. Public Law 99-457, the education of the handicapped amendment, created (in part) a new discretionary program to address the special needs of handicapped infants, toddlers, and their families. An important component of that program is a provision for early identification through "Child Find" programs and early habilitation through development of individualized family service plans. Clearly, audiologists msut be able to provide appropriate clinical services for this important population.

This chapter provides an overview of diagnostic evaluation of hearing loss in infants age birth through 2 years. A child's optimum development critically depends on these early years, and successful habilitation of children with hearing impairment requires diagnosis and intervention during the first 2 years of life.

PREVALENCE OF HEARING IMPAIRMENT IN INFANTS

Prevalence refers to the total number of cases of a condition in a population during a specified period of time (Jacobson and Jacobson, 1987; Moscicki, 1984). Prevalence of hearing loss is greater in infants who are born with or who develop specific health conditions during the newborn period than in infants with an uneventful birth and newborn history (Feinmesser and Tell, 1976; Simmons, 1980).

Most estimates of the prevalence of hearing loss in infants are derived from investigations of the efficacy of newborn hearing screening programs. Feinmesser and Tell (1976) tested 17,731 newborn infants to determine efficacy of behavioral screening for detection of deafness. By age 5 years, 25 of these infants were found to have bilateral hearing impairment of at least a moderate degree. Eighteen of these twenty-five infants were "at risk" for hearing impairment due to prenatal

251

factors (e.g., family history of deafness, parental consanguinity) or perinatal factors (e.g., severe neonatal sepsis, elevated serum bilirubin). Only seven infants had no known condition placing them at risk for hearing impairment.

Simmons (1980) evaluated 12,138 infants by an automated newborn behavioral screening device, the Crib-o-Gram (COG), and obtained firm diagnosis of mild to profound hearing loss in 42 infants. Simmons found a much higher rate of hearing impairment among graduates of an intensive care nursery (31 in 1554 infants tested; 1 : 52) than among graduates of well-baby nurseries (11 in 10,584 infants tested; 1 : 1000).

Neither Feinmesser and Tell nor Simmons obtained follow-up hearing tests in all their study infants. Their data may underestimate true impairment rate because mild hearing impairment or unilateral hearing impairment may have been undetected. Hosford-Dunn et al. (1987) obtained audiologic follow-up of 820 infants who graduated from a neonatal intensive care unit (NICU). They found 97 children with some degree of either unilateral or bilateral hearing impairment (11.8% of all infants followed), and 39 infants with bilateral hearing impairment of moderate (i.e., 45–70 dB HL) degree or greater (4.8% of all infants followed). Health characteristics of infants in intensive care units vary between units, and efforts to determine prevalence in a given intensive care unit should be based on unit-specific samples of infants (Halpern, Hosford-Dunn, and Malachowski, 1987).

Because prevalence is related to number of cases during a specified period of time, prevalence of hearing impairment in infants will vary depending on health conditions in the environment. For example, the rubella epidemic of 1963 through 1965 resulted in a substantial number of deaf infants among children born during these years (Brown, 1986). It is estimated that approximately 10,000 to 20,000 infants were born with hearing loss related to the epidemic (Northern and Downs, 1984). Annual surveys of children receiving special education for handicapping conditions clearly show a marked increase in the number of hearing-impaired students born in 1964 and 1965 (Brown, 1986; Karchmer, 1985).

Ability to predict prevalence of hearing impairment in a population of infants will depend on a variety of factors including specific health characteristics of the infants, and general health conditions in the environment. Factors that result in a neonatal intensive care also result in a high prob-

ability of hearing impairment. Any infant at risk for hearing impairment should receive audiologic follow-up (American Speech-Language-Hearing Association, 1982).

ETIOLOGY OF HEARING IMPAIRMENT IN INFANTS

Many conditions that place an infant at risk for hearing impairment have been identified. These conditions often affect the infant at a very young age. If hearing impairment is not present at birth, it is typically acquired during the first 2 years of life. Although infants with normal hearing at birth may acquire hearing loss in childhood related to some genetic conditions (Konigsmark and Gorlin, 1976) and to certain high-risk conditions (Dahle et al., 1979; Naulty, Weiss, and Herer, 1986; Nieldt et al., 1986; Sell et al., 1985), Simmons (1980) reported that "nearly all, if not all, sensorineural hearing losses in very young children occur before they are discharged from the newborn nursery. . . ."

A number of categorization schemes have been developed to classify etiologies of childhood hearing impairment. One useful scheme is consideration of the nature of the hearing impairment (conductive versus sensory) and the time when the hearing impairment occurred (present at birth, congenital hearing impairment; or developed after birth, acquired hearing impairment). Unless all infants are tested at birth, however, time when hearing loss occurred may be indeterminate in many cases. Most conductive hearing impairments in children are acquired; most sensory hearing impairments are congenital.

CONDUCTIVE HEARING IMPAIRMENT

Acquired

Otitis media is the most common infectious disease of childhood (Bluestone and Klein, 1988), and otitis media with effusion (OME) is the most common cause of acquired conductive hearing loss, affecting an estimated 10 percent of preschool and school-aged children (Northern and Downs, 1984). Otitis media can occur in both normal newborns (Shurin, Pelton, and Klein, 1976) and newborns in intensive care nurseries. In fact, OME has been documented in up to 30 percent of infants in NICUs (Berman, Balkany, and Simmons, 1978; Pestalozza, 1984). Age at first episode of otitis media is important because it is significantly associated with recurrent episodes (Bluestone and Klein, 1988). Research has shown that infants with onset of OME before age 2 months have, on the average, a longer total duration of bilateral effusion than infants with later onset of OME (Marchant et al., 1984). Infants with early onset of OME are at risk for persistent effusion and conductive hearing loss.

The hearing loss typically associated with OME is mild to moderate, fluctuant, unilateral, or bilateral. Although hearing loss associated with OME may be only mild, evidence shows that OME can affect language development and verbal ability, especially in the critical language-learning preschool years (Sak and Ruben, 1982). Teele et al. (1984), for example, reported results of a study of 205 children followed prospectively from birth to age 3. They found that children who had spent prolonged periods with middle ear effusion had significantly lower scores on standardized speech and language tests when compared with children who had spent little time with middle ear disease. Time spent with middle ear effusion in the first 6 to 12 months of life was most strongly associated with poor scores. Recently, the American Academy of Pediatrics Committee on Early Childhood, Adoption, and Dependent Care (1984) recommended assessing hearing and monitoring communication skills development for children with acute otitis media or middle ear effusion, or both, persisting for more than 3 months. Surgical treatment with insertion of tympanostomy tubes should be considered when OME is present for 12 weeks continuously (usually despite antibiotic therapy), or if the child has had more than three episodes of acute suppurative otitis within a 6-month period.

OME in children with preexisting sensory hearing loss is especially problematic. Parents may become confused about the cause of hearing loss and the expected benefits of medical/surgical treatment (Hayes, 1987). Medical/surgical treatment is typically more aggressive for these children to minimize decrease in sensitivity related to OME.

Congenital

Congenital conductive hearing loss is frequently associated with syndromal abnormalities and head and neck anomalies. Congenital aural atresia (absence of an external ear canal) is usually associated with microtia (deformity of the auricle) and often accompanied by developmental anomaly of the middle ear. Common syndromes associated with congenital aural atresia with microtia and congenital conductive or mixed (conductive and sensory) hearing loss, or a combination, include cleft lip and palate, Goldenhar syndrome, Treacher Collins syndrome, Apert's syndrome, Pierre Robin syndrome, and osteogenesis imperfecta (Bergstrom, 1987). Absence of obvious ear abnormality in infants with craniofacial anomalies does not preclude presence of hearing impairment.

Congenital conductive hearing impairment often requires surgical exploration or intervention. For the child with microtia and aural atresia, reconstruction of the pinna is considered for aesthetic reasons, and is not attempted before age 4 years. This procedure is difficult, technical, and staged and usually requires four to six surgical procedures to accomplish an acceptable result. The alternative to surgically reconstructed ears, prosthetic ears, has not met with universal satisfaction due to unpredictable adhesion and local skin irritation in the adhesion area. Recently, use of rare earth magnets to attach aural prostheses has shown considerable promise as an alternative to aural surgical reconstruction.

Reconstruction of the ear canal and middle ear structures depends on (1) degree of abnormality as revealed by computed tomography scans, (2) presence of congenital cholesteatoma in the canal atresia, which might enlarge and displace ossicles or a tympanic remnant and further jeopardize hearing, and (3) success of aural habilitation by amplification. In general, surgical reconstruction of the ear canal does not occur before age 12 to 18 months. An important factor complicating aural reconstructive surgery is possible injury to the seventh (facial) cranial nerve, which usually does not lie in its normal position in children with congenital aural atresia/microtia with associated middle ear anomalies.

SENSORY HEARING IMPAIRMENT

Etiology of hearing impairment is unknown in approximately 30 to 40 percent of children with sensory loss (Brown, 1986). Determining etiology of childhood sensory hearing loss is essential because sensory hearing loss represents a symptom of a disease or syndrome, not a disease unto itself. With appropriate otologic and audiologic evaluation at a very early age, identification of the etiology of hearing impairment should be possible for many children (Bergstrom, 1987).

Congenital

During the 1960s, congenital rubella syndrome was the most commonly identified cause of sensory hearing loss in children (Brown, 1986; Karchmer, 1985). This finding reflects the prevalence of congenital rubella syndrome in children born during the epidemic of 1963 to 1965. Success of the rubella vaccination program has virtually eliminated congenital rubella syndrome as an important cause of childhood hearing loss.

For children born in years other than during a rubella epidemic, heredity is the most commonly reported cause of congenital hearing impairment (Brown, 1986). Bergstrom (1987) in her review of 1048 cases of prelinguistic hearing loss identified 363 cases of sensory hearing loss related to genetic (heredity) factors.

Maternal infections other than rubella associated with congenital hearing loss include cytomegalovirus (CMV), toxoplasmosis, and sexually transmitted diseases. CMV may lead to progressive hearing loss in childhood (Dahle et al., 1979; Gerkin, 1984), and infants known to have congenital CMV should receive audiologic monitoring, at least through their preschool years (Coplan, 1987). Maternal exposure to certain substances or conditions can also be toxic to fetal development and lead to congenital hearing loss (e.g., drugs, alcohol, severe maternal diabetes) (Bergstrom, 1987; Gerkin, 1984; Gerkin and Church, 1987). Perinatal (around the time of birth) conditions that lead to very early onset, if not congenital hearing loss, include very low birth weight (Bergman et al., 1985), anoxia, hyperbilirubinemia, and persistent pulmonary hypertension of the newborn (Naulty et al., 1986, Sell et al., 1985).

Acquired

Meningitis is the most common cause of acquired sensory hearing loss in children. Investigators estimate that approximately 18,000 cases of the most common form of meningitis (*Haemophilus influenzae* type b) occur in the United States each year (Eskola et al., 1987). Depending on the causative organism, between 6 and 30 percent of children with meningitis will develop unilateral or bilateral mild to profound hearing loss (Dodge et al., 1984). Attack rates are highest for infants less than 1 year of age (Schlech et al., 1985). Fortunately, recent development of an effective vaccine

for *H. influenzae* may eventually eliminate meningitis as an important cause of childhood hearing impairment (Eskola et al., 1987).

Other infectious diseases that can result in acquired sensory hearing loss include mumps, measles, chickenpox, and influenza. Children may also acquire sensory hearing loss through trauma and high fever (Brown, 1986).

Otologic Assessment

Because defining etiology of hearing loss is important for determining optimum treatment and for providing adequate parental counseling, infants with sensory hearing loss should receive otologic assessment consisting of (1) thorough exploration of the parents' observation of their infant's behavior, (2) an appropriately designed history and physical examination, and (3) additional medical evaluations.

In the absence of a systematic hearing screening program, parents are the single most important factor in early identification of childhood hearing loss. Recent data indicate that, on the average, parents of hearing-impaired children express concern about their child's auditory behavior approximately 7 months prior to confirming diagnosis, regardless of the child's risk status (Elssmann et al., 1987). All health care providers should be alert to parental observations that suggest hearing loss, even in very young infants.

A thorough otologic history and physical examination for children is based on an extended risk-screening assessment, and specifically probes areas for further investigation. Important areas in the pediatric otologic history are (1) family history, including history of progressive deafness and blindness, (2) maternal factors including exposure to drugs, chemicals, or infectious agents during pregnancy, (3) circumstances of birth, and infant and newborn factors, (4) other health factors such as congenital heart disease, seizures, and accidental trauma including skull fractures, and (5) developmental milestones, especially age of walking and other gait-related behaviors that might reveal abnormal vestibular function.

Additional medical investigations are useful for revealing anatomic abnormalities or for confirming presence of metabolic, infectious, or genetic processes. For example, computed tomography scanning of inner and middle ears permits identification of anatomic anomalies such as Mondini malformation. Serologic studies are useful for detecting congenital syphilis or hypothyroidism, and ophthalmologic consultation is mandated in families with history of progressive blindness to rule out retinitis pigmentosa associated with Usher's syndrome.

The possibility that a child's sensory hearing loss is progressive or fluctuant is especially problematic. Because children often cannot report progression of hearing loss, until proved otherwise, all childhood sensory hearing loss should be considered progressive. A parent's report of apparent "good days" and "bad days" in their child's hearing behavior is very important in suggesting progressive or fluctuant hearing loss. Conditions that result in progressive hearing loss in children include congenital CMV (Dahle et al., 1979), persistent pulmonary hypertension of the newborn (Naulty et al., 1986; Sell et al., 1985), specific genetic conditions (Konigsmark and Gorlin, 1976), and perilymph fistula (Paparella et al., 1987).

Spontaneous perilymph fistula (as opposed to traumatic implosive or explosive injury) has been widely reported by a number of investigators (Grundfast and Bluestone, 1978; Paparella et al., 1987; Petroff, Simmons, and Winzelberg, 1986). Recently, one author (Pashley) reviewed presenting complaints and clinical signs in 34 children with proved fistulas. Fistulas were confirmed in all children by exploratory tympanotomy. On initial presentation, high-frequency sloping sensory hearing loss was present in 26 percent of the children, and an irregular "up and down" pattern of hearing loss across the frequency range was noted in 35 percent of the children. Documented fluctuation or progression in hearing loss was present in 29 percent of the children. Computed tomographic scan of the inner ear in all children revealed the Mondini abnormality in seven (21%). Vestibular signs, including clumsiness, unsteadiness, and late walking occured in 59 percent of patients, and a complaint of spinning or true whirling vertigo was present in 35 percent (all older children). Electronystagmography was abnormal in 35 percent of the children, but most children (59%) could not be evaluated by this test. In general, a clinical picture of documented or suspected progressive or fluctuant sensory hearing loss with vestibular signs warrants the suspicion of spontaneous perilymph fistula. In our series, repair of the fistula resulted in resolution of vestibular signs and stabilization of hearing loss in almost all children.

Depending on the referral route, otologic assessment may precede or follow audiologic evaluation. In either case, audiologic evaluation of infants can occur at any age and should be mandatory for any infant at risk for hearing impairment. Newborn infants can be screened by electrophysiologic procedures, and infants as young as 6 months can be evaluated by sophisticated behavioral test procedures.

AUDIOLOGIC SCREENING OF NEWBORN INFANTS

An entire professional literature is devoted to theories of health screening. In general, several criteria must be met before screening for diseases is applied to a given population (Frankenburg, 1975). Table 12-1 summarizes these criteria as they relate to screening for hearing loss in infants and clearly shows that screening for hearing impairment in infants is warranted (Hall, Kripal, and Hepp, 1988; Northern and Downs, 1984; Ruth, Dey-Sigman, and Mills, 1985).

Downs was one of the first audiologists to promote early identification of hearing impairment through systematic nursery-based screening programs. For more than 25 years, she has advocated for routine and systematic evaluation of newborn infants (Downs and Hemenway, 1969; Downs and Silver, 1972; Downs and Sterritt, 1964, 1967; Northern and Downs, 1984), and her early research provides the foundation for many later studies of newborn hearing screening.

Newborn hearing screening provokes considerable debate. There is little controversy about the importance of early identification of hearing impairment, but considerable disagreement exists about the most efficient approach for hearing loss identification. Two approaches have been widely investigated. One approach, behavioral observation of newborn responses or its variant, automated behavioral evaluation, has been used both for mass screening programs and for screening selected groups of at-risk newborns. The second approach, screening by electrophysiologic procedures, has, in general, been recommended only for at-risk infants. Although published studies indicate that substantially more than 50,000 infants have been screened in various screening programs worldwide (Bhattacharya, Bennett, and Tucker, 1984; Downs and Hemenway, 1969; Feinmesser and Tell, 1976; Murray, Javel, and Watson, 1985; Simmons, 1980), complete consensus on the most appropriate procedure and age at testing has not yet been achieved (Alberti et al., 1985;

TABLE 12-1. CRITERIA FOR SELECTING HEALTH CONDITIONS FOR SCREENING AND APPLICATION TO SCREENING FOR HEARING IMPAIRMENT IN INFANTS

Criteria	Hearing impairment of infants
1. Condition should be prevalent.	1. Infants in well baby nursery: 1 in 1000 Infants in intensive care nursery: 1 in 52 (Simmons, 1980)
2. Condition is serious.	2. Speech and language development, and academic achievement are significantly delayed in hearing-impaired children (Allen, 1986; Osberger, 1986)
3. Screening decreases time to diagnosis.	3. In absence of systematic screening, diagnosis of hearing impairment in infants is delayed to age 18 months or older, and even longer for infants with mild to moderate hearing loss (Elssmann et al., 1987; Stein, Clark, and Kraus, 1983)
4. Diagnostic tests are available to confirm hearing loss in infants who fail screening.	4. Comprehensive diagnostic evaluation is possible in very young infants (American Speech-Language-Hearing Association, 1982)
5. Condition is treatable, and prognosis is improved with early identification.	5. Habilitation, including amplification, can and should begin by age 6 months (American Speech-Language-Hearing Association, 1982)
6. Screening should not harm the infants and should be acceptable to parents.	6. Screening for hearing impairment is noninvasive. Parents express concern about hearing impairment long before they receive appropriate referral for audiologic services (Elssmann et al., 1987)
7. Cost of screening, diagnosis, and treatment is reasonable when compared to cost of delayed diagnosis and treatment.	7. Cost of screening can be controlled by preselecting population to be screened and by minimizing unnecessary follow-up (Hayes and Ringger, 1987; Kileny, 1987; Stein, Ozdamer, Kraus, and Paton, 1987)

Source: From Frankenburg, W. (1975). Principles in selecting diseases for screening. In W. Frankenburg & B. Camp (Eds.), *Pediatric screening tests* (pp. 9–22). Springfield, IL: Charles C. Thomas. With permission.

Durieux-Smith et al., 1985, 1987; Hosford-Dunn et al., 1987; Hyde et al., 1984; Mahoney and Eichwald, 1987; Weber, 1987).

MASS SCREENING

In the 1960s, concerted efforts were made to develop nursey-based mass screening programs (Downs and Hemenway, 1969; Downs and Sterritt, 1964, 1967). These programs were based on observation of the infant's behavioral response to sound. This technique received continuous investigation through the next decade (Feinmesser and Tell, 1976; Mencher and Gerber, 1981). Efforts to reduce variability related to observer bias resulted in development of specific guidelines for test conditions and response detection (Mencher and Gerber, 1981; Northern and Downs, 1984). Despite these improvements, behavioral observation screening programs continued to result in a high incidence of false-negative and false-positive results, and mass screening by behavioral observation is not recommended (American Speech-

Language-Hearing Association, 1982). Citing poor test performance, Jacobson and Morehouse (1984) argued that "the continued use of newborn behavioral screening as a routine procedure must be seriously questioned...." Currently, most investigators favor screening infants at risk for hearing impairment either by automated behavioral response procedures or by electrophysiologic test techniques (Durieux-Smith et al., 1985, 1987; Galambos, Hicks, and Wilson, 1982, 1984; Gorga et al., 1987; Hayes and Ringger, 1987; Hosford-Dunn et al., 1987; Jacobson and Morehouse, 1984).

THE CONCEPT OF "AT RISK"

The concept that conditions during pregnancy, birth, and neonatal life can result in significant morbidity to surviving infants is well established. As early as 1892, a French obstetrician, Pierre Budin, developed "a special department of weaklings" for premature infants (Ensher and Clark, 1986). Infants were admitted to this department because they were at risk for a poor outcome based on prematurity (in Budin's definition, birth weight <2500 g).

In general, two factors contribute to an infant's risk for morbidity: (1) biologic conditions that are consistently associated with developmental disorders (e.g., Down syndrome, Treacher Collins syndrome) and (2) medical conditions that are associated with later impairment (e.g., severe respiratory distress, very low birth weight). Throughout the 1960s, special NICUs were developed to care for newborns at risk for mortality and morbidity.

Downs and Silver (1972) extended the concept of at risk to detection of hearing impairment. They defined five risk factors that placed an infant at risk for hearing impairment and recommended immediate referral for audiologic evaluation for any infant manifesting one of these factors. In 1973, a national committee composed of representatives from audiology/speech pathology, otolaryngology, and pediatrics developed a High-Risk Register that incorporated Downs and Silver's five factors. The committee met again in 1981 and revised and expanded the High-Risk Register to include seven risk factors (American Speech-Language-Hearing Association, 1982; Gerkin, 1984). Table 12-2 lists these factors.

Risk registry devices are useful for restricting the initial population to be tested to those infants with a high probability of hearing impairment (Feinmesser and Tell, 1976). Their principal disadvantage is that 50 percent or more of hearing-impaired children have no known risk factor at the time of birth (Elssmann et al., 1987; Stein, Clark, and Kraus, 1983). If newborn hearing screening is restricted only to infants who manifest risk conditions, then fully 50 percent of hearing-impaired children will not be detected.

SCREENING AT-RISK NEWBORNS

With the exception of positive family history, factors that place an infant at risk for hearing impairment usually also result in risk for other medical or developmental disabilities (Halpern et al., 1987). These infants are typically cared for in the NICU. Within the past decade, many hearing screening programs have been developed to test infants in the NICU. Both automated behavioral approaches and electrophysiologic techniques have been applied to these infants.

TABLE 12-2. FACTORS IDENTIFYING THOSE INFANTS WHO ARE AT RISK FOR HEARING IMPAIRMENT

1. Family history of childhood hearing impairment
2. Congenital perinatal infection (e.g., cytomegalovirus, rubella, herpes, toxoplasmosis, syphilis)
3. Anatomic malformations involving the head and neck (e.g., dysmorphic appearance including syndromal and nonsyndromal abnormalities, overt or submucous cleft palate, morphologic abnormalities of the pinna)
4. Birth weight < 1500 g
5. Hyperbilirubinemia at level exceeding indications for exchange transfusion
6. Bacterial meningitis, especially *Haemophilus influenzae*
7. Severe asphyxia, which may include infants with Apgar scores of 0 to 3 or who fail to institute spontaneous respiration by 10 minutes and those with hypotonia persisting to 2 hours of age

Source: From the American Speech-Language-Hearing Association. Joint Committee on Infant Hearing. (1982). Position statement. *ASHA, 24,* 1017–1018. With permission.

Automated Behavioral Screening

In the United States, the Crib-O-Gram (COG) has received considerable attention as an automated behavioral screening device (Durieux-Smith et al., 1985; Hosford-Dunn et al., 1987; Simmons and Russ, 1974; Webb, Krishnan, and Katzman, 1985). Although originally developed for mass screening purposes, the COG has been used in a number of NICU programs. The COG detects changes in an infant's ongoing movement in response to sound by means of a motion-sensitive transducer placed beneath the infant's mattress. The output of the transducer is routed to a signal-processing system that compares pre- and poststimulus activity and automatically scores response presence. Responses to a number of signals are evaluated to obtain a statistically valid sample. Another automated test procedure, the auditory response cradle, has received investigation in Great Britain (Bennett, 1979; Bennett and Lawrence, 1980; McCormick, Curnock, and Spavins, 1984).

One problem with behavioral screening programs, whether based on behavioral observation or automated response detection, is that relatively intense (i.e., 75–95 dB sound pressure level [SPL]) signals must be used to elicit a response. Newborns typically do not produce reliable responses to signals at lower-intensity levels (Bennett and Lawrence, 1980). Because of these high intensities, infants with mild to moderate sensitivity loss may "pass" a behavioral screening when, in fact, hearing is sufficiently impaired to affect speech and language development (Durieux-Smith et al., 1985).

Other problems also affect successful screening by COG in the NICU. Durieux-Smith et al. (1985) reported that approximately 30 percent of NICU infants with established electrophysiologic thresholds of 30 dB nHL failed the COG (false-positive results), and that 8 in 21 infants with bilateral mild to moderate hearing loss passed the COG (false-negative results). Thirty-two percent of 280 infants tested by COG changed from "pass" to "fail," or vice versa, on COG retest (poor test-retest reliability). Hosford-Dunn et al. (1987) completed follow-up audiologic testing of 483 of 585 infants screened by COG in the NICU. They reported that COG failed to detect 14 of 41 permanent losses (6 were considered significant) and failed 78 infants who had no degree of permanent hearing loss at follow-up. To reduce overreferral based on COG failure, Hosford-Dunn et al. recommended referring only those infants who fail two successive tests.

If COG or any other behavior-based approach is used in the newborn nursery, clinicians must precisely define the degree of hearing impairment that the technique is capable of detecting (Durieux-Smith et al., 1985; Hosford-Dunn et al., 1987). Parents/caregivers must be made to appreciate the difference between passing a hearing screening for any degree of significant hearing loss and passing a hearing screening only for severe or profound hearing loss. If parents do not understand this difference, then identification of mild to moderate hearing loss in infants who pass a behavioral hearing screening may be further delayed because parents are falsely reassured by the nursery-based pass. Although this outcome may be relatively rare, it has potentially tragic results for the infant in question.

Electrophysiologic Screening

For more than 25 years, investigators have studied techniques that measure electrical activity from the auditory system as a means of predicting hearing sensitivity. These evoked potentials are characterized by small amplitudes relative to ongoing electroencephalographic activity and are time locked to the eliciting signal. Development of small laboratory averaging computers in the 1960s permitted evaluation of the clinical utility of these auditory evoked potentials (AEPs). AEPs did not receive attention for screening hearing of newborns until investigators demonstrated that evoked potentials (1) could be reliably recorded in newborn and premature infants, (2) showed a predictable development course, and (3) provided accurate estimation of auditory sensitivity. One component of the family of AEPs, the auditory brainstem response (ABR), demonstrates all these characteristics (Hecox and Galambos, 1974; Salamy and McKean, 1976; Schulman-Galambos and Galambos, 1975, 1979; Starr et al., 1977). The early research reports of ABR in newborn infants were followed by a decade of clinical investigation of the ABR as a newborn hearing screening procedure. Numerous investigators have confirmed the presence of ABRs in premature infants at levels that effectively rule out significant hearing impairment and the technique has achieved widespread acceptance in many NICUs (Durieux-Smith et al., 1985, 1987; Galambos et al., 1982, 1984; Gorga et al., 1987; Hayes and Ringger, 1987; Jacobson and Morehouse, 1984; Ruth et al., 1985).

Several factors must be considered in development of a NICU-based ABR screening program. Among the most important are age and state of the infant at test, test environment, and follow-up strategies.

Age and state of the infant at test are important because the ABR changes rapidly during the first few weeks and months of life, especially for premature infants (Gorga et al., 1987; Lary et al., 1985). In general, threshold and latency of the response decrease and amplitude increases from birth (including premature infants) through about age 18 months (Gorga et al., 1987; Lary et al., 1985; Salamy and McKean, 1976; Schulman-Galambos and Galambos, 1975). Figure 12-1 from Gorga et al. (1987) shows average ABR wave V latencies in premature infants as a function of intensity with conceptional age (gestational age plus chronological age) as the parameter. The figure demonstrates the systematic decrease in response latency with increase in age in premature infants. Although the responses may be observed in premature infants as young as age 28 weeks' gestation (Lary et al., 1985; Starr et al., 1977), most investigators recommend testing infants when they reach postconceptional age 36 weeks or older to avoid false-positive results on the basis of neurodevelopment (Durieux-Smith et al., 1987; Gorga et al., 1987; Hayes and Ringger, 1987). Infant state is an important variable because severe neonatal disease may affect the CNS and compromise predictions of auditory sensitivity based on the ABR (Gorga et al., 1987; Hall et

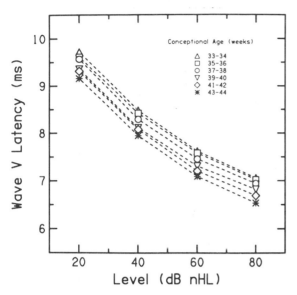

Figure 12-1. Average ABR wave V latencies in premature infants as a function of intensity with conceptional age as the parameter. As conceptual age increases, latency of wave V systematically decreases. (From Gorga, M. P., et al. (1987). Auditory brainstem responses from graduates of an intensive care nursery: Normal patterns of response. *Journal of Speech and Hearing Research, 30,* 311–318. With permission.)

al., 1988; Hayes and Ringger, 1987; Roberts et al., 1982; Stein, Ozdamar, Kraus, and Paton, 1983). Infants should be in a stable physiologic state before their hearing is screened by ABR.

Test environment is important because noise levels in many NICUs may interfere with optimum hearing screening, especially for relatively low intensity level signals (Richmond, Konkle, and Potsic, 1986). Hyde et al. (1984) reported a failure rate of 26 percent on initial ABR screening that was performed in the NICU. On retest in a sound-controlled environment within 24 hours, failure rate dropped to 12 percent, suggesting that the NICU is not an optimal environment for hearing screening. Ambient noise levels in the NICU have been reported to consistently exceed 60 dBA (Hall et al., 1988; Roberts et al., 1982), and this level may interfere with threshold evaluation (Richmond et al., 1986). Some investigators recommend screening all infants in a sound-controlled environment (Gorga et al., 1987), and one equipment manufacturer has attempted to account for fluctuating noise levels in the NICU by automatically halting response averaging when noise levels exceed a certain limit (Kileny, 1987).

Finally, development of appropriate follow-up strategies is essential if nursery-based screening is to be effective. Fria (1985) and Ruth et al. (1985) discuss the important difference between screening for disease and diagnosing disease. Failure on a nursery-based screen requires follow-up evaluation to diagnose hearing loss. Unfortunately, early reports of the ABR as a screening procedure indicated that compliance for follow-up evaluation was often poor (Galambos et al., 1984).

One problem with follow-up based on screening failure is motivating parents/caregivers about importance of diagnostic evaluation (Hayes, 1987). Stein, Ozdamar, Kraus, and Paton (1983) suggested that the difficulty and problems of follow-up could be reduced if the ABR screening protocol were expanded to include threshold and latency measures in infants who failed the initial screening. This procedure could be applied during the screening appointment, thereby reducing costs associated with repeated visits. The information gained from this evaluation would permit treatment of those infants with suspected conductive hearing loss prior to discharge, and possibly reduce need for additional evoked potential follow-up of infants with middle ear effusion. In addition, parental compliance for follow-up might improve if specific information about the nature of the ABR abnormality were provided at the time of screening failure.

Hayes and Ringger (1987) applied this principle to their NICU-based screening program. They obtained threshold and latency measures on infants who failed to demonstrate a response to clicks at 40 dB nHL or lower. Based on these threshold and latency measures, Hayes and Ringger categorized infant's responses by degree of predicted impairment and probable site of dysfunction. They developed three specific follow-up strategies depending on these predictions. For infants with predicted mild conductive loss, they recommended follow-up by behavioral evaluation after medical evaluation and treatment, and when the infant reached developmental age 6 months. For infants with predicted mild sensory, or moderate conductive or sensory loss, or a combination, they recommended follow-up diagnostic assessment, including additional evoked potential measures, following medical evaluation and treatment, and within 2 months of nursery discharge. Finally, for infants with predicted severe sensitivity loss, Hayes and Ringger recommended medical evaluation and diagnostic reevaluation within 1 month of nursery discharge. They found better follow-up compliance in infants whose initial ABR predicted more severe sensitivity loss than in infants whose initial ABR predicted mild conductive dysfunction. Hayes and Ringger concluded that immediate application of the ABR as a diagnostic procedure to infants who fail the nursery-based screening provides information important for development of follow-up strategies and may improve parental compliance for follow-up, at least for infants with potentially more severe hearing impairment.

ABR is a powerful technique for early screening and assessment of hearing in infants. The American Speech-Language-Hearing Association Committee on Infant Hearing (1989) recently published guidelines that recognize this procedure as the optimum approach to newborn hearing screening of infants at risk. If the procedure can become sufficiently low cost, ABR may provide the long sought-for approach to mass screening of newborn infants.

Deferred Screening

Some investigators recommend screening at-risk newborns following discharge from the newborn nursery when the infants reach age 4 months or older (Alberti et al., 1985; Hyde et al., 1984; Mahoney and Eichwald, 1987). These investigators argue that the advantages of deferred screening are

1. The test will be less contaminated by sequelae of severe neonatal illness or by maturational effects.
2. There is an increased likelihood of detecting progressive hearing losses, or hearing losses acquired after the neonatal period.
3. There is better control over test environment and infant state.
4. There is less likelihood of interfering with parental bonding if hearing loss identification is deferred beyond the newborn period.
5. No intervention strategies are known for hearing loss identified in the first few weeks of life (Alberti et al., 1985).

Deferred screening, however, is not optimal in most communities because it results in significant loss to follow-up. Many infants who should receive hearing evaluation do not return under deferred screening schemes. Mahoney and Eichwald (1987), for example, were able to document follow-up hearing evaluation of only 4684 out of 24,082 high-risk infants in a deferred screening program in which all appointments were offered

free of charge. Offering deferred screening as a routine component in total health care has been suggested to improve follow-up compliance (Hosford-Dunn et al., 1987); however, even in countries offering comprehensive, government-sponsored health care for infants and children, follow-up compliance for audiologic evaluation is often not satisfactory (Feinmesser and Tell, 1976).

It is sobering to recall that deferred screening has always been an option, especially after investigators convincingly demonstrated that auditory sensitivity of infants as young as 6-months' developmental age could be accurately assessed by low-cost, sensitive behavioral procedures. Unfortunately, deferred screening programs simply have not achieved acceptable follow-up compliance to warrant their recommendation, especially for infants at risk for hearing impairment. For screening to be effective, easy access to the population to be screened is essential. As noted by Downs and Sterritt (1964) more than 20 years ago, "Not until school age is reached will the child population again be so easily available; any screening program aimed at a later age group would be difficult and expensive in comparison with neonatal screening. . . ."

DIAGNOSTIC AUDIOLOGIC EVALUATION OF INFANTS

Only 7 to 12 percent of all newborns are at risk for hearing impairment (Jacobson and Morehouse, 1984; Mahoney and Eichwald, 1987). Even if all infants at risk received hearing screening in the newborn nursery, the vast majority of infants would receive no systematic evaluation for hearing impairment. Evaluation techniques are available that permit accurate behavioral assessment in infants as young as 6 months of age. A major challenge of pediatric audiology is to bring these procedures into routine use with all normally developing infants.

In general, diagnostic evaluation of infants and young children requires a test battery approach that combines behavioral measures of auditory sensitivity and physiologic measures of middle ear function (Jerger and Hayes, 1976).

BEHAVIORAL EVALUATION

Two behavioral approaches are used to evaluate auditory sensitivity in infants less than 2 years of age. The first approach employs an unconditioned test strategy in which the infant's responses are neither conditioned nor reinforced. This unconditioned procedure, behavioral observation audiometry (BOA), is commonly used to assess infants less than 6-months' developmental age and has received widest application in newborn hearing screening programs (Downs and Hemenway, 1969; Downs and Sterritt, 1964, 1967; Feinmesser and Tell, 1976; Jacobson and Morehouse, 1984; Mencher and Gerber, 1981). The second approach applies systematic conditioning procedures to control the infant's responses. Several conditioned test procedures have been developed, especially for testing children age 3 years and older. For young infants, visual reinforcement audiometry (VRA) is the most effective conditioned test procedure.

Behavioral Observation Audiometry

BOA involves controlled observation of an infant's overt behavioral response to sound. The observation is controlled in that only trained observers perform BOA and only specific behaviors are accepted as a response. No systematic reinforcement is used following responses. In general, BOA is applicable to neonates, very young infants, and older developmentally delayed children who cannot be conditioned by operant conditioning procedures. For newborn infants, suprathreshold stimulation is required to elicit reflexive or arousal responses. Older infants may demonstrate "awareness" or unconditioned head-turn response at reasonably soft stimulus levels (Friedrich, 1985).

BOA has only limited application and cannot reliably estimate auditory sensitivity (Thompson and Folsom, 1981). Because the infant's responses are not controlled by the examiner, assessment of threshold is not possible. BOA, in combination with electrophysiologic measures, may lead to development of an initial clinical impression. It cannot provide definitive diagnostic information, however.

Visual Reinforcement Audiometry

In contrast to BOA, VRA yields precise information about auditory sensitivity in infants as young as developmental age 6 months (Friedrich, 1985). Normally developing infants turn their heads to interesting or novel sounds in their environment. Muir and Field (1979) have demonstrated that these head-turning responses are present at birth, but that neuromotor develop-

ment and control prevent ready observation of these responses. Without systematic reinforcement, these natural head-turning responses habituate to repeated stimulation. By reinforcing these head-turning responses when an infant achieves neuromotor control (at about age 6 months), the response behavior can be controlled and valid estimates of hearing sensitivity can be obtained.

Suzuki and Ogiba (1961) reported results of a conditioning procedure involving the head-turn (localization) in infants. They called this procedure *conditioned orientation reflex* audiometry because it depended on components of the orientation response (alertness and orientation to low-level stimuli). In their procedure, an infant's auditory localization response was followed by presentation of a visual stimulus (lighted doll). The visual stimulus acted to reinforce the naturally occurring localization response. Suzuki and Ogiba reported that conditioned orientation reflex audiometry was successful more than 80 percent of the time for defining hearing sensitivity in children age 1 to 3 years. In the decade following Suzuki and Ogiba's report, several other investigators confirmed the utility of visual reinforcement for auditory localization responses in evaluating hearing sensitivity in young children (Haug, Baccaro, and Guilford, 1967; Liden and Kankkunen, 1969). In general, these early studies suggested that the lower age limit for visual reinforcing procedures was 12 months.

Wilson, Moore, and Thompson (1976) defined sound-field response levels to noise in normally developing infants between 5 and 18 months of age. They presented complex noise in a threshold-seeking paradigm and visually reinforced all appropriate responses. Average response levels for infants from 6 months through 18 months of age were approximately 25 dB SPL, and the tenth and ninetieth percentile points were approximately 20 and 30 dB SPL. Matkin (1977) defined average response levels to warbled tones and speech presented in the sound field by age for infants between 6 months and 36 months. His results are summarized in Figure 12-2. By age 6 to 11 months, infants respond, on the average, at hearing levels of approximately 25 dB, and by age 12 to 17 months, infants respond, on the average, at hearing levels of approximately 20 dB. These results indicate that it is possible to rule out all but a minimal hearing loss in infants as young as age 6 months with the use of VRA.

Behavioral measures provide important quantitative and qualitative information regarding an

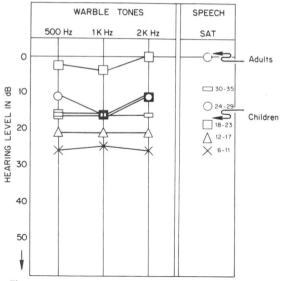

Figure 12-2. Average response levels by age for warble tones and speech presented in the sound field. (From Matkin, N. [1977]. Assessment of hearing sensitivity during the preschool years. In F. Bess [Ed.], *Childhood deafness: Causation, assessment, and management* [pp. 127–134]. New York: Grune & Stratton. With permission.)

infant's hearing status. VRA is the most important procedure for defining hearing sensitivity in infants age 6 months to approximately 3 years. For younger infants, or infants who cannot be conditioned to respond to sound, BOA provides qualitative information. The limitations inherent with BOA, however, suggest that it is best used in combination with measures that do not require the infant's cooperation.

Immittance Audiometry

Because OME is prevalent in infants, it is important to evaluate middle ear status during diagnostic audiologic evaluation. Immittance audiometry provides a rapid, accurate assessment of middle ear function in infants and young children (Northern, 1981; Northern and Downs, 1984). The combination of tympanometry and acoustic reflex measures can provide clinically relevant predictions of middle ear function, and in the case of normal middle ear function, prediction of sensory hearing level (Hall, 1981; Jerger et al., 1974).

Keith (1973, 1975) was one of the first to investigate immittance audiometry (impedance audiometry) in neonates. He reported results of measurement of the compliance, tympanogram, and presence of stapedial (acoustic) reflex in normal newborns less than 152 hours old. Keith con-

cluded that results of impedance audiometry in newborns are not substantially different from results in older children, and that impedance audiometry can be helpful in testing middle ear function in young infants.

In the mid-1970s, debate about the validity of tympanometry in infants less than 7 months old developed. Paradise, Smith, and Bluestone (1976) described results of an experiment comparing tympanometry and otoscopy in children ranging in age from 10 days to 5 years. For children age 7 months and older, there was a high positive correlation between tympanometry and otoscopy. For children less than 7 months, however, tympanometry yielded a distressing number of false-negative results (24 of 40 abnormal ears yielded normal tympanograms). These investigators advised against the use of tympanometry in infants less than 7 months of age.

Most investigators agree that any single component of the acoustic immittance test battery results in only limited diagnostic information (Jerger et al., 1974; Northern, 1981). In contrast, the combination of tympanometry and acoustic reflex measures provides important diagnostic information, even in very young infants. In a study of infants less than 7 months old, Schwartz and Schwartz (1978) reported that tympanometric results were normal in 16 of 20 ears with evidence of effusion, but that acoustic reflexes were absent in all 20 ears. Although a normal tympanogram does not rule out the possibility of effusion in an infant's ear, the combination of a normal tympanogram and normal acoustic reflexes indicates a high probability of normal middle ear function.

In 1974, Jerger et al. reported on the use of acoustic reflex thresholds to predict sensory hearing level. Their report, based on the relationship of threshold for broad-band noise versus threshold for pure tones, has been confirmed by numerous investigators (Hall, 1978, 1981; Margolis and Fox, 1977; Popelka, Margolis, and Wiley, 1976). In general, predictive accuracy varies with age and is best in children (Hall, 1981; Jerger, Hayes, and Anthony, 1978; Silman, Gelfand, and Emmer, 1981). Bennett and Weatherby (1982) have shown that the noise-tone acoustic reflex threshold difference is present in normal neonates. Further research on prediction of auditory sensitivity based on the acoustic reflex in neonates may lead to methods to improve evaluation of hearing impairment in newborns.

In general, immittance audiometry should be applied to evaluation of infants and young children as part of a test battery approach. The individual components of the immittance battery may have only limited value in isolation, but in combination, and in conjunction with other measures of auditory function, tympanometry and acoustic reflex measures yield important information about middle ear function and sensory status. Efforts to define more precisely relationships between tympanometry and acoustic reflex thresholds in neonates may result in additional tools for audiologic evaluation of very young infants.

AUDITORY EVOKED POTENTIALS

With the exception of the ABR, AEPs have only limited application in audiologic assessment of infants. Because most clinically relevant AEPs originate from the central nervous system (CNS), they are affected by neuromaturation and subject state variables such as sleep, sedation, and CNS dysfunction. Neuromaturation and sedation effects are especially problematic in AEP assessment of infants.

As reviewed by Schwartz and Morris in this volume, AEPs are described by their latency from stimulus as early (0–10 msec), middle (15–100 msec), and late (100–500 msec). Initial attempts to develop clinically meaningful AEP procedures concentrated on the late potentials (Goldstein, 1963). These relatively large amplitude potentials can be elicited by pure tone signals at intensity levels approximating behavioral thresholds. Unfortunately, the late potentials exhibit considerable inter- and intrasubject variability in amplitude, latency, and morphology and are significantly influenced by sleep, sedation, and CNS dysfunction.

The middle latency response (MLR) received research attention in the 1970s. Similar to the late response, the MLR can also be elicited by frequency-specific signals at relatively low intensity levels. The developmental aspects of the MLR have not been clearly defined, and several investigators have reported that the MLR is not reliably present in infants (Musiek, Verkest, and Gollegly, 1988; Stein and Kraus, 1987). The important clinical applications of the ABR have stimulated renewed interest in the MLR. As more information about this response becomes available, its clinical importance in evaluation of infants and young children might increase (Jerger, Oliver, and Chmiel, 1988).

A variant of the MLR, the 40-Hz event-related potential, is elicited by presenting signals at a rate of 40 per second. Because the period of the MLR is approximately 25 msec, a 40-Hz rate of stimulation enhances the amplitude of the response by overlapping and summating each successive response. The resultant average is an oscillatory waveform of 40 Hz. The response is subject to fast Fourier transform analysis, hence to objective response detection, and predictions of frequency-specific sensitivity within 5 to 10 dB of behavioral thresholds have been reported (Dauman et al., 1984; Martin and Hayes, 1982). Unfortunately, the 40-Hz event-related potential is significantly influenced by subject state. Martin and Hayes (1982), for example, reported that amplitude of the response decreased and threshold increased when subjects fell asleep during the test procedure. This important disadvantage limits application of the 40-Hz event-related potential in audiologic evaluation of infants.

Presently, the early potentials, and especially the ABR, are the most clinically useful AEPs for assessment of infants and young children. The response can be reliably recorded, and valid estimates of auditory sensitivity are possible based on threshold of the response.

Diagnostic audiologic evaluation of infants and young children requires a test battery approach combining appropriate behavioral procedures and immittance audiometry. For some infants, the ABR should also be used to estimate auditory sensitivity. For infants who cannot be conditioned to behavioral test procedures, the combination of BOA, ABR, and immittance audiometry permits accurate estimation of hearing sensitivity and middle ear function. For infants who can respond to conditioned behavioral test procedures, VRA and immittance audiometry permit definition of auditory sensitivity and middle ear function.

FUTURE DIRECTIONS

It is never "too soon" to test an infant's hearing. Valid and reliable techniques are available that provide information relevant to presence, degree, and nature of hearing impairment in very young infants, even newborns. Delay in identification of hearing loss in any infant because of age or developmental status is not necessary.

To improve early identification, two aspects of infants' assessment need immediate attention. First, tools for assessment, both electrophysiologic and behavioral, need refinement. Although rapid developments in both areas have significantly improved our ability to evaluate very young infants, the job is not complete. Measures are needed that will predict more precisely degree and configuration of hearing impairment to facilitate development of habilitation strategies. Measures are also needed that will reliably assess middle ear function in newborns to improve diagnosis of ear disease. In addition to hearing sensitivity, the effects of prematurity, anoxia, and other health conditions that place an infant at risk on the fragile central auditory system must be considered as early as possible.

The second area needing immediate attention is heightened awareness that infants, even newborns, can receive accurate audiologic assessment. Unless pediatricians, family practitioners, nurses, other health care providers, and parents know that an infant is "never too young" to have hearing tested, unacceptable delays in identification and habilitation will continue to occur (Elssmann et al., 1987). Until mass screening is available for all newborns, early referral from individuals who care for infants must be relied on.

Early identification is possible. It is our responsibility to make it happen.

REFERENCES

Alberti, P., Hyde, M., Riko, K., Corbin, H., & Fitzhardinge, P. (1985). Issues in early identification of hearing loss. *Laryngoscope, 95,* 373–381.

Allen, T. (1986). Patterns of academic achievement among hearing impaired students: 1974 and 1983. In A. Schildroth & M. Karchmer (Eds.), *Deaf children in America* (pp. 161–206). Boston: College-Hill Press.

American Academy of Pediatrics. Committee on Early Childhood, Adoption, and Dependent Care. (1984). *Middle ear disease and language development* (Reprint REX006).

American Speech-Language-Hearing Association. Committee on Infant Hearing. (1989). Audiologic screening of newborn infants who are at risk for hearing impairment. *ASHA, 31,* 89–92.

American Speech-Language-Hearing Association. Joint Committee on Infant Hearing. (1982). Position statement. *ASHA, 24,* 1017–1018.

Bennett, M. (1979). Trials with the auditory response cradle I: Neonatal responses to auditory stimuli. *British Journal of Audiology, 13,* 125–134.

Bennett, M., & Lawrence, R. (1980). Trials with the auditory response cradle II: The neonatal respiratory response to auditory stimuli. *British Journal of Audiology, 14,* 1–6.

Bennett, M., & Weatherby, L. (1982). Newborn acoustic reflexes to noise and pure-tone signals. *Journal of Speech and Hearing Research, 25,* 383–387.

Bergman, I., Hirsch, R., Fria, T., Shapiro, S., Holzman, I., & Painter, M. (1985). Cause of hearing loss in the high-risk premature infant. *Journal of Pediatrics, 106,* 95–101.

Bergstrom, L. (1987). Medical diagnosis of prelinguistic hearing loss. In K. Gerkin & A. Amochaev (Eds.), *Hearing in Infants: Proceedings from the National Symposium.*

Seminars in Hearing, 8, 83–88.

Berman, S., Balkany, T., & Simmons, M. (1978). Otitis media in the neonatal intensive care unit. *Pediatrics, 62,* 198–201.

Bhattacharya, J., Bennett, M., & Tucker, S. (1984). Long term follow up of newborns tested with the auditory response cradle. *Archives of Diseases in Childhood, 59,* 504–511.

Bluestone, C., & Klein, J. (1988). *Otitis media in infants and children.* Philadelphia: Saunders.

Brown, S. (1986). Etiological trends, characteristics, and distributions. In A. Schildroth & M. Karchmer (Eds.), *Deaf children in America* (pp. 33–54). Boston: College-Hill Press.

Coplan, J. (1987). Deafness: Ever heard of it? Delayed recognition of permanent hearing loss. *Pediatrics, 79,* 206–213.

Dahle, A., McCollister, F., Stagno, S., Reynolds, D., & Hoffman, H. (1979). Progressive hearing impairment in children with congenital cytomegalovirus infection. *Journal of Speech and Hearing Disorders, 44,* 220–229.

Dauman, R., Szyfter, W., de Sauvage, R., & Cazals, Y. (1984). Low frequency thresholds with 40 Hz MLR in adults with impaired hearing. *Archives of Otolaryngology, 240,* 85–89.

Dodge, P., Davis, H., Feigin, R., Holmes, S., Kaplan, S., Jubelirer, D., Stechenberg, B., & Hirsch, S. (1984). Prospective evaluation of hearing impairment as a sequela of acute bacterial meningitis. *New England Journal of Medicine, 311,* 869–874.

Downs, M., & Hemenway, W. (1969). Report on hearing screening of 17,000 neonates. *International Audiology, 8,* 72–76.

Downs, M., & Silver, H. (1972). The "A.B.C.D.'s" to H.E.A.R. *Clinical Pediatrics, 11,* 563–565.

Downs, M., & Sterritt, G. (1964). Identification audiometry for neonates: A preliminary report. *Journal of Auditory Research, 4,* 69–80.

Downs, M., & Sterritt, G. (1967). A guide to newborn and infant hearing screening programs. *Archives of Otolaryngology, 85,* 15–22.

Durieux-Smith, A., Picton, T., Edwards, C., Goodman, J., & MacMurray, B. (1985). The crib-o-gram in the NICU: An evaluation based on brain stem electric response audiometry. *Ear & Hearing, 6,* 20–24.

Durieux-Smith, A., Picton, T., Edwards, C., MacMurray, B., & Goodman, J. (1987). Brainstem electric response audiometry in infants of a neonatal intensive care unit. *Audiology, 26,* 284–297.

Elssmann, S., Matkin, N., & Sabo, M. (1987). Early identification of congenital sensorineural hearing impairment. *Hearing Journal, 40,* 13–17.

Ensher, G., & Clark, D. (1986). *Newborns at risk. Medical care and psychoeducational intervention.* Salem, MA: Aspen.

Eskola, J., Peltola, H., Takala, A., Kayhty, H., Hakulinen, M., Karanko, V., Kela, E., Rekola, P., Ronnberg, P., Samuelson, J., Gordon, L., & Makela, P. (1987). Efficacy of *Haemophilus influenzae* type b polysaccharide-diphtheria toxoid conjugate vaccine in infancy. *New England Journal of Medicine, 317,* 717–722.

Feinmesser, M., & Tell, L. (1976). Neonatal screening for detection of deafness. *Archives of Otolaryngology, 102,* 297–299.

Frankenberg, W. (1975). Principles in selecting diseases for screening. In W. Frankenburg & B. Camp (Eds.), *Pediatric screening tests* (pp. 9–22). Springfield, IL: Charles C. Thomas.

Fria, T. (1985). Identification of congenital hearing loss with the auditory brainstem response. In J. Jacobson (Ed.), *The auditory brainstem response* (pp. 317–336). Boston: College-Hill Press.

Friedrich, B. (1985). The state of the art in audiologic evaluation and management. In E. Cherow (Ed.), *Hearing-impaired children and youth with developmental disabilities. An interdisciplinary foundation for service* (pp. 122–125). Washington, DC: Gallaudet College Press.

Galambos, R., Hicks, G., & Wilson, M. (1982). Hearing loss in graduates of a tertiary intensive care nursery. *Ear & Hearing, 3,* 87–90.

Galambos, R., Hicks, G., & Wilson, M. (1984). The auditory brainstem response reliably predicts hearing loss in graduates of a tertiary intensive care nursery. *Ear & Hearing, 5,* 254–260.

Gerkin, K. (1984). The high risk register for deafness. *ASHA, 26,* 17–23.

Gerkin, K., & Church, M. (1987). Fetal alcohol syndrome and hearing loss. In K. Gerkin & A. Amochaev (Eds.), *Hearing in infants: Proceedings from the National Symposium. Seminars in Hearing, 8,* 89–92.

Goldstein, R. (1963). Electrophysiologic audiometry. In J. Jerger (Ed.), *Modern developments in audiology* (pp. 167–192). New York: Academic Press.

Gorga, M., Reiland, J., Beauchaine, K., Worthington, D., & Jesteadt, W. (1987). Auditory brainstem responses from graduates of an intensive care nursery: Normal patterns of response. *Journal of Speech and Hearing Research, 30,* 311–318.

Grundfast, K., & Bluestone, C. (1978). Sudden or fluctuating hearing loss and vertigo in children due to perilymph fistula. *Annals of Otology, Rhinology, and Laryngology, 87,* 761–771.

Hall, J. (1978). Predicting hearing level from the acoustic reflex: A comparison of three methods. *Archives of Otolaryngology, 104,* 601–605.

Hall, J. (1981). Hearing loss prediction by the acoustic reflex in a young population. *International Journal of Pediatric Otorhinolaryngology, 3,* 225–243.

Hall, J., Kripal, J., & Hepp, T. (1988). Newborn hearing screening with auditory brainstem response: Measurement problems and solutions. In D. Worthington (Ed.), *Auditory evoked response measurement in children. Seminars in Hearing, 9,* 15–33.

Halpern, J., Hosford-Dunn, H., & Malachowski, N. (1987). Four factors that accurately predict hearing loss in "high risk" neonates. *Ear & Hearing, 8,* 21–25.

Haug, O., Baccaro, P., & Guilford, F. (1967). The pure-tone audiogram on the infant: The PIWI technique. *Archives of Otolaryngology, 86,* 101–106.

Hayes, D. (1987). Problems in habilitation of hearing-impaired infants. In K. Gerkin & A. Amochaev (Eds.), *Hearing in Infants: Proceedings from the National Symposium, 8,* 181–185.

Hayes, D., & Ringger, J. (1987). *Diagnostic ABR in the NICU.* Paper presented at the X. Biennial International Symposium, International ERA Study Group. Charlottesville, VA.

Hecox, K., & Galambos, R. (1974). Brain stem and auditory evoked responses in human infants and adults. *Archives of Otolaryngology, 99,* 30–33.

Hosford-Dunn, H., Johnson, S., Simmons, B., Malachowski, N., & Low, K. (1987). Infant hearing screening: Program implementation and validation. *Ear & Hearing, 8,* 12–20.

Hyde, M., Riko, K., Corbin, H., Moroso, M., & Alberti, P. (1984). A neonatal hearing screening research program using brainstem electric response audiometry. *Journal of*

Otolaryngology, 13, 49–54.

Jacobson, J., & Jacobson, C. (1987). Application of test performance characteristics in newborn auditory screening. In K. Gerkin & A. Amochaev (Eds.), *Hearing in infants: Proceedings from the National Symposium. Seminars in Hearing, 8,* 133–141.

Jacobson, J., & Morehouse, R. (1984). A comparison of auditory brainstem response and behavioral screening in high risk and normal newborn infants. *Ear & Hearing, 5,* 247–253.

Jerger, J., & Hayes, D. (1976). The cross-check principle in pediatric audiometry. *Archives of Otolaryngology, 102,* 614–620.

Jerger, J., Burney, P., Mauldin, L., & Crump, B. (1974). Predicting hearing loss from the acoustic reflex. *Journal of Speech and Hearing Disorders, 39,* 11–22.

Jerger, J., Hayes, D., & Anthony, L. (1978). Effect of age on prediction of sensorineural hearing level from the acoustic reflex. *Archives of Otolaryngology, 104,* 393–394.

Jerger, J., Oliver, T., & Chmiel, R. (1988). Auditory middle latency response: A perspective. In D. Worthington (Ed.), *Auditory evoked response measurement in children. Seminars in Hearing, 9,* 75–86.

Karchmer, M. (1985). A demographic perspective. In E. Cherow (Ed.), *Hearing impaired children and youth with developmental disabilities. An interdisciplinary foundation for service* (pp. 36–56). Washington, DC: Gallaudet College Press.

Keith, R. (1973). Impedance audiometry with neonates. *Archives of Otolaryngology, 97,* 465–467.

Keith, R. (1975). Middle ear function in neonates. *Archives of Otolaryngology, 101,* 376–379.

Kileny, P. (1987). ALGO-1 automated infant hearing screener; preliminary results. In K. Gerkin & A. Amochaev (Eds.), *Hearing in infants: Proceedings from the National Symposium. Seminars in Hearing, 8,* 125–131.

Konigsmark, B., & Gorlin, R. (1976). *Genetic and metabolic deafness.* Philadelphia: Saunders.

Lary, S., Briassoulis, G., de Vries, L., Dubowitz, L., & Dubowitz, V. (1985). Hearing threshold in preterm and term infants by auditory brainstem response. *Journal of Pediatrics, 107,* 593–599.

Liden, G., & Kankkunen, A. (1969). Visual reinforcement audiometry. *Acta Oto-laryngologica* (Stockholm), 67, 281–292.

Mahoney, T., & Eichwald, J. (1987). The ups and "downs" of high-risk hearing screening: The Utah statewide program. In K. Gerkin & A. Amochaev (Eds.), *Hearing in infants: Proceedings of the National Symposium. Seminars in Hearing, 8,* 155–163.

Marchant, C., Shurin, P., Turcyzk, V., Wasikowski, D., Tutihasa, M., & Kinney, S. (1984). Course and outcome of otitis media in early infancy: A prospective study. *Journal of Pediatrics, 104,* 826–831.

Margolis, R., & Fox, C. (1977). A comparison of three methods for predicting hearing loss from acoustic reflex thresholds. *Journal of Speech and Hearing Research, 20,* 241–253.

Martin, J., & Hayes, D. (1982). *Use of an FFT criterion to identify presence of auditory evoked response (40 Hz ERP) at behavioral threshold.* Paper presented at XVI International Congress of Audiology, Helsinki.

Matkin, N. (1977). Assessment of hearing sensitivity during the preschool years. In F. Bess (Ed.), *Childhood deafness: Causation, assessment, and management* (pp. 127–134). New York: Grune & Stratton.

McCormick, B., Curnock, D., & Spavins, F. (1984). Auditory screening of special care neonates using the auditory response cradle. *Archives of Disease in Childhood, 59,* 1160–1172.

Mencher, G., & Gerber, S. (Eds.). (1981). *Early management of hearing loss.* New York: Grune & Stratton.

Moscicki, E. (1984). The prevalence of "incidence" is too high. *ASHA, 26,* 39–40.

Muir, D., & Field, J. (1979). Newborn infants orient to sounds. *Child Development, 50,* 431–436.

Murray, A., Javel, E., & Watson, C. (1985). Prognostic value of auditory brainstem evoked response screening in newborn infants. *American Journal of Otolaryngology, 6,* 120–131.

Musiek, F., Verkest, S., & Gollegly, K. (1988). Effects of neuromaturation on auditory-evoked potentials. In D. Worthington (Ed.), *Auditory evoked response measurements in children. Seminars in Hearing, 9,* 1–13.

Myklebust, H. (1950). *Your deaf child (a guide for parents)* (p. 80). Springfield, IL: Charles C Thomas.

Naulty, C., Weiss, I., & Herer, G. (1986). Progressive sensorineural hearing loss in survivors of persistent fetal circulation. *Ear & Hearing, 7,* 74–77.

Nield, T., Schrier, S., Ramos, A., Platzker, A., & Warburton, D. (1986). Unexpected hearing loss in high-risk infants. *Pediatrics, 78,* 417–421.

Northern, J. (1981). Impedance measurement in infants. In G. Mencher & S. Gerber (Eds.), *Early management of hearing loss* (pp. 131–149). New York: Grune & Stratton.

Northern, J., & Downs, M. (1984). *Hearing in children* (3rd ed.). Baltimore: Williams & Wilkins.

Osberger, M. (Ed.). (1986). Language learning skills in hearing-impaired students. *ASHA Monograph, 23.*

Paparella, M., Goycoolea, M., Schachern, P., & Sajjadi, H. (1987). Current clinical and pathological features of round window disease. *Laryngoscope, 97,* 1151–1160.

Paradise, J., Smith, C., & Bluestone, C. (1976). Tympanometric detection of middle ear effusion in infants and young children. *Pediatrics, 58,* 198–210.

Pestalozza, G. (1984). Otitis media in newborn infants. *International Journal of Pediatric Otorhinolaryngology, 8,* 109–124.

Petroff, M., Simmons, F., & Winzelberg, J. (1986). Two emerging perilymph fistual "syndromes" in children. *Laryngoscope, 96,* 498–501.

Popelka, G., Margolis, R., & Wiley, T. (1976). The effect of activating signal bandwidth on acoustic reflex thresholds. *Journal of the Acoustical Society of America, 59,* 153–159.

Richmond, K., Konkle, D., & Potsic, W. (1986). ABR screening of high-risk infants: Effects of ambient noise in the neonatal nursery. *Otolaryngology — Head and Neck Surgery, 94,* 552–556.

Roberts, J., Davis, H., Phon, G., Reichert, T., Sturtevart, E., & Marshall, R. (1982). Auditory brainstem responses in preterm neonates: Maturation and follow-up. *Journal of Pediatrics, 101,* 257–263.

Ruth, R., Dey-Sigman, S., & Mills, J. (1985). Neonatal ABR hearing screening. *Hearing Journal, 38,* 39–45.

Sak, R., & Rubin, R. (1982). Effects of recurrent middle ear effusion in pre-school years on language and learning. *Journal of Developmental Behavior and Pediatrics, 3,* 7–11.

Salamy, A., & McKean, C. (1976). Post-natal development of human brainstem potentials during the first year of life. *Electrocochleograhy and Clinical Neurophysiology, 40,* 418–426.

Schlech, W., Ward, J., Band, J., Hightower, A., Fraser, D., & Broome, C. (1985). Bacterial meningitis in the United States, 1978 through 1981. *Journal of the American Medical Association, 253,* 1749–1754.

Schulman-Galambos, C., & Galambos, R. (1975). Brain stem auditory-evoked responses in premature infants. *Journal of Speech and Hearing Research, 18,* 456–465.

Schulman-Galambos, C., & Galambos, R. (1979). Brain stem evoked response audiometry in newborn hearing screening. *Archives of Otolaryngology, 105,* 86–90.

Schwartz, D., & Schwartz, R. (1978). A comparison of tympanometry and acoustic reflex measurements for detecting middle ear effusion in infants below seven months of age. In E. Harford, F. Bess, & C. Bluestone (Eds.), *Impedance screening for middle ear disease in children* (pp. 91–96). New York: Grune & Stratton.

Sell, E., Gaines, J., Gluckman, C., & Williams, E. (1985). Persistent fetal circulation: Neurodevelopmental outcome. *American Journal of Diseases in Childhood, 139,* 86–90.

Shurin, P., Pelton, S., & Klein, J. (1976). Otitis media in the newborn infant. *Annals of Otology, Rhinology, and Laryngology, 85,* 216–222.

Silman, S., Gelfand, S., & Emmer, M. (1987). Acoustic reflexes in hearing loss identification and prediction. In J. Hall (Ed.), *Immittance audiometry. Seminars in Hearing, 8,* 379–390.

Simmons, F. (1980). Patterns of deafness in newborns. *Laryngoscope, 90,* 448–453.

Simmons, F., & Russ, F. (1974). Automated newborn hearing screening, the Crib-o-Gram. *Archives of Otolaryngology, 100,* 1–7.

Starr, A., Amlie, R., Martin, W., & Sanders, S. (1977). Development of auditory function in newborn infants revealed by auditory brainstem potentials. *Pediatrics, 60,* 831–839.

Stein, L., & Kraus, N. (1987). Maturation of the middle latency response. In K. Gerkin & A. Amochaev (Eds.), *Hearing in infants: Proceedings from the National Symposium. Seminars in Hearing, 8,* 93–101.

Stein, L., Clark, S., & Kraus, N. (1983). The hearing-impaired infant: Patterns of identification and habilitation. *Ear & Hearing, 3,* 232–236.

Stein, L., Ozdamar, O., Kraus, N., & Paton, J. (1983). Follow-up of infants screened by auditory brainstem response in the neonatal intensive care unit. *Journal of Pediatrics, 103,* 447–453.

Suzuki, T., & Ogibi, Y. (1961). Conditioned orientation audiometry. *Archives of Otolaryngology, 74,* 192–198.

Teele, D., Klein, J., Rosner, B., & the Greater Boston Otitis Media Study Group (1984). Otitis media with effusion during the first three years of life and development of speech and language. *Pediatrics, 74,* 282–287.

Thompson, G., & Folsom, R. (1981). Hearing assessment of at-risk infants. *Clinical Pediatrics, 20,* 257–261.

Webb, K., Krishnan, V., & Katzman, G. (1985). Newborn hearing screening using the Crib-o-Gram. *Archives of Otolaryngology — Head and Neck Surgery, 112,* 420–422.

Weber, H. (1987). Ten years of searching for the hearing-impaired infant in rural Colorado. In K. Gerkin & A. Amochaev (Eds.), *Hearing in Infants: Proceedings from the National Symposium. Seminars in Hearing, 8,* 149–154.

Wilson, W., Moore, J., & Thompson, G. (1976). *Sound-field auditory thresholds of infants utilizing visual reinforcement audiometry (VRA).* Paper presented at the American Speech-Language-Hearing Association annual meeting, Houston.

CHAPTER 13

Balance Disorders ("The Dizzy Patient")

Neil T. Shepard • *Steven A. Telian*

When consideration is given to the spectrum of patients that have difficulties associated with the "balance system," not all will have complaints of "dizziness" or true vertiginous experiences. Therefore, the classification of "dizzy patient," as in the title, reflects only a subpopulation of patients experiencing balance and gait disorders. In order to provide accurate assessment and proper management of patients with balance disorders, a broad frame of reference is needed. The patients that are referred to an otologist and then undergo objective studies of vestibular and balance system function have a wide range of descriptive complaints. These may include vertigo or less classic symptoms ranging from linear vexion, pulsion, lightheadedness, unsteadiness to clumsiness that should not be considered as all the same.

The emphasis of the chapter will reflect this expanded concept of balance and gait disorders. Because of limited space, a comprehensive treatment of balance disorders, for which entire texts have been written (Baloh and Honrubia, 1983; Barber and Sharpe, 1988), is not possible in this setting. Instead, the authors will present a general review of balance system physiology from a functional approach to provide a picture of the integrated system. Specific details of vestibular, oculomotor, and postural control physiology will be referred to other sources. General pathophysiology of the balance system will be followed by details of the evaluation of balance disorder patients. In discussion of management, the reader will be introduced to the use of balance retraining/compensation and habituation therapy program.

BALANCE SYSTEM PHYSIOLOGY

POSTURAL CONTROL

The maintenance of upright posture while sitting or more important, when standing requires an alignment of the body's center of mass (with the gravity vector) positioned over the available support surface (typically the feet when standing unassisted) (Figure 13-1). A major goal of the postural control portion of the balance system is to quickly determine perturbations in the center of mass away from its desired location and the rapid onset of corrective muscular reaction. Independently and in combination, the body uses sensory input and automatic muscle response to accomplish this goal by producing particular muscle responses to specific stimulus inputs (called *stimulus-coded response pairing*) (Figure 13-2). The input of visual, vestibular, and somatosensory systems provides the avenues by which external stimuli (visual image movements or body accelerations, or both) are coded to produce a muscle response (Allum and Pfaltz, 1985; Forssberg and Nashner, 1982; Horak and Nashner, 1986; Nashner, 1979, 1983, 1987; Nashner and Berthoz, 1978). The muscle responses are learned and stereotyped relative to the stimulus as long as the environmental context remains unchanged. For example, a person standing on a flat surface (larger than the foot) that suddenly jerks forward causing a backward sway provides for visual (moving environment), vestibular (linear and angular acceleration), and somatosensory (an opening plan-

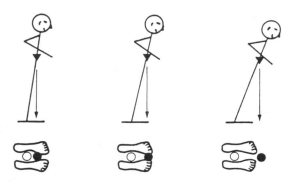

Figure 13-1. Cartoon illustrating maintenance of center of mass (triangle) over the support surface in alignment with gravitational pull. (Adapted from Nashner, L. M. [1987]. *A systems approach to understanding and assessing orientation and balance disorders.* Paper on advances in diagnosis and management of balance disorders. NeuroCom International. With permission.)

tar flexion movement of the ankle angle giving muscle stretch receptor stimulation) inputs. As shown in Figure 13-3A, a repeatable sequential contraction of the tibialis anterior, quadriceps, and abdominal musculature causes recovery, bringing the body back into the upright position from the backward sway. This stimulus-coded response is highly repeatable as long as the support surface and the size of the perturbing movement remain the same. If the patient is asked to stand on a surface narrower than the foot length and the same movement of the surface is exe-

cuted, giving the same sensory input cues, the muscle response (shown in Figure 13-3B) is entirely changed. The new stimulus-coded response pair uses the old stimulus with a new muscle response, resulting in movement at the hips for maintenance of stance. In this example the only change was the environmental context, that is, the size of the support surface relative to the length of the foot (Diener, Horak, and Nashner, 1988; Horak and Nashner, 1986; Nashner, 1985).

Although changes in environmental context cause appropriate changes in the harmonious responses to the three input cues, they may also be placed in direct conflict with one another. Under this situation, it is theorized that as the visual and somatosensory inputs are compared to the information from the vestibular end organ, congruent information is maintained and conflicting information is selectively suppressed (Barin, 1987). Time is required for this process to take place. The effects of these sensory conflicts are analyzed during this interval because of the automatic reaction from the stereotyped muscle response pairing to a common stimulus. An example of this is experienced when sitting in a stationary vehicle and the car alongside begins to move. The reflex is to step on the brake in response to a false sensation of

Figure 13-2. Schematized representation of the stimulus-coded response pairing in the balance system. The sensory inputs of vision, vestibular end organ, and somatosensory at the ankle are shown on the left with muscle response on the right. (Developed by NeuroCom International, With permission.)

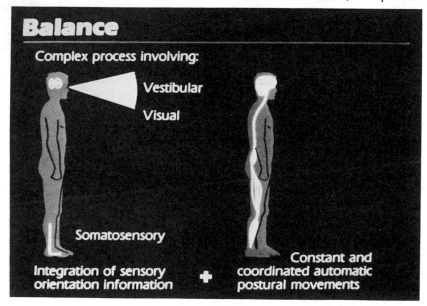

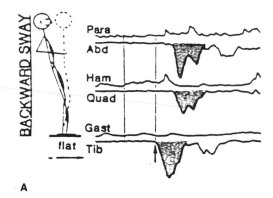

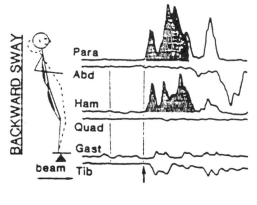

Figure 13-3. A. Induced backward sway of the patient with rectified surface EMG responses shown from the various muscle groups. B. Same size of perturbation inducing backward sway, but the patient is now standing on a beam instead of a flat, firm surface. Muscle responses to recover from the sway are shown. Abd, abdominal musculature; Gast, gastrocnemius; Ham, hamstring; Para, paraspinal muscles; Quad, quadriceps; Tib, tibialis anterior. (Adapted from Horak, F. B., & Nashner, L. M. [1986]. Central programming of postural movements: Adaptation to altered support-surface configurations. *Journal of Neurophysiology, 55*[6], 1369–1381.)

backward motion. This example of linear vexion (perception of linear motion when none is taking place) illustrates sensory conflict between the visual input and the actual body and head movement. The optokinetic visual input gave the incorrect perception of motion, triggering a learned automatic, although an incorrect, response. In a short time it is apparent that backward motion is not taking place, and the brake is released. If the event repeats almost immediately, the incorrect response is not produced. Sensory conflicts are numerous during normal activities. Although many primarily involve the visual input, they certainly also occur through the somatosensory pathways (standing or walking on an irregular or compressive surface, e.g., a soft rug, mud, or gravel). The normal balance system handles these conflicts with only minor disruptions in activity because of the automatic stimulus-coded response pairing within a given context. This ability to modify one's muscle response behavior for a constant stimulus given changing context conditions reflects the adaptive-learning properties of the system. This is a characteristic that allows for an alteration in the stimulus-coded response pair in order to change an erroneous response to a given stimulus following an initial stimulus presenta-

tion. This was demonstrated in a study (Nashner and Grimm, 1978) in which the dominant cue (change in ankle angle) (Allum, 1983; Diener et al., 1984; Keshner, Allum and Pfaltz, 1987) was presented without the usual concomitantly forward-induced sway by tilting the toes up (Figure 13-4). Therefore, if the typical muscle response to a closure of the ankle angle (dorsiflexion maneuver) is selected, a destabilizing reaction is produced. The body is pulled backward in the absence of forward sway, instead of producing a forward motion to compensate for the toes being tilted upward. If muscle electromyogram activity is recorded from the principal muscle groups of the lower limbs, the expected stimulus-coded response to a toes-up condition is initially the same as that for induced forward sway — gastrocnemius followed by hamstring contraction. This is followed, after some delay, by the contraction of the tibialis and then the quadriceps in order to counteract the automatic but incorrect destabilizing muscle activity. As this test condition is repeated over five trials, the strength of the gastrocnemius and the hamstring response progressively decreases, leaving only the correct adaptive response from the tibialis and the quadriceps. This adaptive learning capability demonstrates the plasticity of the postural control portion of the balance system as well as its context dependency. It is hypothesized that a large number of muscle response combinations could be used at any time for any given stimulus-context condition. Thus, the goal of rapid reaction time is best served by comparative consideration of actual performance versus desired performance through a limited set of response actions that are contingent on the stimulus-context conditions (Nashner and McCoullum, 1985). In other words, one does not have to

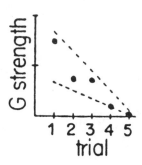

Figure 13-4. Result of sudden dorsiflexion maneuver of the ankle joint without concomitant forward sway. The associated rectified EMG responses from monitored muscle groups are shown in the middle panel for five repeated trials. The panel on the right shows the change in strength (adaption) of gastrocnemius over the five trials. G, gastrocnemius; H, hamstring; T, tibialis anterior; Q, quadriceps. (Adapted from Nashner, L. M., & Grimm, R. J. [1978]. Clinical applications of the long loop motor control analysis in intact man: Analysis of multiloop dyscontrols in standing cerebellar patients. *Neurophysiology, 4,* 300–319.)

consciously consider each response to select the optimal combination of muscles to use.

EYE MOVEMENT CONTROL

Functional control of eye movements associated with the balance system can be divided into major categories. The control of eye movements independent of head motion (ocular motor control), and that coordinated with head movements (ocular motor and vestibulo-ocular reflex [VOR] control), provide perceptions of motion relative to the environment. They also make it possible to focus on objects in the visual field in a precise manner when the target, the person, or both are in motion.

VESTIBULO-OCULAR REFLEX

The VOR system provides for compensatory eye movements in response to angular and linear accelerations of the head. If the head is rotated to the right in an accelerating movement, a compensatory eye movement to the left is produced. As the movement is continued and the eye approaches the physical limits of the orbit, the VOR compensatory motion is transiently interrupted by a rapid corrective movement (saccade) of the eye in the direction of rotation. This saccade activity, which is not part of the VOR, results from the position of the eye in the orbit, which activates the saccade control system (Baloh and Honrubia, 1983). Continued acceleration will produce repeated alternating compensatory (slow) and saccadic (fast) eye movements. This pattern is referred to as *jerk nystagmus*. The compensatory movement is called the *slow-phase component* with the saccadic activity called the *fast-phase component* (Figure 13-5). By convention the jerk nystagmus produced is named by the direction of the fast-phase component. Therefore, the eye response in rotation to the right is referred to as *right beating*

jerk nystagmus. This response results from stimulation of the horizontal semicircular canals. Analogous activity can be noted for rotation in other planes of motion stimulating the other semicircular canals or for linear acceleration events. Detailed discussions of the anatomy and physiologic considerations in the production of the VOR are published elsewhere (Baloh and Honrubia, 1983; Doslak, Dell'Osso, and Daroff, 1982; Gacek, 1980; Pulaski, Zee, and Robinson, 1981; Ryu, 1986; Schwarz, 1986; Zee, 1978). The major goal of the VOR is to maintain a foveal image (image focused on the area of the retina giving the clearest vision)

Figure 13-5. Cartoon demonstrating the vestibulo-ocular reflex (VOR) compensatory movement of the eyes to the left for an angular acceleration to the right. Corrective saccade movement of the eyes in the direction of rotation that interrupts the VOR is also shown.

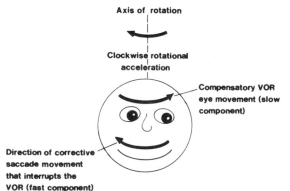

for a visual target of interest during head movements. An additional goal of the vestibular end-organ mechanism is to provide information about change in velocity of movement (acceleration/deceleration) rather than simply detecting whether or not movement is occurring. The system is unresponsive to very low accelerations (< 0.016 degree/second) or situations of constant velocity (zero acceleration).

OCULOMOTOR CONTROL SYSTEM WITH AND WITHOUT THE VESTIBULO-OCULAR REFLEX

The control of eye movements when motionless and the perception of movement when traveling at a constant velocity depend on three interacting oculomotor control systems: smooth pursuit, saccade, and optokinetic. The latter is the one that provides for sensations of movement during constant velocity (or very low accelerations) and produces eye movements in the form of jerk nystagmus like those of the VOR. For example, most have had the experience of traveling on a plane during a smooth flight at a constant velocity with no sensation of motion unless they look out the window. Both the perception of motion and the sensation of speed increase as the objects outside the window come closer to the aircraft. This is the *optokinetic system effect*. Optokinetic stimulation is accomplished by having large objects move across the visual field as a result of a moving visual field or a stationary visual field with movement of the observer (Figure 13-6) (Kubo et al., 1981; Rahko, 1984; Ventre, 1985; Zasorin et al., 1983). The sensations produced by optokinetic stimulation can be strong enough to cause all of the (vegetative) symptoms of motion sickness including emesis without ever having the subject move. The optokinetic stimulus is most often the one in conflict with the other sensory inputs, such as in the example of the inappropriate application of the car brake given previously. The special effect of motion that most individuals experience in large-screen theaters and simulated "space rides" at amusement parks is generated through optokinetic stimulation. The ability of the optokinetic system to provoke sensations of motion when the body is not moving, as well as provide indications of movement when the head is in constant velocity or very low acceleration, seems to be accomplished by interaction with the vestibular system. This is speculated to

take place at the level of the vestibular nucleus through a modulation of the primary afferent input from the semicircular canals and not by direct influence on the semicircular canals themselves (Cohen et al., 1981; Waespe, Cohen, and Raphan, 1983, 1985; Zee et al., 1981). In effect, the optokinetic system extends the ability to perceive motion during times when the vestibular end organ is unable to provide accurate information.

The smooth pursuit and saccade systems, although controlling eye movement, do not provide the sensations of motion resulting from optokinetic stimulations. Many investigators studying the oculomotor control systems suggest that the optokinetic nystagmus, made up of slow and fast alternating components, is the combination of both the smooth pursuit system (for the slow component) and the saccade system (for the fast component) in addition to a separate optokinetic system (Baloh and Honrubia, 1983; Honrubia, Baloh, and Khalili, 1989). The smooth pursuit system maintains the visual image on the retina (on the fovea) during a tracking (following) movement of the eyes. In order for this system to function, the target motion must be predictable with a frequency under approximately 1.5 Hz with peak velocity less than 120 degrees/second (this varies depending on the actual trajectory of the target) (Lisberger, Morris, and Tychsen, 1987; Robinson, 1968; Zee, 1984; Zee, Leigh, and Mathieu–Millaire, 1980). The goal of this system overlaps with the VOR in maintaining a foveal image since it operates with the head motionless and the target moving, with the target motionless and the head in motion, and when both are moving together. Although the VOR is not activated at very low frequencies, the use of the smooth pursuit system coupled with the VOR allows for accurate tracking of a stationary or moving object when the head is in motion over a frequency range of less than 0.001 to 5.0 Hz (Schwarz, 1986).

The functional goal of the saccadic system is to provide for rapid replacement of a visual image of interest onto the fovea. When the head is stationary and the target frequency or speed exceeds the limits of the smooth pursuit system, saccadic movements begin to appear. These are rapid eye movements that reposition the target on the fovea, stimulated by "retinal slip" of the image toward the periphery of the retina. The less predictable the motion of the target is, or the more the limits of the smooth pursuit system are exceeded, more saccadic catch-up activity is required. Certainly, when the head is in motion (with or without con-

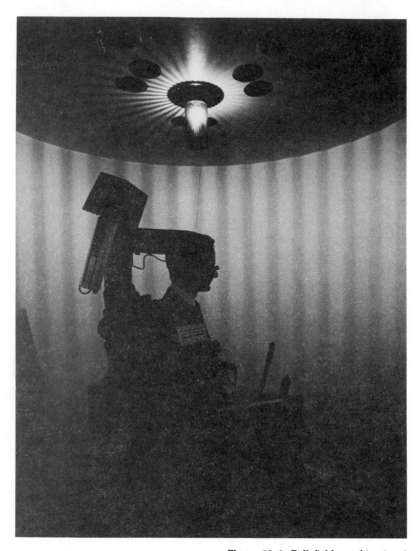

Figure 13-6. Full field optokinetic stimulus that can be rotated with the patient still, the patient rotated with the stripes stable, or both moved simultaneously. (From Oviatt, D. [1988, Spring]. Cutting through the fog of silence. *Advance,* University of Michigan Medical Center, p. 16. With permission.)

comitant target motion), the saccadic activity appears to be essential to maintain visual fixation (Cohen, and Buttner–Ennever, 1984; Cohen et al., 1985).

Saccadic eye movements then are stimulated not only by voluntary tracking of targets but also make up the fast-phase component of optokinetic jerk nystagmus and the jerk nystagmus resulting from stimulation of the semicircular canals.

Functional activities of the vestibulo-ocular and oculomotor portions of the balance system similar to those of the postural control system, but in this case response musculature, are that of the extraocular muscles. Stimulus-coded response pairs govern the VOR and the oculomotor control sys-

tems and show similar properties of context dependency and adaptive learning plasticity (Furst, Goldberg, and Jenkins, 1987; Melvill, Berthoz, and Segal, 1984; Melvill and Mandl, 1981, 1983; Paige, 1983).

A knowledge of the physiology of the balance system as just outlined sets the framework for understanding the various types of objective measures needed to evaluate the pathologic changes seen in the balance disorder patient.

BALANCE SYSTEM PATHOLOGY

ACUTE PATHOLOGIC PROCESS

Dysfunction of the balance system, especially vertigo of acute onset, usually originates from pathology associated with either the vestibular nerve or the peripheral vestibular labyrinth. This results in asymmetric input to the vestibular nuclei, which produces a hallucination of persistent angular motion (vertigo) and jerk nystagmus with its fast component beating toward the side with the higher rate of neural activity (Figure 13-7). In the acute phase, the nystagmus is present despite visual fixation (attempted suppression of nystagmus through the smooth pursuit system), which reflects only the strength of the nystagmus rather than indicating pathology in the central vestibular pursuit system. As the lesion becomes chronic, the nystagmus is typically observed only when visual fixation is eliminated, such as in the dark or with the use of special glasses (Frenzel lenses) that prevent the patient from focusing. The nystagmus can also be observed by recording the eye movements using electrodes near the eyes. This process is electronystagmography (ENG) and provides a means of tracking eye movements behind closed lids or in a darkened environment by measuring changes in eye position indicated by

Figure 13-7. Cartoon illustrating the perception of rotational movement to the right with an acute reduction in activity of the left horizontal semicircular canal. Eye movement deviation to the left (slow component) by activation of the VOR and the saccadic interruption (fast component) moving the eyes back to the right as shown.

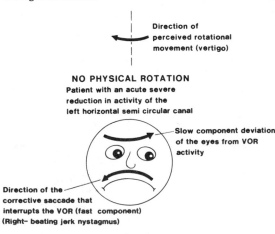

the polarity of the natural corneal-retinal potential relative to each electrode (Barber and Stockwell, 1980).

Pathology affecting the balance system is certainly not limited to the peripheral system (involving labyrinth or cranial nerve VIII, or both). Changes in the central vestibular system including the vestibulo-ocular pathways, the vestibulospinal system, or the extravestibular portions integrating the total balance system can produce a number of different complaints, which can vary from unsteadiness or ataxia with no indication of vertigo or motion intolerance to severe vertiginous episodes. The report of true vertigo is less frequent when the peripheral vestibular system is not involved.

CENTRAL COMPENSATION

A unique feature of the balance system is its ability to compensate for peripheral system pathology resulting in asymmetries, provided the effecting lesion is stable over time or varying very slowly (Igarashi, 1984; McCabe and Sekitani, 1972; Pfaltz, 1983; Takahashi, Uemura, and Fujishiro, 1984; Takemori et al., 1984). The compensation process results from activity in the vestibulo-ocular pathways in the cerebellum and the brainstem. The process of reestablishment of symmetric firing rates at the level of the vestibular nuclei is accomplished without modulating the neural input to the vestibular nuclei from the peripheral system. Although many details of this process are known, the precise mechanism remains a mystery (Courjon et al., 1982; Schwarz, 1986). From empiric data and animal studies, it appears that the compensation process is enhanced by head movement but inhibited by preexisting or concomitant central vestibular pathway involvement (Igarashi et al., 1978, 1979; Mathog and Peppard, 1982). Medications that cause central nervous system suppression, such as those typically used for acute symptoms of vertigo, are probably counterproductive (Bernstein, McCabe, and Ryu, 1974; Ishikawa and Igarashi, 1984, 1985; Matsunaga, Shiraishi, and Kubo, 1983; McCabe, Sekitani, and Ryu, 1973; Pykko et al., 1984; Peppard, 1986; Ryu et al., 1984; Sekitani, McCabe, and Ryu, 1971; Zee, 1985). It is also suspected that above age 65 years, the likelihood of complete compensation is reduced (Norré and Beckers, 1988; Stelmach and Worringham, 1985; Woollacott, Shumway–Cook, and Nashner, 1986).

Slower adaptive processes also occur for central vestibular lesions (Strong et al., 1984). This delay is illustrated in stroke and head injury patients in whom numerous abnormalities of the balance system are often demonstrated, with or without indications of peripheral involvement.

In general the patients requiring extensive, continuing medical care are those in whom the compensation process has been ineffective. This results from lesions of the peripheral or central systems that are unstable, such as seen in repeated insults from Ménière's disease, chronic suppurative middle ear disease, perilymphatic fistula, and vascular events including migraine headaches and ischemia. Another major group of patients in whom compensation may fail resulting in ongoing symptoms are those with injury to the portions of the central nervous system that are required to participate in the process. It is also possible to have the process of compensation be successfully completed after which the patient may undergo a decompensation process. The original symptoms then recur because of systemic illness, use of various medications, surgical procedures, or simply with aging. One other factor that may hinder the patient's recovery is psychiatric disease, which may complicate a severe balance disorder (Brightwell and Abramson, 1975; Jacob, 1988; Jacob et al., 1985; Rigatelli et al., 1984). Depression, anxiety, and occasionally frank panic attacks many times intensify the subjective symptoms out of proportion to the extent of the actual lesion. This complication introduces an extra dimension in general patient management.

BALANCE AND GAIT DISORDER EVALUATION

The evaluation of the balance disorder patient consists of several major components: history of presenting symptoms, otologic and neurologic physical examination, and laboratory studies.

HISTORY

The history of presenting symptoms is often the most important component in the diagnostic process. Although this is typically done by the managing physician, it should also be done by the person performing the balance function studies. This additional history can and should serve as a cross check and will influence the interpretation of the balance studies. In general, the information gathered should include a record of the onset of symptoms and their characteristics, the progression of symptoms over time, details of the current symptoms, predisposing past medical history, and the use of medications. An example of the requisite information is shown in Figure 13-8. Detailed discussions of what historical information is useful and suggested interpretations are provided elsewhere (Baloh and Honrubia, 1983).

LABORATORY STUDIES

Because of the intimate relationship of the vestibular end organ and the cochlea, audiometric evaluations are an essential part to the work-up for a balance disorder patient. Typically pure tone and speech audiometry are adequate to establish coexisting auditory pathology. The use of auditory brainstem response is appropriate when asymmetries in hearing or unexplained peripheral vestibular findings are present. Coexisting auditory pathology is a strong lateralizing indicator in patients with peripheral vestibular dysfunction.

Metabolic and radiographic studies are typically used to identify various pathologic processes that may account for the balance dyfunction complaints. It is fairly common for all of these studies to be within normal limits in patients with balance disorders, especially those involving the labyrinth.

The purposes of the balance function studies are threefold and are outlined in Table 13-1. The most traditional purpose is that of site of lesion localization, which may result in recommendations concerning involvement by other medical disciplines. Until recently, little or no assessment of the patient's functional capabilities or recommendations concerning rehabilitation have been provided. Table 13-2 shows the various activities for a complete modern balance function study, which will fulfill the purpose outlined. These activities are accomplished through a variety of studies that require the use of relatively expensive, newly available technology. Although the use of this new technology has led to a better understanding and assessment of the balance system, the principles of the testing can be accomplished many times, if only qualitatively, without the use of these expensive units. Thus, the principles of the basic balance function study can be pursued by any laboratory, regardless of size. The discussion to follow will be limited to an overview of each of the tests including their use for specific target populations and the expected information.

DATE: MAH:

EXAMINER: NAME:

REFERRING PHYSICIAN: D.O.B.:

U OF M BALANCE TESTING CENTER
PATIENT HISTORY AND SX

ONSET: (DATE OF ONSET; SUDDEN VS GRADUAL; PAST HX.)

CHARACTERISTICS: (OBJECTIVE VS SUBJECTIVE VERTIGO, R OR L; SPELLS OR CONTINUOUS SX.)

IF IN SPELLS: (FREQUENCY; DURATION; SX BETWEEN ATTACKS; SX SPONTANEOUS OR MOTION PROVOKED.)

IF CONTINUOUS: (UNSTEADY; LIGHTHEADED; AND/OR VERTIGO.)

PREDISPOSING FACTORS: (YES/NO)

HEAD INJURY: _____   NECK INJURY: _____   OTOTOXIC DRUGS: _____   TOXIC CHEM: _____

FLU/VIRUS: _____   MIGRAINE SELF: _____   MIGRAINE FAM: _____   D.M. SELF: _____

D.M. FAM: _____   EYE DISEASE: _____   HYPERTENSION: _____   PERIPHERAL VASC: _____

HEART DISEASE: _____   NEUROMUSCULAR: _____   ORTHOPEDIC: _____   BAROTRAUMA: _____

AUDITORY SX: (AS AD AU EQ NN)

TINNITUS: _____   IF AU, TINNITUS GREATER IN: _____

AURAL FULLNESS: _____   IF AU, FULLNESS GREATER IN: _____

PERCEIVED HEARING LOSS; SUDDEN: _____   FLUCTUANT: _____   GRADUAL: _____

EAR SURGERY: (CIRCLE ONE) AS   AD   AU   NONE

PROCEDURES:

POSITIONING SX: (CIRCLE ALL THAT APPLY)

LAY DOWN FROM SITTING	SIT UP FROM LAYING	ROLL R OR L IN BED
STAND UP FROM SITTING	TURN HEAD R OR L	BEND OVER
STRAIGHTEN FROM BENDING	LOOK UP OR DOWN	

OTHERS: (DESCRIBE)

MOTION INTOLERANCE:

CAR SICKNESS (NOW, AND PAST HX.)	SX ON ELEVATORS OR ESCALATORS
SX IN STORE AISLES	SX WHILE STANDING NEAR TRAFFIC

OTHERS: (DESCRIBE)

MISCELLANEOUS:

INCREASE IN SX OR FREQUENCY/DURATION OF ATTACKS WITH PHYSICAL EXERTION:

OSCILLOPSIA:

LOSS OF CONSCIOUSNESS:

FALLING (OR SX OF IMMINENT FALL, OR DIRECTION):

NUMBNESS OR TINGLING IN FACE OR EXTREMITIES:

VISUAL SX:

MEMORY LAPSE:

NERVOUSNESS SCALE:

CURRENT MEDICATIONS:

DISABILITY SCALE: (CIRCLE ONE)

0 NO DISABILITY, NEGLIGIBLE SYMPTOMS.

1 NO DISABILITY, BOTHERSOME SYMPTOMS.

2 MILD DISABILITY, PERFORMS USUAL DUTIES, SYMPTOMS INTERFERE WITH SOCIAL ACTIVITIES.

3 MODERATE DISABILITY, DISRUPTS USUAL DUTIES.

4 RECENT SEVERE DISABILITY, ON MEDICAL LEAVE OR HAD TO CHANGE JOB.

5 LONG TERM SEVERE DISABILITY, UNABLE TO WORK FOR EXTENDED PERIOD.

Figure 13-8. Suggested two-part history form for information to be taken during the balance function studies.

**TABLE 13-1. PURPOSE OF
BALANCE FUNCTION ASSESSMENT**

1. Site of lesion information relative to the various
   components of the balance system:

Inputs	Outputs	Neural pathways
Vestibular end organs	Muscular contractions	Vestibulo-ocular
Vision	Vegetative symptoms	Vestibulospinal
Somatosensory	Perceptions	Oculomotor
		Vestibulo — "other"
		Visual — "other"

2. Functional capabilities of patient relative to
   a. correlation to expressed symptoms
   b. static and dynamic maintenance of stance
   c. predictions of potentially troublesome
      environmental conditions (risk for falls)

3. Recommendations for use of and potential effectiveness
   of habituation and balance retraining exercise/
   therapy programs

**TABLE 13-2. COMPLETE BALANCE
FUNCTION ASSESSMENT**

1. Spontaneous and positionally related abnormal eye
   movements

2. Relative sensitivity of vestibular end organs

3. Evaluation of vestibular end organ (via VOR) across
   a broad-frequency and acceleration range

4. Oculomotor capabilities across a normal physiologic
   range of stimuli (saccade, pursuit, and optokinetic
   systems)

5. Vertical semicircular canal and otolith organ function

6. Functional characterization of the total system
   including
   a. integration of three sensory inputs and various
      strategies for their use
   b. coordination of musculature of lower limbs under
      dynamic conditions
   c. environmental risks for falls

ELECTRONYSTAGMOGRAPHY

ENG has come to refer to a procedure involving a series of subtests during which eye movement recordings are made to gain information about the function of portions of the peripheral and central vestibular system. From the previous discussion of oculomotor control, it follows that eye movements serve as a "window" into the functioning of the vestibular and the oculomotor control systems. Details of the techniques of ENG testing and interpretation of the detailed findings are provided through other sources (Baloh, Honrubia, and Sills, 1977; Baloh, Solingen, Sills, and Honrubia, 1977; Barber and Sharpe, 1988; Barber

and Stockwell, 1980; Furman, Wall, and Kamerer, 1988; Jacobson and Henry, 1989; Jacobson and Means, 1985; Kumar, 1981; O'Neill, 1987; Proctor et al., 1986; Sills, Baloh, and Honrubia, 1977; Stockwell, 1983; Wetmore, 1986).

The ENG is useful for all patients with balance dysfunction, although protocols may have to be adjusted to suit the particular needs of an individual, dictated by age, anxiety level, and physical condition. Spontaneous, nonprovoked eye movements (spontaneous nystagmus) and eye movements provoked by changes in the orientation of the vestibular end organ relative to the gravitational field (positional nystagmus) are recorded. Effects of rapid positioning into a specific head position (Hallpike maneuver) are typically part of the ENG and were designed to provide evidence for one specific condition — benign paroxysmal positional vertigo and nystagmus. Although oculomotility evaluations are part of the traditional ENG, these will be discussed separately. The last part of the ENG evaluation involves a measure of the responsiveness of the horizontal semicircular canal on each side. This is performed through caloric irrigations. These irrigations can be performed by open- or closed-loop water irrigation or through air insufflation. The purpose of the irrigation is to produce a change in the temperature of the endolymph fluid within the horizontal canal in one receptor organ at a time. This causes asymmetric activity resulting in nystagmus and perception of circular motion (vertigo) in most normal individuals. The eye movement response from stimulation of one side is compared to that from the other to give a measure of relative sensitivity. This is the only method of selective determination of unilateral sensitivity presently available. Other methods of end-organ stimulation provoke both right- and left-side responses simultaneously.

Interpretation of abnormal eye movements during the ENG suggests possible lesion sites in the peripheral vestibular or central vestibular-ocular pathways, or both. The ENG is a physiologic test, not one of the functional abilities of the patient. Nevertheless, the results serve many times as an explanation for symptoms the patient may be experiencing. The detection of abnormal from normal or artifactual eye movement activity is a pattern recognition task requiring an experienced interpreter. In many cases the abnormalities found will be generally nonlocalizing; however, based on the characteristics of the eye movements, patient history, and other balance function studies, the probability of peripheral versus central involvement may be predicted (Kumar and Sutton, 1984; Kumar, Mafee, and Torok, 1982; Lambert, 1986; Stockwell, 1983; Takemori, Aiba, and Shizawa, 1981). The use of the phrase *peripheral vestibular system involvement* must not be interpreted to indicate a lesion in the vestibular labyrinth unless other supporting evidence of inner ear involvement is present, such as cochlear hearing loss. The ENG findings indicating peripheral lesion site can *not* differentiate between the labyrinth, cranial nerve VIII, or the vestibular nucleus portion of the brainstem. A localizing tool similar to auditory brainstem response testing for the vestibular system is desirable but not yet available.

It is important to appreciate the limitations of the ENG, especially since it is the most frequently used modality for balance function evaluation (Kileny and Kemink, 1986; Kileny, McCabe, and Ryu, 1980; Takemori, Moriyama, and Totsuka, 1979). The principal limitation is that a normal ENG evaluation may rule out certain pathologies but does not necessarily indicate a normally functioning balance system. Many aspects of the balance system that may contribute to patient symptoms are not evaluated with an ENG. The reciprocal problem is encountered when caloric irrigations produce no response from either periphery. This finding should *not* be interpreted to indicate completely nonfunctioning peripheral vestibular systems. Vestibular function, like the auditory system, has frequency-specific characteristics over which it functions. Calorics stimulate only the low-frequency, low-intensity (angular acceleration equivalent) end of this spectrum (Fernandez and Goldberg, 1971; Honrubia et al., 1982; Kamerer and Furman, 1988; Schwarz, 1986). Consequently, absent caloric responses are often seen in patients who have not suffered a complete loss of function. Finally, the ENG evaluation does not provide for testing of the capacity for integration of all sensory input information (vision, vestibular, and somatosensory) used by the balance system, and it does not test the patient's ability to handle conflicting information. Both of these issues are critical in assessing the overall state of functional capacity.

As an example of the evaluation process being described, all the associated test findings on patient JM will be presented. The patient's chief complaint and presenting history indicate a 72-year-old man with sudden onset of symptoms of dysequilibrium and constant unsteadiness in June of 1987. Symptoms are prominent when standing or attempting to walk and reduced when sitting or lying. Patient denies vertigo or lightheadedness. Onset of symptoms were 2 days postdischarge from a hospital following treatment for endocarditis with 21 days of intravenous gentamycin. The patient reports diagnosed peripheral neuropathy (condition that reduces proprioception sensitivity) affecting both hands and feet. Past medical history reveals a left hip replacement within 2 months before this visit and unoperated cataract in the right eye. Aural fullness and fluctuant and progressive perceived loss of hearing were reported associated with the left ear.

The results of the ENG evaluation on 4/7/89 indicated right beating spontaneous nystagmus that was sporadic in occurrence with slow-phase velocity of 2 to 3 degrees/second. Right beating positional nystagmus was present in 6 of 11 positions tested with slow-phase velocity of 2 to 4 degrees/second considered to be of clinical significance by published criteria (Stockwell, 1983). Patient responded only to ice water calorics showing responses less than 9 degrees/second with a calculated 36 percent weaker response for irrigation to the right compared to those to the left. These results were interpreted to indicate a bilateral weakness. The percentage difference can be misleading when the absolute slow-phase velocities are low (< 10 degrees/second) as in this case, and the absolute difference between the calorics was only 4.6 degrees/second. The 36 percent difference could simply reflect a predisposition to right beating nystagmus as indicated with the spontaneous and positional results. By patient history the most likely periphery for greater involvement would be the left and not the right. Although the indications for peripheral involvement may provide an explanation for the patient's expressed symptoms, the other factors of hip replacement, peripheral neuropathy, and reduced visual acuity may certainly be contributing to the overall condition. The extent of these other factors is not revealed with the ENG.

OCULOMOTILITY STUDIES

These tests are designed to evaluate the oculomotor pathways for functions of gaze, smooth pursuit tracking, saccade movement, and optokinetic nystagmus, all without vestibular end-organ stimulation. They are traditionally performed as part of the ENG; however, with the recent advent of computerized ENG analysis, a more thorough and quantitative assessment of the oculomotor tasks can be made.

In general these studies are useful in all patients for whom the ENG would be used. The four tests provide the only dedicated portion of the balance testing that gives information about the central vestibular system, principally brainstem and cerebellar pathways.

Abnormal findings on any of these studies imply pathology of the central pathways. Usually smooth pursuit tracking and optokinetic responses are the most sensitive to lesions, but the abnormalities are nonlocalizing to specific areas within the oculomotor pathways. Although gaze and saccade testing are less sensitive, they are more site specific relative to brainstem and cerebellar pathways. Saccade testing, when evaluated by a program that can provide measures of maximum saccade velocity, latency to onset of saccade after target movement, and the accuracy of the movement for various subtended arcs of target motion, can suggest specific lesions of the cerebellar vermus or the parapontine reticular formation of the brainstem (Abel and Barber, 1981; Baloh, Honrubia, and Sills, 1977; Barber and Stockwell, 1980; Bogousslavsky and Meienberg, 1987; Gresty, Page, and Barratt, 1984; Koenig, Dichgans, and Dengler, 1986; Leigh and Zee, 1982; Ranalli, Sharped, and Fletcher, 1988; Sharpe, Herishanu, and White, 1982; Simons and Buttner, 1985; Stockwell, 1983; Yee et al., 1982; Zee and Leigh, 1983; Zee and Robinson, 1978).

Increased sensitivity of the smooth pursuit tracking test is achieved by stressing the pursuit system using progressively higher frequencies and target speeds. This unfortunately also increases the major limitation with this procedure, that is, age-related deterioration of performance. Therefore, it is important to have age-related norms for pursuit performance. This test, like that of saccades, is best performed using computerized systems that allow for the detailed calculations in order to quantify performance.

The oculomotility results for patient JM indicate normal formal saccade results and normal optokinetic nystagmus, examples of each are given in Figures 13-9 and 13-10, respectively. Pursuit tracking (Figure 13-11) shows a combination of saccadic catch-up manuevers (patient's eye falling behind the target and a saccade maneuver is used to replace the image on the fovea Figure 13-11B) mixed with saccade movements that lead the target (anticipating target position instead of following target per instructions Figure 13-11A). The results demonstrate central vestibulo-ocular path-

way involvement yet are probably explainable on the basis of changes associated with age.

SINUSOIDAL HARMONIC ACCELERATION TEST (ROTATIONAL CHAIR TESTING)

The vestibular end organ operates over a range of frequencies and accelerations with calorics providing a low-frequency, low-acceleration (equivalent) stimulus. The use of rotational chair testing has developed as a means for stimulating the horizontal semicircular canal over a range of frequencies and accelerations. The commercially available devices provide for computer-controlled movement, recording of eye activity, and analysis of eye movements relative to chair (head) movement. The typical mode of chair movement is sinusoidal, hence the name *sinusoidal harmonic acceleration*. The acceleration stimulus activates the VOR and is repeated for multiple cycles at a given frequency with the slow-phase eye movements averaged and analyzed by comparison to head movement (Baloh et al., 1982; Hamid et al., 1986; Hess, Baloh, and Honrubia, 1985; Hirsch, 1986; Honrubia, Jenkins, Misner, Baloh, Yee, and Lau, 1984; Honrubia, Jenkins, Baloh, Yee, and Lau, 1984; Istil, Hyden, and Schwartz, 1983; LeLiever, Calhoun, and Correia, 1984; Wall, Black, and Hunt, 1984). Three specific parameters are evaluated:

1. *Phase* provides information about the position of the eyes relative to the position of the head.
2. *Gain* is the ratio of the averaged peak slow-component eye velocity to the averaged peak head velocity.
3. *Asymmetry* is a measure of the difference in averaged peak slow-component eye velocity resulting from acceleration to the right versus acceleration to the left, expressed in percentage.

The test is also a physiologic, not functional evaluation, but is felt to provide information beyond that gathered from the ENG, especially related to the status of compensation. This evaluation is critical in individuals for whom calorics are either significantly reduced, absent, or ambiguous due to significant anatomic differences in the external or middle ear anatomy. From some preliminary work comparing performance of various bal-

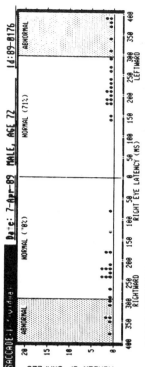
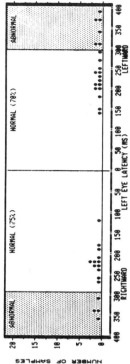
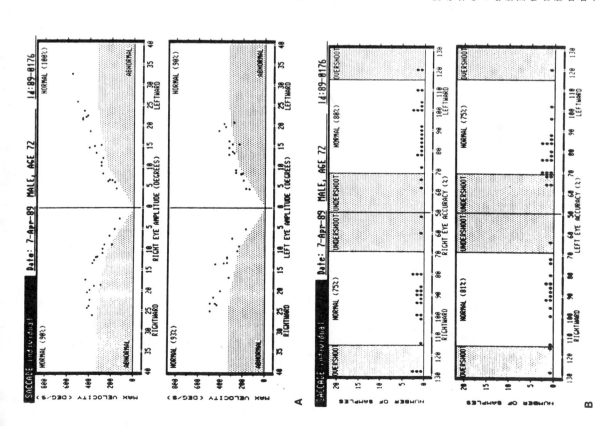

Figure 13-9. Random saccade testing results from patient JM are illustrated and interpreted as normal. *A.* Maximum saccade velocity for each saccade movement analyzed is plotted versus the subtended arc movement of the eyes in degrees. This is shown for right eye (top panel) and the left eye (bottom panel) separately for eye movements rightward and leftward. The stippled area represents abnormal velocities. The number in parentheses indicates the percentage of saccade movements with normal velocities. *B.* Plot of the number of saccade movements versus a measure of accuracy of the eye excursion relative to the target movement. *100%* indicates eye movement equal to target movement with under- and overshoot areas indicated. Display of individual eye activity same as in A. *C.* Plot of the number of saccade movements versus the latency to onset of the eye movement following the target movement. Display of individual eye activity same as A. (From ICS Medical Corporation. With permission.)

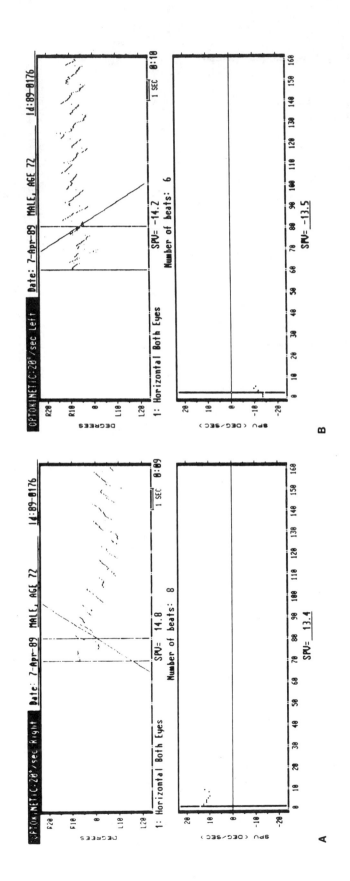

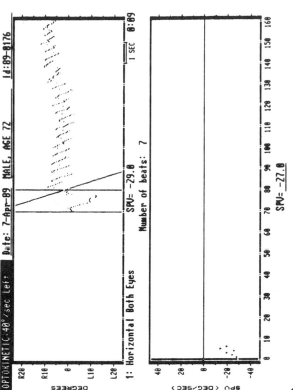

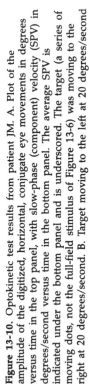

D with the display the same as described in A. C. Target moving to the right at 40 degrees/second with the display the same as described in A. D. Target moving to the left at 40 degrees/second with the display the same as described in A. These results are interpreted as normal since symmetry in SPV is demonstrated for each speed and the SPV average increases by a factor of 2 as the target speed was increased. (From ICS Medical Corporation. With permission.)

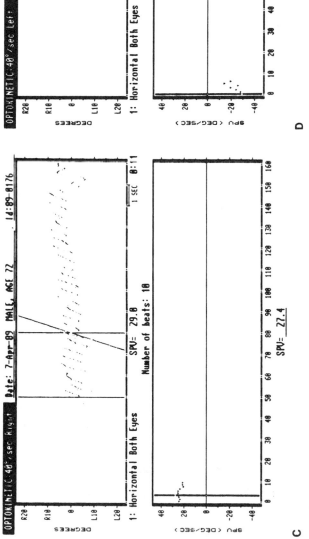

C

Figure 13-10. Optokinetic test results from patient JM. A. Plot of the amplitude of the digitized, horizontal, conjugate eye movements in degrees versus time in the top panel, with slow-phase (component) velocity (SPV) in degrees/second versus time in the bottom panel. The average SPV is indicated under the bottom panel and is underscored. The target (a series of moving dots, not the full-field stimulus of Figure 13-6) was moving to the right at 20 degrees/second. B. Target moving to the left at 20 degrees/second

282

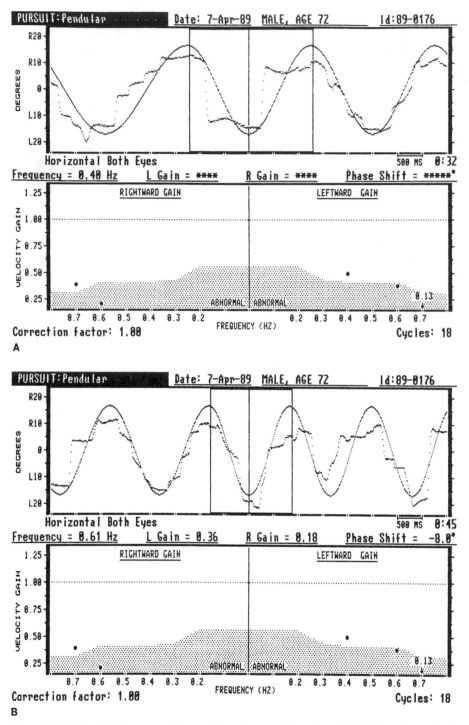

Figure 13-11. Results from smooth pursuit tracking test for patient JM. A. Plot of amplitude of the conjugate, horizontal eye movements in degrees versus time in the top panel. The bottom panel plots velocity gain (velocity of the patient's eye movements divided by the velocity of the target) versus frequency of target movement for rightward and leftward target excursions. A target frequency of 0.4 is illustrated. B. A target frequency of 0.61 is shown with the remainder of the display the same as A. Discussion of these results is given in the text. (From ICS Medical Corporation. With permission.)

ance function studies, a full rotary chair study, consisting of four or five test frequencies, may not be routinely necessary (Shepard et al., 1987). The complete study has its maximum usefulness for (1) patients in whom caloric results are uncertain or unobtainable; (2) pediatric patients, infants, and others with mental age under 10 years; and (3) patients requiring pre- and posttreatment evaluation or for whom serial vestibular testing is necessary such as when ototoxic drugs are given. Test-retest reliability appears superior to ENG alone. In general abnormal findings with this evaluation usually relate to peripheral vestibular system function, whereas central vestibular status must be evaluated through other tests.

Information about the high-frequency activity of the vestibular end organ can be obtained, at least

qualitatively, by having the passive head movement accomplished with the chair system. An auditory stimulus such as a metronome can provide the timing to produce different frequencies of horizontal rotation. Technology now exists permitting recording and analysis of resulting eye movements as described in the literature (Fineberg, O'Leary, and Davis, 1987). Typically, when qualitative substitutes are made for tests such as rotational chair, validity and test-retest reliability may be expected to suffer. This should not preclude the use of qualitative substitute methods, but one must recognize the care needed during interpretation and the limitations of the conclusions.

For case JM the rotational chair findings are given in Figure 13-12. These demonstrate significant reduction in the slow-phase eye velocity (indicated by low gain) for frequencies of rotation from 0.02 to 0.32 Hz. The slow-component eye velocity increases to within the normal range (gain within ± two standard deviations) for frequencies of 0.64 and 1.28 Hz. These findings are interpreted to indicate a severe reduction in VOR suggestive of bilateral peripheral weakness; however, they clearly indicate residual function in at least one periphery. It is important that a virtual absence in caloric response, as was demonstrated on the ENG, not be interpreted as totally absent function of the peripheral system. It is clear now that although a severe reduction in VOR is present at the lower frequencies, the system's sen-

Figure 13-12. Rotational chair results on patient JM. A. Plot of both phase (circles) and gain (squares) versus frequency of the sinusoidal chair rotation with peak velocity of 50 degrees/second for each frequency tested. Phase values are given in degrees on the left ordinate with the gain (eye slow-component velocity divided by chair velocity) on the right ordinate. The lines give the ± two standard deviation limits for phase (P---P) and gain (G---G). B. Plot of asymmetry, the percentage of difference between right and left slow-component velocity versus test frequency. The lines represent ± two standard deviation limits. Phase and asymmetry measures are not valid for gain values less than 0.1. A discussion of the results is given in the text. (From Neurokinetics, Inc. With permission).

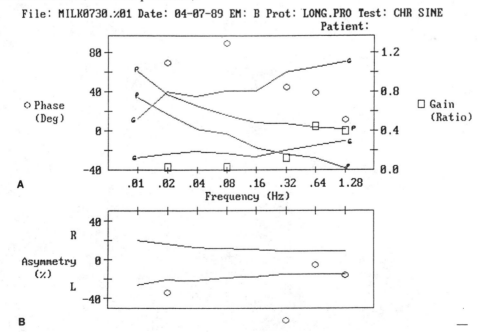

sitivity returns to within normal limits as the test frequency is increased, enhancing the prognosis for compensation over time.

DYNAMIC POSTUROGRAPHY

All of the above tests provide primarily physiologic data with little specific quantitative functional evaluation. Further, ENG and rotational chair evaluations deal only with isolated parts of the balance system and do not assess the system as a whole. The use of posturography has been proposed to fill this void by providing quantitative assessment of postural stability during stance. Clinical observations and recordings of static postural control (eyes open or closed Romberg and tandem Romberg testing) have been used for many years (Black, Wall and O'Leary, 1978; Norré and Forrez, 1983; Wall and Black, 1983; Wolfson et al., 1986; Yoneda and Tokumasu, 1986). Although this provides some information about the use of all three sensory inputs for maintenance of stance with and without vision, no controlled, systematic disruption in foot somatosensory cues is possible using standard Romberg testing. In addition, performance during sensory conflict situations cannot be evaluated. So, although beginning the evaluation of postural control, the Romberg test falls short of a complete test of sensory organization abilities and coordinated muscles re-

sponses during both static and dynamic (induced sway) conditions. Among the other arguments for expansion of the evaluation of postural function is the suggestion that the gait problems seen in the elderly may result from deterioration of the postural control system (Woollacott, 1988). The concept of dynamic postural testing has recently begun gaining acceptance for clinical use. This provides for measurement of body sway (reflecting postural stability) during two distinct protocols. One assesses coordination of the muscle reactions to induced forward and backward sway, and the other analyzes the ability to maintain equilibrium during changing sensory input conditions (Figures 13-13 and 13-14) (Black and Nashner, 1984; Black et al., 1988; Black, Wall, and Nashner, 1983; Nashner, 1983; Nashner, Friedman, and Wusteney, 1988). The monitoring of sway is done through a dual force-plate system on which the

Figure 13-13. Platform translations for the movement coordination portion of dynamic posturography. The movement shown on the left induces forward sway with a variety of parameters calculated during the patient's recovery. The induced sway (forward as shown or backward) is done at three increasing perturbation sizes of the brief horizontal translations (three trials are given at each perturbation size). The cartoon on the right shows the platform movement to test for adaptation. The platform suddenly tilts the toes up in five successive trials or down in five trials. (Developed by NeuroCom International, Inc. With permission.)

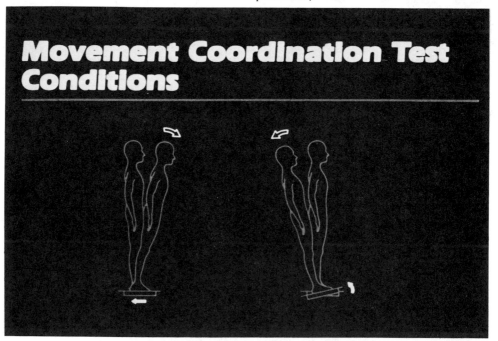

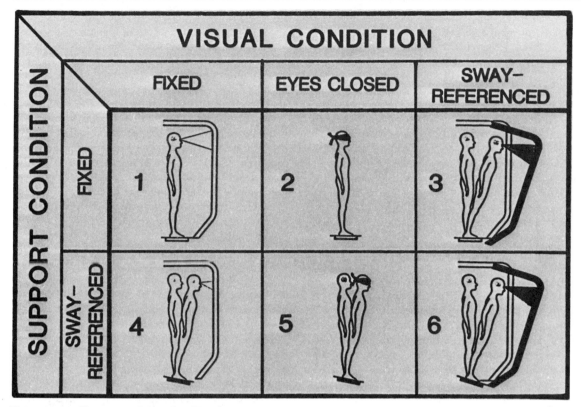

VISUAL CONDITION

SUPPORT CONDITION

FIXED / EYES CLOSED / SWAY–REFERENCED

FIXED — 1, 2, 3

SWAY–REFERENCED — 4, 5, 6

Figure 13-14. Six test conditions for the sensory organization portion of dynamic posturography. In the top three conditions, accurate foot somatosensory cues are available to the patient in all of the tests. The first and second conditions are simply eyes open and eyes closed Romberg tests, each performed one time with a 20-second trial. Condition 3 provides for orientationally inaccurate visual information (visual conflict) in that if the patient sways anterior or posterior, the visual surrounding moves with the patient. In conditions 4, 5, and 6, inaccurate foot somatosensory cues are provided by tilting the platform equal to the patient's anterior/posterior sway. Then for each of these conditions (4, 5, and 6), the same visual variations are tested as in conditions 1, 2, and 3. Therefore, in conditions 5 and 6, the only accurate input cue is vestibular end-organ information. In conditions 3 through 6, three 20-second trials of each are tested. (Developed by NeuroCom International, Inc. With permission.)

patient stands. The dynamic aspects of the testing involve introduction of perturbation of balance by jerks of the support surface either forward or backward. The sensory conflict inputs are accomplished through a technique whereby patient sway is stabilized relative to visual and somatosensory cues as illustrated in Figure 13-14. This provides a moving visual field synchronized with the anterior/posterior sway of the patient at low frequencies of sway, which becomes out of phase at higher frequencies. In either case, the visual in-

formation received by the patient is not of functional use in maintaining stance and in fact conflicts with the information being obtained by the vestibular end-organ and the foot somatosensory cues. Similar disruption in the ankle angle is done by having the force plate tilt toes down or up coincident with swaying forward or backward. During either movement coordination or sensory organization protocols, the body movement reflected by force changes at the feet are analyzed to provide records of the patient's reaction.

Since this is the only test that provides for a direct assessment of the functional abilities of the balance system as a whole and analysis of the stimulus-coded responses of the postural control system, it seems appropriate to include this evaluation for all patients with balance complaints. The specific nature of findings seems highly population dependent. For example, patients with compensated peripheral lesions who have mild motion-provoked symptoms typically show normal findings. In contrast, patients with ongoing complaints of disequilibrium, in whom the ENG and rotational chair evaluations may indicate completed compensation, may show abnormalities that would demonstrate continued dysfunction. Therefore, posturography adds a third dimension to the evaluation of compensation complementing the ENG and the rotational chair tests.

Interpretation of the results from the movement coordination portion are used to implicate possible pathology in the long-loop pathway system. Basically, the long-loop system involves the afferent neural pathways from the muscle stretch receptors in the ankles, through the spinal column connections into the brainstem, as well as the efferent motor neurons. Although influenced by vestibular end-organ activity and cortical input, the major input in this reflex appears to be the changes in the ankle angle (Allum and Pfaltz, 1985). Of importance is the information about extravestibular portions of the balance control system that may be contributing to the patient's symptoms. In addition, information about weight bearing and strength reactions to induced sway is available and may help one understand the patient's symptoms of balance dysfunction.

The sensory organization portion provides useful guidance relative to pathology in the vestibular system but does not distinguish between peripheral or central lesions. This portion, like the movement coordination test, is primarily a functional evaluation. The interpretation of the data usually involves the identification of abnormal patterns of performance. The most common patterns are abnormalities on test conditions 5 and 6, or 2, 3, 5, and 6, or 4, 5, and 6 (refer to Figure 13-14). These provide information about how well patients are able to use the sensory information available to them. This information may also suggest environmental conditions in which the patient is at risk for a fall.

To capitalize on the plasticity of the balance system discussed earlier, the results from dynamic posturography will direct attention to specific areas of functional deficit that may be addressed by balance retraining therapy program. In addition, counseling relative to difficult environmental situations and precautionary activities for these conditions can take place. Despite being new on the clinical scene, dynamic posturography holds promise as a strong, functionally oriented tool for the assessment of postural control in balance disorder patients.

As with rotational chair, ways exist to reproduce qualitatively the sensory organization protocol when the test equipment is unavailable (Horak, 1987; Shumway–Cook and Horak, 1986). Various means of quantifying anterior/posterior sway may be substituted for the force plate; however, there are uncertainties in interpretation under these conditions.

A summary of the dynamic posturography results for case JM are presented in Figures 13-15 and 13-16 with sensory organization and movement coordination findings, respectively. The sensory organization results demonstrate a pattern of visual and vestibular dysfunction. This indicates the patient's inability to use the vestibular system information alone for the maintenance of stance indicated by six falls out of six trials on test conditions 5 and 6 (see Figures 13-14 and 13-15). Additionally two falls out of three trials on condition 4 indicate the lack of use of accurate visual information when available. The results demonstrate the patient's reliance on accurate foot somatosensory cues for maintenance of stance. The vestibular dysfunction is commonly seen and most probably explained by the previous results indicating a severe bilateral peripheral weakness. The visual dysfunction may result from a reduction in use of visual information because of decreased acuity due to cataract development, especially in the right eye.

The movement coordination findings (Figure 13-16) demonstrate abnormal weight bearing and a strength asymmetry showing little use of the left foot and leg during recovery from forward- or backward-induced sway. This is explained by the patient's recent left hip replacement. The results also demonstrate significant difficulty in adapting to sudden changes in foot support surface orientation from flat to foot inclined up or down by 4 degrees.

The patient's history and test findings collectively suggest severe bilateral peripheral vestibular system involvement, with residual function remaining secondary to ototoxic drug administration. Indications for central vestibular system involvement are noted but are most probably explained by changes associated with age. Posturography findings are consistent with severe vestibular system involvement, decreasing visual acuity and orthopedic problems. Increased risks for falls would be anticipated when attempting to walk over compressible, irregular, or ramplike surfaces, especially in a visually compromised environment.

MANAGEMENT OF THE BALANCE DISORDER PATIENT

Care of the balance disorder patient may involve short-term use of vestibular suppressant medication for acute symptoms, up to a long-term, multidisciplinary, medical/surgical, and balance therapy approach. It is not within the scope of this

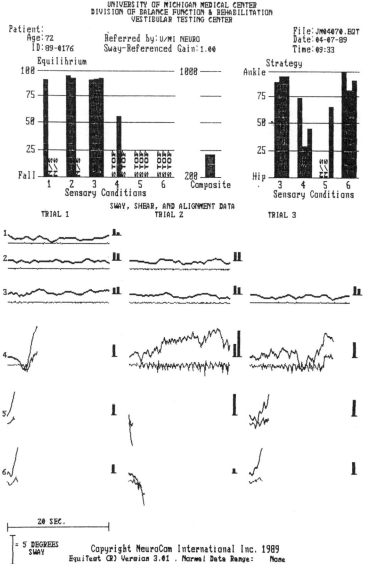

Figure 13-15. Sensory organization results for patient JM. The bar graph in the upper left shows the results on each of the six test conditions. The equilibrium score is a percentage figure with *100%* indicating no sway and *Fall* indicating the patient swayed to their theoretic limit of stability. A *STOP* indicates the operator terminated that trial prior to completion because the patient took a step to prevent a fall or actually began a fall. The composite bar graph is a mathematical combination of the six test condition results. The bar graph on the right presents a measure of the amount of shear or horizontal force that is applied by the foot against the support surface. A strategy score of 100% (Ankle) is seen with virtually no shear force. A score of 0% (Hip) indicates significant shear force. The three columns in the bottom half of the figure are for trials 1, 2, or 3 for each of the six test conditions. The top line presents the actual anterior/posterior sway amplitude in degrees over the 20-second interval. The second trace is the activity in the shear force transducer over the 20 seconds. See text for interpretation of results. (From NeuroCom International, Inc. With permission.)

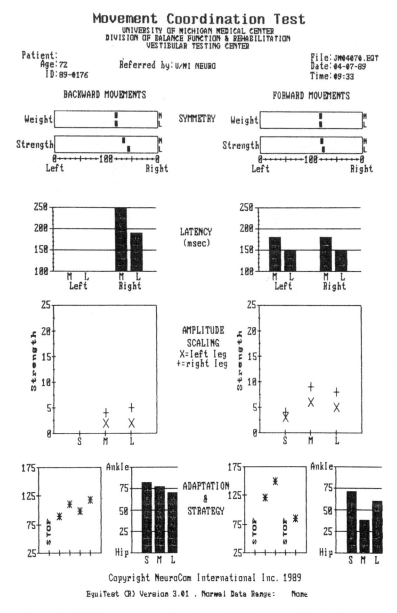

Movement Coordination Test
UNIVERSITY OF MICHIGAN MEDICAL CENTER
DIVISION OF BALANCE FUNCTION & REHABILITATION
VESTIBULAR TESTING CENTER

Patient:
Age: 72
ID: 89-0176

Referred by: U/MI NEURO

File: JM04070.EQT
Date: 04-07-89
Time: 09:33

Figure 13-16. Movement coordination results for patient JM are shown. The column of results on the left presents findings for backward translations of the platform inducing forward sway. The column on the right shows results for forward translations inducing backward sway. Weight and strength at the top give a percentage symmetry measure of weight bearing on each foot and leg and the strength of each foot and leg during the translations. The latency bar graphs show latency to onset of force reaction against the support surface to recover from the medium (M) and large (L) platform translations. The amplitude scaling graphs plot strength of reaction for right and left legs individually versus the small (S), medium, and large support surface translations. The adaptation and strategy graphs plot a measure of force against the surface versus trials 1 through 5 for toes tilted up (left column) and tilted down (right column). The bar graph for the adaptation and strategy portion is as described for strategy in Figure 13-17. (From NeuroCom International, Inc. With permission.)

chapter to comprehensively review the medical/ surgical management of these disorders (Graham, Sataloff, and Kemink, 1984; Hughes, 1981; Kemink and Graham, 1985; McElveen et al., 1988; Paparella and Sajjadi, 1988; Seltzer and McCabe, 1986; Shelton and Simmons, 1988; Zee, 1988). A brief discussion of the usefulness of a balance retraining and habituation therapy program is useful since it is a relatively novel approach with little information available at present in the literature.

The balance therapy programs in operation typically involve two specific areas of concentration. The first involves the use of habituation exercises in an effort to reduce or eliminate motion-provoked symptoms under certain conditions. The efficacy of this portion of therapy has been recognized for many years (Brandt and Daroff, 1980; Hecker, Haug, and Herndon, 1974). This approach has been adjusted and customized to target a broader scope of patients than the traditional use of Cawthorne exercises for benign paroxysmal positional vertigo (Norré, 1984, 1987; Norré and Becker, 1988; Norré and De Weerdt, 1980; Takemori, Ida, and Umezu, 1985). The second area of concentration is that of balance and other functional deficit retraining. More specifically this involves direct attempts to modify patients' postural control in order to correct particular functional deficits detected on formal dynamic posturography or similar informal functional evaluations (Leigh, 1988; Tangeman and Wheeler, 1986). Both of these goals are typically approached with exercise activities customized to the needs of the patient.

Predictive criteria for identifying patients who will benefit from such a program and the general prognosis for those patients are not yet available. Clinical trials for patients with "pure" peripheral vestibular system lesions and stroke or head injury patients are in progress. These will define indicators to predict when this treatment approach should be used as a sole modality and when it is best combined with medical or surgical treatment. The general goals of the balance rehabilitation program at The University of Michigan are shown in Table 13-3. When describing the program to patients emphasis is placed on number 4. Preliminary results and conclusions from the first year of a 2-year project are shown in Figures 13-17, 13-18, and Tables 13-4 and 13-5 (Telian et al., 1989). Tables 13-4 and 13-5 show the preliminary distribution of patients into those receiving limited and substantial benefit. As the project progresses, these distributions may indeed change.

The project goals are (1) to assess the efficacy of such a therapy program in reducing symptoms and in teaching patients how to manage symptoms associated with balance and gait disorders;

TABLE 13-3. GOALS FOR BALANCE RETRAINING/ COMPENSATION AND HABITUATION PHYSICAL THERAPY PROGRAM

1. Improve compensation for peripheral and/or central balance system lesions.
2. Cause habituation to rapid movements for which the vestibular system is responding in an abnormal manner.
3. Reduce environmental risks for falls via retraining of balance and postural control under static and dynamic conditions.
4. Educate the patient in techniques for managing their balance disorder — therapy is not a "cure."

Figure 13-17. A. Definitions for each of the six categories of disability. B. Bar graph illustrates the number of patients with a particular disability score both pre- and posttherapy. A shift toward lower disability scores posttherapy is clearly shown. (Adapted from Telian et al. [In press].)

DISABILITY SCALE

0	No disability - negligible symptoms
1	No disability - bothersome symptoms
2	Mild disability - performing usual duties
3	Moderate disability - disrupts usual duties
4	Recent severe disability - medical leave
5	Established severe disability

A

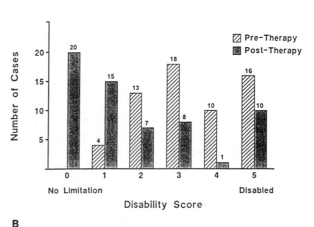

B

RESPONSE GROUP

A   Complete resolution of symptoms

B   Marked improvement/mild symptoms

C   Mild improvement/persistent symptoms

D   No improvement

E   Worse

A

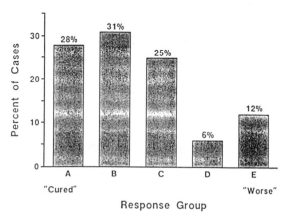

B

Figure 13-18. A. Definitions for each of the five response groups based on posttherapy symptoms relative to pretherapy symptoms. B. The percentage of patients in each of the response groups posttherapy is illustrated by the bar graph. (Adapted from Telian, S. A., et al. [In press]. Habituation therapy for chronic vestibular dysfunction: Preliminary results. *Otolaryngology — Head & Neck Surgery.*)

TABLE 13-4. LIMITED RESULTS OF VESTIBULAR HABITUATION THERAPY

Mixed central peripheral lesions

Head injury

Unstable peripheral lesions

Bilateral peripheral lesions

Objective measures uncompensated

Established disability

Source: Adapted from Telian, S. A., et al. (In press). Habituation therapy for chronic vestibular dysfunction: Preliminary results. *Otolaryngology — Head & Neck Surgery.*

TABLE 13-5. EXCELLENT RESULTS OF VESTIBULAR HABITUATION THERAPY

Stable unilateral peripheral lesions

Postoperative decompensation

Objective measures compensated

Isolated central nervous system lesions?

Recent disability

Source: Adapted from Telian, S. A., et al. (In press). Habituation therapy for chronic vestibular dysfunction: Preliminary results. *Otolaryngology — Head & Neck Surgery.*

and (2) to correlate presenting symptoms, pertinent medical history, medical diagnosis, objective test findings, age, and other factors with therapy outcome. This will help to build a profile for referral and prognosis for patients participating in a balance therapy program. In general the preliminary findings are quite encouraging (Figures 13-17 and 13-18). Anecdotally, the program may have a dramatic impact on the problems experienced by patients, even when other modalities have failed. The major goal is to define how this program will perform in a large population of balance disorder patients.

Patient JM is being managed by referral for balance retraining therapy with specific goals to (1) increase use of accurate visual information to assist with balance, supplementing use of somatosensory information; (2) increase use of residual vestibular system information; (3) provide counseling on how to predict what environmental situations may pose difficulties and how to circumvent the problems; and (4) reduce sensitivity to rapid head movements that occur in three specific planes of motion. In addition the patient has been referred to an otologist for follow-up concerned with his reported progressive loss of auditory sensitivity on the left.

CONCLUSION

This abbreviated overview of balance function and assessment should at the least impress on the reader the complexity of the system and the difficulties inherent in the evaluation of such a system. Although substantial diagnostic and therapeutic advances have been achieved, considerable need still exists for basic science and clinical investigation directed toward the evaluation and treatment of balance disorders.

REFERENCES

Abel, S., & Barber, H. O. (1981). Measurement of optokinetic nystagmus for otoneurological diagnosis. *Annals of Otology, Rhinology, and Laryngology,* (Suppl. 79), *90*(1), 1–12.

Allum, J. H. (1983). Organization of stabilizing reflex responses in tibialis anterior muscles following ankle flexion perturbations of standing man. *Brain Research, 264,* 297–301.

Allum, J. H., & Pfaltz, C. R. (1985). Visual and vestibular contributions to pitch sway stabilization in the ankle muscles of normals and patients with bilateral peripheral vestibular deficits. *Experimental Brain Research, 58,* 82–94.

Baloh, R. W., & Honrubia, V. (1983). *Clinical neurophysiology of the vestibular system.* Philadelphia: F. A. Davis.

Baloh, R. W., Honrubia, V., & Sills, A. (1977). Eye-tracking and optokinetic nystagmus. Results of quantitative testing in patients with well-defined nervous system lesions. *Annals of Otology, Rhinology, and Laryngology, 86,* 108–114.

Baloh, R. W., Sills, A. W., & Honrubia, V. (1977). Patients with peripheral and central vestibular lesions. *Annals of Otology, Rhinology, and Laryngology, 86* (Suppl. 43), 24–30.

Baloh, R. W., Solingen, L., Sills, A. W., & Honrubia, V. (1977). Effect of different conditions of ocular fixation. *Annals of Otology, Rhinology, and Laryngology, 86* (Suppl. 43), 1–6.

Baloh, R. W., Yee, R. D., Jenkins, H. A., & Honrubia, V. (1982). Quantitative assessment of visual-vestibular interaction using sinusoidal rotatory stimuli. In V. Honrubia & M. A. B. Brazier (Eds.), *Nystagmus and clinical approaches to the patient with dizziness* (pp. 231–237). New York: Academic Press.

Barber, H. O., & Sharpe, J. A. (Eds.). (1988). *Vestibular disorders.* Chicago: Year Book.

Barber, H. O., & Stockwell, C. W. (1980). *Manual of electronystagmography.* St. Louis: C. V. Mosby.

Barin, K. (1987). Human postural sway responses to translational movements of the support surface. *Proceedings of the Ninth Annual Conference of the IEEE Engineering in Medicine and Biology Society,* 0745–0747.

Bernstein, P., McCabe, B. F., & Ryu, J. H. (1974). The effect of diazepam on vestibular compensation. *Laryngoscope, LXXXIV*(2), 267–272.

Black, F. O., & Nashner, L. M. (1984). Vestibulo-spinal control differs in patients with reduced versus distorted vestibular function. *Acta Oto-laryngologica* (Stockholm), (Suppl. 406), 110–114.

Black, F. O., Shupert, C. L., Horak, F. B., & Nashner, L. M. (1988). Abnormal postural control associated with peripheral vestibular disorders. *Progress in Brain Research, 76,* 263–275.

Black, F. O., Wall, C., & Nashner, L. M. (1983). Effects of visual and support surface orientation references upon postural control in vestibular deficient subjects. *Acta Oto-laryngologica* (Stockholm), *95,* 199–210.

Black, F. O., Wall, C., & O'Leary, D. P. (1978). Computerized screening of the human vestibulospinal system. *Annals of Otology, Rhinology, and Laryngology, 87,* 853–860.

Bogousslavsky, J., & Meienberg, O. (1987). Eye movement disorders in brain-stem and cerebellar stroke. *Archives of Neurology, 44,* 141–148.

Brandt, T., & Daroff, R. B. (1980). Physical therapy for benign paroxysmal positional vertigo. *Archives of Otolaryngology, 106,* 484–485.

Brightwell, D. R., & Abramson, M. (1975). Personality characteristics in patients with vertigo. *Archives of Otolaryngology, 101,* 364–366.

Cohen, B., & Buttner-Ennever, J. A. (1984). Projections from the superior colliculus to a region of the central mesencephalic reticular formation (cMRF) associated with horizontal saccadic eye movements. *Experimental Brain Research, 57,* 167–176.

Cohen, B., Matsuo, V., Fradin, J., & Raphan, T. (1985). Horizontal saccades induced by stimulation of the central mesencephalic reticular formation. *Experimental Brain Research, 57,* 605–616.

Cohen, B., Volker, H., Raphan, T., & Dennett, D. (1981). Velocity storage, nystagmus, and visual-vestibular interactions in humans. *Annals of the New York Academy of Sciences,* 421–433.

Courjon, J. H., Flandrin, J. M., Jeannerod, M., & Schmid, R. (1982). The role of the flocculus in vestibular compensation after hemilabyrinthectomy. *Brain Research, 239,* 251–257.

Diener, H. C., Dichgans, J., Guschlbauer, B., & Mau, H. (1984). The significance of proprioception on postural stabilization as assessed by ischemia. *Brain Research, 296*(1), 103–109.

Diener, H. C., Horak, F. B., & Nashner, L. M. (1988). Influence of stimulus parameters on human postural responses. *Journal of Neurophysiology, 59*(6), 1888–1904.

Doslak, M. J., Dell'Osso, L. F., & Daroff, R. B. (1982). Alexander's law: A model and resulting study. *Annals of Otology, Rhinology, and Laryngology, 91,* 316–322.

Fernandez, C., & Goldberg, J. M. (1971). Physiology of peripheral neurons innervating semicircular canals of the squirrel monkey. II. Response to sinusoidal stimulation and dynamics of peripheral vestibular system. *Journal of Neurophysiology, 34,* 661–673.

Fineberg, R., O'Leary, D. P., & Davis, L. (1987). Use of active head movements for computerized vestibular testing. *Archives of Otolaryngology — Head and Neck Surgery, 113,* 1063–1065.

Forssberg, H., & Nashner, L. M. (1982). Ontogenetic development of postural control in man: Adaptation to altered support and visual conditions during stance. *Journal of Neuroscience, 2*(5), 545–552.

Furman, J. M. R., Wall, C., & Kamerer, D. B. (1988). Alternate and simultaneous binaural bithermal caloric testing — a comparison. *Annals of Otology, Rhinology, and Laryngology, 97,* 359–364.

Furst, E. J., Goldberg, J., & Jenkins, H. A. (1987). Voluntary modification of the rotatory induced vestibulo-ocular reflex by fixating imaginary targets. *Acta Oto-laryngologica* (Stockholm), *103,* 232–240.

Gacek, R. R. (1980). Neuroanatomical correlates of vestibular function. *Annals of Otology, 89,* 2–5.

Goodhill, V., & Harris, I. (1979). Examination of the dizzy patient. In V. Goodhill (Ed.), *Diseases, deafness, and dizziness* (pp. 226–246). Hagerstown, MD: Harper & Row.

Graham, M. D., Sataloff, R. T., & Kemink, J. L. (1984). Titration streptomycin therapy for bilateral Ménière's disease: A preliminary report. *Otolaryngology — Head and Neck Surgery, 92*(4), 440–447.

Gresty, M., Page, N., & Barratt, H. (1984). The differential diagnosis of congenital nystagmus. *Journal of Neurology, Neurosurgery, and Psychiatry, 47,* 936–942.

Hamid, M. A., Hughes, G. B., Kinney, S. E., & Hanson, M. R. (1986). Results of sinusoidal harmonic acceleration test in one thousand patients: Preliminary report. *Otolaryngology — Head and Neck Surgery, 94*(1), 1–5.

Hecker, H. C., Haug, C. O., & Herndon, J. W. (1974). Treatment of the vertiginous patient using Cawthorne's vestibular exercises. *Laryngoscope, 84*(11), 2065–2072.

Hess, K., Baloh, R. W., & Honrubia, V. (1985). Rotational testing in patients with bilateral peripheral vestibular disease. *Laryngoscope, 95,* 85–88.

Hirsch, B. E. (1986). Computed sinusoidal harmonic acceleration. *Ear & Hearing, 7*(3), 198–203.

Honrubia, V., Baloh, R. W., & Khalili, R. (1989). Subjective and oculomotor responses during interaction of smooth pursuit with optokinetic and vestibular stimuli. *Abstracts of the Twelfth Midwinter Research Meeting.* St. Petersburg, FL: Association for Research in Otolaryngology.

Honrubia, V., Jenkins, H. A., Baloh, R. W., & Lau, C. G. Y. (1982). Evaluation of rotatory vestibular tests in peripheral labyrinthine lesions. In V. Honrubia & M. A. B. Brazier (Eds.), *Nystagmus and vertigo: Clinical approaches to the patient with dizziness* (pp. 57–67). New York: Academic Press.

Honrubia, V., Jenkins, H. A., Baloh, R. W., Yee, R. D., & Lau, C. G. Y. (1984). Vestibulo-ocular reflexes in peripheral labyrinthine lesions: I. Unilateral dysfunction. *American Journal of Otolaryngology, 5*, 15–26.

Honrubia, V., Jenkins, H. A., Minser, K., Baloh, R. W., & Yee, R. D. (1984). Vestibulo-ocular reflexes in peripheral labyrinthine lesions. II. Caloric testing. *American Journal of Otolaryngology, 5*, 93–98.

Horak, F. B. (1987). Clinical measurement of postural control in adults. *Journal of American Physical Therapy Association, 67*(12), 1881–1885.

Horak, F. B., & Nashner, L. M. (1986). Central programming of postural movements: Adaptation to altered support-surface configurations. *Journal of Neurophysiology, 55*(6), 1369–1381.

Hughes, G. B. (1981). A new decade of surgery for vertigo. *American Journal of Otolaryngology, 2*(4), 391–401.

Igarashi, M. (1984). Vestibular compensation: An overview. *Acta Oto-laryngologica* (Stockholm), (Suppl. 406), 78–82.

Igarashi, M., Levy, J. K., Reschke, M., Kubo, T., & Watson, T. (1978). Locomotor dysfunction after surgical lesions in the unilateral vestibular nuclei region in squirrel monkeys. *Archives of Otorhinolaryngology, 221*, 89–95.

Igarashi, M., Levy, J. K., Takahashi, M., Alford, B. R., & Homick, J. L. (1979). Effect of exercise upon locomotor balance modification after peripheral vestibular lesions (unilateral utricular neurotomy) in squirrel monkeys. *Advances in Oto-Rhino-Laryngology, 25*, 82–87.

Ishikawa, K., & Igarashi, M. (1984). Effect of diazepam on vestibular compensation in squirrel monkeys. *Archives of Otorhinolaryngology, 240* 49–54.

Ishikawa, K., & Igarashi, M. (1985). Effect of atropine and carbachol on vestibular compensation in squirrel monkeys. *American Journal of Otolaryngology, 6*, 290–296.

Istil, Y., Hyden, D., & Schwartz, D. W. F. (1983). Quantification and localization of vestibular loss in unilaterally labyrinthectomized patients using a precise rotatory test. *Acta Oto-laryngologica* (Stockholm), *96*, 437–445.

Jacob, R. G. (1988). Panic disorder and the vestibular system. *Psychiatric Clinics of North America, 11*(2), 361–374.

Jacob, R. G., Moller, M. B., Turner, S. M., & Wall, C. (1985). Otoneurological examination in panic disorder and agoraphobia with panic attacks: A pilot study. *American Journal of Psychiatry, 142*(6), 715–720.

Jacobson, G. P., & Henry, K. G. (1989). Effect of temperature on fixation suppression ability in normal subjects: The need for temperature- and age-dependent normal values. *Annals of Otology, Rhinology, and Laryngology, 98*, 369–372.

Jacobson, G. P., & Means, E. D. (1985). Efficacy of a monothermal warm water caloric screening test. *Annals of Otology, Rhinology, and Laryngology, 94*, 377–381.

Kamerer, D. B., & Furman, J. M. R. (1988). Rotational responses of patients with bilaterally reduced caloric responses. Uppsala, Sweden: Barany Society Meeting.

Kemink, J. L., & Graham, M. D. (1985). Hearing loss with delayed onset of vertigo. *American Journal of Otology, 6*(4), 344–348.

Keshner, E. A., Allum, J. H. J., & Pfaltz, C. R. (1987). Postural coactivation and adaptation in the sway stabilizing responses of normals and patients with bilateral vestibular deficit. *Experimental Brain Research, 69*, 77–92.

Kileny, P., & Kemink, J. (1986). Artifacts and errors in the electronystagmographic (ENG) evaluation of the vestibular system. *Ear & Hearing, 7*(3), 151–156.

Kileny, P., McCabe, B., & Ryu, J. H. (1980). Effects of attention-requiring tasks on vestibular nystagmus. *Annals of Otology, Rhinology, and Laryngology, 89*, 9–12.

Koenig, E., Dichgans, J., & Dengler, W. (1986). Fixation suppression of the vestibulo-ocular reflex (VOR) during sinusoidal stimulation in humans as related to the performance of the pursuit system. *Acta Oto-laryngologica* (Stockholm), *102*, 423–431.

Kubo, T., Igarashi, M., Jensen, D., & Wright, W. (1981). Eye-head coordination and lateral canal block in squirrel monkeys. *Annals of Otology, Rhinology, and Laryngology, 90*, 154–157.

Kumar, A. (1981). Diagnostic advantages of the Torok monothermal differential caloric test. *Laryngoscope, 91*, 1679–1694.

Kumar, A., & Sutton, D. L. (1984). Diagnostic value of vestibular function tests: An analysis of 200 consecutive cases. *Laryngoscope, 94*, 1435–1442.

Kumar, A., Mafee, M., & Torok, N. (1982). Anatomic specificity of central vestibular signs in posterior fossa lesions. *Annals of Otology, Rhinology, and Laryngology, 91*, 510–515.

Lambert, P. R. (1986). Nonlocalizing vestibular findings on electronystagmography. *Ear & Hearing, 7*(3), 182–185.

Leigh, J. (1988). Management of oscillopsia. In H. O. Barber & J. A. Sharpe (Eds.), *Vestibular disorders* (pp. 201–211). Chicago: Year Book.

Leigh, R. J., & Zee, D. S. (1982). The diagnostic value of abnormal eye movements: A pathophysiological approach. *Johns Hopkins Medical Journal, 151*, 122–135.

LeLiever, W. C., Calhoun, K. H., & Correia, M. J. (1984). Diagnostic accuracy of rotation testing vs. standard vestibular test battery — a long-term study. *Laryngoscope, 94*, 896–900.

Lisberger, S. G., Morris, E. J., & Tychsen, L. (1987). Visual motion processing and sensory-motor integration for smooth pursuit eye movements. *Annual Review of Neuroscience, 10*, 97–129.

Mathog, R. H., & Peppard, S. B. (1982). Exercise and recovery from vestibular injury. *American Journal of Otolaryngology, 3*, 397–407.

Matsunaga, T., Shiraishi, T., & Kubo, T. (1983). Differential effects of diazepam upon vestibulo- and visual-oculomotor responses in the rabbit. *Acta Oto-laryngologica* (Stockholm), (Suppl. 393), 33–39.

McCabe, B. F., & Sekitani, T. (1972). Further experiments on vestibular compensation. *Laryngoscope, LXXXII*(3), 381–396.

McCabe, B. F., Sekitani, T., & Ryu, J. H. (1973). Drug effects on postlabyrinthectomy nystagmus. *Archives of Otolaryngology, 98*, 310–313.

McElveen, J. T., Shelton, C., Hitselberger, W. E., & Brackmann, D. E. (1988). Retrolabyrinthine vestibular neurectomy: A reevaluation. *Laryngoscope, 98*, 502–506.

Melvill, J. G., & Mandl, G. (1981). Motion sickness due to vision reversal: Its absence in stroboscopic light. *Annals of the New York Academy of Sciences, 374*, 303.

Melvill, J. G., & Mandl, G. (1983). Neurobionomics of adaptive plasticity: Integrating sensorimotor function with environmental demands. In J. E. Desmedt (Ed.), *Motor control mechanisms in health and disease*. New York: Raven Press.

Melvill, J. G., Berthoz, A., & Segal, B. (1984). Adaptive modification of the vestibulo-ocular reflex by mental effort in darkness. *Experimental Brain Research, 56,* 149.

Nashner, L. M. (1979). Organization and programming of motor activity during postural control. In R. Granit & O. Pompeiano (Eds.), *Progress in brain research* (Vol. 50, pp. 177–184). New York: Elsevier/North-Holland.

Nashner, L. M. (1983). Analysis of movement control in man using the movable platform. In J. E. Desmedt (Ed.), *Motor control mechanisms in health and disease* (pp. 607–619). New York: Raven Press.

Nashner, L. M. (1985). Strategies for organization of human posture. In M. Igarashi & F. O. Black (Eds.), *Vestibular and visual control on posture and locomotor equilibrium* (pp. 1–8). Houston: Seventh International Symposium of International Society of Posturography.

Nashner, L. M. (1987). A paper on advances in diagnosis and management of balance disorders: *A systems approach to understanding and assessing orientation and balance disorders*. Portland, OR: NeuroCom International.

Nashner, L., & Berthoz, A. (1978). Visual contribution to rapid motor responses during postural control. *Brain Research, 150,* 403–407.

Nashner, L. M., & Grimm, R. J. (1978). Clinical applications of the long loop motor control analysis in intact man: Analysis of multiloop dyscontrols in standing cerebellar patients. *Neurophysiology, 4,* 300–319.

Nashner, L. M., & McCoullum, G. (1985). The organization of human postural movements: A formal basis and experimental synthesis. *Behavioral and Brain Sciences, 8,* 135–172.

Nashner, L. M., Friedman, J., & Wusteney, E. (1988). Dynamic posturography assessment of patients with peripheral and central vestibular system deficits: Correlations with results from other clinical tests. Sweden: Barany Society Meeting.

Norré, M. E. (1984). Treatment of unilateral vestibular hypofunction. In W. J. Oosterveld (Ed.), *Otoneurology* (pp. 23–39). New York: Wiley.

Norré, M. E. (1987). Rationale of rehabilitation treatment for vertigo. *American Journal of Otolaryngology, 8,* 31–35.

Norré, M. E., & Beckers, A. (1988). Benign paroxysmal positional vertigo in the elderly. Treatment by habituation exercises. *Journal of the American Geriatrics Society, 36,* 425–429.

Norré, M. E., & De Weerdt, W. (1980). Treatment of vertigo based on habituation. *Journal of Laryngology and Otology, 94,* 689–696.

Norré, M. E., & Forrez, G. (1983). Evaluation of the vestibulospinal reflex by posturography. New perspectives in the otoneurology. *Acta Oto-Rhino-Laryngologica Belgica, 37*(5), 679–686.

O'Neill, G. (1987). The caloric stimulus. *Acta Oto-laryngologica* (Stockholm), *103,* 266–272.

Paige, G. D. (1983). Vestibuloocular reflex and its interactions with visual following mechanisms in the squirrel monkey. II. Response characteristics and plasticity following unilateral inactivation of horizontal canal. *Journal of Neurophysiology, 49,* 152.

Paparella, M. M., & Sajjadi, H. (1988). Endolymphatic sac revision for recurrent Ménière's disease. *American Journal of Otology, 9*(6), 441–447.

Peppard, S. B. (1986). Effect of drug therapy on compensation from vestibular injury. *Laryngoscope, 96,* 878–898.

Pfaltz, C. R. (1983). Vestibular compensation. Physiological and clinical aspects. *Acta Oto-laryngologica* (Stockholm), *95,* 402–406.

Proctor, L., Glackin, R., Shimizu, H., Smith, C., & Lietman, P. (1986). Reference values for serial vestibular testing. *Annals of Otology, Rhinology, and Laryngology, 95,* 83–90.

Pulaski, P. D., Zee, D. S., & Robinson, D. A. (1981). The behavior of the vestibulo-ocular reflex at high velocities of head rotation. *Brain Research, 222,* 159–165.

Pykko, I., Schalen, L., Jantti, V., & Magnusson, M. (1984). A reduction of vestibulo-visual integration during transdermally administered scopolamine and dimenhydrinate. *Acta Oto-laryngologica* (Stockholm), (Suppl. 406), 167–173.

Rahko, T. (1984). Optokinetic nystagmus. *Acta Ophthalmologica* (Suppl. 161), 153–158.

Ranalli, P., Sharped, J. A., & Fletcher, W. A. (1988). Palsy of upward and downward saccadic, pursuit, and vestibular movements with a unilateral midbrain lesion: Pathophysiologic correlations. *Neurology, 38*(1), 114–122.

Rigatelli, M., Casolari, L., Bergamini, G., & Guidetti, G. (1984). Psychosomatic study of 60 patients with vertigo. *Psychoter. Psychosom., 41,* 91–99.

Robinson, D. A. (1968). The oculomotor control system: A review. *Proceedings of the Institute of Electronic and Electrical Engineers, 56*(6), 1032–1049.

Rubin, W. (1982). Harmonic acceleration tests as a measure of vestibular compensation. *Annals of Otology, Rhinology, and Laryngology, 91,* 489–492.

Ryu, J. H. (1986). Anatomy of the vestibular end organ and neural pathways. In C. Cummings, J. Fredrickson, L. Harker, C. Krause, & D. Schuller (Eds.), *Otolaryngology — head and neck surgery* (Vol. 3, chap. 142). St Louis: C. V. Mosby.

Ryu, J. H., Babin, R. W., Liu, C., & McCabe, B. F. (1984). Effects of ketamine on the adaptive responses of second-order der vestibular neurons of the cat. *American Journal of Otolaryngology, 5,* 262–265.

Schwarz, D. W. F. (1986). Physiology of the vestibular system. In C. Cummings, J. Fredrickson, L. Harker, C. Krause, & D. Schuller (Eds.), *Otolaryngology — head and neck surgery* (Vol. 3, chap. 144). St Louis: C. V. Mosby.

Sekitani, T., McCabe, B. F., & Ryu, J. H. (1971). Drug effects on the medial vestibular nucleus. *Archives of Otolaryngology, 93,* 581–589.

Seltzer, S., & McCabe, B. F. (1986). Perilymph fistula: The Iowa experience. *Laryngoscope, 94,* 37–49.

Sharpe, J. A., Herishanu, Y. O., and White, O. B. (1982). Cerebral square wave jerks. *Neurology, 32,* 57–62.

Shelton, C., & Simmons, F. B. (1988). Perilymph fistula: The Stanford experience. *Annals of Otology, Rhinology, and Laryngology, 97,* 105–108.

Shepard, N. T., Turner, R. G., Vaillancourt, P., & Bauman, M. (1987). *Performance evaluation of tests for balance function assessment.* Paper presented at the Association for Research in Otolaryngology midwinter meeting, Clearwater, FL.

Shumway–Cook, A., & Horak, F. B. (1986). Assessing the influence of sensory interaction on balance. Suggestion from the field. *Journal of American Physical Therapy Association, 66*(10), 1548–1550.

Sills, A. W., Baloh, R. W., & Honrubia, V. (1977). Results in normal subjects. *Annals of Otology, Rhinology, and Laryngology, 86* (Suppl. 43), 7–23.

Simons, B., & Buttner, U. (1985). The influence of age on optokinetic nystagmus. *Psychiatry and Neurological Sciences, 234,* 369–373.

Stelmach, G. E., & Worringham, C. (1985). Sensorimotor

deficits related to postural stability. Implications for falling in the elderly. *Clinics in Geriatric Medicine, 1*(3), 679–691.

Stockwell, C. W. (1983). *ENG Workbook.* Baltimore: University Park Press.

Strong, N. P., Malach, R., Lee, P., & Van Sluyters, R. (1984). Horizontal optokinetic nystagmus in the cat: Recovery from cortical lesions. *Developmental Brain Research, 13,* 179–192.

Takahashi, M., Uemura, T., & Fujishiro, T. (1984). Recovery of vestibulo-ocular reflex and gaze disturbance in patients with unilateral loss of labyrinthine function. *Annals of Otology, Rhinology, and Laryngology, 93,* 170–175.

Takemori, S., Aiba, T., & Shizawa, R. (1981). Visual suppression of caloric nystagmus in brain-stem lesions. *Annals of the New York Academy of Sciences,* 846–854.

Takemori, S., Ida, M., & Umezu, H. (1985). Vestibular training after sudden loss of vestibular functions. *ORL; Journal of Oto-Rhino-Laryngology and its Related Specialties, 47,* 76–83.

Takemori, S., Maeda, T., Seki, Y., & Aiba, T. (1984). Vestibular compensation after sudden loss of inner ear or vestibular nerve functions. *Acta Oto-laryngologica* (Stockholm), (Suppl. 406), 91–94.

Takemori, S., Moriyama, H., & Totsuka, G. (1979). The mechanism of inhibition of caloric nystagmus by eye closure. *Advances in Oto-Rhino-Laryngology, 25,* 208–213.

Tangeman, P. T., & Wheeler, J. (1986). Inner ear concussion syndrome: Vestibular implications and physical therapy treatment. *Topics in Acute Care and Trauma Rehabilitation, 1*(1), 72–83.

Telian, S. A., Shepard, N. T., Smith–Wheelock, M., & Kemink, J. L. (In press). Habituation therapy for chronic vestibular dysfunction: Preliminary results. *Journal of Otolaryngology — Head and Neck Surgery.*

Ventre, J. (1985). Cortical control of oculomotor functions. I. Optokinetic nystagmus. *Behavioural Brain Research, 15,* 211–226.

Waespe, W., Cohen, B., & Raphan, T. (1983). Role of the flocculus and paraflocculus in optokinetic nystagmus and visual-vestibular interactions: Effects of lesions. *Experimental Brain Research, 50,* 9–33.

Waespe, W., Cohen, B., & Raphan, T. (1985). Dynamic modification of the vestibulo-ocular reflex by the nodulus and uvula. *Science, 228,* 199–202.

Wall, C., & Black, F. O. (1983). Postural stability and rotational tests: Their effectiveness for screening dizzy patients. *Acta Oto-laryngologica* (Stockholm), *95*(3–4), 235–246.

Wall, C., Black, F. O., & Hunt, A. E. (1984). Effects of age, sex, and stimulus parameters upon vestibulo-ocular responses to sinusoidal rotation. *Acta Oto-laryngologica* (Stockholm),

98, 270–278.

Wetmore, S. J., (1986). Extended caloric tests. *Ear & Hearing, 7*(3), 186–190.

Wolfson, L. I., Whipple, R., Amerman, P., & Kleinberg, A. (1986). Stressing the postural response. A quantitative method for testing balance. *Journal of the American Geriatrics Society, 34,* 845–850.

Woollacott, M. H. (1988). Posture and gait from newborn to elderly. In B. Amblard, A. Berthoz, & F. Clarac (Eds.), *Posture and gait. Development, adaptation and modulation* (pp. 3–12). Amsterdam: Elsevier.

Woollacott, M. H., Shumway–Cook, A., & Nashner, L. M. (1986). Aging and posture control: Changes in sensory organization and muscular coordination. *International Journal of Aging and Human Development, 23*(2), 97–114.

Yee, R. D., Baloh, R. W., Honrubia, V., & Jenkins, H. A. (1982). Pathophysiology of optokinetic nystagmus. In V. Honrubia & M. A. B. Brazier (Eds.), *Nystagmus and vertigo: Clinical approaches to the patient with dizziness* (pp. 251–275). New York: Academic Press.

Yoneda, S., & Tokumasu, K. (1986). Frequency analysis of body sway in the upright posture. Statistical study in cases of peripheral vestibular disease. *Acta Oto-laryngologica* (Stockholm), *102,* 87–92.

Zasorin, N. L., Baloh, R. W., Yee, R. D., & Honrubia, V. (1983). Influence of vestibulo-ocular reflex gain on human optokinetic responses. *Experimental Brain Research, 51,* 271–274.

Zee, D. S. (1978). The organization of the brainstem ocular motor subnuclei. *Notes and Letters,* 384–385.

Zee, D. S. (1984). New concepts of cerebellar control of eye movements. *Otolaryngology — Head and Neck Surgery, 92,* 59–62.

Zee, D. S. (1985). Perspectives on the pharmacotherapy of vertigo. *Archives of Otolaryngology, 111,* 609–612.

Zee, D. S. (1988). The management of patients with vestibular disorders. In H. O. Barber & J. A. Sharpe (Eds.), *Vestibular disorders* (pp. 254–274). Chicago: Year Book.

Zee, D. S., & Leigh, R. J. (1983). Disorders of eye movements. *Neurologic Clinics, 1*(4), 909–928.

Zee, D. S., & Robinson, D. A. (1978). A hypothetical explanation of saccadic oscillations. *Annals of Neurology, 5,* 405–414.

Zee, D. S., Leigh, R. J., & Mathieu–Millaire, F. (1980). Cerebellar control of ocular gaze stability. *Annals of Neurology, 7,* 37–40.

Zee, D., Yamazaki, A., Butler, P., & Gucer, G. (1981). Effects of ablation of flocculus and paraflocculus on eye movements in primates. *Journal of Neurophysiology, 46*(4), 878–899.

CHAPTER 14

Auditory Test Strategy

Martyn L. Hyde • M. Jean Davidson • Peter W. Alberti

THE PROBLEM

There are many pressures to create or to adopt new procedures but it is difficult to discard old favorites. The result is an accumulating morass of tests, yet the audiologist or otologist must evaluate, select, and interpret these in a rational, quantitative manner. Currently, this is a very difficult task, because of an inadequate scientific basis.

Evidence of this problem is clear. In otoneurologic assessment, J. Jerger (1983) emphasized "the importance of a test battery approach," a view echoed by many in the *Handbook of Clinical Audiology* (Katz, 1985). In contrast, Turner, Frazer, and Shepard (1984a) stated that "the test battery concept is flawed," and Schwartz (1987a) criticized the use of "test batteries that have limited purchase power." A dialogue between Miller (1987) and Schwartz (1987b) emphasized the differing opinions. Furthermore, scrutiny of published data on many audiologic tests reveals significant deficiencies. For example, after evaluation of the auditory brainstem response (ABR) as a hearing assessment tool for infants, the U.S. National Research Council Committee on Hearing, Bioacoustics and Biomechanics (CHABA, 1987) noted the "inadequacy of current data," thirteen years after the seminal report (Hecox and Galambos, 1974).

Obviously, the state of the art is unsatisfactory. Several factors have contributed to this situation: Audiology is a young, rapidly evolving, multidisciplinary field, so lack of depth in some source areas is inevitable; careful scientific reflection is difficult in an environment that demands instant productivity; also, the entire domain of clinical decision making is quite complicated, and is undergoing vigorous development in many diverse areas of application.

The goal of this chapter is to encourage and facilitate a critical and quantitative approach to the evaluation and selection of auditory tests. Both formal and informal procedures will be considered, and the discussion will relate to "classic" diagnostic audiology and to issues regarding therapy. Helpful concepts and techniques are available within the body of knowledge known as clinical decision analysis (CDA). Good introductory texts are by Sackett, Haynes, and Tugwell (1985) and by Sox, Blatt, Higgins, and Marton (1988); more detail is available from Weinstein and Fineberg (1980); a primary source is the journal *Medical Decision Making*. Here, a brief outline of terminology and decision goals will lead to an explanation of the basic principles of CDA. Finally, illustrative clinical problem areas will be discussed.

THE DIAGNOSTIC PROCESS

WHAT IS DIAGNOSIS?

Diagnosis is a common human activity, in fields ranging from medicine through weather forecasting to defense systems (Swets, 1988). Concepts of disease and diagnosis have a fascinating history (King, 1982). Here, diagnosis is considered a means to appropriate management and involves allocating the individual to one of several categories that are distinct and meaningful in terms of therapy or prognosis. This is a broad definition that facilitates the application of decision analytic terminology and principles to a wider range of audiologic activities.

It is important to distinguish a *disorder,* which is an anatomic, physiologic, or biochemical derangement, an *illness,* which is the cluster of symptoms and signs, and a *predicament,* which is the overall personal and social situation of the patient (Sackett et al., 1985). Also, there are useful distinctions between *impairment,* which is abnormality of structure or function, *disability*, which is the consequent restriction of ability to perform an activity with a normal manner or range, and *handicap*, which is the resulting lack of fulfillment of a role considered normal for the particular individual (World Health Organization, 1980). An example is a 40 dB loss of pure tone sensitivity (impairment), an ensuing inability to understand speech in noise (disability), and incapacity to continue work as a presidential press officer (handicap).

WHAT IS A TEST?

A very broad definition of a test is useful because a consistent analytic approach can be applied, regardless of whether the data arise from a simple observation or a complex procedure. Noting a symptom can be thought of as a test, and so can informal observations during the clinical encounter. Here, any discrete, deliberate act of data collection will be considered as a test. This means that the decision analytic approach can be applied to almost any element of audiologic assessment. Classic audiologic diagnostic tests are an important part of the overall spectrum of tests, but they are only a part.

WHAT IS STRATEGY?

From the Greek *strategia*, meaning "the office of a general," the word suggests the devising or employment of plans toward a goal. A plan implies a structured decision making process. The goal must be explicit and its achievement should be verifiable. The line between strategy and tactics is often vague, but here, the conduct of a single test will be considered to be a tactical matter, whereas the placing of that test in a goal-oriented context is the domain of strategy.

PURPOSES OF TESTING

Reasons to test can be clinical or nonclinical, and although the clinical rationale is of paramount importance, nonclinical factors may influence the strategy (Epstein and McNeil, 1985). Clinical reasons for testing that is diagnostic in the broad sense noted earlier fall into four general and interrelated areas:

1. To detect dysfunction and gauge its severity
2. To determine therapy and monitor its effectiveness

3. To aid in prognosis
4. To contribute to scientific knowledge

Other influences may include the use of tests as "therapy," confusion between the amount of testing and the quality of care, belief in testing folklore, economic factors, fear of malpractice suit, professional gamesmanship, and financial gain. Clinical decision analysis usually addresses clinical rationale for testing, although in principle the techniques can address any material aspect.

DIAGNOSTIC THINKING

How do good clinicians think, and why are some better than others? The modern approach, which dates from the late 1950s (Ledley and Lusted, 1959), is concerned with exactly how a diagnosis is achieved, the goals being to quantify and improve the process, as well as to determine how best to teach it. Other forces promoting quantitative analysis include the trend toward computer-assisted decision support and pressures of economic accountability. Despite resistance, clinical thought processes are becoming less and less mysterious. There is growing recognition that explicit logical or mathematical formulation of the steps in diagnostic decision making can be productive for all concerned (Macartney, 1987).

Four diagnostic approaches are commonly recognized:

1. *Exhaustive* (mindless completeness), involving a myriad of clinical observations and tests, followed by sifting to uncover a diagnosis. This approach is used by inexperienced clinicians, but is discarded after the accumulation of experience and judgment.
2. *Gestalt* (pattern recognition), involving rapid realization that the presentation fits a previously experienced pattern and diagnosis. This process is not sequential and may involve subtle clues. It is common in experienced clinicians, especially in straightforward cases.
3. *Algorithmic*, involving multiple, branching paths of unambiguous decisions and outcomes, especially useful in complex situations.
4. *Hypothetico-deductive*, wherein a short list of potential diagnoses is formed rapidly and then progressively refined using the results of clinical and paraclinical tests.

The hypothetico-deductive approach is by far the most important (Sackett et al., 1985), but they are not mutually exclusive. For example, an initial stage of pattern recognition may lead to hypothesis formation, and the resoluton of alternative hypotheses may be done algorithmically.

THE PROBABILITY REVISION MODEL

The hypothetico-deductive process inevitably includes uncertainty and the most convenient conceptual framework for this is probability theory. Another possibility is the use of categorical (absolute, definite) decision rules (e.g., if this is true, then do that) that do not involve probability; indeed, many computerized "expert systems" use this method of rule-based decision making. However, when clinical reasoning is expressed using probability, a very extensive body of techniques and knowledge can be brought to bear.

The commonest model is *Bayesian probability revision*, wherein at any point in the assessment of the patient there is a set of plausible diagnoses (disease states), each with a probability. Prior probabilities are those in place before any particular test, and those in place after the test result is known are posterior probabilities, which may in turn form the priors for the next test. Prior and posterior probabilities are related by Bayes' formula (see Appendix). In this model, the patient is conceptualized as an evolving list of probabilities. Clinical observations and formal tests are used to revise this list so that some of the diagnoses are eliminated or so that one diagnosis becomes almost certain.

CLINICAL DECISION ANALYSIS

A strategy can be defined as a set of tests and associated decision rules, for example: Do test A and if the result is positive do test B. The concern is to select the best tests and to form strategies that are efficient and effective. To do this, there must be a way of quantifying performance. Questions such as whether a particular test is good or bad, or whether one test is better than another, are absolutely fundamental. CDA is the body of techniques concerned with test performance analysis and with design and quantitative evaluation of testing and therapeutic strategies. It has been applied to many medical and paramedical areas (Pauker and Kassirer, 1987). CDA is most useful for complex problems involving weighing of competing options under conditions of uncertainty, but its basic principles are relevant to even the simplest situations. Some of these principles will be presented now.

A clear distinction will become apparent between performance measures that are intrinsic to tests themselves, known as test operating characteristics, and other measures that are concerned with the effect of tests when they are used in some specific context. A given test with given operating characteristics may be adjusted and used in different ways, depending on the goal and the situation. This distinction is not always apparent from the literature.

Of course, CDA has its own jargon, and it is somewhat ironic that within CDA there is much variety of terminology and symbology, often of a parochial nature. Here, an attempt has been made to follow a classic, mainstream epidemiologic approach.

TEST OPERATING CHARACTERISTICS

THE DECISION MATRIX

The simplest decision model allows only two "disease" states (D− and D+), such as normal or hearing impaired, cochlear or retrocochlear. A test to distinguish these states yields a dichotomous (binary) outcome such as pass (T−) or fail (T+). The combination of test outcome and disease state form a 2 × 2 table often called a decision matrix, which has a standard format shown in Table 14-1. All situations with a binary truth and a binary decision can be expressed in this way. Any single test result is called true positive, true negative, false positive, or false negative. The corresponding cell entries TP, TN, FP, and FN are the numbers of cases falling into each cell, given some total number n.

Several useful ratios can be defined in terms of cell frequencies in the decision matrix, and are listed in Table 14-1. For example, the number of disease negative patients is TN+FP, so the ratio FP/(TN+FP) is the proportion of disease negative patients who test positive, otherwise known as the false positive rate, or FPR. When n is very large, these ratios tend toward the actual outcome probabilities; for small n, the observed ratios are statistical estimates of the true probabilities and are subject to sampling error.

TABLE 14-1. THE 2 × 2 DECISION MATRIX
(CONTINGENCY TABLE) AND ASSOCIATED VARIABLES

	Disease Positive D+	Disease Negative D–		
Test Positive T+	True Positive TP	False Positive FP		
Test Negative T–	False Negative FN	True Negative TN		

Total number of cases	$N = TP + FN + FP + TN$
Number with disease	$TP + FN$
Number without disease	$FP + TN$
True positive rate (TPR, sensitivity)	$TP / (TP + FN)$
False negative rate (FNR)	$FN / (TP + FN)$
True negative rate (TNR, specificity)	$TN / (FP + TN)$
False positive rate (FPR)	$FP / (FP + TN)$
Efficiency (accuracy)	$(TP + TN) / N$
Positive predictive value (PPV)	$TP / (TP + FP)$
Negative predictive value (NPV)	$TN / (FN + TN)$

The disease state may be establishable unequivocally, for example, by serology, histology, or surgery. Often, some test is considered to be definitive and is called a gold standard; when it is evaluated against the true disease state, FN and FP rates are negligible. There may be no gold standard, but even when there is, it is often difficult, expensive, unpleasant, hazardous, or unavailable. Thus, alternative tests are sought and evaluated against the gold standard. For example, ABR testing might be evaluated using magnetic resonance imaging (MRI) as the gold standard for presence or absence of an acoustic tumor.

SENSITIVITY AND SPECIFICITY

These are the most popular operating characteristics. Sensitivity, or the true positive rate (TPR), is the probability of a positive test when disease is present. The left matrix column in Table 14-1 defines the only two possible outcomes when disease is present, so sensitivity and the FNR must sum to unity (1.0). The specificity, or true negative rate (TNR), is the probability of a negative test when disease is absent; specificity and the FPR must also sum to unity. For a perfect test, both sensitivity and specificity are 1.0, and both the FPR and FNR are zero. For a useless (random) test such as tossing a coin, they are both 0.5.

There is no way to derive probabilities that refer to different disease states from one another without more information. For example, the sensitivity reveals nothing about the specificity. To specify the matrix, at least one probability from each

disease state is required. To be given either sensitivity or specificity alone is not very useful if the goal is to evaluate test performance. For example, suppose a test were positive in all of 100 patients with a certain disorder. The sensitivity estimate is 1.0, but that is not much use if the test also would fail most of a disease-negative group. In short, to quantify test performance usefully, estimates of both sensitivity and specificity must be provided.

What can be said, if both quantities are indeed available? Consider test X, with sensitivity and specificity of 0.8 and 0.7, respectively. Test Y, with values of 0.95 and 0.90, for example, would be considered excellent, and is obviously better than X. But, what about test Z, with values of 0.9 and 0.6? Is it better than test X? This is not so easy, and the problem arises because there are *two* numbers to consider, for each test; the preference is clear only if one of the quantities is held constant, or if the difference between tests is in the same direction for both. The test efficiency, defined in Table 14-1 as the overall proportion of correct outcomes, might be the answer, but only if there is no difference in the importance of FP and FN errors. This is not usually the case, so this efficiency is not very useful. To pursue a better measure of test goodness, deeper insight into the test process is needed.

A STATISTICAL MODEL OF THE TEST VARIABLE

A powerful model that is widely applied postulates an underlying continuous test variable,

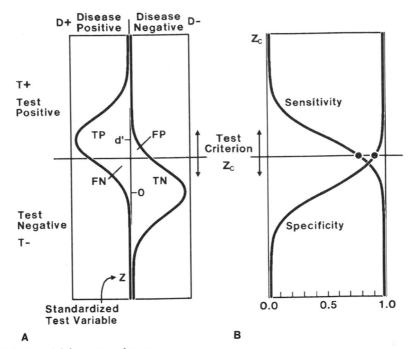

A   **B**

Figure 14-1. Statistical model for test performance. (A) The distributions of the test variable are plotted vertically, to correspond with the format of the 2 × 2 matrix in Table 14-1. The D− and D+ distributions have means of zero and d', respectively. Both are normal (Gaussian), with unit variance and SD. The variable z is related to the actual test variable x by $z = (x - m)/s$, where m and s are the mean and SD of x for D−. The criterion for test positivity (operating point), z_c, can be positioned anywhere, with consequent changes in the four areas shown. (B) Any single position of the criterion yields a value for test sensitivity and specificity (*solid circles*). As the criterion is changed, these measures vary inversely.

either explicit or implicit. Measurements of this variable will have some statistical distribution over a population of D− persons, and this distribution will be similar but shifted for D+ persons. It is also assumed that the distributions are of statistically normal (Gaussian) form, with the same variance but different means (Figure 14-1A). In statistical jargon, this is a normal, equal-variance (NEV) model. The range of the test variable is partitioned by the test operating point (decision criterion), to give the positive and negative test outcomes. The areas under the distributions correspond to the four basic probabilities in the decision matrix.

Inspection of Figure 14-1A reveals that as the operating point changes, the sensitivity and specificity vary inversely. The exact relationship is shown in Figure 14-1B. The form and separation

of the distributions are fixed and governed by the phenomena underlying the test measurements, but operating characteristics such as the sensitivity and specificity are adjustable variables governed by both the underlying distributions *and* the choice of operating point. This severely limits the usefulness of a single pair of sensitivity and specificity values, both for quantifying test performance or for comparing tests. For example, two versions of the same test may give entirely different values because of differences in operating point, either intentional or unintentional. Alternatively, two tests with apparently different performance may, in fact, be expressing the same intrinsic quality of performance, if differences in operating point were taken into account.

THE RELATIVE OPERATING CHARACTERISTIC

Description

How can the complete test performance be expressed? Figure 14-1 reveals that as the operating point increases, both sensitivity (TPR) and the FPR decrease. A graph of the sensitivity against the FPR is called a relative operating characteristic (ROC; Figure 14-2A). The historical term was receiver operating characteristic, now restricted for use in the area of signal detection (Swets, 1988).

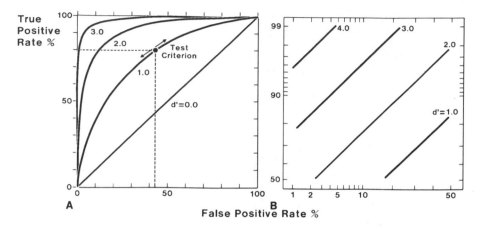

Figure 14-2. (A) Relative operating characteristics (ROCs) for several values of the parameter d'. At any value of d', the associated ROC expresses the trading relationship between the sensitivity (true-positive rate) and the false-positive rate (1.0 specificity). (B) The upper left quadrant of (A) replotted with double normal probability axes. Such axes are linear in units of the standard normal deviate, so they are nonlinear in probability, giving better resolution of the most important region of the full ROC plane in (A). Suitable graph paper is available as #41,453 from the Codex Book Co., Norwood, MA. Note that the ROCs are now linear.

For detailed exposition of the ROC and its application in the evaluation of diagnostic systems, see Metz (1978), Swets and Pickett (1982), and Swets (1988).

A single operating point gives one sensitivity/FPR pair and one point on the ROC, so the entire curve expresses the continuum of test performance for all possible values of operating point. In Figure 14-2A, various ROCs are shown, indexed by the parameter d' (d prime); the larger d', the more the ROC extends into the upper left corner of the plane. The perfect test has unity TPR for all nonzero FPR, and d' is infinite; the useless test, such as tossing a coin, generates the dotted diagonal, and d' is 0.0. With reference to the statistical model of Figure 14-1, d' is the distance between the means of the D− and D+ distributions; in terms of the raw (unstandardized) test variable, d' is the number of standard deviations between the means. When d' is zero, there is no difference between the two distributions, and the sum of sensitivity and specificity is unity, which defines the diagonal line in Figure 14-2A.

Figure 14-2B shows the important, upper left quadrant of Figure 14-2A, but replotted with axes that are linear in the so-called standard normal deviate (a normally distributed variable with zero mean and unit variance), so they are nonlinear in probability. This has the effect of expanding the probability regions of particular interest, close to 0.0 and 1.0. Moreover, for the NEV model (see Figure 14-1), all ROCs are now linear with unity slope (1.0, 45 degrees). Every ROC has its associated value of d', and the measure d' is a very useful indicator of the goodness of a test. It is a single number, and is independent of the operating point. This is appropriate, because changing a test

operating point does not make the test intrinsically more or less accurate; the only way to alter the d' of a test is to modify the test in such a way as to increase the separation of the D− and D+ distributions, or reduce their variance.

Another measure of the goodness of a test is the area under the ROC, known as A (formally A_z), which ranges between 0.5 for a useless test and 1.0 for a perfect test (see Figure 14-2A). For the binormal linear ROCs such as have just been described, d' and A are related by:

$$z(A) = d'/1.4142$$

where z(A) = the standard normal deviate that corresponds to a probability equal to A.

For example, if d' is 1.0, z(A) equals 0.7071, and normal distribution tables give a value of 0.76 for A. It is possible to interpret A as the percentage of correct decisions in a paired comparison (two-alternative forced choice) task: If the decision maker were presented with pairs of test results, one of each from the D− and D+ distributions, the result from D+ would be correctly identified in a proportion of cases equal to A. Table 14-2 shows some relationships between sensitivity, specificity, d', and A.

TABLE 14-2. SELECTED VALUES THAT ILLUSTRATE THE RELATIONSHIPS AMONG SENSITIVITY, SPECIFICITY, d', AND A_z

		Sensitivity						
Specificity		0.50	0.60	0.70	0.80	0.90	0.95	0.99
0.50	d'	0.00	0.25	0.52	0.84	1.28	1.64	2.33
	A_z	0.50	0.57	0.64	0.72	0.82	0.88	0.95
0.60		0.25	0.50	0.77	1.09	1.53	1.89	2.58
		0.57	0.64	0.71	0.78	0.86	0.91	0.96
0.70		0.52	0.77	1.04	1.36	1.80	2.16	2.85
		0.64	0.71	0.77	0.83	0.90	0.94	0.98
0.80		0.84	1.09	1.36	1.68	2.12	2.48	3.17
		0.72	0.78	0.83	0.88	0.93	0.96	0.99
0.90		1.28	1.53	1.80	2.12	2.56	2.92	3.61
		0.82	0.86	0.90	0.93	0.96	0.98	0.995
0.95		1.64	1.89	2.16	2.48	2.92	3.28	3.97
		0.88	0.91	0.94	0.96	0.98	0.99	0.998
0.99		2.33	2.58	2.85	3.17	3.61	3.97	4.66
		0.95	0.96	0.98	0.99	0.995	0.998	0.999

Measurement

The production of ROCs is usually straightforward; often, test operating points are explicit, numerical, and easily altered. For example, if the latency difference between waves I and V of the ABR were used as a test for acoustic tumor detection, the operating point might be an interval of 4.5 msec, larger values yielding a positive result. Given ABR measurements in two groups, namely those proven to have a tumor and those proven not to have a tumor, the ROC is generated simply by estimating the sensitivity and FPR for several values of the criterion. When there is no explicit, numerical test variable, a rating method may be used. For example, the likelihood of successful use of a hearing aid might be rated on a scale from very unlikely to almost certain, on the basis of an array of formal and informal data. Given subsequent evidence of actual success or failure with the aid, an ROC could be constructed by varying a scale point used to form a binary prediction of success or failure by partitioning the rating scale. Examples of an implicit variable and operating point occur in basic pure tone threshold testing; here, the patient has an internal representation of tonal loudness, and there is an operating point for the binary decision to respond or not. Reinstructing the patient to respond "even if you are not sure," is an attempt to lower the operating point.

Having obtained several pairs of sensitivity and FPR values, the points can be plotted on the plane of Figure 14-3; a line can be fitted by eye, or via a computer program (Swets and Pickett, 1982). The values of d' or A can be estimated, and procedures exist for placing confidence limits on these estimates and for significance testing of differences between estimates (Swets and Pickett, 1982).

Validity of the NEV Model

If the variances of the distributions for D− and D+ are unequal, the ROC depends on both the distance between the means and the variance ratio. Most commonly, the variance is larger for the D+ distribution, which causes the ROC slope to be less than unity on the binormal plot. Variance equality (homogeneity) can sometimes be restored by a transformation of the data, such as taking the square root or logarithm of all measurements. The other assumption, that of normal distributional form, is based mainly on an appeal to the central limit theorem, namely that any variable that is a sum of many underlying variables will tend to be normally distributed. It is often reasonable, and the ROC remains roughly linear on a binormal plot even for quite non-normal underlying distributions (Swets, 1988). Tranformations which homogenize variance often improve normality (Snedecor and Cochran, 1980).

Evaluation of Tests

When the NEV model is valid, *all* information about intrinsic test performance is contained in d'.

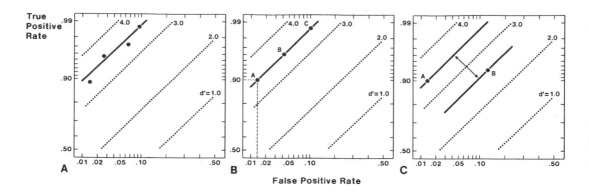

Figure 14-3. Uses of the ROC plane. (A) Fitting an ROC to several pairs of TPR and FPR values, which might arise from a single study in which the test criterion was varied, or from several studies with different criteria. (B) Inferring the entire ROC, and therefore the TPR and FPR at specific points such as B and C, from a single experimentally determined point, A. (C) Comparison of the accuracy of two tests, giving results A and B, in terms of the differences in d' (*arrow*). Note that any inferences based on a single TPR/FPR pair must be made with due caution.

The value of d' can be deduced from a single sensitivity and FPR pair (see Appendix); the single point serves to define the entire ROC, and the sensitivity and FPR (hence, the specificity) for *any* operating point can be derived easily (Figure 14-3). Under NEV conditions, the evaluation or comparison of tests can be based entirely on d' (or A). Graphically, the comparison of two tests is a matter of determining the intersection of their ROCs with the minor diagonal of the ROC plane; the closer to the top left corner, the higher d' and the better the test. Of course, it is still necessary to consider the statistical significance of observed differences.

The use of a single sensitivity/FPR pair to deduce the entire ROC is vulnerable to violation of the NEV assumptions, and any inferences from such a procedure should be treated cautiously, unless there is direct evidence that the equal variance assumption is valid or can be made so by transformation. When deriving d' and ROCs from available source data, the assumption can often be tested directly if there is an explicit variable such as ABR wave latency; one way is to compute sample variances and test them with an F (variance ratio) test. On the other hand, when working with published summary data, such as sensitivity and specificity, there may be little choice but to make the variance assumption in the dark. Whatever the situation, the more points used to estimate the ROC, the better.

If the equal-variance assumption is drastically violated, then d' loses much of its value, because it no longer summarizes all of the information in the ROC. The ROC slope will be different from unity and there is no unique value of d'. A single ROC data point is no longer sufficient test accuracy. The measure A can be calculated either from

an empirical ROC curve plotted on the unit plane of Figure 14-2A, or by the implicit formula:

$$z(A) = a \bullet b/(1 + b^2)^{1/2}$$

where a and b = the intercept and (nonunity) slope, respectively, of the ROC in the binormal plane of Figure 14-2B.

These parameters are expressed in units of the standard normal deviate (Swets and Pickett, 1982). In this situation of unequal variances, A is still a valid measure of test accuracy.

It is possible that ROCs for two tests may cross, and if they do, then neither d' nor A will be an adequate tool for test comparison: The fact is that neither test is superior over the entire range of operating points. The question of superiority is meaningful only if a particular FPR is specified, at which the sensitivities may be compared directly.

All in all, the measure A is probably the most useful index of the accuracy of a test, but for an introductory development, d' has the advantage of a more obvious relationship to the underlying data model.

Whatever performance measure is used, proper account must be taken of statistical principles. The values determined by experiment are estimates, and their utility will depend upon good experimental design and adequate sample size. Use of statistical confidence limits is essential, but is frequently overlooked, perhaps because such limits reveal clearly the limited precision that is often achieved. For example, statistical tables of confidence limits on binomial proportions indicate that, for a sensitivity estimate of 0.8, the 95 percent confidence interval for the true sensitivity is from 0.66 to 0.90, even with a sample size of 50 cases of confirmed disease (Beyer, 1968).

INDEFINITE TEST RESULTS

The ROC can be viewed as an extension of the 2 × 2 decision matrix concept, for a set of values of the operating point. Whether a single matrix or an ROC curve is being considered, there is a problem concerning test results that are neither normal nor abnormal; that is, they may be intermediate or uninterpretable. They are not handled consistently in the literature; indeed, they are curiously rare. If reported, they may be excluded from analysis, or considered to be positive when calculating specificity, or negative when calculating sensitivity. The lack of consistency is a serious source of discrepancy between studies. Furthermore, for a test to be useful, it must be applicable and must give determinate results most of the time. This problem has been examined by Simel, Feussner, Delong, and Matchar (1987), who suggested an extension of the decision matrix to six cells, with modified estimates of sensitivity and specificity. ROC concepts can be applied to these modified estimates.

THE LIKELIHOOD RATIO

Some measurements are naturally dichotomous (binary), but when there is a range of test results, to impose the dichotomy is artificial. Loss of information occurs when a variable of interval or ratio strength is forced into ordinal or nominal categories; the fewer the categories the greater the loss, which arises from inability to distinguish measurements within any category. The 2 × 2 matrix is dichotomous, but it is often desirable to account for at least several categories of test outcome.

The likelihood ratio (LR) is a test operating characteristic that is applicable to *any* test outcome, ranging from a dichotomy to a continuous variable. The LR of a given test outcome is the ratio of probabilities that that outcome would occur in the D+ and D− states. For a dichotomous decision, the LR of a positive test (LR+) equals TPR/FPR, that is, sensitivity/(1−specificity). The LR of a negative test (LR−) equals FNR/

TNR, or (1−sensitivity)/specificity; thus the LRs can be determined from the sensitivity and specificity, and vice versa.

For a useless test, the sensitivity equals the FPR, so both LR+ and LR− equal unity. Suppose a test has sensitivity and specificity both equal to 0.90, then LR+ is 9.0 and LR− is 0.11. The bigger LR+ is, the better, the perfect test having an infinite LR+. The smaller LR− is, the better, the perfect test giving zero. In terms of the statistical model, the LR is the ratio of areas under the D+ and D− distributions, to the right (LR+) or left (LR−) of the operating point (see Figure 14-1A). In the case of multiple or continuous test outcomes, there is no positive or negative result, only the set of test outcomes and their associated LRs.

While the LR is not yet as familiar as sensitivity and specificity, it has several advantages (Sackett et al., 1985). The 2 × 2 decision matrix can be extended to multiple disease states without difficulty, but there is no simple and generalized extension to multiple test outcomes. In the latter situation, the LR is a simple and potentially more powerful approach, because no loss of information due to dichotomization is involved. Other advantages of the LR will be noted later. A possible disadvantage is the apparent lack of a well established analogue to the ROC, to express the effects of criterion change, for a binary test. Further development is required, and in the interim, it seems reasonable to use both approaches in tandem.

COMBINATIONS OF TESTS

Operating Characteristics

The measures considered so far apply to single tests, but tests often occur in combinations. The overall characteristics of the combination are determined by the characteristics of the component tests and the combinatorial decision rules. Consider two tests, X and Y. The combination options are:

1. Do X, then do Y only on the X+ patients. Overall positive is positive on both.
2. Do Y, then do X only on the Y+ patients. Overall positive is positive on both.
3. Do X and Y. Overall positive is positive on both.
4. Do X and Y. Overall positive is positive on either.

A combination is called a *series* procedure when overall positivity requires positivity for all tests, and a *parallel* procedure when a positive result on any of the tests is sufficient. Thus, cases 1, 2, and 3 are all series, and case 4 is parallel. A series is called sequential if doing one of the tests depends on the outcome of another, as for 1 and 2; procedures which are not sequential are simultaneous. The major advantage of sequential procedures is the ability to stop. Table 14-3 shows the sensitivity and specificity of the combinations, and it is the criterion for overall positivity that matters for these parameters, not the manner in which the tests are done. Thus, 1 and 2, which are sequential, give the same results as 3, which is a simultaneous series, and these are all distinct from 4, which is the only parallel procedure. With a series rule, the overall sensitivity is always less than that of any single test, but the specificity will be greater than that of any single test. A parallel rule yields the opposite results. The total number of tests differs among the three series procedures and can be reduced most effectively by using the test with the highest specificity first. The likelihood ratios for the various combinations can be derived by substituting the overall sensitivity and specificity into the LR formulae given earlier.

Just as for a single test, the sensitivity and specificity of a combination have a trading relationship: Sensitivity can only be increased at the expense of specificity, and vice versa. By combining statistically independent tests, the combination cannot have both sensitivity and specificity better than the best of the tests in the combination. Thus, the rationale for using a combination must be based on either cost-benefit considerations (see later) or inability to adjust the best single test to give the desired performance characteristics. If the characteristics of the individual tests are adjustable, as is usually the case, it can be shown that a sequential procedure is formally superior (Doubilet and Cain, 1985).

The formulae given in Table 14-3 are correct if the tests are statistically independent, that is, if outcomes of one test are not influenced by the outcomes of the other. In classic diagnostic testing, this assumption is likely to be true only if the tests access different aspects of the underlying pathophysiology. Usually, however, positive correlation (concordance, convergence) between tests is expected. In this case, the formulae of Table 14-3 will overestimate the changes in sensitivity and specificity when tests are combined. For example, if two tests are perfectly positively correlated, then the characteristics of the combination are identical to those of any one of the tests, and the combination is absolutely pointless, at least from the performance standpoint.

If there are available probability estimates for all combinations of outcome for several tests, then not only can the independence of tests be tested but also the correct combination characteristics can be derived using conditional probabilities (Sackett et al., 1985). For two tests, what is required for a complete solution is a 2×2 cross-tabulation of the outcomes for tests X and Y, in both disease positive and disease negative persons. These combinatorial principles may be extended to complex strategies with many types of combination and decision rule, but the probability expressions can become cumbersome, especially if all correlations between tests are considered. For a more detailed discussion of the performance of test combinations, see Turner (1988).

The Trouble with Parallel Rules

Parallel rules can be hazardous. For example, take a set of five central auditory tests with a parallel rule for abnormality. Let them access unrelated pathophysiologic phenomena, which is what they are supposed to do, and let their outcomes be binary and statistically independent. Let all the tests be used with operating points at the 90th percentile of the range of results in disease-free individuals, which is a common (but flawed) definition of abnormality. Then, the probability of any single normal patient being called abnormal

TABLE 14-3. PERFORMANCE OF COMBINATIONS OF TWO STATISTICALLY INDEPENDENT TESTS

Positivity criterion	Overall sensitivity	Overall specificity	Expected no. of tests
1. X then Y	seX • seY	spX + spY − spX • spY	N[1 + p • seX + (1 − p) • (1 − spX)]
2. Y then X	seX • seY	spX + spY − spX • spY	N[1 + p • seY + (1 − p) • (1 − spY)]
3. X and Y	seX • seY	spX + spY − spX • spY	2N
4. X or Y	seX + seY − seX • seY	spX • spY	2N

se = sensitivity; sp = specificity.

equals $(1 - 0.9^5)$ or 0.41, that is, it is quite likely. Suppose further that five such patients are seen in a week. The probability that all five patients will be correctly labelled is 0.59^5, or 0.07; that is, there is a 93 percent chance of calling at least one of five normal patients abnormal, which should be alarming. The problem arises partly from the decision to call a normal person abnormal outside the 90th percentile, but more importantly test combinations should not be assembled without due regard for the laws of probability.

THE INTERPRETATION OF TESTS

The outline of test operating characteristics is now complete. Using those tools, test performance can be quantified and summarized, and tests can be evaluated meaningfully. However, these measures reveal little about the goals of testing and the impact of test results.

CHANGING THE PROBABILITIES

In the Bayesian probability revision model the effect of testing is to change the probability of disease; recall that here, the word disease is being used very generally. The case of many diseases can be handled by extension of the methods to be presented for a single disease.

Tests change the prior (pre-test) probability of disease into the posterior (post-test) probability, and it is the latter that governs the clinical impact of the test. Certain posterior probabilities are very important, and are known as rule-out and rule-in thresholds (Pauker and Kassirer, 1980; Sackett et al., 1985). To dismiss a disease, its probability must fall below a rule-out threshold, typically less than 0.1. Conversely, to decide that a disease is present, its probability must exceed a rule-in threshold, typically above 0.9. Ideally, these thresholds are explicit, but they always exist at least implicitly, and their levels will reflect the consequences of errors. For example, if a fatal illness can be cured only if identified early, then a rule-out threshold for that diagnosis may be set very low. Conversely, if a treatment is hazardous or very expensive, the rule-in threshold may be very high. In general, the goal of testing is to rule in or rule out diseases as efficiently as possible.

Given some particular test result, the posterior probability is determined by two factors: the operating characteristics of the test, and the prior probability of disease. Thus, a test can be conceived as something that operates on prior probability to produce posterior probability, with the operating characteristics affecting the amount of probability change. The proportion of diseased individuals within some defined population is called the disease prevalence, and for any individual selected at random from that population, the prevalence equals the prior probability of disease. Here, the two terms are equivalent, and may refer to extant probabilities at any stage in the clinical assessment. The precise relationships between prevalence, test operating characteristics, and posterior probabilities will now be explored.

PREDICTIVE VALUE OF A TEST RESULT

The sensitivity and specificity are conditional probabilities of particular test results, given the disease state, but in the clinical situation the disease state is unknown, and the major task is to estimate the conditional probability of disease, given the test result. This is the converse of the information provided by sensitivity and specificity, which are per se more relevant to research because the usual research method is to examine test results from groups of patients with known disease status.

Indices which are more useful in the clinical situation can be defined with reference to the 2 × 2 decision matrix of Table 14-1. Earlier, only the columns were considered, but when the matrix is conceived to be obtained by sampling, its rows have meaning in probability terms. Thus, TP/(TP + FP) estimates the probability of disease given a positive test, also known as the positive predictive value (PPV), and TN/(TN + FN) is the negative predictive value (NPV). Thus, the posterior probability of disease equals the PPV when the test is positive and $(1 - NPV)$ when the test is negative. If the test is useless, the PPV equals the prevalence.

It should be noted that the FN and FP rates were defined earlier as the complements of sensitivity and specificity, respectively. There is not universal agreement about this; for example, the FPR is sometimes defined as the complement of the PPV (Fleiss, 1981). This unfortunate situation makes it essential to determine which definition is in use.

In the Bayesian concept of conditional probability, sensitivity, for example, is the probability of event A (T+) given event B (D+), and the posterior probability of disease (PPV) is the probability of B given A. These are related by Bayes' formula, so the importance of operating characteristics such as sensitivity and specificity is not only as tools for evaluating tests, but also that in the clinical decision situation, they permit posterior probabilities to be derived from given priors (see Appendix). Table 14-4 shows some combinations of prevalence, sensitivity, specificity, likelihood ratio, and PPV. These relationships can be used to answer very important questions such as: Given a prevalence of 0.1, what combinations of sensitivity and specificity will give a PPV of at least 0.9, that is, so as to rule in the disease, given a positive test?

USING LIKELIHOOD RATIOS

Like sensitivity and specificity, the LR is defined in terms of test outcome probabilities given the disease states, but via Bayes' formula it permits derivation of posterior probabilities from priors. The LR formulation is simpler than that using sensitivity and specificity. The LR has a straightforward relationship to prior and posterior *odds* for disease. The relationship of odds and probabilities is: odds equal probability/(1 − probability), or conversely: probability equals odds/(odds + 1).

Given this, it is easy to show that: posterior odds equal prior odds × LR+, which is just another way of stating Bayes' formula. Thus, it is easy to calculate the posterior probability of disease, given the prevalence and the LR for the test result. When a sequence of tests is used, the elegance of this approach is even more obvious, because the posterior odds from test 1 become the prior odds for test 2, and so on. As a result, the odds after the Nth test are simply the initial prevalence times the product of the LRs for each test result. This is true provided that either the tests are statistically independent, or the LRs are the appropriate conditional ratios (Sackett et al., 1985).

These simple LR formulations of the effect of a test or a series of tests are an attractive alternative to the direct use of sensitivity and specificity. For example, the earlier question relating a prevalence of 0.1 to a PPV of 0.9 is handled very easily: the prior odds are 0.1/0.9 equals 1 : 9, and the target posterior odds are 0.9/0.1 or 9 : 1, so the required LR+ is 81. To see if a particular test with a given sensitivity and specificity is adequate, the LR+ would be calculated and compared with the required value. Ideally, though, the LR values or functions for the test would have been provided, as part of its specification.

TABLE 14-4. SELECTED VALUES THAT ILLUSTRATE THE RELATIONSHIPS AMONG TEST SENSITIVITY, SPECIFICITY, LIKELIHOOD RATIOS, AND PREDICTIVE VALUES FOR VARIOUS LEVELS OF DISEASE PREVALENCE (PRE-TEST PROBABILITY)

Sens	Spec	LR+	LR−	0.01 PPV	0.01 NPV	0.05 PPV	0.05 NPV	0.10 PPV	0.10 NPV	0.50 PPV	0.50 NPV
0.80	0.80	4.00	0.250	0.039	0.997	0.174	0.987	0.308	0.973	0.800	0.800
	0.90	8.00	0.222	0.075	0.998	0.296	0.988	0.471	0.976	0.889	0.818
	0.95	16.0	0.211	0.139	0.998	0.457	0.989	0.640	0.977	0.941	0.826
	0.99	80.0	0.202	0.447	0.998	0.808	0.989	0.899	0.978	0.988	0.832
0.90	0.80	4.50	0.125	0.043	0.999	0.191	0.993	0.333	0.986	0.818	0.889
	0.90	9.00	0.111	0.083	0.999	0.321	0.994	0.500	0.988	0.900	0.900
	0.95	18.0	0.105	0.154	0.999	0.486	0.994	0.667	0.988	0.947	0.905
	0.99	90.0	0.101	0.476	0.999	0.826	0.995	0.909	0.989	0.989	0.908
0.95	0.80	4.75	0.063	0.046	0.999	0.200	0.997	0.345	0.993	0.826	0.941
	0.90	9.50	0.055	0.088	0.999	0.333	0.997	0.514	0.994	0.905	0.947
	0.95	19.0	0.053	0.161	0.999	0.500	0.997	0.679	0.994	0.950	0.950
	0.99	95.0	0.051	0.490	0.999	0.833	0.997	0.913	0.994	0.990	0.952
0.99	0.80	4.95	0.013	0.048	0.999	0.207	0.999	0.355	0.999	0.832	0.988
	0.90	9.90	0.011	0.091	0.999	0.343	0.999	0.524	0.999	0.908	0.989
	0.95	19.8	0.011	0.167	0.999	0.510	0.999	0.688	0.999	0.952	0.990
	0.99	99.0	0.010	0.500	0.999	0.839	0.999	0.917	0.999	0.990	0.990

LR+ = sens/(1 − spec); LR− = (1 − sens)/spec; PPV = p • sens/[p • sens + (1 − p) • (1 − spec)]; NPV = (1 − p) • spec/[(1 − p) • spec + p • (1 − sens)].

THE RATIONALE FOR CHOICE OF TEST

Relationships between prior and posterior probabilities are shown in Figure 14-4, which is very important. The performance of acoustic reflex tests in the detection of acoustic tumor would yield such curves, assuming a d' of about 2.0 (Turner, Shepard, and Frazer, 1984). The deviation from the unit-slope line of the useless test reflects the change in probability. For a given operating point, the test will yield two curves as the prevalence changes: one for T+ and the other for T−. At any prevalence, the separation of the two curves is a measure of test impact, which may take values between zero and unity. In general, this distance is largest at moderate prevalence. Individual differences from the unit-slope line show that when prevalence is low, T+ changes the probability more than T− does, whereas at high prevalence the negative result has more effect.

Figure 14-5 shows probability curves for several sets of operating characteristics. Given T+, specificity has more effect than sensitivity, especially when prevalence is low. Given T−, sensitivity has more effect than specificity, especially when prevalence is high. Thus, when the goal is to rule in a particular diagnosis, a test with high specificity is needed. When the goal is to rule out the diagnosis, a test with high sensitivity is needed. When prevalence is high, a positive test tends to confirm disease, but a negative test is not very helpful in ruling it out. When the prior probability is low, a negative test tends to rule out disease, but a positive test is not very helpful to confirm it.

All of this emphasizes the dynamic view of tests. Not only is test performance adjustable, changing the sensitivity and specificity or the likelihood ratios by manipulating the operating point, but also the appropriateness and impact of the test will depend upon the goal and context of its use. Is it intended to rule in or rule out? Is the situation one of low or moderate prevalence? In general, the development of an optimal testing strategy requires optimization of the individual test operating points and the manner in which the tests are combined. Typically, the early stages of assessment involve a filtering process which increases the prevalence to a moderate value, at which point a test with a good LR+ (about 10 or more) could rule the disease in at the 0.9 level, and a test with a good LR− (about 0.1 or less) could rule it out at the 0.1 level.

ESTIMATION OF PREVALENCE

The importance of prevalence is now clear. It is essential to gather prevalence estimates for all disorders of interest in a specific clinical milieu. These

Figure 14-4. The effect of a test result (T+ or T−) on disease probability. For T+ the posterior (posttest) probability is the positive predictive value; for T−, it is the complement of the negative predictive value. These curves apply for sensitivity and specificity of 0.85. The diagonal shows a useless test, one that does not change the probability, for which the sensitivity and specificity sum to unity. Rule-in and rule-out thresholds are also shown.

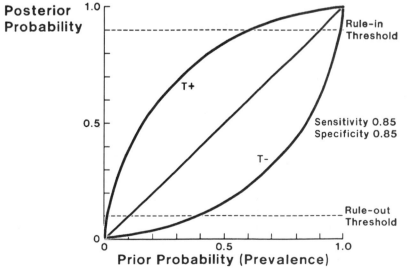

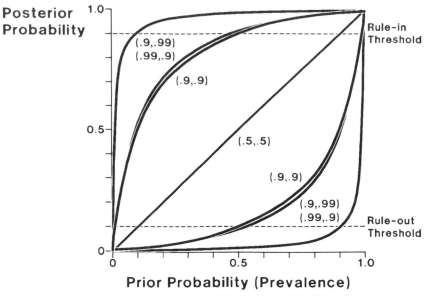

Figure 14-5. Probability functions for several pairs of values (*bracketed*) for sensitivity and specificity. These curve families define the impact of a test, in terms of the Bayesian probability revision model. Note the marked effects of specificity for the upper (T+) curves, and of sensitivity for the lower (T−) curves.

can be obtained from published data or local experience. Published data must be scrutinized to ensure that the disease definition and target population are appropriate. Estimation from local experience can be either formalized or not; the best method is to adopt a rigorous definition of the target disease and to observe the accumulation of cases over some predetermined time period. Each new case can be used to update the prevalence estimate. Account must be taken of changes over time in referral base or in any other patient selection criteria. For rare diseases, this experiential approach is impractical. In the absence of concrete data, clinicians can use subjective probability estimates, but caution is required, here. Physicians, for example, tend to overestimate disease prevalence and are generally reluctant to update their beliefs (Dolan, Bordley, and Mushlin, 1986). There is also little agreement on the meaning of such terms as *rare, common,* and the like, which have no real place in science (Nakao and Axelrod, 1983).

OPTIMIZATION OF TESTS AND STRATEGIES

Up to this point, the concern has been mainly with probabilities: first, the probabilities of test results, given disease states, followed by the (Bayesian) probabilities of disease, given test results. Tests can be compared, and the impact of a test can be evaluated, but there are several cru-

cial questions that require one more step: the assignment of costs or utilities to the outcomes of decisions.

OPTIMIZATION OF TEST OPERATING POINT

Suppose some binary test is considered for use because it has a good d' and a positive result is likely to lead to rule-in decision, given a known prevalence. How should the operating point be selected? Borrowing from statistical decision theory, the problem is solved by assigning specific quantitative "utility" to the various decision outcomes. The optimal operating point is that which maximizes the long-term expected utility, which is a sum of utilities weighted by their associated probabilities. Utilities can reflect many things, such as dollar costs of procedures and therapies, risk and benefit, morbidity, quality of life, outcome preference ratings, life expectancy, and so on. One approach is to assign dollar costs to all aspects of the decision outcomes and then to proceed to minimize the expected cost, and this is sometimes known as cost-benefit analysis. There are many options, with their associated terminologies (Sackett et al., 1985; Weinstein and

Fineberg, 1980) but the essence of it all is maximization or minimization of a weighted sum.

Sometimes it is difficult to assign the costs or utilities, and it might be thought that the assignment is artificial or arbitrary. However, the very concept of optimizing a decision under uncertainty actually *demands* a value structure. If the value system is not known then the decision cannot be optimized. This is an unpalatable but unavoidable conclusion. It can be speculated that clinicians often adopt implicit utilities that may be difficult to express, but that influence their decision behavior, nevertheless.

Consider the simplest possible example: optimizing a binary test, with costs assigned only to the FP and FN errors. Figure 14-6 shows the situation, and it can be derived that the test operating point that maximizes utility (minimizes cost) is given implicitly by the equation:

$$LR+ = (CFP/CFN) \cdot (1-p)/p$$

where LR+ = the likelihood ratio,
p = the prior probability,
CFP and CFN = the costs of FP and FN errors, respectively.

A slightly more elaborate equation includes the cost of correct decisions. The cost of the test itself, the test *overhead* cost, does not affect the choice of operating point, but it affects the cost of any strategy involving the test.

The consequences of this equation are quite reasonable and easy to visualize in terms of the statistical model in Figure 14-1. Moving the operating point (test criterion) upward increases

the LR+ (equals TPR/FPR) because the FP area (probability) decreases faster than the TP area, whereas moving downward decreases the ratio. Increasing CFP or reducing prevalence increases the optimal LR+, so the criterion moves upward, giving a smaller FPR (high specificity needed). On the other hand, increasing the prevalence or CFN reduces the optimal LR+, and a move downward is needed (high sensitivity desired). In the event that errors are equally costly, the optimal operating point is chosen such that the likelihood ratio equals the prior odds against disease.

The bottom line is that in order to optimize a test it is necessary to know the costs of errors, or at least the cost ratio, as well as the prevalence of the disorder of interest. Because both the outcome costs and the prevalence of disorder are a function of the strategic context of the test, such as at which point in a test sequence it is to be done, it follows that it is impossible to generalize about what the optimal point should be. The notion that there is some invariant optimal decision criterion for any audiologic test is incorrect.

DECISION TREE ANALYSIS

It is now appropriate to consider the optimization of strategies, of which tests are only elements. This problem introduces the full procedure of clinical decision analysis. The formal CDA approach is as follows (Sackett et al., 1985):

1. Develop a decision tree, which is a flow diagram indicating all the pertinent courses of action, and their consequences.
2. Assign probabilities to the branches from terminal chance nodes.
3. Assign utilities to all of the possible outcomes.
4. Calculate the expected utilities for each node on the tree, using branch utilities weighted by probabilities. Working back toward the beginning of the tree is called "folding back."
5. Select the decision path giving the highest overall expected utility.
6. Test the analysis to see whether the answer changes, given plausible alterations in probability or utility. This is known as *sensitivity analysis*, and is an important tool (Pauker and Kassirer, 1987).

Figure 14-6. Optimization of the operating point of a binary test. The circles indicate nodes at which probabilistic (nonpredetermined) events occur. The outcome probabilities and associated costs of false-positive (CFP) and false-negative (CFN) errors are indicated. The optimal test-operating point minimizes the expected cost.

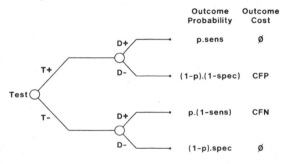

Expected Cost = CFP.(1−p).(1−spec) + CFN.p.(1−sens)

Consider Figure 14-7A, which shows a decision tree for the fundamental problem of whether or

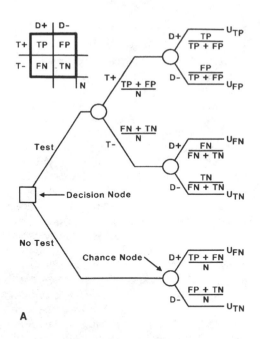

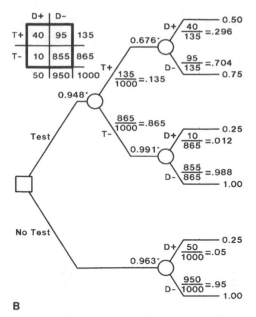

A

B

Figure 14-7. The decision tree and matrix for the test/no test problem. (A) Generic, indicating probability expressions and utilities. (B) A numeric example; the starred numbers at the chance nodes are the expected utilities.

not to perform a test. The best outcome is that the patient is free of disease and has not been labelled as disease positive; next, the patient is disease free but is labelled as disease positive, with attendant costs of anxiety, further testing, or treatment; next, the patient has the disease and knows it, but benefits from therapy; worst, the patient has the disease, does not know it, and does not receive therapy. Assign, for example, utilities of 1.0, 0.75, 0.50, and 0.25 to these four outcomes. Let the prevalence be 0.05, and let the test have sensitivity 0.8 and specificity 0.9. A simple way to decide whether or not to test is to solve the problem numerically, using a 2 × 2 decision matrix. One way to determine the required table elements is to allocate 1000 patients, say, to the column totals dictated by the prevalence (in this case 50 and 950) and then work out the cells using the sensitivity and specificity. The results are shown in Figure 14-7B. Given this, is it better to test or not?

In the non-test strategy, all patients are told they are disease free. The probability of disease is the prevalence, and so the expected utility is 0.05 × 0.25 + 0.95 × 1.0, which equals 0.9625. The other strategy is more complicated, and yields an expected path utility of 0.948. Therefore, it is better in the long run not to administer this test. If there were concern that the prevalence might actually be higher than 0.05, a sensitivity analysis could be done, calculating the results for a plausible range of prevalence increase. For p equals 0.10, for exam-

ple, the conclusion is the same, because the expected utilities are now 0.962 and 0.90. Thus, the sensitivity analysis confirms the stability of the decision, and for this problem, the optimal strategy is not to test.

A simpler analysis arises if only error costs are used. In general it is better not to test unless the cost ratio CFP/CFN is less than the posterior odds for disease, given a positive test; to prove this makes a good, basic exercise, and the proof is given in the Appendix.

CDA offers a way of pruning decision trees to give a clinical algorithm or *protocol*, which is a set of specified operations usually in the form of a structured sequence of observations and formal tests, and usually expressed as a logical flow chart. The protocol tree is distinct from the decision tree of CDA, in that the protocol *specifies* activity, whereas the decision tree identifies possible activities. The protocol embodies consistent test strategy and is an excellent tool for the promotion of high-quality clinical activities. Wherever possible, detailed protocols should be formulated and obeyed. Clear, general methodologic guidelines for protocol formulation are available (Pass, Komaroff, and Ervin, 1982).

CURRENT SITUATION

At this point, the basic tools with which to evaluate, compare, and optimize tests and to build strategies have been outlined. Several audiologic areas will now be used to illustrate and elaborate these ideas. In general, there has been only very limited penetration of CDA techniques into audiology, and so at present it is difficult to locate or to derive from the literature the information needed to evaluate tests and strategies in a complete and quantitative manner. The need for further studies exhibiting proper attention to statistical, epidemiologic and decision theoretic principles is acute.

ACOUSTIC TUMOR DIAGNOSIS

The detection of acoustic tumor (AT) has been a focus of classic diagnostic audiology for many years. Early detection and early surgical removal reduce the morbidity associated with both the disease and the surgical treatment. Large tumors impinge upon brainstem and cerebellar structures, giving greater operative difficulty and risk.

The general prevalence of AT may be as high as 1 percent, but most are very small and asymptomatic; the prevalence of symptomatic AT is about 1 : 100,000. About 90 percent of all cerebellopontine angle (CPA) tumors are AT, the remainder being mostly meningiomas. Initial symptoms and signs vary greatly, but both the emphasis upon early detection and advances in testing methods have resulted in diagnosis at a stage when hearing loss is often the only presenting physical finding. See Hart, Gardner, and Howieson (1983) for a detailed review of first reported symptoms, presenting complaints, and symptoms at diagnosis.

BACKGROUND

Many strategies have been proposed for AT detection, and there are large differences in practice on a continental, national, and regional basis, as well as radical changes in strategies over time. There has been more published work with a CDA flavor in this area than for any other audiologic topic. Although now dated, Hart and Davenport (1981) examined the performance of audiologic, vestibular, and radiologic tests and analyzed various protocols using methods of decision theory, including costs. S. Jerger (1983) introduced some principles of decision analysis, and she applied them to several tests individually and in combination, emphasizing the trading relationship between sensitivity and specificity when constructing test combinations with series and parallel decision rules. A combination of acoustic reflexes, PI-PB and Bekesy Comfortable Loudness gave a sensitivity of 1.0 under a parallel rule, and a specificity of 1.0 under a series rule, which raises an interesting problem: if either sensitivity or specificity is 1.0, it is impossible to compute d' using a single-point algorithm, because such a value is not obtainable under the NEV model. The data Jerger presented were estimates obtained in 20 patients with AT and 20 with cochlear disease. With that sample size, the 95 percent confidence interval for sensitivity or specificity is 0.83 to 1.0. If 0.85, say, were the true value of sensitivity, then with the stated specificity of 0.55, the estimated d' is only 1.2. Thus, it is feasible that performance is very mediocre indeed, despite the perfect sample score. This underlines the importance of large samples and the use of confidence intervals.

The dependency of posterior probability (PPV) on prior probability (prevalence) is a very important matter. Jerger warned about this but went on to estimate PPV in the group of 40 subjects with a controlled prevalence of 0.5. This is a much higher value than typically would be encountered clinically, even in a tertiary center. Given the sensitivity and specificity, or the likelihood ratios, and as Schwartz (1987a) has noted, it is easy to recalculate the PPV for realistic prevalences; this leads to a much less flattering picture for some of the classic audiologic tests, as should be expected from their indifferent d'. However, another important point is that a mediocre test should not normally be used at all, once the filtering process of observations and preliminary tests has raised the prevalence to somewhere in the region of 0.5. At that point, definitive radiology would be appropriate, and a test that could neither rule in nor rule out the tumor would be almost futile.

Jerger also stressed the dependency of ROC methods upon the validity of assumptions, and this cautious approach is certainly wise. However, the current view is that certain aspects of ROC analysis can be quite robust and useful in a wide variety of fields, despite massive violation of the normality assumption, as well as inhomogeneous variances (Swets, 1988).

Turner and his colleagues (Turner and Nielsen, 1984; Turner et al., 1984) published a series of articles dealing with some aspects of the CDA approach, oriented toward the area of AT diagnosis. They combined the results from many studies, giving average values for sensitivity and specificity for many tests, and then computed d' using the NEV model (which they called Gaussian, equal variance, or GEV). Tests were then ranked by d', and ABR testing had by far the best performance of any audiologic test.

Turner took the interesting position of treating d' as a variable, when the ROC did not have unity slope. The present authors' view is that when the NEV model is not valid, d' calculations based upon it will be incorrect, and this is not really a matter of variation in d'. Under such conditions, single-point estimates of d' are suspect; more than one sensitivity and specificity pair is needed, to determine the ROC. Preferably, about four or five points should be used, and the ROC can then indicate operating points with specific FP rates.

Dobie (1985) discussed critically several of the points raised by Turner and colleagues, and gave a cogent description of the use of cost benefit analysis to select and optimize tests for AT. Recently, Turner (1988) gave a detailed analysis of the principles of constructing test protocols with known performance, at least in terms of sensitivity and specificity. Appropriately, Turner pointed out the current lack of information regarding statistical independence, or otherwise, for audiologic tests in this area. Until such data are provided, analyses of strategies involving combinations of audiologic tests will only yield approximate solutions.

NEW OPERATING POINT OR NEW TEST?

Even for a single test, such as the ABR, there is much variation on reported performance. Some of this is due to differences in the operating point of the test, and some to changes in the intrinsic quality of the test, as reflected in the underlying statistical model. These effects must be distinguished carefully. ABR testing provides a very convenient example of this widespread problem.

Suppose ABR testing were simplified so that the test variable is the interaural latency difference for ABR wave V, known as IT_5 or ILD V. This is a continuous variable, with the diagnostic dichotomy created by the operating point; increase in ILD V beyond the operating point leads to the T+ decision. Selters and Brackmann (1979) gave a scattergram of raw data points, which is a very informative format for publication of data, permitting analysis by the reader. For an ILD V criterion of 0.2 msec, the reported sensitivity and false positive rate were 0.98 and 0.24, respectively, giving a single-point d' estimate of 2.75. Figure 14-8

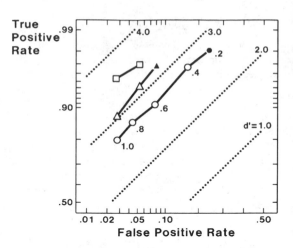

Figure 14-8. ROCs for the detection of acoustic tumor using the ABR interaural wave V latency difference. Circles = latency not corrected for hearing loss; various test criteria are indicated. Triangles = corrected by 0.1 msec per 10 dB of loss at 4 kHz above 50 dB HL. Squares = corrected by 0.1 msec of loss per 5 dB above 55 dB at 4 kHz. (Derived from the data of Selters and Brackmann [1979].)

shows that the ROC derived from their data has excellent linearity and unit slope.

Selters and Brackmann, referring only to a single point (the solid circle) on the ROC, noted the high FPR and suggested a latency correction of −0.1 msec for every 10 dB, or fraction thereof, of pure tone hearing loss above 50 dB at 4 kHz. For the same abnormality criterion (0.2 msec), this "corrected ILD V" gives a sensitivity of 0.97 and a FPR of 0.08, leading to a single-point d' of 3.25. The associated ROC, in Figure 14-8, is shifted towards the upper left corner. Without latency correction, the FPR of 0.08 could have been obtained by altering the criterion to about 0.6 msec, but only at the cost of a substantial decrease in sensitivity. The use of corrected ILD V constitutes a real change in the test itself; the correction transforms the underlying variable so as to increase the effective distance between the nontumor and tumor distributions. It achieves this primarily by reducing the variance of the test variable, for the nontumor distribution.

Further analysis of Selters and Brackmann's raw data reveals that it is possible to improve the latency correction scheme. For example, a correction of 0.1 msec per 5 dB above 55 dB at 4 kHz gives the third ROC in Figure 14-8; here, the d' is about 3.6, which is excellent performance. This can be improved even further by more elaborate schemes, such as taking the patient's age and gender into account. These d' can be compared with the average of 2.9 for the ABR according to the review by Turner and colleagues (1984), covering a mixture of ABR abnormality criteria. Curiously, the very recent audiologic literature continues to include articles evaluating ABR performance that are based on uncorrected ABR measures.

It was noted earlier that when disease prevalence is low, it is the specificity of the test that is most influential for increasing the posterior probability of disease, given a positive test. For a typical AT prevalence of about 0.01, using the best ROC in Figure 14-8, the more conservative abnormality criterion shown yields an FPR of about 0.025 and a probability change from 0.01 to about 0.28, the likelihood ratio being about 38. The more liberal criterion gives an FPR of 0.055, a likelihood ratio of about 18, and a posterior probability of about 0.15.

DISEASE SEVERITY

The acoustic tumor is not a dichotomous disease; tumor size affects both test performance and prevalence estimates. As patients present earlier and earlier for assessment, so the situation is created in which prevalence and test operating characteristics interact. An extensive review was given by Hart, Gardner, and Howieson (1983), and in Table 14-5 are compared selected sensitivity, specificity, likelihood ratio, d', and A_z data derived from that study and from the review of Turner, Shepard, and Frazer (1984). As might be expected, test performance is clearly poorer for small tumors.

CHANGING GOLD STANDARDS

The nature of the gold standard test (GS) has a major effect on the utility structure of AT assess-

ment strategies. Years ago, the GS was iophendylate posterior fossa myelography and its morbidity was one factor that prompted the use of elaborate filtering protocols to raise the prevalence to a high value, prior to performing the myelography. The more recent introduction of air-contrast computed tomography (CT), a procedure with excellent sensitivity and good specificity (even for small tumors), allowed AT rule-out with less morbidity. Thus, patients can be referred to air CT at lower probabilities of disease than was reasonable for iophendylate myelography. The recent widespread implementation of magnetic resonance imaging (MRI) is a new factor; technical advances are rapid, and MRI is likely at least to equal air CT in terms of operating characteristics, even in its noninvasive form without the use of contrast agents (Curati, Graif, Kingsley, et al., 1986). However, MRI is an expensive procedure, so the key issues now are overhead costs and availability. In general, pressures for health cost containment are likely to ensure continuing interest in effective audiologic strategies for prevalence enhancement.

It can be quite difficult to obtain valid performance estimates for procedures that may qualify as gold, or near gold, standards. The only arbiter is the definitive procedure, which in the case of AT is surgery and pathologic report; the cost of unnecessary surgery can be high, and there is a tendency to rely on lesser indicators or to allow the outcome of the procedure in question to influence the decision about surgery. Also, when error rates are very low, increasingly large and diverse samples are required to specify those rates with acceptable precision. Third, there are phases in the evaluation and use of all tests, not just potential gold standards, and these may have very marked effects when error rates are small; early on, there is a tendency to study the tests in very clear examples of the target disease, and with nor-

TABLE 14-5. OPERATING CHARACTERISTICS FOR THREE TESTS COMMONLY USED IN THE DIAGNOSIS OF ACOUSTIC TUMORS

| Test | All tumors | | | | | | Small tumors | | | | | |
	Sens	Spec	LR+	LR−	d'	A	Sens	Spec	LR+	LR−	d'	A
ABR[a]	0.96	0.91	10.7	0.044	3.09	0.986	0.91	0.91	10.1	0.099	2.68	0.971
ABR[b]	0.95	0.89	8.6	0.056	2.87	0.979						
AR[a]	0.84	0.90	8.4	0.178	2.27	0.946	0.77	0.90	7.7	0.256	2.02	0.924
AR[b]	0.84	0.85	5.6	0.188	2.03	0.925						
ENG[a]	0.87	0.68	2.7	0.191	1.60	0.855	0.57	0.68	1.8	0.632	0.65	0.677
ENG[b]	0.85	0.67	2.6	0.224	1.48	0.853						

ABR = auditory brainstem response; AR = acoustic reflex absence or decay; ENG = caloric testing with electronystagmography. Derived from [a]Hart, Gardner, and Howieson (1983), and [b]Turner, Shepard, and Frazer (1984). Note the effect of tumor size, and that the test accuracy measure A takes slightly different values from the A' used by Turner et al.

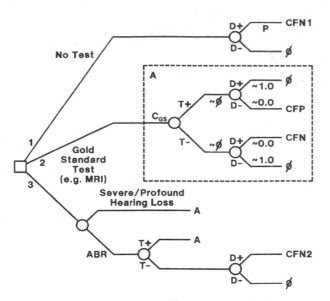

Figure 14-9. A decision tree for acoustic tumor detection.

mal controls. Ultimately, the test will be used on a spectrum of disease severity, with diverse competing pathologies; under those conditions, the test performance may be very much poorer. This is one reason why so many tests are adopted enthusiastically but are eventually discarded.

SPECIFIC STRATEGIES

Suppose that some body of preliminary investigation yields patients who are candidates for a particular strategy for detection of AT. The first issue is whether all those patients are equivalent. The *index of suspicion* is a facet of clinical judgment that could be viewed as a prevalence modifier and might be taken into account in the test strategy; however, despite attempts to standardize this index in a numerical form (Windle-Taylor, Dhillon, Kenyon, and Morrison, 1984), there has been little formal analysis of this problem from a decision theoretic standpoint. Here, it will be assumed that all patients suspected of AT are essentially equivalent, in terms of their probability of disease. A decision tree for their evaluation is shown in Figure 14-9.

Strategy 1: Do Not Test

The cost of this strategy arises primarily from FN error of probability p, where p equals the AT prevalence in the suspect group. In D+ patients, treatment will be delayed, with attendant costs of both pre-treatment morbidity and possible changes in the treatment outcome. These costs are

not well understood, but one approach is via the legal view as might arise in a malpractice suit. The expected cost per patient is p × CFN, so the prevalence is crucial; it depends on the criteria for suspicion and the referral base, and will probably lie between 0.01 and 0.05 for AT. If CFN were set at 1,000,000 units, a modest malpractice award if the units are dollars, the expected cost per patient lies between 10,000 and 50,000. This is really an incremental cost associated with failure to diagnose early, because those patients who have tumors will ultimately have to be tested and treated. To set the costs rationally, detailed information about the relationships between surgical timing and outcomes would be required.

Strategy 2: Give Everyone the Gold Standard

Presuming that error rates are negligible for the GS, the expected cost per patient is the overhead cost of the test, comprising the true cost of the test itself, plus the cost of morbidity due to it. For AT, nowadays, test mobidity is low, so what matters is the actual cost of air CT or MRI, or perhaps a combination of the two. In this example, the cost will be set at 1000 units. This strategy is clearly better than the first, unless prevalance or the cost of false negatives is much lower than suggested.

Strategy 3: A One-Test Filter

It appears that in terms of operating characteristics, the ABR is the best filter for the MRI. One strategy is to use the ABR for all suspects, and do the GS on only ABR-positives. The first problem is that the ABR is affected by end-organ dysfunction. What is the diagnostic value of a flat ABR tracing in a dead ear, and what are the limits of the latency correction process? Thus, some proportion of patients cannot be tested satisfactorily with the ABR, and that proportion will depend on local variables. A complication is that there is no clear point, in terms of hearing loss, at which ABR testing suddenly becomes useless; this is a complex matter involving details of etiology, severity, type, and contour of hearing loss.

In this example, the strategy will bifurcate, using the ABR if the pure tone audiogram gives 80 dB HL or better at 2 kHz, bilaterally. In the authors' milieu, this would mean that about 10 percent of suspects could not be tested by ABR. The simplest thing to do is send all such cases for the GS; another strategy would be to substitute some nonaudiologic test, such as electronystagmography (d' 1.5, down to 0.7 for small tumors, according to Hart et al., 1983) or tomograms of the internal auditory canal (d' 2.1), for ABR in the 10 percent of cases.

Consider the cost analysis for the simpler case of 90 percent ABR, 10 percent direct to the GS. The results suggest that, at prevalence p, use of the ABR will reduce overall average costs unless the cost of a false negative error is greater than about (20/p) times the overhead cost difference of the GS and ABR. If the respective costs are 1000 and 250, and the prevalence is 0.01, then the ABR sequence is cheaper unless the false negative cost is over 1,000,000. The cost solution depends more strongly on the sensitivity of the ABR than its specificity. Inclusion of an IAC tomogram in the non-ABR path would be optimized and costed in exactly the same way as done for the ABR path.

Other Strategies

The analysis of whether to interpose some even cheaper audiologic test X, as a filter for the ABR, follows similar but slightly more elaborate logic than that used when interposing the ABR before the GS. The series combination sensitivity can only be worse than that of the best component (see Table 14-3), and for the AT, FN errors are

costly, so X must have its operating point adjusted to give high sensitivity. For the series sensitivity to be at least 0.90, given that ABR sensitivity is about 0.96, the series equations indicate that test X must have a sensitivity of at least 0.94. Coupling this with a modest specificity requirement of 0.75 leads to a minimum required d' of 2.23, which is higher than that of most, if not all, the tests in the classic audiologic battery for AT. Even if such a test were found, the FNR is at least doubled, and one in four patients will go on to have an ABR test. Thus, it is difficult to make a good case for any other audiologic "special test" filter for the ABR. A possible candidate is acoustic reflex tests, with d' derived from published data of about 1.4 to 2.1. Using the largest of these, with the operating point set to give a sensitivity of 0.94, the specificity will be about 0.71. The cost balance is dominated by the increase in FNR from 0.04 to 0.10, versus the saving because only 29 percent of patients receive ABR testing. The most favorable situation for interposing acoustic reflex testing is one of low prevalence and high overhead cost ratio. A complete appreciation of the impact would require analysis of the full decision tree. There are many other questions that might be explored, such as that of finding an optimal combination if ABR testing is not available.

Many authors have favored a parsimonious sequential strategy with ABR testing as an element (Barr, Brackmann, Olson, and House, 1985; Cashman and Nedzelski, 1983; Turner et al., 1984; Turner, 1988). The present authors support strongly the principle of parsimony but as yet are unaware of any complete optimization according to the principles of CDA. It is likely that there is no universally optimal strategy: The analytic solution will depend upon many local factors, including prevalence, overhead and error costs, clinical resources and constraints.

EARLY AUDIOLOGIC ASSESSMENT OF THE HIGH-RISK INFANT

The next illustrative problem to be considered is early diagnosis of hearing loss in infancy, along the lines suggested by the American Academy of Pediatrics' Joint Committee on Infant Hearing (1982). It is argued that detection, quantification, and management of hearing loss often do not occur sufficiently early, and that this delay compromises development of communication skills. Early detection and management of the hearing impaired infant is thought to be important for minimizing sequelae. The Joint Committee recommended the use of a high-risk register, followed by audiologic testing of those at risk. The target suggested was to initiate habilitation before the age of six months, wherever possible.

Clinical programs for early audiologic assessment of high risk infants are now quite widespread, especially in North America. This is due mainly to the application of the ABR, which has become a very popular tool in this area. Behavioral assessment can be inaccurate in the first year of life, and careful distinction is required between the thresholds of responsivity and of hearing sensitivity. This problem is acute if carefully controlled conditioning is not feasible, such as in the first few months, or in certain neurologically impaired infants (Wilson and Thompson, 1984). Automated behavioral techniques of interest include the Auditory Response Cradle (Davis, 1984) and the Crib-O-Gram (COG). For a general review, see Swigart (1986).

BACKGROUND

There has been little application of CDA principles, although several descriptions of the decision matrix and predictive value concepts are available (e.g., Fria, 1985; Jacobson and Jacobson, 1987; Kenworthy, 1987). Some of the limitations of research in the area of infant ABR assessment were noted by Murray, Javel, and Watson (1985) and in the CHABA (1987) report. Specifically from the CDA viewpoint, major areas of need involve better specification of the target disorder, and better estimates of both prevalence and the operating characteristics of various tests. With respect to the last, more extensive follow-up data for validation of tests performed in early infancy are required. It is essential to follow those who pass and those who fail, otherwise operating characteristics cannot be derived. Typically, only failures are followed, yielding an estimate of the positive predictive value; this reveals nothing about the NPV, so the prevalence, sensitivity, specificity, ROC, and likelihood ratios remain a mystery. Also, the conclusions of studies in which the proportion of cases followed is small are highly suspect; there is no guarantee at all that those who were followed are representative.

EARLY DIAGNOSIS

This area of infant assessment is a good example of efforts at early diagnosis, which is a distinct type of activity, requiring special considerations (Sackett et al., 1985). Much of audiologic assessment involves the symptomatic patient, wherein the mandate of the clinician is to do no harm, but there is no implied guarantee of effective therapy. Early diagnosis, on the other hand, usually means presymptomatic diagnosis by a screening or case-finding strategy. Here, there is an implied commitment to ameliorate or cure. Important issues are:

1. Does the illness have sufficient prevalence or incidence?
2. Is the burden of disability sufficiently great?
3. Does early diagnosis really improve the outcome?
4. Will patients comply with therapeutic regimens?
5. Are follow-up and management facilities sufficient and effective?
6. Is the program acceptable in cost-benefit terms?

It might be argued that infants cannot complain of hearing loss and so society must act aggressively on their behalf, but especially in screening programs involving new techniques, the opportunity for both waste and even harm is considerable. For example, will a parent of a child who was screened negative at 3 months of age be less likely to seek prompt advice about an apparent hearing problem at age 1 year? The issues listed reflect quite clearly some of the CDA aspects that have been introduced and warrant careful consideration.

There is considerable evidence that hearing loss has deleterious effects on development of the central auditory pathways and on the development of communicative skills, but there is as yet no unequivocal demonstration of the existence of a critical period beyond which these effects can be redressed. However, because of the widespread implementation of early assessment programs it may now be difficult to study this problem by a randomized prospective trial of early intervention. There may be little choice but to continue to resort to retrospective studies, with all their inherent weaknesses. Nevertheless, there is a need for rigorous application of decision analysis and in particular, cost-benefit studies, in this area.

DISEASE DEFINITION

Quantitative definition of the target disorder is a prerequisite for the evaluation and selection of test strategies, and for consideration of disease probabilities. Here, the target disorder is hearing loss, an entity which is much more complex and common than an acoustic tumor. Hearing loss is multivariate, the pure tone audiogram comprising many data items. At any frequency, there is a continuum of disease severity. Also, unilaterality or bilaterality of the loss and its type and etiology add to the complexity of disease definition. All of this must be considered when trying to detect and measure the disease.

It is natural to simplify by categorizing or even dichotomizing the spectrum of hearing losses. One way is to define what is normal and then call everything else abnormal. However, there is no clear understanding of what constitutes normal hearing sensitivity in a young infant. It is difficult to unravel responsivity and stimulus audibility in behavioral testing paradigms. ABR results suggest that the peripheral sensitivity of a young infant can be as good or better than that of a normal adult.

It can be argued that the real issue here is not whether the child has a sensitivity threshold that satisfies some definition of normal, but whether there will be significant compromise of the acquisition of speech and language skills. However, the quantitative relationship between the impairment, namely pure tone sensitivity loss, and the disability, namely compromised speech and language acquisition, is not established. In the past, the focus was on severe bilateral sensory hearing loss (SHL), with its indisputable sequelae. Nowadays, the debate is about just how little hearing loss should be considered unacceptable. There is the complication that factors such as socioeconomic status might influence the consequences of any given impairment.

GOLD STANDARD

There is no GS test for hearing loss in the first year of life, so determination of the accuracy and validity of any test proposed for audiometric use in that period is not straightforward. Audiometry at an age when accurate behavioral testing is feasible might be considered a GS, but in some children, such as those who have multiple neurologic handicaps, this approach may never yield reliable data. Another difficulty with a deferred GS is that if the hearing status changes in the period between early testing and definitive testing, the estimates of error rates for the early test will be inflated. If a test is viable in both infants and adults, as the ABR is, an alternative is to extrapolate adult validity to the young infant, but this has obvious dangers due to the implicit assumptions. Clearly, to compare ABR results in early infancy and at a later date does not validate early ABR testing, but does give limited information about test-retest reliability.

PREVALENCE

If some hearing test is to be administered soon after birth, then the prevalence of disease at birth is likely to be a good estimator of the pre-test probability of disease. Prevalence at birth is often incorrectly referred to as incidence (Hennekens and Buring, 1987). The prevalence of severe SHL in newborns is widely assumed to be about one per thousand live births (Martin, 1982; Schein and Delk, 1974), and this defines the prior probability of disease. Its exact value depends on the hearing loss criterion, and may be as high as 15 per 1000 for hearing loss of any degree. Detailed and accurate information on this is impossible to obtain at present, because of the lack of a GS test. In general, the results of any attempt to measure the prevalence of hearing loss will depend on many variables such as time (e.g., in relation to epidemic cycles, health care developments, and age at test), place (e.g., geographic, local health care standards, and survey or referral base), and method (e.g., behavioral, electrophysiologic, criteria, etc.) (Davidson, Hyde, and Alberti, 1989).

HIGH-RISK GROUPS

Attention is often directed toward infants at risk for hearing loss, and membership of a high-risk group can be conceived as a test that enhances prevalence. A risk register is a combination of binary subtests with a parallel decision rule. The risk factor "birth weight under 1500 g" is one such subtest: The test variable is birth weight and 1500 g is the operating point (decision criterion). By varying the operating point and determining the proportion of cases with hearing loss in the at-risk and nil-risk groups, an ROC can be derived. The factor "familial childhood hearing impairment" is also a binary test, the operating point being perhaps a function of the closeness of the familial tie. Usually, the register outcome is also binary: at risk or not. The parallels between risk register and acoustic tumor suspicion index are clear, and undoubtedly information is lost by dichotomizing the subtests and overall outcome.

The manner in which the information required to compile the risk register is collected is crucial for its operating characteristics, and varies greatly in cost and validity, according to local factors and effort expended. For example, the answer "no" for some factor is only informative if the answer "yes" was sought with sufficient diligence, and this may be a major source of discrepancy between studies. Some measures, such as birth weight, are well-defined and easy to access. Others, such as familial hearing loss, can be much more taxing: The accuracy of recall can vary greatly, and the quality of the answers may depend greatly on the skill and perceptiveness of the questioner. This is a matter of changing the effective d' of the register factor, not its operating point.

In some centers, the practice is to screen groups such as all neonatal intensive care graduates, many of whom will have at least one of the Joint Committee risk factors. This policy of evaluating a logistically distinct group can be very convenient, and the conventional risk data may or may not be gathered. Again, attendance in NICU can be conceived as a binary test. The length of stay in intensive care may be a convenient quantitative index of risk, and could serve to define an operating point. There are, of course, babies at risk who do not receive intensive care, such as those with a familial factor, so the sensitivity of such a test as this is clearly limited.

CONTINUOUS DISEASE AND TEST VARIABLES

In the case of acoustic tumor, a slight extension of the concept of dichotomous disease was considered, namely, the matter of tumor size. When hearing loss is the target disorder, however, there is a full numeric scale of disease severity that has at least some interval strength. Couple this with the continuous scales produced by tests such as the ABR, that essentially provide numerical estimates of the true hearing sensitivity, and the situation seems far removed from that of the 2 × 2 decision matrix. How are such situations to be analyzed?

One approach is to impose dichotomies and use the techniques developed previously, and this is often very revealing. A disease dichotomy in terms of normal or abnormal hearing sensitivity (when measurable reliably) is one choice, but if, for example, it were known that the development of communication skills is compromised for impairments greater than 30 dB, then that level would be the basis for a hearing loss dichotomy more directly oriented towards actual disability. Then, the ability of various tests to predict the disease categories might be examined by also dichotomizing the test variable, and using the 2 × 2 matrix approach. This could be done for various values of the disease criterion. Here, it is important to define the disease criterion independently of the test characteristics, because to base the definition of disease on some preconceived notion of what the test can do will flatter the test.

What if there is no reasonable dichotomy of disease? Multiple categories of both disease severity and test outcome can be handled by a larger decision matrix. Although the basic concepts of sensitivity and specificity, or the likelihood ratio, can no longer be applied as described earlier, the goodness of the test can be expressed in other ways, such as by correlation or regression coefficients. In fact, all cases ranging from the 2 × 2 situation through to continuous disease and test variables can be conceptualized in the same (Bayesian) way, namely, in terms of the conditional distribution of disease states, given the various test outcomes. The 2 × 2 matrix is merely the simplest possible example of this, and the other end of the scale is a multivariate scattergram. The complexity of the analytic techniques varies greatly for the different situations, but the conceptualization is consistent.

For continuous variables, or discrete variables with many possible values, a scattergram of the test and disease variables, or the test and gold standard values, is usually an informative way to present the data. Regression analysis of the GS variable on the test variable is appropriate, to quantify predictive accuracy; note that the regression of y on x is not the same as that of x on y. If the GS outcome is dichotomous, and the test outcome is continuous, then logit regression analysis is appropriate, whereas if the GS is dichotomous and the set of predictive variables includes dichotomous and continuous types, the logistic regression is needed (Fleiss, 1981).

SPECIFIC STRATEGIES

Various strategies for early diagnosis of hearing loss were described in Swigart (1986). Consider the common approach of using the ABR in infants who are positive on a typical high-risk register. The register is a test, and as was noted previously, the sensitivity of a series combination of tests is governed by that of the weakest link. Here, the weak link is the register, for which typical operating characteristics are not impressive; for example, the sensitivity seems to be about 0.5 (Riko, Hyde, and Alberti, 1985). The specificity is roughly 0.90 to 0.95, because about 1 in 10 to 1 in 20 babies is on the register. This gives a d' of as little as about 1.3, which is very modest. Fria (1985) considered that the sensitivity of the ABR may be as high as 0.98, with specificity of about 0.90 to 0.95. These correspond to a d' of well over 3.0, which is about as good as the ABR when used otoneurologically. Even if the very high sensitivity were correct, the series combination with the register would yield overall sensitivity and specificity values of 0.49 and 0.99, with a d' of about 2.3. Still a very good (overall) test performance, but with an operating point which is probably inappropriate in cost-benefit terms because of the high FN rate.

Why not simply increase the sensitivity of the register, by altering its operating point? This is not straightforward. The decision rule for the register subtests (factors) is already as lax as possible, positivity on any one of the subtests being sufficient for register positivity. The criteria for the subtests could be made less stringent, such as by increasing the low birth weight criterion to 2000 g, and the resulting overall operating point might be more appropriate; the basic tradeoff is between the cost of doing more ABR tests and having fewer FN errors. Of course, if there is no register factor at all that correlates with disease, as might be the case for recessive familial impairment, there is a constraint on the tradeoff. The principles for analysis of this simple strategy of filtering with a risk register are the same as those outlined earlier, for the acoustic tumor problem of filtering with ABR before definitive radiology.

When a behavioral screening test is interposed between the risk register and the ABR, the effect on combination performance depends strongly upon the degree of hearing loss that is considered to be clinically significant, because the sensitivity of behavioral tests improves as the loss

severity increases. If the goal is to detect minimal hearing loss on the grounds that it can indeed compromise communication skills, then the use of any behavioral screen seems undesirable (Jacobson and Morehouse, 1984). Following a report by Johnsen, Bagi, and Elberling (1983), there is accumulating evidence that the otoacoustic emissions discovered by Kemp (1978) may be a viable test preceding the ABR. If, on the other hand, the goal is to detect only moderate to severe losses, the behavioral filter is more reasonable. For further analysis of operating characteristics for various test strategies, see Turner (1988).

Prager, Stone, and Rose (1987) reported a cost effectiveness analysis of ABR and COG testing in NICU graduates based on review of several studies. They defined the target disease as hearing loss which is "permanent, bilateral, and of sufficient severity so as to require amplification," a vague but popular criterion in the primary literature. A prevalence of 2 percent was used, which is representative, and the sensitivity and specificity values adopted were 1.0 and 0.86 for the ABR and 0.75 and 0.71 for COG. The testing cost per infant detected was 50 to 100 percent higher for COG than for BERA, despite a test overhead cost ratio of about 1 : 5.5. False negatives were not assigned a cost, but were treated as a distinct outcome variable, in terms of which the ABR was clearly superior. The actual cost per infant detected by the ABR was $5,000 to $10,000.

Whatever the actual test series, current risk factors are a major limitation on overall sensitivity. Given that no sufficiently cheap, objective, and sensitive test yet exists, the logical target of research and strategic implementation is the group that are missed by the register. This comprises about 50 percent of all children with at least moderate SHL, and probably a higher percentage if milder or unilateral losses are also targeted. Preschool case finding and information programs for both parents and physicians are obvious strategies. The otoacoustic emissions procedure may prove to be viable as a general screening tool.

CONCLUDING REMARKS

Clinical decision analysis can and should be applied much more vigorously, even routinely, to many aspects of clinical audiology. The techniques can be beneficial for both diagnosis and therapeutic problem solving. CDA is not a panacea for all ills, but even if an optimal strategy cannot be deduced and translated into a concrete protocol, systematic and critical examination of goals, test performance, and outcome utilities are likely to yield new insights.

There have been sporadic applications and explanations of certain aspects of CDA in the audiologic literature, some of these being of high quality, but the majority of published work still does not reflect consideration of statistical, epidemiologic, and decision theoretic principles. This has had a serious limiting effect on both the quality of clinical practice and the general rate of progress within the discipline. It is to be hoped that these techniques will increase rapidly their foothold in audiology.

CDA itself requires much further development work and dissemination. One of the reasons why the ROC, for example, has not yet found a wider audience is that it has not been explained and publicized adequately. Articles about its power and generality, such as that recently by Swets (1988), will help to redress this. Also, there is an onus on those who have, or aspire to, leadership roles in audiologic research to explore, use, and teach such techniques more effectively.

The notion of a test as a fixed, immutable entity should be discarded in favor of the test as a continuum. Techniques that reflect this, such as the ROC, should be adopted routinely, and this itself would have a profound impact on the nature and value of published data. Specifically, there is a need for more explicit definition and manipulation of operating points. A corollary of this is the need for less predigestion of published data. Provision of source data permits the audience to perform their own analyses, as well as to make more informed decisions about the availability and representativeness of the data. Here, tools such as the scattergram or multiple-category crosstabulation are highly effective.

For the clinical audiologist, the strategic approach has few limitations. For example, lack of validity for a published claim about some test can be viewed as a disease, the prevalence of which is perhaps as high as 0.5, even in prestigious journals. A high index of suspicion on the part of the clinician is necessary and appropriate, when testing such claims for validity. Definitive tests for lack of credibility are readily available (Sackett et al., 1985), and the effects of using these tests will be remarkable.

Furthermore, the audiologist can set about gathering local prevalence data, estimating test per-

formance characteristics, evaluating utilities and applying the techniques outlined earlier. This will contribute towards the building of a more solid foundation for clinical practices. These activities should be considered to be a natural and integral part of a dynamic and evolving profession.

APPENDIX

BAYES' FORMULA

Let P(A/B) denote the probability of event A, given that event B has occurred, that is, the conditional probability of A, given B. Let the complement of B be denoted by B−, so that P(B) + P(B−) = 1.0. Then, Bayes' formula can be expressed as:

$$P(B/A) = P(A/B) \bullet P(B)/[P(A/B) \bullet P(B) + P(A/B-) \bullet P(B-)]$$

In the context of the 2 × 2 decision matrix, the prior probability of disease is denoted as P(D+), or p, and the posterior probability of disease given a positive test is P(D+/T+), which is the positive predictive value (PPV) of the test result. The sensitivity is P(T+/D+) and the specificity is P(T−/D−). Thus, Bayes' rule yields:

$$P(D+/T+) = sens \bullet p/[sens \bullet p + (1 - spec) \bullet (1 - p)]$$

Given the prior probability, sensitivity, and specificity, the posterior probability can be derived either by using the above expression or using published graphs and tables (Benish, 1987).

Another form of Bayes' rule is the odds-likelihood ratio form:

$$Posterior\ odds = likelihood\ ratio \times prior\ odds$$
$$P(D+/T+)/[1 - P(D+/T+)] = LR+ \bullet [p/(1 - p)]$$
where LR+ = P(T+/D+)/P(T+/D−) = sens/(1 − spec)

This is actually an easier approach if the likelihood ratio is provided, because of the very simple relationship between odds and probabilities. See this text, and a nomogram (Sackett et al., 1985).

DEDUCTION OF d' AND A

The problem is to deduce d', given a single pair of values for sensitivity and specificity. This is done using tables of the cumulative standard normal distribution F(z), in reverse. These tables come in several forms, the simplest being such that F(0.0) = 0.5. Suppose the sensitivity and specificity are 0.8 and 0.9, respectively. The procedure is to find the values of z that give F(z) equal to 0.8 and 0.9 in the body of the tables, and then sum these values of z. Thus, 0.8 corresponds to a z of 0.84, and 0.9 to a z of 1.28. The sum is 2.12, which is the estimated d'. The associated single-point estimate of the areal measure A is the value of F(z) given that z = d'/1.4142, that is, z = 2.12/1.4142 = 1.5, so A = 0.9332. This A takes slightly different values from the A' described by Turner and Nielsen (1984).

TO TEST OR NOT

Consider only FP and FN error costs, denoted as CFP and CFN. The non-test path has expected cost p • CFN, where p is the prevalence. The test path has expected cost

$$(1 - spec) \bullet (1 - p) \bullet CFP + p \bullet (1 - sens) \bullet CFN$$

The test should be used if:

$$(1 - spec) \bullet (1 - p) \bullet CFP + p \bullet (1 - sens) \bullet CFN < p \bullet CFN$$

thus,

$$(1 - spec) \bullet (1 - p) \bullet CFP/CFN - p \bullet sens < 0$$

and therefore

$$CFP/CFN < [p/(1 - p)] \bullet [sens/(1 - spec)]$$

the right-hand side of which is the product of the prior odds for disease and the likelihood ratio for a positive test, namely, the posterior odds for disease.

ACKNOWLEDGMENTS

The authors thank Krista Riko, Director of Mount Sinai and Toronto General Hospitals' Otologic Function Unit, for useful discussions. Support is acknowledged from the Medical Research Council of Canada, the Ontario Ministry of Health, and the Saul A. Silverman Family Foundation.

REFERENCES

American Academy of Pediatrics. Joint Committee on Infant Hearing. (1982). Position statement. *Pediatrics, 70,* 496–497.

Barr, D. M., Brackmann, D. E., Olson, J. E., & House, W. F. (1985). Changing concepts of acoustic neuroma diagnosis. *Archives of Otolaryngology 111,* 17–21.

Benish, W. A. (1987). Graphic and tabular expression of Bayes' Theorem. *Medical Decision Making, 7,* 104–106.

Beyer, W. H. (1968). Table of limits on binomial proportions. In W. H. Beyer (Ed.), *Handbook of tables for probability and statistics.* Boca Raton, FL: CRC Press.

CHABA. (1987). Brainstem audiometry of infants. *ASHA, January 1987,* 47–55.

Cashman, M., & Nedzelski, J. M. (1983). Cerebellopontine angle lesions and audiological test protocol. *Journal of Otolaryngology, 12,* 180–186.

Curati, W. L., Graif, M., Kingsley, D., King, T., Schultz, C., & Steiner, R. (1986). MRI in acoustic neuroma: A review of 35 patients. *Neuroradiology, 28,* 208–214.

Davidson, J., Hyde, M. L., & Alberti, P. W. (1989). Epidemiologic patterns in childhood hearing loss: A review. *International Journal of Pediatric Otolaryngology, 17,* 239–266.

Davis, A. (1984). Detecting hearing impairment in neonates — the statistical decision criterion for the auditory response cradle. *British Journal of Audiology, 18,* 163–168.

Dobie, R. A. (1985). The use of relative cost ratios in choosing a diagnostic test. *Ear & Hearing, 6,* 113–116.

Dolan, J. G., Bordley, D. R., & Mushlin, A. I. (1986). An evaluation of clinicians' subjective prior probability estimates. *Medical Decision Making, 6,* 216–223.

Doubilet, P. M., & Cain, K. C. (1985). The superiority of sequential over simultaneous testing. *Medical Decision Making, 5,* 447–451.

Epstein, A. M., & McNeil, B. J. (1985). Physician characteristics and organizational factors influencing use of ambulatory tests. *Medical Decision Making, 5,* 401–414.

Fleiss, J. L. (1981). *Statistical methods for rates and proportions.* New York: Wiley.

Fria, T. J. (1985). Identification of congenital hearing loss with the auditory brainstem response. In J. T. Jacobson (Ed.), *The auditory brainstem response* (pp. 317–334). Boston: College-Hill Press.

Hart, R. G., & Davenport, J. (1981). Diagnosis of acoustic neuroma. *Neurosurgery, 9,* 450–463.

Hart, R. G., Gardner, D. P., & Howieson, J. (1983). Acoustic tumors: Atypical features and recent diagnostic tests. *Neurology (NY), 33,* 211–221.

Hecox, K., & Galambos, R. (1974). Brainstem auditory evoked responses in human infants and adults. *Archives of Otolaryngology, 99,* 30–33.

Hennekens, C. H., & Buring, J. E. (1987). *Epidemiology in medicine.* Boston: Little, Brown.

Jacobson, J., & Jacobson, C. (1987). Principles of decision analysis in high risk infants. *Seminars in Hearing, 8,* 133–141.

Jacobson, J., & Morehouse, R. (1984). A comparison of ABR and behavioral screening in high risk and normal newborn infants. *Ear & Hearing, 5,* 247–253.

Jerger, J. (1983). Strategies for neuroaudiological evaluation. *Seminars in Hearing, 4,* 109–120.

Jerger, S. (1983). Decision matrix and information theory

analyses in the evaluation of neuroaudiologic tests. *Seminars in Hearing, 4*, 121–132.

Johnsen, N. J., Bagi, P., & Elberling, C. (1983). Evoked emissions from the human ear. III. Findings in neonates. *Scandinavian Audiology, 12*, 17–24.

Katz, J. (1985). *Handbook of clinical audiology*. Baltimore: Williams & Wilkins.

Kemp, D. T. (1978). Stimulated acoustic emissions from within the human auditory system. *Journal of the Acoustical Society of America, 64*, 1386–1391.

Kenworthy, O. T. (1987). Identification of hearing loss in infancy and early childhood. In J. G. Alpiner & P. A. McCarthy (Eds.), *Rehabilitative audiology: Children and adults* (pp. 18–43). Baltimore: Williams & Wilkins.

King, L. S. (1982). *Medical thinking: A historical preface*. Princeton, NJ: Princeton University Press.

Ledley, R. S., & Lusted, L. B. (1959). Reasoning foundations of medical diagnosis. *Science, 130*, 9–21.

Macartney, F. J. (1987). Logic in medicine. *British Medical Journal, 295*, 1325–1331.

Martin, J. A. M. (1982). Aetiological factors relating to deafness in the European community. *Audiology, 21*, 149–158.

Metz, C. E. (1978). Basic principles of ROC analysis. *Seminars in Nuclear Medicine, VIII*, 283–298.

Miller, M. H. (1987). Comment on "Neurodiagnostic audiology: Contemporary perspectives." *Ear & Hearing, 8*, 314.

Murray, A., Javel, E., & Watson, C. (1985). Prognostic validity of auditory brainstem evoked response screening in newborn infants. *American Journal of Otolaryngology, 6*, 120–131.

Nakao, M. A., & Axelrod, S. (1983). Numbers are better than words: Verbal specifications of frequency have no place in medicine. *American Journal of Medicine, 74*, 1061–1065.

Pass, T. M., Komaroff, A. L., & Ervin, C. T. (1982). Categorical approaches to clinical decision support. In B. T. Williams (Ed.), *Computer aids to clinical decisions* (Vol. 1, pp. 95–138). Boca Raton, FL: CRC Press.

Pauker, S. G., & Kassirer, J. P. (1980). The threshold approach to clinical decision making. *New England Journal of Medicine, 302*, 1109.

Pauker, S. G., & Kassirer, J. P. (1987). Decision analysis. *New England Journal of Medicine, 316*, 250–258.

Prager, D. A., Stone, D. A., & Rose, D. N. (1987). Hearing loss screening in the neonatal intensive care unit: Auditory brainstem response versus Crib-O-Gram; a cost-effectiveness analysis. *Ear & Hearing, 8*, 213–216.

Riko, K., Hyde, M. L., & Alberti, P. W. (1985). Hearing loss in early infancy: Incidence, detection and assessment. *Laryngoscope, 95*, 137–145.

Sackett, D. L., Haynes, R. B., & Tugwell, P. (1985). *Clinical epidemiology: A basic science for clinical medicine*. Boston:

Little, Brown.

Schein, J. D., & Delk, M. T. (1974). *The deaf population of the United States*. Silver Spring, MD: National Association of the Deaf.

Schwartz, D. M. (1987a). Neurodiagnostic audiology: Contemporary perspectives. *Ear & Hearing, 8* (Suppl. 4), 43S–48S.

Schwartz, D. M. (1987b). Reply to Miller. *Ear & Hearing, 8*, 314.

Selters, W. A., & Brackmann, D. E. (1979). Brainstem electrical response audiometry in acoustic tumor detection. In W. F. House & C. M. Luetje (Eds.), *Acoustic tumors: Vol. 1: Diagnosis* (pp. 225–236). Baltimore: University Park Press.

Simel, D. L., Feussner, J. R., Delong, E. R., & Matchar, D. B. (1987). Intermediate, indeterminate and uninterpretable diagnostic test results. *Medical Decision Making, 7*, 107–115.

Snedecor, G. W., & Cochran, W. G. (1980). *Statistical methods*. Iowa State University Press.

Sox, H. C., Blatt, M. A., Higgins, M. C., & Marton, K. I. (1988). *Medical decision making*. Boston: Butterworth.

Swets, J. A. (1988). Measuring the accuracy of diagnostic systems. *Science, 240*, 1285–1293.

Swets, J. A., & Pickett, R. M. (1982). *Evaluation of diagnostic systems: Methods from signal detection theory*. New York: Academic Press.

Swigart, E. (1986). *Neonatal hearing screening*. Boston: College-Hill Press.

Turner, R. G. (1988). Techniques to determine test protocol performance. *Ear & Hearing, 9*, 177–189.

Turner, R. G., & Nielsen, D. W. (1984). Application of clinical decision analysis to audiological tests. *Ear & Hearing, 5*, 125–133.

Turner, R. G., Frazer, G. J., & Shepard, N. T. (1984). Formulating and evaluating audiological test protocols. *Ear & Hearing, 5*, 321–330.

Turner, R. G., Shepard, N. T., & Frazer, G. J. (1984). Clinical performance of audiological and related diagnostic tests. *Ear & Hearing, 5*, 187–194.

Weinstein, M. C., & Fineberg, H. V. (1980). *Clinical decision analysis*. Philadelphia: Saunders.

Wilson, W. R., & Thompson, G. (1984). Behavioral audiometry. In J. Jerger (Ed.), *Pediatric audiology* (pp. 2–44). Boston: College-Hill Press.

Windle-Taylor, P.C., Dhillon, R. S., Kenyon, G. S., & Morrison, A. W. (1984). Acoustic neuroma suspicion index: An aid to investigation and diagnosis. *Laryngoscope, 94*, 1464–1467.

World Health Organization. (1980). *International classification of impairments, disabilities and handicaps*. Geneva: WHO.

Index

Index

Metz test. *See* Acoustic reflex
Microtia, 91, 163, 198, 253
Middle ear, 161–162
  and ABR, 172–173
  and audiologic findings in atypical conductive
    hearing impairments, 183–193
  and audiologic management of patients with
    pathology in, 193–195
  clinical examination of, 162–163
  disorder and immittance patterns, 119, 120–122
  glossary of terms about, 197–198
  and immittance, 166–169
  infections and toxins, 90, 100–101, 120, 122,
    164–165, 179, 183, 192–193, 198, 274
  negative pressure in, 122
  otoscopy of, 164–166
  patterns of audiometric findings in, 173–183
  and pure tone audiometry, 169–172
  surgery, 85–86
Middle latency response (MLR), 64, 263
Migraine headache, 274
Mondini's dysplasia, 87, 92
Mucinous fluid, 100
Mueller speaking tube, 72
Multiple sclerosis (MS), 37, 38, 39, 104–105, 134
Mumps, 102, 254
Myelography, 313

Necrosis, 198
Negative deflection, 169
Negative predictive value (NPV), 305
Neonatal intensive care unit (NICU), 252, 257,
  258–260, 318, 319
Neoplasms and growth, 94–99. *See also* Acoustic
    neuromas
  acoustic tumors, 96–98
  brainstem gliomas, 98–99
  cholesteatoma, 95, 165, 166, 192, 197, 200
  glomus tumors, 95–96
  keratosis obturans, 95
  meningiomas, 98, 217, 311
  osseous tumors, 99
  osteomas and exostoses, 70, 94–95, 164, 198
  squamous cell carcinomas, 96
Neurilemoma, solitary and multiple, 96–97
NEV, 299, 300, 301–303, 311, 312
Nicolet Enhancer I, 150–151
Noise
  electrical, 157
  hearing loss due to, 86, 127, 201, 203
  patient, with ABR, 156–157
  as signal type, 56, 64
  unwanted background, 151–152
Noise detection threshold (NDT), 41
Noise interference level (NIL), 41
Normal, equal-variance (NEV) model, 299, 300,
  301–303, 311, 312
NPV, 305

Nystagmus. *See* Vertigo
  jerk, 271, 273
  positional, 276

Occlusion effect, 73, 198
Ocular motor control, 270
Oculomotility studies, 277–278
Odds, 306
Operating point, 299–303, 307, 308–309, 311,
  312–313, 315, 318, 320
Optokinetic system effect, 271
Optokinetic visual input, 269
Organ of Corti, 162
Oscillator, 55, 56
Osseous tumors, 99
Ossicular chain defects, 71, 83, 122, 161, 166,
  169, 179, 183, 187
Osteomas, 70, 94, 164, 198
Osteoradionecrosis with infection, 85
Otitis
  externa, 70, 163, 164, 198
  media, 90, 100–101, 120, 122, 164–165, 179,
    183, 192–193, 198, 274. *See also* Fluid
Otoacoustic emissions, 319
  with effusion, infant, 252–253, 262
Otolaryngology, 5, 67, 71, 72
Otologic examination, 67–74
  and the facial nerve, 73
  immittance audiometry in, 74
  and main complaint, 69
  and patient history, 69–70
  physical, 70–71
  radiography and laboratory tests in, 73–74
  and taste, 73
  with tuning fork, 71–73
Otology, 67
Otomycosis, 164
Otorrhea, 69
Otosclerosis, 71, 106, 161, 162, 166, 183, 198,
  205–206
  cochlear, 183, 206, 209–211
Ototoxicity, 76, 77–79, 201
  and aminoglycosides, 78, 89–90, 212
  and aspirin, 89
  and carbon monoxide poisoning, 90–91
  and *cis*-platinum, 90
  and diuretics, 90
  and middle ear infections, 90
Overhead cost, 309

Paracusia Willisii, 69
Paradoxial ipsilateral ear effect, 238
Paragangliomas, 95–96
Parallel procedure, 304–305, 311
Parkinson's disease, 239
Pediatric Speech Intelligibility (PSI) test, 243
Pendred's syndrome, 87, 200
Perichondritis, 70, 99, 163